Canine
Rehabilitation &
Physical
Therapy

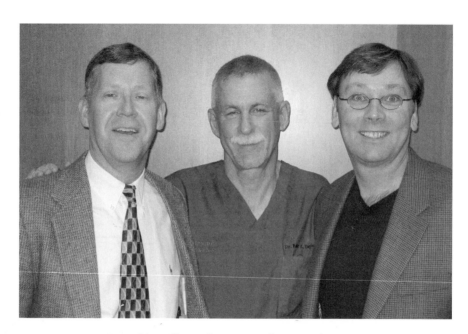

Darryl L. Millis, Robert A. Taylor, David Levine

Canine Rehabilitation & Physical Therapy

Darryl L. Millis, MS, DVM, DACVS, CCRP
Associate Professor of Orthopedic Surgery
Department of Small Animal Clinical Sciences
College of Veterinary Medicine
University of Tennessee
Knoxville, Tennessee

David Levine, PT, PhD, DABPTS (Orthopaedics), CCRP
UC Foundation Professor of Physical Therapy
The University of Tennessee at Chattanooga
Chattanooga, Tennessee

Adjunct Associate Professor
Department of Small Animal Clinical Sciences
The University of Tennessee College of Veterinary Medicine

Adjunct Professor
Department of Clinical Sciences
North Carolina State University College of Veterinary
   Medicine

Robert A. Taylor, MS, DVM DACVS, CCRP
Alameda East Veterinary Hospital
Denver, Colorado

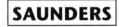

An Imprint of Elsevier

SAUNDERS

An Imprint of Elsevier

11830 Westline Industrial Drive
St. Louis, Missouri 63146

CANINE REHABILITATION AND PHYSICAL THERAPY ISBN 0-7216-9555-8

NOTICE

Veterinary Medicine an ever-changing field. Standard safety precautions must be followed, but as new research and clinical experience broaden our knowledge, changes in treatment and drug therapy may become necessary or appropriate. Readers are advised to check the most current product information provided by the manufacturer of each drug to be administered to verify the recommended dose, the method and duration of administration, and contraindications. It is the responsibility of the licensed prescriber, relying on experience and knowledge of the patient, to determine dosages and the best treatment for each individual patient. Neither the publisher nor the authors assume any liability for any injury and/or damage to persons or property arising from this publication.

International Standard Book Number: 0-7216-9555-8

Publishing Director: Linda L. Duncan
Senior Editor: Liz Fathman
SeniorDevelopmental Editor: Jolynn Gower
Publishing Services Manager: John Rogers
Senior Project Manager: Beth Hayes
Designer: Gail Hudson

Printed in the United States of America

Last digit is the print number: 9   8   7   6   5   4   3   2

Contributors

Caroline P. Adamson, MSPT
Director, Physical Rehabilitation Services
Colorado Canine Sports Medicine/Rehabilitation
    Clinic
Alameda East Veterinary Hospital
Denver, Colorado

Brian S. Beale, DVM, DACVS
Gulf Coast Veterinary Specialists
South Houston, Texas

John Bevan, DVM
Surgical Intern
Gulf Coast Veterinary Specialists
Huston, Texas

Albert S. Dorn, MS, DVM, DACVS
Professor of Small Animal Surgery
Department of Small Animal Clinical Sciences
University of Tennessee
Knoxville, Tennessee

Daniel Q. Estep, PhD, CAAB
Vice President
Animal Behavior Associates, Inc.
Littleton, Colorado

Robert Gillette, DVM
College of Veterinary Medicine
Auburn University
Auburn, Alabama

Maria H. Glinski, DVM, CA
Animal Rehabilitation and Fitness Center
Aiken, South Carolina

Siri Hamilton, PT, LVT
Knoxville, Tennessee

Kristinn Heinrichs, PhD, PT, SCS, ATC, CSCS
Peak Sports Performance International
Savannah, Georgia

Michael Hoelzler
Resident in Small Animal Surgery
Department of Small Animal Clinical Sciences
University of Tennessee
Knoxville, Tennessee

Lovetta Immel, MSPT
Savannah, Georgia

Janna Johnson, DVM
Allpets Clinic
Boulder, Colorado

Angela Lewelling, PTA
Clinical Associate
Department of Small Animal Clinical Sciences
University of Tennessee
Knoxville, Tennessee

Denis Marcellin-Little, MS, DEDV, DACVS, DECVS
Associate Professor of Orthopedic Surgery
Department of Clinical Sciences
College of Veterinary Medicine
North Carolina State University
Raleigh, North Carolina

Laurie McCauley, DVM
Lake Villa, Illinois

Lin McGonagle, MSPT, LVT
Genoa, New York

Ann Marie Manning, DVM, DACVECC
Angell Memorial Animal Hospital
Boston, Massachutsetts

Murphy, Nancy, PT
Ketchum, Idaho

Cheryl Riegger-Krugh, PhD, PT
Health Sciences Center
University of Colorado
Denver, Colorado

Lauren M. Rittenberry, PT
Knoxville, Tennessee

Paul Shealy, MS, DVM
Veterinary Specialists of the Southeast
North Charleston, South Carolina

Janet E. Steiss, DVM, PhD, PT
Associate Professor
Department of Biomedical Sciences
College of Veterinary Medicine
Nursing and Allied Health
Tuskegee University
Tuskegee, Alabama

Amanda Sutton, MSCP, SRP, Grad Dipl Phys
Harestock Stud
Kennel Lane
Littleton, Nr. Winchester
Hampshire, UK

**William B. Thomas, DVM, MS, DACVIM
(Neurology)**
Associate Professor of Neurology and
    Neurosurgery
Department of Small Animal Clinical Sciences
University of Tennessee
Knoxville, Tennessee

Joseph P. Weigel, MS, DVM, DACVS
Associate Professor of Surgery
Department of Small Animal Clinical Sciences
University of Tennessee
Knoxville, Tennessee

James (Ned) Williams, DVM, DACVS
Carolina Veterinary Specialists
Greensboro, North Carolina

Acknowledgments

When writing a textbook in a new area that incorporates two separate professions, there are many challenges to overcome and people to thank. I would like to especially thank Dave and Bob for the humor and expertise that each offered in this project, despite busy schedules and the many demands in their everyday lives. Thanks are also in order to the many physical therapists and veterinarians who have helped move the field forward and provided kind words and encouraged our efforts. I would be remiss if I did not thank my colleagues and co-workers at the University of Tennessee for helping me during this time to make the process bearable by providing help and support in the clinics and laboratory. I would especially like to thank my family for putting up with me over the past 2 years; my wife Linda who has always encouraged and supported my efforts, regardless of how daunting they might seem; my son Christopher who was always asking when I would be done writing my "story"; my son Nicholas who thought it was cool to write a book and has already shown his own talent at writing and illustrating; and my parents George and Adeline who made all of this possible by encouraging and supporting me from the very beginning. Finally, I would like to thank my patients, past and present, for allowing me to learn about and try new methods of rehabilitation, to help the future patients.

Darryl L. Millis

Many thanks are owed when a book 5 long years in the formation is finally completed. So many people have generously given their time and thoughts to help me, and all cannot be listed; however, a few special people should be thanked by name for their support and encouragement: My co-editors and friends, Darryl and Bob who are not only exceptional surgeons but exceptional people. The many contributors who have helped to keep this work spirited and always enjoyable. My colleagues, students, and patients/clients at UTC, UTCVM, and many other clinics. I continue to learn everyday from all of you. Old friends, like Kevin and Ivan, who have kept me laughing for the last 20 years, and new friends like Denis who do likewise. To many family members across this country who remind me of what family means, and to the memory of many others like Diane, Phil, and Marie, who will always be with me. My parents, Jack and Marie, to whom I owe much. Because of them I grew up thinking that everyone was unselfish, open, honest, and compassionate. Their strong work ethic and loyalty have been indispensable life lessons. My children Lauren Allyn, Sarah Marie, and Hadley Christian who are too young to read but like pictures of the "doggies" anyway. My best friend, my bride, my Allison—who somehow understands me completely and supports me wholly. And to the one who was with me before I was born.

David Levine

The field of veterinary physical therapy is growing both in interest and in the numbers of veterinarians, physical therapists, students of both professions and the general public. I would like to acknowledge the many fine canine athletes and working dogs that I have had the privilege to help return them to full function and athleticism. There are many clients and colleagues who have helped and encouraged our efforts in the past many years. Melanie Cody, PT, and Merry Lester, PT, were early collaborators, colleagues, and peers whose encouragement and faith in our efforts helped us in our initial canine physical therapy efforts. My two co-editors have devoted many hours of toil and effort to help further the discipline, and we gratefully acknowledge their efforts.

Robert A. Taylor

Preface

Individuals involved in veterinary medicine and surgery have witnessed remarkable progress in their ability to diagnose and treat problems that, in the recent past, would have been untreatable. Total hip replacement in the dog, laparoscopic procedures, arthroscopic surgery and the widespread use of sophisticated imaging modalities such as magnetic resonance imaging, computed tomography, and real-time ultrasonic imaging are daily occurrences in veterinary medicine. With the availability of these sophisticated diagnostic techniques, the expectations for enhanced functional results have grown.

Human physical therapy is an internationally recognized discipline, and the positive efforts of postsurgical and postinjury rehabilitation have been documented and recognized in human health care. Relatively little attention has been given to veterinary patients afflicted with similar conditions. There is profound interest on the part of veterinary caregivers to learn about and provide rehabilitation and therapy following surgery, illness, or injury. Techniques used in human physical therapy are being adapted for use in small animal patients.

The purpose of this textbook is to provide a basic understanding of physical therapy techniques and interventions for dogs. Most professional programs in veterinary medicine do not provide training in physical therapy. Educational programs in physical therapy do not include evaluation and treatment of animals. These factors have resulted in a need for close collaboration between veterinarians, physical therapists, and veterinary technicians to provide optimal evaluation and treatment of animal patients. Currently, these collaborative efforts and relationships are being used to create treatment protocols for many types of neurologic, and musculoskeletal injuries in animals. In this book, we hope to amalgamate the knowledge that physical therapists, veterinarians, and veterinary technicians possess to allow a faster and more complete recovery from debilitating conditions.

It is with these goals in mind that this volume was conceived and written. We foresee the time when veterinary physical therapy will be a recognized discipline and all animal patients, their owners, and veterinary caregivers will benefit.

Contents

Section V

PHYSICAL THERAPY FOR SPECIFIC DIAGNOSES

Canine
Rehabilitation &
Physical
Therapy

INTRODUCTION TO PHYSICAL REHABILITATION

■ Chapter 1

History of Canine Physical Rehabilitation

Lin McGonagle and Robert A. Taylor

History of Canine Physical Rehabilitation

The idea of applying rehabilitation principles and techniques to animals is not new. In fact, many of the treatment protocols for humans were developed and continue to be developed using animal models.[1-7] The use of dogs as a research model has linked traditional physical therapy practice and veterinary medicine. Currently, protocols that have been developed and studied in humans undergoing rehabilitation are being adapted for use in animal physical rehabilitation. Higher owner expectations combined with increased sophistication and technical abilities of veterinary surgeons have resulted in greater interest in physical therapy and rehabilitation.

Interest in the practice of canine rehabilitation in the United States gained momentum in the late 1980s and throughout the 1990s as a result of the influence of classic texts, national presentations by the American Physical Therapy Association (APTA) and American Veterinary Medical Association (AVMA), and the formation of the Animal Physical Therapist Special Interest Group within the APTA. In the past 10 years public demand and awareness have increased the need for research activity.[8-13] Many veterinarians have felt a need to improve postoperative patient care, because, traditionally, preoperative management, diagnostic procedures, and surgical treatment have been emphasized. The results seen with humans undergoing intensive postoperative rehabilitation have caused many veterinarians to rethink patient management strategies, so that postoperative rehabilitation, once overlooked, is now becoming more common in veterinary practice.

The APTA position statement and the AVMA "Guidelines for Alternative and Complementary Veterinary Medicine" have provided some initial guidelines for the field of animal physical therapy. Each professional organization has recognized the other and has published guidelines for collaborative working relationships.

The APTA House of Delegates adopted a position statement in June 1993 regarding animal physical therapy, which states that the APTA "endorses the position that physical therapists may establish collaborative, collegial relationships with veterinarians for the purposes of providing physical therapy services or consultation."[14]

The "Guidelines for Alternative and Complementary Veterinary Medicine" were adopted in July 1996 by the AVMA House of Delegates.[15] The document, which defined veterinary physical therapy as "the use of noninvasive techniques, excluding veterinary chiropractic, for the rehabilitation of injuries in non-human animals," established the following guidelines:

Veterinary physical therapy should be performed by a licensed veterinarian or, where in accordance with state practice acts, by (1) a licensed, certified, or registered veterinary or animal health technician educated in veterinary physical therapy or (2) a licensed physical therapist educated in non-human animal anatomy and physiology. Veterinary physical therapy performed by a non-veterinarian should be performed under the supervision of, or referral by, a licensed veterinarian who is providing concurrent care. Veterinary physical therapy performed by non-veterinarians should be limited to the use of stretching; massage; stimulation by use of low-level lasers, electrical sources, magnetic fields, and ultrasound; rehabilitative exercises; hydrotherapy; and applications of heat and cold.

New guidelines were adopted by the AVMA House of Delegates in 2001.[16] They evaluated several medical approaches described by the terms "complementary," "alternative," and "integrative" and collectively described them as Complementary and Alternative Veterinary Medicine (CAVM). Examples of CAVM include aromatherapy; Bach flower remedy therapy; energy therapy; low-energy photon therapy; magnetic field therapy; orthomolecular therapy; veterinary acupuncture, acutherapy, and acupressure; veterinary homeopathy; veterinary manual or manipulative therapy (similar to osteopathy, chiropractic, or physical medicine and therapy); veterinary neutraceutical therapy; and veterinary phytotherapy.

The basic concept behind these new guidelines was to emphasize that CAVM should be held to the same standards as traditional veterinary medicine, including validation of safety and efficacy by the scientific method. In addition, the guidelines state that "The AVMA believes veterinarians should ensure that they have the requisite skills and knowledge for any treatment modality they may consider using." Finally, another pertinent point is that "The quality of studies and reports pertaining to CAVM varies; therefore, it is incumbent on a veterinarian to critically evaluate the literature and other sources of information. Veterinarians and organizations providing or promoting CAVM are encouraged to join with the AVMA in advocating sound research necessary to establish proof of safety and efficacy." Although the field of small animal rehabilitation is relatively new as compared with other areas of CAVM, it is encouraging that a number of studies have already indicated its benefit in treating several conditions. In addition, other studies have evaluated modalities and the responses of tissues to rehabilitation following injury.

Journals and books have provided information on animal physical rehabilitation for more than 20 years. Ann Downer has described hydrotherapy and rehabilitation of long bone fractures.[17] Contributions were made during the 1980s relating to general principles of physical rehabilitation in small animals[18-21] and postoperative management of the neurosurgical patient.[22]

Although these articles have increased awareness of physical rehabilitation as a treatment option in veterinary medicine, "Postsurgical physical therapy: the missing link," by Taylor,[9] captured the interest of the veterinary community. Throughout the remainder of the 1990s, the number of publications increased. Topics included cranial cruciate ligament rupture and rehabilitation,[9,10,23] postoperative management of spinal surgery in the dog,[22] and management considerations for trauma patients.[24] Collaboration of veterinarians and physical therapists has increased, resulting in publications regarding physical rehabilitation for the critically ill patient.[25,26] It is clear that the dissemination of information has strengthened the ties between veterinarians and physical therapists and increased support for the efficacy of rehabilitation approaches in animal care.

Several books have helped shape the field of animal physical rehabilitation. *Physical Therapy for Animals: Selected Techniques* by Downer[17] influenced professionals as early as 1978. *Canine Sports Medicine and Surgery*[27] added to the growing field of sports medicine and discussed the role of physical rehabilitation in treating injuries of dogs.

In the mid-1980s topics relating to physical rehabilitation of canine athletes were presented at several annual meetings of the International Greyhound Symposium. Since then many other veterinarians and physical therapists have lectured and presented continuing education and research findings at more than 50 regional, national, and international human and veterinary conferences.

In August 1999 the First International Symposium for Physical Therapy and Rehabilitation in Veterinary Medicine was sponsored by and held at Oregon State University. More than 300 participants from 21 countries met over 4 days to present clinical and research findings and to share ideas. This meeting focused entirely on animal physical rehabilitation and brought the professions of veterinary medicine and physical therapy together to exchange information and share ideas. The Second International Symposium for Physical Therapy and Rehabilitation in Veterinary Medicine was held in 2002 at the University of Tennessee.

Worldwide Animal Rehabilitation and Physical Therapy Associations

Veterinarians and physical therapists in many countries have been sharing information and working together for many years. There are professional organizations for animal physical rehabilitation in at least 10 countries: Australia, Canada, Finland, Germany, The Netherlands, New Zealand, South Africa, Sweden, the United Kingdom, and the United States. In many of these countries, the groups are formally recognized by their respective national physical therapy associations. Box 1-1 provides a brief history of these organizations and contact information.

Although there is robust interest in the area of canine physical rehabilitation at local, national, and international meetings, there is no formal association for both veterinarians and physical therapists in the United States. Physical rehabilitation is gaining greater acceptance in veterinary medicine, and, as it is integrated into veterinary curricula, it will continue to grow. Currently, physical rehabilitation rotations and instruction are available at a number of veterinary colleges and physical therapy programs as a part of the professional curriculum.

■ ■ ■ **BOX 1-1** Animal Physical Rehabilitation Organizations of Selected Countries (Official Names)

Australia
Australian Animal Physiotherapy Association
Recognized by the Australian Physiotherapy Association (http://www.physiotherapy.asn.au/)

Canada
Canadian Horse and Animal Physiotherapy Association (CHAP)
First organized in 1994
Currently applying for national recognition by the Canadian Physiotherapy Association (http://www.physiotherapy.ca/)
E-mail: chap@animalptcanada.com
Website: http://www.animalptcanada.com/

Finland
Association of Animal Physiotherapy
Founded in 1997
Recognized as a subgroup of the Finnish Association of Physiotherapists (http://www.fysioterapia.net)

The Netherlands
Nederlandsee Verening voor Fysiotherapie bij Dieren (NVFD)
(Dutch Animal Physical Therapy Association)
Founded in 1989
Recognized by the Dutch Ministry of Agriculture since 1992
Address: Hindelaan 56, 1216 CW Hilversum, The Netherlands

South Africa
South African Association of Physiotherapists in Animal Therapy (SAAPAT)

In the 1970s Winks Greene, PT, promoted working with animals, and in 1984 he opened the Natal Equine Therapy Centre.
SAAPAT first organized in 1988
Gained official recognition in 1998 as a special interest group of the South African Society of Physiotherapy

Sweden
The Association of Registered Physiotherapists of Veterinary Medicine
Founded in 1995
Became a section member of the Swedish Association of Registered Physiotherapists in 1996

United Kingdom
Association of Chartered Physiotherapists in Animal Therapy (ACPAT)
1966 Veterinary Surgeon's Act—permits animal physiotherapy treatment
In 1988 ACPAT recognized by the Chartered Society of Physiotherapists (http://www.csp.org.uk/)
E-mail: secretary@acpat.org.uk
Website: http://www.acpat.org.uk/

United States
Animal Physical Therapist Special Interest Group
Officially recognized by the American Physical Therapy Association (http://www.apta.org) since 1998
Website: http://www.orthopt.org/sigs/animal_pt_sig

Future Trends

Physical rehabilitation in small animal practice has become increasingly common and will continue to become more accepted as the scientific literature evolves. In many orthopedic and neurologic conditions, physical rehabilitation is becoming commonplace as a means to enhance recovery, as it is in human medicine and surgery. Wellness and preventive medicine such as physical rehabilitation for weight reduction and for maintenance of muscle strength and cardiorespiratory fitness is also emerging as a trend among pet owners.

REFERENCES

1. Daily L et al: The effects of microwave diathermy on the eye of the rabbit, *Am J Ophthalmol* 35:1001-1017, 1952.
2. Douglas WW, Malcolm JL: The effect of localized cooling on conduction of cat nerves, *J Physiol* 130:53-71, 1955.
3. Lehman JF, Brunner GD, Martinis AJ: Ultrasonic effects as demonstrated in live pigs with surgical metal implants, *Arch Phys Med Rehabil* 40:483-488, 1959.
4. Nadasdi M: Inhibition of experimental arthritis by athermic pulsing shortwave in rats, *Am J Orthop* 2:105-107, 1960.
5. Ely TS et al: Heating characteristics of laboratory animals exposed to ten centimeter microwaves, *Biol Eng* 11:123-137, 1964.
6. Jezdinsky J, Marek J, Ochonsky P: Effects of cold and heat therapy on traumatic oedema of rat hind paw, *Acta Univ Palacki Olomuc Fac Med* 66:185-201, 1973.
7. Michalski WJ, Sequin J: The effect of muscle cooling and stretch on muscle spindle secondary endings in the cat, *J Physiol* 253:341-356, 1975.
8. Bocobo C et al: The effect of ice on intra-articular temperature in the knee of the dog, *Am J Phys Med Rehabil* 70:181-185, 1991.
9. Taylor RA: Postsurgical physical therapy: the missing link, *Compend Cont Educ Pract Vet* 14:1583-1594, 1992.
10. Johnson JM et al: Rehabilitation of dogs with surgically treated cranial cruciate ligament-deficient stifles by use of electrical stimulation of muscles, *Am J Vet Res* 58:1473-1477, 1997.
11. Millis DL, Levine D: The role of exercise and physical modalities in the treatment of osteoarthritis, *Vet Clin North Am Small Animal Pract* 27:913-930, 1997.
12. Steiss JE, Adams CC: Effect of coat on rate of temperature increase in muscle during ultrasound treatment of dogs, *Am J Vet Res* 60:76-80, 1999.
13. Levine D, Millis DL, Mynatt T: Effects of 3.3 MHz ultrasound on caudal thigh muscle temperature in dogs, *Vet Surg* 30:170-174, 2001.
14. *Position on physical therapists in collaborative relationships with veterinarians,* American Physical Therapy Association House of Delegates 06-93-20-36 (Program 32), 1993.
15. Guidelines for alternative and complementary veterinary medicine. In *AVMA directory,* Schaumburg, Ill, 2000, American Veterinary Medical Association.
16. Guidelines for Complementary and Alternative Veterinary Medicine, AVMA Policy Statements and Guidelines, 2001, American Veterinary Medical Association, Schaumburg, Ill.
17. Downer AH: *Physical therapy for animals: selected techniques,* Springfield, Ill, 1978, Charles C Thomas.
18. Tanger CH: Physical therapy in small animal patients: basic principles and application, *Compend Cont Educ Pract Vet* 10:933-936, 1984.
19. Moore M, Rasmussen J: Physical therapy in small animal medicine. I. *Compend Cont Educ Pract Vet* 4:199-203, 1981.
20. Moore M, Rasmussen J: Physical therapy in small animal medicine. II. *Compend Cont Educ Pract Vet* 5:262-266, 1981.
21. Mann FA, Wagner-Mann C, Tagner CH: Manual goniometric measurement of the canine pelvic limb, *J Am Animal Hosp Assoc* 24:189-194, 1988.
22. Sikes R: Postoperative management of the neurosurgical patient, *Problems Vet Med* 3:467-477, 1989.
23. Millis DL et al: A preliminary study of early physical therapy following surgery for cranial cruciate ligament rupture in dogs, *Vet Surg* 26:434, 1997.
24. Payne JT: General management considerations for the trauma patient, *Vet Clin North Am Small Anim Pract* 25:1015-1029, 1995.
25. Manning AM, Ellis DR, Rush J: Physical therapy for critically ill veterinary patients. I. Chest physical therapy, *Compend Cont Educ Pract Vet* 19:675-689, 1997.
26. Manning AM, Rush J, Ellis DR: Physical therapy for critically ill veterinary patients. II. The musculoskeletal system, *Compend Cont Educ Pract Vet* 19:803-807, 1997.
27. Bloomberg MS, Dee JF, Taylor RA: *Canine sports medicine and surgery,* Philadelphia, 1998, WB Saunders.

Regulatory and Practice Issues for the Veterinary and Physical Therapy Professions

Albert S. Dorn, Nancy Murphy, and David Levine

Definition of Physical Therapy

A definition of physical therapy has been developed by the American Physical Therapy Association (APTA) and has recently been amended. In this model definition, physical therapy includes examining and evaluating patients with impairments, functional limitations, disability, and other health-related conditions to determine a diagnosis, prognosis, and intervention. Some examples of areas that may be examined include aerobic capacity, arousal, cognition, assistive and supportive devices, barriers, ergonomics, gait, balance, pain, posture, prosthetic requirements, and range of motion.[1]

Physical therapists also alleviate impairments and functional limitations by designing, implementing, and modifying therapeutic interventions. Some examples of these activities include therapeutic exercise, functional training, manual therapy techniques, electrotherapeutic modalities, and patient-related instruction. Physical therapists are also involved with helping to prevent injury, impairments, functional limitations, and disability, and with the promotion and maintenance of fitness, health, and quality of life in all age populations. Physical therapists accomplish these tasks in a variety of situations, including patient consultation, education, and research.

Definition of Veterinary Medicine

The practice of veterinary medicine is described in the directory of the American Veterinary Medical Association (*AVMA Directory*) in a section entitled The Model Practice Act (Act).[2] The Act has been periodically updated and revised, and in the current version (Section 2, paragraph 8), the practice of veterinary medicine means:

(a) to diagnose, treat, correct, change, relieve, or prevent animal disease, deformity, defect, injury, or other physical or mental conditions; including the prescription or administration of any drug, medicine, biologic, apparatus, application, anesthetic, or other therapeutic or diagnostic substance or technique, and the use of any manual or mechanical procedure for artificial insemination, for testing for pregnancy, or for correcting sterility or infertility or to render advice or recommendation with regard to any of the above.

(b) to represent, directly or indirectly, publicly or privately, an ability and willingness to do an act described in subsection (a).

(c) to use any title, words, abbreviation, or letters in a manner or under circumstances which induce the belief that the person using them is qualified to do any act described in subsection (a).

(d) to apply principles of environmental sanitation, food inspection, environmental pollution control, animal nutrition, zoonotic disease control, and disaster medicine in the promotion and protection of public health.[2]

In the Model Practice Act the description, application, and relationship of physical therapy and other alternative and complementary therapies to the current practice of veterinary medicine are vague and unclear. In an attempt to more clearly describe the relationship of physical therapy and other modalities to the practice of veterinary medicine, the AVMA has written and established Guidelines for Alternative and Complementary Veterinary Medicine. These guidelines describe the potential use and application of these therapies for veterinary patients.[3]

Alternative and Complementary Veterinary Medicine

The AVMA Guidelines for Alternative and Complementary Veterinary Medicine (Guidelines), approved in 1996, address topics such as veterinary acupuncture and acutherapy, veterinary chiropractic, veterinary physical rehabilitation, massage therapy, veterinary homeopathy, veterinary botanical medicine, nutraceutical medicine, and holistic veterinary medicine. The guidelines specifically related to physical rehabilitation and massage therapy are as follows:

PREAMBLE

Veterinary medicine, like all professions, is undergoing changes with increasing rapidity. Additional modalities of diagnosis and therapy are emerging in veterinary and human medicine. These guidelines reflect the current status of the role of these emerging modalities within the parameters of veterinary medicine for use in providing a comprehensive approach to the health care of nonhuman animals. Use of these modalities is considered to constitute the practice of veterinary medicine. Any exceptions will be indicated in the following guidelines. Such modalities should be offered in the context of a valid Veterinarian-Client-Patient Relationship. It is recommended that appropriate client consent must be obtained. Educational programs for veterinarians and veterinary technicians are available for many of the modalities. It is incumbent upon veterinarians to pursue education in their proper use. It should be borne in mind that because the emergence and development of these modalities is a dynamic process, as time passes, the following descriptions may need to be modified. In fact, the updated guidelines adopted by the AVMA House of Delegates in 2001 state that "The AVMA believes veterinarians should ensure that they have the requisite skills and knowledge for any treatment modality they may consider using."

Veterinary Physical Rehabilitation

Veterinary physical rehabilitation is the use of noninvasive techniques, excluding veterinary chiropractic, for the rehabilitation of injuries in nonhuman animals. Veterinary physical rehabilitation performed by non-veterinarians should be limited to the use of stretching; massage therapy; stimulation by use of low-level lasers, electrical sources, magnetic fields, and ultrasound; rehabilitative exercises; hydrotherapy; and applications of heat and cold. Veterinary physical rehabilitation should be performed by a licensed veterinarian or, where in accordance with state practice acts, by a licensed, certified, or registered veterinary or animal health technician educated in veterinary physical rehabilitation or a licensed physical therapist educated in non-human animal anatomy and physiology. Veterinary physical rehabilitation performed by a non-veterinarian should be performed under the supervision of, or referral by, a licensed veterinarian who is providing concurrent care.[3]

Massage Therapy

Massage therapy is a technique in which the therapist uses only his or her hands and body to massage soft tissues. Massage therapy on non-human animals should be performed by a licensed veterinarian with education in massage therapy or, where in accordance with state veterinary practice acts, by a graduate of an accredited massage school who has been educated in non-human animal massage therapy. When performed by a non-veterinarian, massage therapy should be performed under the supervision of, or referral by, a licensed veterinarian who is providing concurrent care.[3]

The development of the AVMA Guidelines for Alternative and Complementary Veterinary Medicine is a recognition by the veterinary profession that other health care professionals have information and knowledge that may benefit veterinary patients. Veterinarians should not hesitate to seek the help, advice, and expertise of others to improve the care and management of their patients. When this expertise, assistance, and advice is sought, however, the responsibility for the care, diagnosis, treatment, and management of the patient remains with the attending veterinarian, and a veterinarian–client–patient relationship will be established.

The Veterinarian–Client–Patient Relationship

The concept of the veterinarian–client–patient relationship (VCPR) was introduced by the AVMA a few years ago to clearly describe the relationship of the veterinarian to clients (the owners) and patients served by the profession. This VCPR is the basis for professional interactions and has become part of a variety of official AVMA documents, including the Principles of Veterinary Medical Ethics, the Model Practice Act, and the Guidelines for Veterinary Prescription Drugs. The Guidelines for Alternative and Complementary Veterinary Medicine also refer to the VCPR, and because these modalities are considered to be part of the practice of veterinary medicine, they should be offered only in the context of a valid VCPR.

As stated in the Principles of Veterinary Medical Ethics,[4] the VCPR is the basis for interaction among veterinarians, owners, and patients. A VCPR exists when all of the following conditions have been met:

1. The veterinarian has assumed responsibility for making clinical judgments regarding the health of the animal(s) and the need for medical treatment, and the client has agreed to follow the veterinarian's instructions.
2. The veterinarian has sufficient knowledge of the animal(s) to initiate at least a general or preliminary diagnosis of the medical condition of the animal(s). This means that the veterinarian has recently seen and is personally acquainted with the keeping and care of the animal(s) by virtue of an examination of the animal(s), or by medically appropriate and timely visits to the premises where the animal(s) are kept.
3. The veterinarian is readily available, or has arranged for emergency coverage, for follow-up evaluation in the event of adverse reactions or the failure of the treatment regimen.

The Principles additionally state that when a VCPR exists, veterinarians must maintain medical records, which should contain information on the diagnosis, care, and treatment of patients.[4]

The Principles also discuss the termination of the VCPR, which would apply when professional services are no longer assumed by the veterinarian or no longer needed by the client. Veterinarians may terminate a VCPR under certain conditions, and they have an ethical obligation to use courtesy and tact in discharging this responsibility. Guidelines for terminating the VCPR are as follows:

1. If there is no ongoing medical condition, veterinarians may terminate a VCPR by notifying the client that they no longer wish to serve that patient and client.

2. If there is an ongoing medical or surgical condition, the patient should be referred to another veterinarian for diagnosis, care, and treatment. The former attending veterinarian should continue to provide care, as needed, during the transition.

The Principles state that clients may terminate the VCPR at any time.[4]

Guidelines for Referrals

The expansion and growth of knowledge, the emergence of specialization, and the use of the services and expertise of other health care professionals have necessitated the increased use of referrals in veterinary medicine. Referrals are to be encouraged among veterinarians, and the Guidelines for Referrals[5] approved by the AVMA in 1990 should be followed when referrals are used. These referral guidelines are summarized and paraphrased as follows:

Definitions

The *referring veterinarian* is the veterinarian who was in charge of the patient at the time of the referral. The *receiving veterinarian* or the *referral veterinarian* is the veterinarian to whom a patient is sent either by referral or for consultation. A *consultation* is a deliberation between two or more veterinarians concerning the diagnosis of a disease and the proper management of the case. A referral is the transfer of responsibility of diagnosis, care, and treatment from the referring veterinarian to the receiving veterinarian, and a new VCPR is established with the receiving veterinarian.

In these descriptions and definitions, the assumption is made that referrals and consultations may occur only between veterinarians. The Guidelines for Referrals do not address a situation in which the individual who is referring or receiving the patient is not a veterinarian. If these Guidelines for Referrals apply only to veterinarians, then other health care professionals may not actually accept or recommend referrals without the involvement of a veterinarian and the establishment of a valid VCPR. However, when a treatment modality such as physical therapy is required, a referral directly to a therapist may be appropriate. In that instance, specific written instructions and orders must accompany the referral. Because of the necessity of a valid VCPR, other health care professionals who might be involved in the diagnosis, care, and treatment of veterinary patients must work closely with veterinarians so a valid VCPR will be established and maintained.

Method of Referral

When a referral is being considered, communication among veterinarians and other health care professionals is essential. Communications may occur by letter, telephone, direct contact, or other means, and the most appropriate method of communication should be determined by the individuals involved. The referring veterinarian should provide the receiving veterinarian with all the appropriate information pertinent to the case before or at the time of the first contact with the patient or the owner. When the referred patient has been examined and a diagnosis has been established, the referring veterinarian should be promptly informed of those findings. Information provided should include diagnosis, proposed care, treatment plans, and other recommendations. If the patient undergoes a prolonged treatment or hospitalization, then immediately upon discharge of the patient the referring veterinarian should receive a detailed and complete report, preferably written, and should be advised as to continuing care of the patient or termination of the case. Each veterinarian involved in the case is entitled to collect fees for service, care, and treatments for professional services, and fee splitting is not allowed.[4]

All licensed veterinarians may receive referrals, and referring veterinarians may refer to whomever they believe appropriate for the situation. Referrals should occur in a timely manner, and veterinarians who solicit or encourage referrals should abide by the AVMA Principles of Veterinary Medical Ethics. The receiving veterinarian should provide only services or treatments relative to the referred condition and should consult the referring veterinarian if other services or treatments are needed.

When referrals are made to other health care providers who may not be licensed veterinarians, the same standards and guidelines must apply. Other health care professionals (non-veterinarians) who are involved with the care and treatment of veterinary patients cannot assume a valid VCPR, and therefore the ultimate responsibility for diagnosis, care, and treatment of the patient remains with the referring veterinarian, as a VCPR must be in effect at all times.

State Practice Acts: Veterinary Medicine and Physical Rehabilitation

Although interest in and support for the unique practice of veterinary physical rehabilitation is growing nationally, each state individually regulates the standards for both veterinary medicine and physical therapy through the respective practice acts for each profession. Both the APTA and the AVMA have adopted positions and policies that support animal physical rehabilitation.[3,6]

These organizations are not the regulatory bodies for the disciplines of physical therapy or veterinary medicine. The practice of veterinary medicine and that of physical therapy are regulated by respective practice acts for each state, and it is the responsibility of individuals who practice veterinary physical therapy to understand the legal issues related to both the veterinary and physical therapy practice acts of their respective states before pursuing this specialized discipline. Individuals practicing veterinary physical rehabilitataion who fail to comply with the rules and regulations of the respective state practice acts could be practicing both veterinary medicine and physical therapy without a license and might be subject to investigation, warning, disciplinary action, or criminal prosecution.

Veterinary Medicine

The veterinary practice acts are often vague when referring to the practice of veterinary physical rehabilitation. One exception is the Idaho Veterinary Practice Act, which lists physical therapy under "therapeutic options and alternative therapies" and states that such therapy "may be performed by assistants under the indirect supervision of a licensed veterinarian." This act further states that "before any therapeutic option or alternative therapy is performed on an animal by a veterinary technician or allied health professional, a veterinarian must first perform a diagnostic evaluation of the patient to rule out the use of conventional forms of veterinary medicine."[7]

In the state of Pennsylvania, both the State Board of Veterinary Medicine and the State Board of Physical Therapy are regulated by the same administration.[8] This arrangement allows for a clear understanding of the regulatory issues affecting both veterinarians and physical therapists when members of either profession are interested in veterinary physical rehabilitiaton. However, individuals practicing their respective professions in that state must be licensed by the regulatory board of their respective profession.

Physical Therapy

The physical therapy practice acts of many states include variable wording for authorizing and sanctioning the application of physical therapy techniques and procedures to animals and to the *direct access* of owners to physical therapy services. Currently, 21 states use the word *human* or *human being,* 4 additional states use the word *person,* and 3 states use the word *individual* in their physical therapy practice acts. This wording may be a problem for physical therapists who wish to practice veterinary physical therapy in those states, because the state practice acts may actually prohibit physical therapists from providing care to animals. Obtaining continuing education units or credits for courses in animal rehabilitation may also be problematic if the state physical therapy board does not accept this area of practice as legal. Direct access to physical therapy by human patients is an intriguing issue, in that 31 states permit direct access to "physical therapy evaluation and treatment" without a physician referral, and another 13 states permit direct access to "physical therapy evaluation only" without a physician referral. In the states that allow direct access of human patients to physical therapy, a physical therapist does not have to act with a physician to initiate physical therapy modalities; however, such direct access is not allowed for veterinary patients because of the definitions of veterinary practice and the necessity for a valid VCPR.[2] The APTA has published all of the physical therapy state practice acts.[9]

Because of the growing interest in animal rehabilitation and physical therapy, the Animal Physical Therapist Special Interest Group (APTSIG) within the Orthopedic Section of the APTA has collected information regarding the state practice acts and animal physical therapy. This information is intended to identify which state practice acts discuss animal rehabilitation and physical therapy, and which state practice acts include the words *humans, people,* or *persons,* which might limit the practice of animal rehabilitation and physical therapy in those states. The APTSIG is also collecting information regarding the veterinary practice acts in all states.

In some states the terms *physical therapy* and *physical therapist* are "protected terms," and therefore only licensed practitioners of physical therapy in those jurisdictions may lawfully represent themselves as physical therapists or state that they provide physical therapy services. Veterinarians or veterinary technicians practicing physical therapy on animals in these jurisdictions should state that they provide physical rehabilitation, or rehabilitation, to avoid potential conflicts, unless they employ a physical therapist or physical therapist assistant in their practice.

The physical therapy state practice act of New Mexico is currently the only physical therapy practice act that specifically addresses veterinary physical therapy, and in that act a doctor of veterinary medicine (DVM) is described as a "primary health care provider."[10] This statement occurs in the section of the practice act pertaining to direct care (access) requirements for physical therapists. In this practice act a "primary health care provider" is defined as

. . . a health care professional acting within the scope of his or her license who provides the first level of basic or general health care for individual's health needs including diagnostic and treatment services and includes: Physician (M.D., D.O., D.P.M.), Doctor of Veterinary Medicine (D.V.M.), etc.

The state physical therapy practice act of New Mexico further defines direct care requirements as follows:

A physical therapist shall not accept a patient for treatment without an existing medical diagnosis for the specific medical or physical problem made by a licensed primary care provider, except for those children participating in special education programs . . . and for acute care within the scope of the practice of physical therapy . . .

The act continues to define direct care requirements with the following statement:

When physical therapy services are commenced under the same diagnosis, such diagnosis and plan of treatment must be communicated to the patient's primary health-care provider at intervals of at least once every sixty (60) days, unless otherwise indicated by the primary care provider. Such communication will be deemed complete as noted in the patient's medical record by the physical therapist.[10]

Fundamentally, the New Mexico state physical therapy practice act allows a physical therapist to obtain referrals from a veterinarian and to have direct access to veterinary physical therapy patients who are in need of acute care physical therapy, as long as communication occurs between the veterinarian and the physical therapist within 60 days of initiating treatment and regularly every 60 days thereafter. Interestingly, the New Mexico veterinary practice act also states that because a physical therapist must work under direct supervision of a veterinarian, the fee for physical therapy services must be paid to the licensed veterinarian or licensed veterinary facility.

This is an example in which the practice acts for veterinary medicine and physical therapy are apparently in conflict. Although some state physical therapy acts allow the treatment of animals by physical therapists, the veterinary practice acts in those states may not allow the same degree of freedom; therefore it is important for the physical therapist and the veterinarian to understand both the physical therapy and the veterinary practice acts in the states where they are working. Although the veterinary practice acts in most states do not address the subjects of who may perform veterinary physical rehabilitation and direct access to patients by physical therapists, the veterinary profession has been careful to monitor who may practice veterinary medicine. State veterinary boards have been active in restraining the practice of veterinary medicine without a license, and the AVMA, through various councils and committees, has promoted the importance of the VCPR. These activities ensure that a veterinarian is the primary health care provider who manages the diagnosis, care, and treatment of the veterinary patients. In addition, the association with professions to enhance and improve the quality of veterinary care has been encouraged by the veterinary profession, and these relationships allow for a role of other health care professionals such as physical therapists in the improvement of such care.

Collaborative Relationships Between the Professions

In 1993 the APTA House of Delegates approved and adopted a position statement concerning collaborative relationships between physical therapists and veterinarians. This position statement reads as follows:

The American Physical Therapy Association endorses the position that physical therapists may establish collaborative, collegial relationships with veterinarians for purposes of providing physical therapy services or consultation. Physical therapists are the provider of choice for the provision of physical services regardless of the client. A collegial relationship is advantageous to the client.[6]

On the national level, collegial relationships have been established between physical therapists and veterinarians for several years with a national liaison between the AVMA and the APTA. National meetings, such as the First Symposium on Rehabilitation and Physical Therapy in Veterinary Medicine, which was held at Oregon State University (OSU) in August 1999, are another example of the growing collaboration between the two professions. Other international collaborative organizations have been formed to foster the growth and document the status of veterinary physical rehabilitation in other nations. In some countries such as the United Kingdom and the Netherlands, physical therapists have been performing veterinary physical therapy in collaboration with veterinarians for many years, and the experiences of practitioners in these countries are being shared and exchanged.

There are many ways for physical therapists and veterinarians to work together. Veterinary colleges could employ physical therapists to provide appropriate care and therapy to patients requiring rehabilitation. Faculty from universities with colleges of veterinary medicine and physical therapy departments could work together to provide clinical service, teaching, and research activities that would benefit students and faculty members from both disciplines. Veterinary hospitals and clinics could employ physical therapists with either full-time or part-time appointments, or these hospitals could consult with physical therapists as needed. In jurisdictions where permitted, physical therapists could establish veterinary rehabilitation therapy practices and solicit referrals from veterinarians in accordance with the state practice acts. Other venues where physical therapists might work include zoos, wildlife rehabilitation centers and parks, and canine and equine performance centers, exhibitions, and rodeos.

When collaborative relationships are initiated between veterinarians and physical therapists, the veterinarian must first establish a VCPR and then develop a care and treatment plan after a diagnosis is confirmed. This information must be communicated to the physical therapist, preferably in writing, before the physical therapy is initiated. Such communications are analogous to writing "doctor's orders" in a medical record. The physical therapist may wish to perform an independent evaluation and confirm a course of treatment in conjunction with the veterinarian. If opinions differ on the appropriate diagnosis and course of treatment, these differences should be negotiated in a professional manner. After the treatment plan is initiated, contacts and communications should continue between the physical therapist and the veterinarian regarding the progress and response of the patient throughout the course of therapy. As in human medicine, in which the physician is ultimately responsible for the patient, the veterinarian must be ultimately responsible for the care and treatment of the patient, because a VCPR must be maintained.

Risk Management for Physical Therapy and Veterinary Professionals

As physical therapists are finding new opportunities for professional services, including veterinary medicine, participation in these situations opens new questions about conduct and professional practice. There is no doubt that physical therapists have knowledge and skills that can benefit veterinary patients, but the legal and ethical issues regarding these collaborative relationships sometimes are unclear. Both the AVMA and the APTA have been supportive of these collaborative relationships; however, many states do not recognize these activities as falling within the scope of physical therapy. For this reason, physical therapists who choose to practice with animals in any professional capacity should be certain that they are acting in compliance with the physical therapy and veterinary medical practice acts in the states where they are working.

As stated earlier, the APTSIG has established a liaison program to assist members with an interest in rehabilitation for animals. The goal of this program is to obtain copies of the various state veterinary medical and physical therapy practice acts and to produce a resource directory of individuals interested in

veterinary rehabilitation. A national liaison coordinator for this program has been identified. While this liaison program is being established, interested individuals should contact appropriate licensing boards for clarification of questions.

The following guidelines are recommended when physical therapy practitioners are interested in practicing veterinary rehabilitation:

1. If the physical therapy practice act includes language that limits the practice to humans by using terminology such as *humans, people,* or *persons,* then practicing on animals may be in violation of that specific practice act. If the term *patient* is used, the language of that practice act may be permissive, and the physical therapist should check with the state licensing board about the exact wording and the current interpretation.
2. After reviewing the state physical therapy practice act, if the wording is still unclear, the physical therapy practitioner should contact the state licensing board for written clarification or consult with an attorney for a legal opinion.
3. If the activities of interest are clarified in the state practice act (and are within the scope of physical therapy practice as defined by the APTA), one should be able to obtain professional liability insurance for these activities. If activities are specifically excluded in the state practice act, it is unlikely that professional liability insurance will provide coverage or protection for potential litigation.
4. Physical therapist assistants (PTAs) who are providing veterinary physical rehabilitation also need to be aware of their state practice act regarding their practicing under the supervision of a licensed physical therapist. This does not necessarily mean on-site supervision; however, it does mean that the physical therapist has seen the patient and decided on a plan of care before the PTA initiates treatment. If they are performing animal rehabilitation under the supervision of a veterinarian, but not calling it physical therapy, this may be permitted based on the veterinary practice act in that individual state.
5. If a state precludes either PTs or PTAs from practicing veterinary physical therapy based on the state's practice act, the PTs or PTAs still may be able to work

under the direct supervision of a veterinarian, but should not call their practice physical therapy; rather they should term it *physical rehabilitation, animal rehabilitation, canine* or *equine rehabilitation,* or something similar. The choice to do this would still have the potential to be in violation of the state practice act and would need to be examined on an individual basis.

Veterinary practice acts in most jurisdictions are quite clear on the issues of the definition of veterinary practice, access to veterinary patients, and who may practice veterinary medicine. In all cases, the establishment of a VCPR is mandatory, and this rule necessitates that a physical therapist who is involved with an animal patient work closely with the veterinarian who has established the VCPR with that owner and patient. Otherwise, a physical therapist practicing on that animal could be in violation of a state veterinary practice act. When a VCPR has been established and followed, any potential legal issues should be minimized.

The following guidelines are recommended when veterinary practitioners are interested in practicing veterinary physical therapy:

1. If the term *physical therapy* or *physical therapist* is a protected term in that state, the term *physical rehabilitation, rehabilitation,* or a similar term should be used.
2. If a veterinary technician, physical therapist, or physical therapist assistant is to provide the veterinary physical rehabilitation, supervision by a veterinarian may be defined differently state by state, and the veterinarian should review this, especially if the individual is providing care off-site, such as in home visits.

Reimbursement and Remuneration for Services

The reimbursement for professional services is another issue that must be resolved when there are collaborative relationships between veterinarians and physical therapists. Both health care professionals are entitled to an appropriate fee, which should be based on the services rendered with consideration for education and training of the health care provider. If the physical therapist is an employee of a veterinarian, the fee for the animal rehabilitation may be included in the total charges for veterinary services. Because the physical therapist is an employee, that individual would be paid directly by the veterinary clinic where employment occurs and services are rendered.

If the physical therapist is self-employed or an independent contractor, a veterinarian could arrange a referral or consultation directly with a physical therapist; however, a VCPR would have to originate and be maintained with the attending veterinarian. In that instance, a separate or direct billing arrangement for veterinary physical therapy services could be appropriate if all involved parties are in agreement.

If the physical therapist is an employee of another health care provider, then that provider could charge the veterinarian or the owner directly, depending on the financial arrangements negotiated at the onset of the treatment plan. The attending veterinarian would be ultimately responsible for the diagnosis, care, and treatment of the patient and would have to write instructions or orders to the health care provider and physical therapist affiliated with that provider. The physical therapist would be an employee of the health care provider and would be paid by that entity.

The physical therapist is entitled to a reasonable fee for services rendered. If a veterinarian refers a patient to another veterinarian, physical therapist, or health care provider, the original veterinarian is not allowed to accept part of the professional fee for the referral of the patient and owner. Such an arrangement is called *fee splitting* or a *kickback*; it is unethical and would be in violation of the Principles of Veterinary Medical Ethics.[4]

In conclusion, the affiliations and collaboration between physical therapists and veterinarians will continue to grow with benefits for patients, owners, veterinarians, and physical therapists. With evolution and additional collaborative experiences in the discipline of animal physical rehabilitation, the specific roles of physical therapists and veterinarians will be clarified as well. Communication and cooperation between the professions of veterinary medicine and physical therapy, the APTA and AVMA, and the respective licensing boards of each state are necessary to successfully integrate physical therapy into the practice of veterinary medicine.

REFERENCES

1. Guide to physical therapy practice, ed 2, *Phys Ther* 81:21-22, 2001.
2. Model Practice Act. In *AVMA directory,* Schaumburg, Ill, 2000, American Veterinary Medical Association.

3. Guidelines for Alternative and Complementary Veterinary Medicine. In *AVMA directory,* Schaumburg, Ill, 2000, American Veterinary Medical Association.

4. Principles of Veterinary Medical Ethics. In *AVMA directory,* Schaumburg, Ill, 2000, American Veterinary Medical Association.

5. Guidelines for Referrals. In *AVMA directory,* Schaumburg, Ill, 2000, American Veterinary Medical Association.

6. Position on physical therapists in collaborative relationships with veterinarians, American Physical Therapy Association House of Delegates 06-93-20-36 (Program 32), 1993.

7. Idaho Veterinary Practice Act, Idaho Board of Veterinary Medicine, Boise, Idaho (1997), Idaho Code 54-2103 (26) and Board Rules IDAPA 46.01.01100.03.d.xv.

8. State Board of Veterinary Medicine and State Board of Physical Therapy, Professional and Vocational Standards, Department of State, Pennsylvania Code, Harrisburg, Pann (1998).

9. www.apta.org/govt_affairs/state/state_practice.

10. State of New Mexico Physical Therapy Board, Regulation and Licensing Department, Statutes and Regulations (1997), Title 16, Chapter 20, Part 10.

■ C h a p t e r 3

Conceptual Overview of Physical Therapy, Veterinary Medicine, and Canine Physical Rehabilitation

■ David Levine and Caroline P. Adamson

The purpose of this chapter is to provide a conceptual framework outlining the general practice of canine physical rehabilitation and physical therapy. Background information regarding the professions of physical therapy and veterinary medicine is included to assist professionals from each discipline to understand the history, educational requirements, and current practice of each other's profession. How to effectively bridge the gap between the physical therapy and veterinary professions is addressed, with models for collaborative practice outlined.

Physical Therapy as a Profession

History of the Physical Therapy Profession in the United States

Physical therapy began in the United States in the early 1900s and focused on treatment of acute anterior poliomyelitis, which reached its peak during the first two decades of the twentieth century. At this time physical therapy was not a true occupation; however, the foundations for the profession were developed. Some of these early applications of physical therapy included exercise, massage, and certain physical agent modalities.[1] The need for physical rehabilitation during and immediately following World War I served to further enhance the emerging field of physical therapy. From its origins, physical therapy has focused on restoring maximal function to individuals with disabilities.

Formal training in physical therapy began around 1918 and was developed by cooperative efforts between the office of the Surgeon General and personnel in civilian institutions.

Individuals who completed these training courses were given the title of Reconstruction Aides, the earliest title of physical therapists.[1] Many of these individuals worked in the military during this time. The first national organization was the American Women's Physical Therapeutic Association, which was founded in 1921. In 1922 this name was changed to the American Physiotherapy Association, and in 1947 to the American Physical Therapy Association (APTA).[1] Throughout the 1940s physical therapy continued to evolve and focused on treating patients who had contracted polio or those injured in World War II. This was a period of major growth in physical therapy, and because of the shortage of physical therapists, many more had to be trained during this time. From the 1940s to the present, physical therapy has gradually become a more autonomous and scientifically based profession. Physical therapy is an accepted medical intervention, and approximately 750,000 people are treated by physical therapists in the United States each day.[2]

THE AMERICAN PHYSICAL THERAPY ASSOCIATION

The American Physical Therapy Association (APTA) is a national professional organization representing more than 66,000 physical therapists, physical therapist assistants, and students in the United States.[3] Membership in the APTA is not mandatory for physical therapists practicing in the United States, and currently more than 90,000 physical therapists are providing health services in the United States.

Major responsibilities of the APTA are monitoring and improving physical therapy edu-

14

cation, practice, and research, and educating the general public about the role of physical therapy in healthcare. The APTA political action committee is one of the 10 largest healthcare political action committees in the nation.

Physical therapists practice in many settings including hospitals, school systems, private practices, extended care facilities and nursing homes, home health agencies, academic institutions, research centers, and government agencies. The APTA has 19 specialty sections, which represent various areas in physical therapy. These include acute care/hospital clinical practice, administration, aquatic physical therapy, cardiopulmonary, clinical electrophysiology, community home health, education, geriatrics, hand rehabilitation, health policy legislation, neurology, oncology, orthopedics, pediatrics, private practice, research, sports physical therapy, veterans' affairs, and women's health. A physical therapist may become board certified by the American Board of Physical Therapy Specialties (Diplomate, ABPTS) in one of seven areas (Cardiopulmonary, Clinical Electrophysiology, Geriatrics, Neurology, Orthopaedics, Pediatrics, and Sports Physical Therapy).

The orthopedic section of the APTA houses the animal physical therapist special interest group, which was formed in 1998 and has quickly grown to more than 400 members. The goals of this group are to:

- Promote physical therapy
- Share information
- Collaborate with other health professionals
- Develop educational programs
- Foster research
- Create guidelines for practice
- Encourage appropriate legislative changes
- Establish a national network
- Protect professional practice

PHYSICAL THERAPIST AND PHYSICAL THERAPIST ASSISTANT EDUCATION

The current entry-level physical therapy degree is a master's or doctoral degree. In the past, the entry-level degree was a bachelor's degree. The APTA supports changing the entry-level degree to the doctoral level by the year 2020. There are approximately 160 APTA-accredited physical therapy educational programs in the United States, which graduate roughly 4500 physical therapists each year. Every physical therapist must pass

a national licensing examination. Additional requirements for practice vary from state to state.

Physical Therapist Assistants complete a 2-year associate's degree from an APTA-accredited program. This training prepares them to provide therapeutic interventions that have been delegated by their supervising physical therapist, but assistants cannot evaluate or prescribe treatment. Requirements for licensure vary from state to state, as do the continuing education requirements.

Educational backgrounds of both physical therapists and physical therapist assistants do not include any formal training in the rehabilitation of animals. Animal anatomy may be studied during undergraduate education, but most likely this will be anatomy of the cat. Application of physical therapy to animals is not included in standard curricula; however, a few physical therapy programs now offer an elective course in this area.

Veterinary Medicine as a Profession

History of the Veterinary Profession

The first college of veterinary medicine was established at Lyon, France. The first college of veterinary medicine in the United States was established at Iowa State University in the 1800s. The initial emphasis in veterinary medicine was on agricultural production and livestock. Gradually the emphasis on the treatment of individual animals shifted to herd management. The emergence of companion animals as members of the family, combined with the shift in agricultural demand, has resulted in the development of small-animal and equine practice as the predominant emphasis in veterinary medicine. Furthermore, the explosion of knowledge in small-animal medicine and surgery, combined with the era of specialization, has resulted in improved healthcare for pets. One area that has been neglected until recently is the rehabilitation of animals with chronic ailments and following surgery. The goals of this new area are to increase function, to improve the ultimate outcome of patients following major surgery, and to enhance the quality of life.

The American Veterinary Medical Association

The national professional organization that represents the approximately 64,000 veterinarians in the United States is the American Veterinary Medical Association (AVMA).[4] The AVMA is responsible for evaluating and credentialing veterinary medical education, administering the national board examination for veterinarians, and overseeing the various specialty colleges. The American College of Veterinary Surgeons (ACVS); American College of Veterinary Internal Medicine (ACVIM), neurology subspecialty; and American College of Veterinary Emergency and Critical Care (ACVECC) are specialty colleges whose members are likely to treat patients that may benefit from rehabilitation. Examples of other related organizations include the American Academy of Veterinary Acupuncture and the American Veterinary Chiropractic Association.

Veterinarians undergo broad training that includes studying diseases of large, small, and exotic animals. Currently there are no specialty organizations for veterinary physical therapy or rehabilitation. Training in this area is relatively limited, although a number of colleges now offer courses or lectures in physical rehabilitation.

Veterinary and Veterinary Technician Education

Veterinarians usually have an average of 4 years of undergraduate education, followed by 4 years of professional curriculum at an AVMA-approved college. Currently there are 29 approved colleges of veterinary medicine in the United States and Canada graduating approximately 2100 veterinarians yearly.[4] Veterinarians are required to pass board examinations in order to practice. Some graduate veterinarians pursue additional training in the form of general internships and residencies in specialties. Specialty certification requires an internship or equivalent training, completion of a formal 2- to 3-year residency program, publication and research requirements, and successful completion of a certifying examination. There are currently 18 specialties recognized by the American Veterinary Medical Association.

Veterinary Technicians complete at least 2 years at an AVMA-accredited program and receive at least an associate's degree. In approximately 40 states and provinces, veterinary technicians are certified, regis-

tered, or licensed.[5] Candidates are tested for competency through an examination which may include oral, written, and practical portions. A state board of veterinary examiners or the appropriate state agency regulates this process. A national examination is available; however, requirements vary by individual states. Veterinary technician specialty organizations recognized by the North American Veterinary Technician Association (NAVTA) are the Academy of Veterinary Emergency and Critical Care Technicians, and the Academy of Veterinary Technician Anesthetists.[6]

Veterinary and veterinary technician programs do not typically include any course work in physical therapy. Although most veterinarians and veterinary technicians have a basic understanding of the rehabilitation process, they have not participated in any formal training in this area. Application of physical therapy to animals is not included in the standard curricula; however, a few veterinary programs now offer an elective course in this area.

Continuing Education

Continuing education is essential to gain the knowledge in the reciprocal field that practitioners need to effectively perform canine rehabilitation and physical therapy. Some ways of accomplishing this are attending continuing education courses, self study, attending meetings of the other profession, volunteering with members of the other profession, and attending related courses such as animal training, handling, and behavior.

A number of courses are offered in this area throughout the world. The First International Symposium on Rehabilitation and Physical Therapy, which was held at Oregon State University in 1999, helped to bring the professions of physical therapy and veterinary medicine together in a professional meeting. Research has been identified as critical to bridge the gap between professions and to establish the efficacy of physical therapy protocols and treatment. There are certificate programs in the United States, the Netherlands, and the United Kingdom.

PHYSICAL THERAPY
EVALUATION/INTERVENTION

Physical therapy encompasses a spectrum of services for humans, including evaluation, intervention, assessment, consultation, education, and research.[2]

Evaluation includes taking a history, evaluation of body systems to be certain that physical therapy is the appropriate medical intervention, and a variety of tests and measurements in order to determine a diagnosis, prognosis, and intervention. Physical therapists assess aerobic capacity and endurance, joint motion and integrity, muscle strength, arousal and cognition, need for assistive and adaptive devices, cranial nerve integrity, environmental barriers, body mechanics, gait, locomotion, balance, skin integrity, motor function, neuromotor development and sensory integration, orthotic, protective and prosthetic devices, pain, posture, reflexes, circulation, and edema.[2]

Physical therapists alleviate impairment and functional limitation by designing, implementing and modifying therapeutic interventions that include the following[2]:

- Therapeutic exercise (ROM, aerobic conditioning, gait training, aquatic therapy, muscle strengthening, balance, coordination, posture, motor control)
- Manual therapy techniques (joint mobilization and manipulation, massage, remodeling scar tissue)
- Wound management (dressings, topical agents, debridement, modalities, oxygen therapy)
- Airway clearance techniques (postural drainage, percussion, vibration, shaking)
- Orthotic and prosthetic intervention
- Electrotherapeutic modalities (electrical stimulation, laser)
- Thermal modalities (superficial heat and cold, and deep heat including ultrasound and diathermy)

Some of the common goals of physical therapy treatment are to decrease pain, improve muscle strength, retard atrophy, decrease swelling, decrease muscle spasm, increase the rate of tissue healing, remodel scar tissue, and improve function and independence in activities of daily living. Prevention of injury, impairment, functional limitation, and disability is also part of physical therapy. This includes promoting and maintaining fitness, health, and quality of life in all age populations.

BRIDGING THE GAP BETWEEN PHYSICAL THERAPY AND VETERINARY MEDICINE

Traditional Physical Therapy and Veterinary Models of Practice

Physical therapists commonly practice by referral from a physician, although more than 30 states currently allow direct access to a physical therapist, meaning that a physical therapist practicing in these states may see a patient without physician referral. Additionally some states allow direct access for evaluation only, meaning that after the evaluation is complete, the patient must still see a physician to allow treatment to begin. In this model, the physical therapist will typically relate to the physician what their findings were to expedite the initiation of treatment. As discussed in Chapter 2, the veterinary practice acts in most states require the physical therapist to work under the direct supervision of a veterinarian, thus precluding a physical therapist from direct access in the care of veterinary patients.

Veterinarians in general practice see a variety of patients with various conditions. In some cases, a referral to a specialist is made for treatment requiring advanced procedures and equipment. In most cases the referred patient is returned to the referring veterinarian for follow-up care and any general patient concerns. Veterinary technicians assist with the diagnostic and treatment procedures under the direction of the veterinarian.

Team Approach to Rehabilitation

The individuals listed in Box 3-1 may be involved in a practice offering animal rehabilitation.

The attending veterinarian is often the primary person responsible for decisions regarding appropriate rehabilitative care. Depending on the injury and repair, specific recommendations are given to the person responsible for the rehabilitation. Precautions to therapy, especially exercises, must be clearly communicated. When veterinarians initiate physical therapy in their practices, the initial sessions should be performed with all team members present, as differences in terminology may cause confusion and possibly result in injury. For example, performing range of motion (ROM) exercises may have different meaning to veterinarians, owners, and physical therapists. Communication and documentation between the team members is critical, and forms such as those illustrated later in this chapter provide an easy way to facilitate this.

The team approach involves a group evaluation or an assessment of the same patient by two or more clinicians within a short period. A core group of clinicians—for example, a veterinarian and a physical therapist, and veterinary technician—is identified as the initial team. The initial team then documents their findings, meets, and decides together the most effective plan for intervention. The core group may request additional evaluations by other experts on the team on an individual case basis. The appropriate clinicians are chosen to initiate the intervention plan. The team reviews the progress of the client periodically. One member of the team is responsible for follow-up after discharge.

This team approach allows for a variety of perspectives on healthcare issues. The team offers the client a detailed interdisciplinary assessment as well as the most cost-efficient method of providing services to resolve or treat the problem.

■ ■ ■ **BOX 3-1**   List of Individuals Contributing to Animal Rehabilitation

- Referring veterinarian
- Veterinary specialist (surgeon, neurologist, internist, emergency and critical care veterinarian)
- Rehabilitation veterinarian
- Physical therapist on staff or as a consultant
- Animal behaviorist
- Nutritionist
- Anesthesiologist
- Acupuncturist
- Veterinary technician
- Physical therapist assistant
- Support staff
- Owner

Collaborative Model for Practice

A proposed model for canine physical rehabilitation is outlined in Figure 3-1 and is based on a similar model for humans.

Documentation

Documentation should provide clear communication between all of the parties involved in the animal's care including the veterinarian, the referring veterinarian if applicable, the person responsible for the physical rehabilitation, and in some cases, the owner. Because documentation is a critical form of communication, all patient files should be updated and documented at each physical rehabilitation treatment. Notes should be written in a clearly understandable, legible manner. An important characteristic of documentation is that the information should be easily obtained in a short period of time. A physical rehabilitation chart should give easy access to pertinent information such as functional status, ROM, treatment given, and patient progress. Because terminology differs between professions, a glossary is included at the end of this book. An example of one difference is the directional term anterior-posterior (A-P) used in human medicine versus cranial-caudal used in veterinary medicine. A treatment given once daily would be qd in the human field, but sid in the veterinary profession.

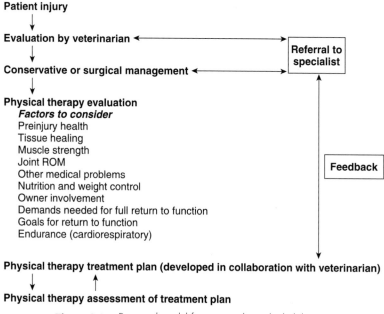

Figure 3-1   Proposed model for canine physical rehabilitation.

Terms such as closed kinetic chain exercises (when the limb is in a weight-bearing position, such as in the weight-bearing or stance phase of walking) are not typically discussed in the veterinary field.

Documentation is also important from a legal perspective, as a record of the animal's condition and a clear documentation of the procedures performed. An example might be an animal that has just completed a therapy session in which it demonstrated weight-bearing on the affected extremity 75% of the time at a slow walk, and had a stifle ROM of 50 degrees flexion and 150 degrees extension that was documented in the medical record. If this animal presents with non–weight-bearing lameness at the next treatment with a ROM of 60 degrees flexion and 130 degrees extension, that would lend support to the idea that the animal had been injured, not during therapy, but rather in its cage, during a walk, or by some other means. Regardless of the mechanism of injury, the documentation may protect the therapist from fault, and also alert the therapist to contact the veterinarian. When an animal's status has changed, an evaluation by the veterinarian is necessary before therapy continues.

Another purpose of documentation is to verify the benefits of the treatment. The progress of the animal may be determined so that alterations can be made to the treatment protocol to further enhance recovery. Careful documentation and record keeping also provide a valid base for research. Conducting periodic chart audits can assist patient care in a variety of ways, including ensuring that all pertinent and necessary information is included, and that the treatment protocol is appropriate for the diagnosis.

The physical therapy chart should include the following key pieces of information:
1. A relevant medical history
2. The history of the present illness, including the attending veterinarian's referral information containing any precautions or contraindications for therapy, and treatment to be given
3. Any objective information such as ROM, function, girth measurements, lameness scores
4. Primary problems to be addressed and goals for the treatment
5. The treatment itself in as much detail as possible
6. The response to treatment

Examples of documentation forms in this chapter include the following:
1. Client information form (Figure 3-2)
2. Referral form (Figure 3-3)
3. Physical rehabilitation evaluation form (Figure 3-4)
4. Orthopedic evaluation form (Figure 3-5)
5. Neurologic evaluation form (Figure 3-6)
6. Daily flowsheet form (Figure 3-7)
7. Referral letter (Figure 3-8)

NEW CLIENT INFORMATION

Owner's name	
Address	
Home phone	
Work phone	
Veterinarian/surgeon	
Date of surgery/injury	

PATIENT INFORMATION:

Name	
Breed	
Age	
Sex	
Color	
Spayed/neutered	

PATIENT HISTORY:

Rabies vaccination	
Past medical history	
Previous surgery	
Allergies	
Special diet/medication	
Previous activity level	
History of present illness	
Treatment since injury/surgery	
Owner's goals	

Figure 3-2   Client information form.

CANINE REHABILITATION CLINIC

Referral Form

Client_____ Patient_____ Date_____

Breed_____ Sex_____ Age_____ Weight_____

Referring veterinarian/clinic:_____

Clinical condition:_____ Onset/Sx date:_____

Special instructions/precautions_____
_____
_____
_____
_____
_____

Frequency and duration: _____Times per day for _____days

☐ Board until _____ Drop off: ☐ MWF ☐ Other_____

☐ T/Th

Plan: ☐ Evaluate and treat

☐ Hot pack   ☐ Gait training

☐ Cryotherapy   ☐ Massage

☐ Ultrasound   ☐ Joint mobilizations

☐ Electrical stimulation   ☐ Weight-bearing/weight shifts

☐ Therapeutic exercise   ☐ Passive range of motion

☐ Hydrotherapy   ☐ Neuromuscular reeducation

☐ OTHER:_____

DVM Siguature_____

Figure 3-3   Referral form.

PHYSICAL THERAPY INITIAL EVALUATION

Patient's name:	
Date:	

PHYSICAL EXAMINATION:

Skin/incisions:		Color/temp:	
Heart rate:		Respirations:	

POSTURE/GAIT:

General observation:			
Preop/injury lameness:	Walk:	Trot:	
Postop/injury lameness:	Walk:	Trot:	
Standing limb position:		Sitting limb position:	

Circumference (cm):	70% femur	80% humerus	Joint line	Other
Affected:				
Unaffected:				
Other:				

RANGE OF MOTION:
Joint(s): Aff/Unaff

Joint(s): Aff/Unaff	Flexion	Extension	AB/adduction	Varus/Valgus	Other
Hip:					
Stifle:					
Hock:					
Shoulder:					
Elbow:					
Carpus:					
Other:					

PALPATION:

Forelimb	
Hind limb	
Spine	
Other	

SPECIAL TESTS:

Neurologic:	
Orthopedic:	
Functional:	
Other:	

Figure 3-4   Physical rehabilitation evaluation form.

TREATMENT:

Modalities:	Manual:	Therex:
Interferential current	Massage	Gait training
Neuro-muscular electrical stimulation	Joint mobilization	Aquatic
	Passive range of motion	Functional
		Swiss ball
Other stim		Foam roll
Ultrasound	Other:	Owner education
Ice		Protocol review
Heat		Other:
Other		

ASSESSMENT/GOALS:

Decrease pain	
Decrease edema	
Increase weight-bearing	
Independent home exercise program	
Return to previous function	
Other	

PLAN:

Return visit	
Call for follow-up	
Call DVM	
Other	

DVM Signature _____

Figure 3-4 cont'd   Physical rehabilitation evaluation form.

CANINE ORTHOPEDIC REHABILITATION
EVALUATION FORM

Patient_____ Client_____ Date_____

Breed_____ Age_____ Sex_____ Date of Sx/onset_____

Referring vet/clinic:_____ Diagnosis_____

History:_____
_____
_____
_____

Medications:_____
Client's goals_____
_____
Functional mobility_____
_____

OBJECTIVE
Involved limb: RF   LF   RR   LR

Range of motion:

Forelimb	R	L	**Rear limb**	R	L
Shoulder			Hip		
1. Flexion _____/_____			1. Flexion _____/_____		
2. Extension _____/_____			2. Extension _____/_____		
Elbow			Stifle		
1. Flexion _____/_____			1. Flexion _____/_____		
2. Extension _____/_____			2. Extension _____/_____		
Carpus			Hock		
1. Flexion _____/_____			1. Flexion _____/_____		
2. Extension _____/_____			2. Extension _____/_____		
			Other _____/_____		

*Visual inspection/palpation:*_____
_____
_____
_____
_____

Pain score:
0 = No pain on palpation of joint
1 = Mild pain; palpation completed
2 = Moderate pain; palpation completed with obvious discomfort noted
3 = Severe pain; palpation not completed
4 = Pain too severe; restraint/sedation needed to palpate

Limb circumference:
Muscle mass:
Affected_____ Unaffected_____
Femur length _____cm   _____cm
70% of length _____ cm   _____cm
Girth   _____ cm   _____cm

Joint effusion:
Affected_____ Unaffected_____
Patellar tendon_____ cm   _____cm
2" above   _____ cm   _____cm
2" below   _____ cm   _____cm

Figure 3-5   Orthopedic evaluation form.

Gait analysis:

Orthopedic lameness

Degree of lameness (stance)	Degree of lameness (walk)	Degree of lameness (trot)
0 = Normal stance	0 = No lameness/weight-bearing on all strides observed	0 = No lameness/weight-bearing on all strides observed
1 = Slightly abnormal stance (partial weight-bearing)	1 = Mild subtle lameness with partial weight-bearing	1 = Mild subtle lameness with partial weight-bearing
2 = Moderately abnormal stance (toe-touch weight-bearing)	2 = Obvious lameness with partial weight-bearing	2 = Obvious lameness with partial weight-bearing
3 = Severely abnormal stance (holds limb off the floor)	3 = Obvious lameness with intermittent weight-bearing	3 = Obvious lameness with intermittent weight-bearing
4 = Unable to stand	4 = Full non–weight-bearing lame	4 = Full non–weight-bearing lame

Post-operative limb use

Degree of limb use (stance)	Degree of limb use (walk)	Degree of limb use (trot)
0 = Normal stance	0 = No lameness	0 = No lameness
1 = Slightly abnormal stance (partial weight-bearing)	1 = Lame but weight-bearing on >95% of strides	1 = Lame but weight-bearing on >95% of strides
2 = Moderately abnormal stance (toe-touch weight-bearing)	2 = Lame but weight-bearing on >50% and <95% of strides	2 = Lame but weight-bearing on >50% and <95% of strides
3 = Severely abnormal stance (holds limb off the floor)	3 = Lame but weight-bearing on >5% and <50% of strides	3 = Lame but weight-bearing on >5% and <50% of strides
4 = Unable to stand	4 = Non–weight-bearing lame or weight-bearing on <5% of strides	4 = Non–weight-bearing lame or weight-bearing on <5% of strides

Gait deviations:_____
_____
_____
_____

*ASSESSMENT*_____
_____
_____
_____

*PLAN OF CARE*_____
_____
_____
_____

Therapist Signature_____

Figure 3-5 cont'd   Orthopedic evaluation form.

**CANINE NEUROLOGIC/SPINAL REHABILITATION
EVALUATION FORM**

Client_____ Patient_____ Date_____

Breed_____ Age_____ Sex_____ Date of Sx/Onset_____

Referring vet/clinic:_____ Diagnosis_____

History:_____

_____

_____

Prior surgeries:_____

Follow-up visit:_____ Medications:_____

Client's goals:_____

OBJECTIVE
Involved area(s) : RF   LF   RR   LR   Spine_____

Mental status: Alert   Depression   Stuporous   Comatose   Aggressive   Fearful   Disoriented

*Palpation/postures:*_____

_____

_____

_____

_____

Active movements:

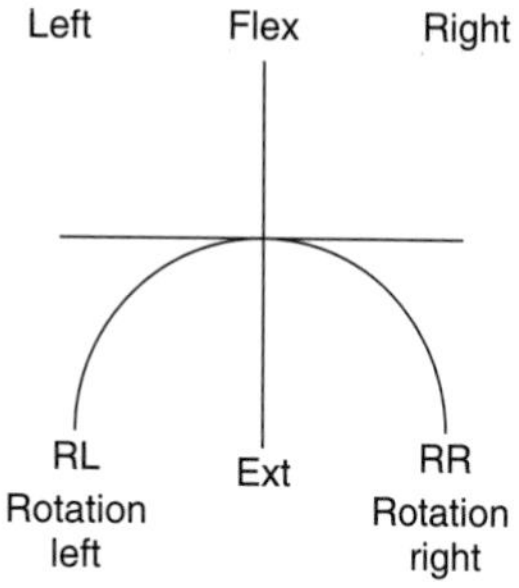

Left   Flex   Right

RL   Ext   RR
Rotation   Rotation
left   right

KEY:
Affected Body Segment
X Tender
O Center of pain
≡ Spasm
/// Guarding
* Reflex contraction
° ROM

Limb circumference:
Muscle mass:
Affected_____   Unaffected_____
Femur length_____cm   _____cm
70% of length_____cm   _____cm
Girth   _____cm   _____cm

Figure 3-6   Neurologic evaluation form.

Gait analysis:
Involved limb(s):_____

Degree of deficit (stance)   Degree of deficit (walk)   Degree of deficit (trot)

_____   _____   _____

5 = Normal strength and coordination
4 = Can stand to support;   **minimal paraparesis** and ataxia
3 = Can stand to support but frequently stumbles and falls;   **mild paraparesis** and ataxia

2 = Unable to stand to support; when assisted, moves
    limbs readily but stumbles and falls frequently;
    moderate paraparesis and ataxia

1 = Unable to stand to support; slight movement when
    supported
    severe paraparesis

0 = Absence of purposeful movement; **paraplegia** or **tetraplegia**

Deviations:_____
_____
_____

Proprioception: (+ intact; − absent)

RF	LF	RR	LR

Spinal reflexes:
Key: 0 = Absent
      +1 = Depressed
      +2 = Normal
      +3 = Exaggerated
      +4 = Clonus
      NE = Not examined

Crossed extensor: _____ Forelimb
  + Present   _____ Hind limb
  − Absent

Forelimb	RF	LF	RR	LR
Flexor reflex				
Biceps (C6-C8)				
Triceps (C7-T2)				
Ext carpi rad (C7-T1)				
Deep pain				
Hind limb				
Flexor reflex				
Patella (L4-L6)				
Cranial tibial (L6-L7)				
Gastrocnemius (L7-S1)				
Sciatic (L6-S1)				
Perineal (S1-S3)				
Deep pain				
Cutaneous trunci				

ASSESSMENT_____
_____
_____

PLAN OF CARE_____
_____
_____

Therapist Signature_____

Figure 3-6 cont'd   Neurologic evaluation form.

**CANINE ORTHOPEDIC REHABILITATION
FLOWSHEET**

PATIENT NAME:_____ CLINICAL CONDITION:_____ SX DATE:_____

CLIENT NAME:_____

TIME	Date	Date	Date	Date	Date

Reassessment: Date / /

ROM   Shoulder   R_____   Hip   R_____   Weight-bearing status:_____

              L_____   L_____   Gait analysis:_____

        Elbow   R_____   Stifle   R_____   _____

              L_____   L_____   *Proprioception:*   OTHER:_____

        Carpus   R_____   Hock   R_____   _____

              L_____   L_____   RF   LF   RR   LR   _____

Limb circumference   **PLAN:**_____

Affected limb _____ Unaffected limb _____   Reflexes: R   L   _____

              _____   _____   Forelimb flexor   _____

              _____   _____   Rear limb flexor   _____

                                                  Patellar   _____

Therapist Signature_____

Figure 3-7   Daily flowsheet form.

CANINE REHABILITATION CLINIC

{Date}

{Address}

Dear Dr. { },

Thank you for referring "Star" to Physical Therapy at The Canine Rehabilitation Clinic and Veterinary Hospital. Star has been treated for 3 days with ultrasound to help resolve the contracture of the digits of the right forelimb and the underwater treadmill to help regain full function of the left hind limb. We are encouraging Star to use the leg in a buoyant environment to avoid exacerbating the contracture; second, the thermal effects of the water will help with improving joint mobility, and finally, the resistant property of the water will help to strengthen the muscles of the limb. I have also reiterated to her owner, Diane, to take Star for short walks (no more than 10 to 15 minutes at a time) no more than 2 to 3 times per day (on the off days from physical therapy).

Dr. Smith has left a message outlining the rehabilitation process and changes in medications to avoid further GI upset for Star. So far, we have seen no adverse reactions to the medications.

Again, thank you for this referral. We will continue physical therapy for 2 days this week and will provide the owner with a home care program to continue strengthening activities for Star. We expect that she will have progressive improvement.

Please do not hesitate to call if you have any questions or concerns: {Phone number}.

Sincerely,

Figure 3-8   Referral letter.

REFERENCES

1. *Healing the generations: a history of physical therapy and the American Physical Therapy Association.* Lyme, Conn, 1995, Greenwich Publishing Group.
2. The guide to physical therapist practice, ed 2 *Phys Ther* 81:21-22, 2001.
3. What is APTA? https://www.apta.org/about/whatisapta, 2001.
4. About the American Veterinary Medical Association. http://www.avma.org/membshp/about.asp, 2001
5. North American Veterinary Technician Association: A regulated profession. http://www.navta.net 2001.
6. Veterinary Technician Specialties. http://www.navta.net/specialties.htm, 2001.

BASIC CONCEPTS OF VETERINARY MEDICINE

Chapter 4

Canine Behavior

Daniel Q. Estep

Several things must occur to achieve the goals of physical rehabilitation. First, there must be effective communication between the person doing the rehabilitation and the canine patient. Second, the patient must be motivated to engage in the therapy. Third, the rehabilitation must be performed in a humane way. Finally, the entire process must be safe for the therapist and the patient. For these things to occur, the therapist must understand what motivates dogs and how to communicate with them.

Clearly, working with dogs is different from working with human patients. Dogs do not communicate in the same fashion as people, and different things motivate dogs. After the communication and motivational systems of dogs are appreciated and understood, working with dogs in a rehabilitation setting may be more pleasant, effective, humane, and safe. The goals of this chapter are to explain these systems and understand how they can be used to benefit the therapist and the patient.

The Communication System of Dogs

Communication occurs when one animal (or person) sends a signal that changes the behav-

ior of another animal (or person).[1] Signals may be behaviors such as a stare, sounds such as a laugh, an odor produced by the animal, or even a touch or caress.[2] Dogs use a variety of sensory channels to send their signals. They depend heavily on vision, using visual displays and changes in body postures. Examples include showing of the teeth or lowering of the ears. Dogs use a variety of sounds to communicate. These include howls, whines, whimpers, and barks. Dogs depend heavily on olfactory communication, but because human olfaction is so poor, very little is known about it. It is known that the reproductive state of a dog can be communicated by smell, as can the individual identity of the animal. Touch is not often considered when canine communication is discussed, but it can be very important. Licking of another dog's muzzle, for example, can communicate something very specific to another dog. It is obvious that a bite can change the behavior of the dog or person who receives it, and it is also a form of communication.

The therapist should be aware of a few rules of animal communication.[3] First, animals tend to emphasize or exaggerate their signals when they communicate so that they may be easily perceived. They may try to make them stand out (e.g., howling loudly); they may repeat their signals (e.g., repeatedly barking); or they may use multiple signals to communicate the same thing (e.g., growling and showing the teeth at the same time). Animals often do all of these things when they signal.

Second, the signals tend to be stereotyped, being consistent from time to time and from individual to individual, so there is no confusion about the meaning. A growl by a Chow Chow is very similar to a growl by a Labrador Retriever. Finally, signals that mean very different things have very different forms. For example, the stiff, upright posture of an offensively threatening dog is almost opposite in form from the hunched, cowering posture of a submissive dog (see Figure 4-1, p. 34).

Miscommunication and Anthropomorphism

Communication systems have evolved to allow animals within the same species to communicate effectively with each other. Except in rare situations, they have not evolved to allow different species to communicate. As a result, different species, such as human beings and dogs, may not understand what the other species is trying to communicate. Miscommunication can be inefficient and dangerous to the individuals involved. For example, dogs often bite people when humans do not recognize that a dog is threatening them.

The natural tendency of people who are interacting with dogs is to interpret dog signals as if they were human signals. There is also a tendency for people to assume that dogs engage in a particular behavior for the same reasons as people. This attribution of human characteristics to nonhumans is called anthropomorphism. It can result not only in miscommunication, but also in inappropriate treatment of animals.[4] For example, a person who believes that a dog is house soiling out of spite may punish the dog after the fact when the cause is really fear or separation anxiety. In this case, punishment is totally inappropriate. For these reasons, it is important that people working with animals be very careful observers of animal behavior and that they understand the motivations of the animal. Without careful observation, a person may miss subtle signals given by the animal and misinterpret what is seen.

From the animal's perspective, a phenomenon similar to anthropomorphism also occurs. Dogs and other animals may interpret human behavior as if we were members of their species. This attribution of animal characteristics to humans by animals is called zoomorphism. In fact, it seems that most animals that have been reared around people and are well socialized tend to zoomorphize. Most dogs tend to view people as strange-looking dogs. They direct canine communication signals to us as if we were dogs, and they tend to interpret our behavior toward them as if we were giving dog signals and not human signals. One implication of this is that our behavior toward dogs may not be interpreted in the way we intend. By understanding dog communication signals and adjusting our behaviors so that we give more dog-appropriate signals, we may make our communication much more effective.

Reading the Body Language and Sounds of Dogs

Understanding the communication signals of dogs is important not only to allow us to communicate more effectively with them, but for another reason as well. Animals reveal their motivations and emotions through their behaviors. If we can understand what emotions and motivations a dog is experiencing, we can predict what the dog may do next and adjust things accordingly. By making changes in our behavior and the environment, we can make further interactions safe and influence the dog to do the things that we want it to do. For example, if there are signs that a dog you are about to handle is fearful, adjustments may be made to reduce the fear and make things safer and more efficient for you, and more humane and comfortable for the dog.

There are several key features that should be the focus of attention when evaluating canine behavior. These include general body position, piloerection, the orientation of the animal to you or others, tail position, ear position, the showing of teeth, facial muscle contraction around the mouth, opening of the eyes and dilation of pupils, and orientation of the eyes. Also listen for vocalizations such as barks or whines.

General Body Position

Evaluate whether the dog is standing up or lying down. Is it standing stiffly erect, or hunched over with head lowered? Is the dog oriented directly facing you, or is it oriented away from you? Is the dog shaking or shivering? Is it moving or trying to move, or is it immobile?

Piloerection (Hair Raising)

Is the hair on the back standing up or is it lying down flat? Not all dogs demonstrate piloerection. Some only raise the hair on their backs between their shoulders; others may raise the hair all the way down the back, including the tail.

Tail Position and Movement

Is the tail standing straight up like a flag pole, or is it tucked down between the legs, or somewhere in between? Is the tail moving from side to side? If so, how fast is it moving?

Ear Position

Are the ears up and facing forward, or are they rotated backward so that they lie flat against the skull? Are they somewhere in between? Ear position is not always easy to read because of the variability in the ears of dogs. Dogs with erect ears such as German Shepherds are much easier to read than flop-eared dogs such as Cocker Spaniels. Dogs that have cropped ears such as some Doberman Pinschers or American Pit Bull Terriers may also be very difficult to read.

Eyes

Are the eyes staring without movement, are they scanning the environment in a relaxed way, or are they darting around rapidly? Is the dog staring directly at you, or at another animal or person? Are the eyelids wide open so that the sclera may be seen, or are they somewhat closed? Are the pupils dilated or constricted?

Mouth

Is the mouth open or closed? Are the teeth showing? If so, are the lips retracted vertically so that only the front teeth and canine teeth are seen, or are they refracted horizontally so that the back teeth are seen as well? If the mouth is closed, do the skin and muscles around the mouth seem relaxed, or tense and wrinkled? Sometimes dogs will wrinkle the skin of the upper lip and expose the teeth without opening the mouth. Is the

dog yawning repeatedly or licking its lips repeatedly?

Sounds

Listen for sounds made by the dog such as barks, howls, growls, whimpers, whines, yelps, or screams. Some sounds, such as growls, may be very low in volume and must be listened for closely.

It is important to note that dogs vary enormously in how they give behavioral signals. Some dogs, for example, have no tails or tails that have been surgically docked. There is little to be gained from looking at tail posture or movement in these dogs. There is even a great deal of variation in tailed dogs regarding how high a dog holds its tail or moves its tail. It is also important to understand that body postures and motivations are dynamic and can change quickly. The animal must be monitored continuously for changes in behavior. It is helpful to observe many dogs to learn how to identify the signals indicating their behavior. Videotapes of dog behavior may also be valuable. One videotape describes canine body postures and shows the features described above and how to interpret them.*

Interpreting the Body Language and Sounds of Dogs

The emotions and motivations of dogs may be inferred from changes in their behavior. In some cases these behaviors are intended as communication signals, such as a growl. In other cases, they are not intended as communication, but still reveal the emotions and motivations of a dog. An example might be a dog that is shaking with fear.

Box 4-1 describes the specific body posture elements and sounds that will be most commonly seen in rehabilitation settings. There is great variability among dogs, and not all dogs display all of the elements. There is no single element that reliably indicates a dog's motivation or intentions. To correctly assess a dog, all of the elements must be observed and evaluated. In addition, the more a dog is handled by the therapist, the more familiar a pattern of behavior becomes, making it somewhat easier to evaluate a patient's behaviors and intentions.

Canine behavior: body postures. Videotape available from Animal Care Training, Denton, Texas.

■ ■ ■ **BOX 4-1**   Communication Signals Used by Dogs to Convey Behaviors

---

Fearful or submissive dogs will usually display:
- Crouched body posture, or lying down, especially rolled over on the back exposing the belly. Dog will usually try to move away from the source of the fear
- Tail tucked between the legs
- Ears pinned back against the skull
- Eyes wide open to expose the sclera, avoidance of direct eye contact
- Lips may be retracted exposing the teeth in a submissive grin
- Whining, whimpering, or yelping
- Shaking, panting, urinating, or defecating
- If the fear continues, the dog may become defensively threatening
- Dogs in pain may show these characteristics as well

Defensively threatening dogs will usually display a mixture of offensive and fearful characteristics:
- Crouched body posture
- Piloerection may occur
- May or may not be directly oriented toward the subject of the threat
- Tail usually down
- Ears may be pinned back
- Eyes not directly staring. May look away from subject of threat, or alternate between staring and avoidance of contact
- Teeth bared in horizontal retraction of lips
- May be growling, barking, whining, whimpering, or yelping
- Dog may whip its head around quickly as if to grab or bite whatever is frightening it
- If these threats do not stop the fear, the dog may snap without making contact or may bite

Offensively threatening dogs will usually display one or more of the following:
- Standing up tall with a stiff body posture, oriented toward the subject of the threat
- Piloerection along the dorsum
- Tail straight up in a vertical line; it may be wagging slowly
- Ears up and forward or pricked forward
- Direct eye contact or staring
- Teeth bared with vertical retraction of the lips
- Barking and/or growling
- Lunging, chasing, or jumping at the target of the aggression
- Snapping the teeth at the target without making contact
- If these threats do not alter the target's behavior, the dog may hit the person with his mouth or bite

Dogs experiencing conflicting emotional or motivational states will display:
- Displacement or irrelevant behaviors such as frequent yawning, licking of the lips, grooming, or sleeping
- Ambivalent behaviors—alternating between different motivational states such as fear and friendliness or submission and defensive threat
- Redirected behaviors—behaviors directed at other animals or people not directly involved with the animal. Redirected aggression is especially dangerous for others in the area if a dog is aggressively motivated but cannot get to the original target

Dogs experiencing pain or distress will display:
- Shaking, panting, urination, or defecation
- Whining, whimpering, yelping, or screaming
- Avoidance or attempts to escape the distressing situation or thing
- Defensive threats or aggression
- Displacement yawning, lip-licking, or grooming
- Fearful responses such as a crouched body posture, wide-open eyes, avoidance of direct eye contact, tucked tail, or ears laid back
- Withdrawal from activities or refusing to move

Figures 4-1 and 4-2 illustrate the body postures and facial displays of dogs organized by different motivational states. The handler must be aware of the fact that aggression or threat by dogs can be offensively or defensively motivated. In offensively threatening dogs, such as those protecting food or toys, there is very little fear and the body postures all tend to make the dog look bigger and to show its weapons (teeth). In defensively threatening dogs, there are both offensive components and fearful components. Defensive aggression occurs most often when a dog is frightened or in pain and believes it is trapped or cornered. In therapeutic situations it will be more likely that defensive threats

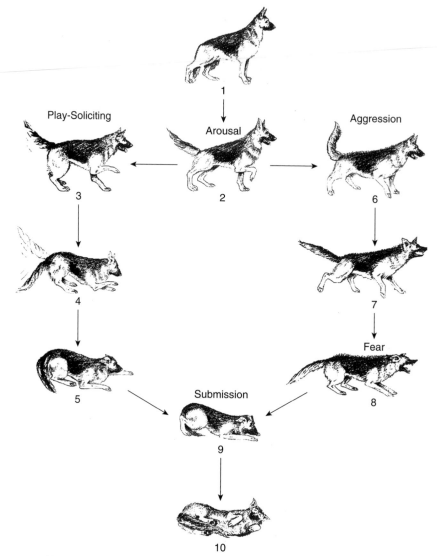

Figure 4-1   General body postures of dogs. Dog 1 shows a relaxed dog. Dog 2 is alert. Dog 3 shows playful behavior. Dogs 4 and 5 show increasing fear and submission. Dog 6 displays offensive aggression. Dog 7 shows mixed motivations of offensive and defensive aggression. Dog 8 shows defensive aggression. Dogs 9 and 10 show fear and/or submission. (From Overall KL: *Clinical behavioral medicine for small animals*, St Louis, 1997, Mosby.)

and aggression will be seen rather than offensive threats and aggression.

In Fig. 4-1, dog 1 is standing in a relaxed position. Dog 2 is aroused or alert to something in the environment, but is not aggressive. Dog 3 shows a play solicitation with no fear or aggressive motivation. Dogs 4 and 5 are demonstrating increasing submission and fear. Dog 6 is demonstrating offensive threats, while dog 8 is showing defensive threats. Dog 7 is demonstrating ambivalent behavior and a mixture of offensive and defensive signals. Threats are signals that let others know that outright aggression (a bite) is likely to

follow, unless something changes. Dog 9 shows submission and fear, and dog 10 shows even stronger fear and submission. Submissive postures are signals that let others know that the dog is not a threat. This usually diminishes threats or aggression from others.

Figure 4-2 shows the facial postures of dogs in greater detail. Dog 1 is alert to something in the environment. Dogs 2 and 3 show increasing offensive aggression. Dogs 4 and 7 show increasing fear and submission with no aggression. Dogs 5, 6, and 8 show mixtures of aggressive and fear motivations and interme-

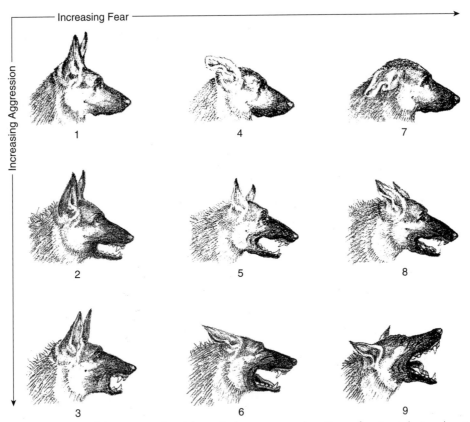

Figure 4-2   Facial postures of dogs. Figures from left to right show increasing fear. Figures from top to bottom show increasing aggressive motivation. Dog 1 is an alert dog. Dog 3 is offensively aggressive. Dog 7 is fearful and/or submissive. Dog 9 is defensively aggressive. All others are intermediate in fear and/or aggression. (From Overall KL: *Clinical behavioral medicine for small animals,* St Louis, 1997, Mosby.)

diate behaviors. Dog 9 shows defensive threat, a mixture of aggression and fear.

In therapy sessions, the handler is likely to see dogs that are fearful, in pain, or distressed, or those experiencing conflicts of motivation or emotion. Defensively aggressive dogs may sometimes be seen. Rarely are offensively aggressive dogs seen. Dogs become fearful in therapy as a result of previous experiences that have produced pain, fear, or discomfort. They may display conflict behavior because conflicting emotions or motivations have been elicited at the same time, such as pain, anxiety, fear, defensive aggression, or the motivation to escape. Defensive aggression is most often elicited when the dog experiences pain or fear in therapy or similar past situations. Offensive aggression is likely only if the dog is disturbed when it has something of value, such as food, a treat, or a toy, and the dog perceives a threat that it will be stolen or taken away. It may also occur as a means of protecting its owner or the dog's territory.

Influencing the Behavior of Dogs

There may be several reasons why you as a therapist may wish to influence the behavior of a patient in therapeutic situations. The most obvious is to encourage the patient to actively engage in the therapy or exercise. Another is that you may want to reduce the fearfulness of a dog so that it is more comfortable in therapy. Yet another is to reduce the defensiveness of a dog to make the situation safer for people interacting with the patient. The behavior of dogs undergoing therapy can be influenced in several ways.

The behavior of a dog in your presence depends on several factors. The first is the health status, motivation, emotional state, predispositions, genetic composition, and prior experiences of the dog. The second factor is the nature of the situation, and where and how the encounter occurs. A dog in a familiar place, such as its home, will behave differently than if it is in a strange place. The third factor is your behavior in the situation. Animals respond to your behavior as if you were a member of their species. Dogs interpret your behavior as if you were giving dog signals.

The handler has little control over dog-related factors. The dog's health status, genetic predispositions, temperament, and prior experiences are beyond your control. The therapeutic situation may also be beyond your control because factors such as where the therapy is performed may be limited. Even so, small changes in the environment could influence the outcome of the session. For example, if seeing others through a window distracts the patient, covering the window may help.

The one factor that is most controllable is the behavior of the handler in the therapy situation. Because the dog will be reading your behavior just as you are trying to read its behavior, your responses may change the dog's motivation and emotional state. These ultimately influence the effectiveness and comfort of the therapy for the patient and the safety for you and others.

Fear in your patient may be reduced or eliminated if you can associate the therapy with strong positive rewards. This may greatly influence the outcome of the therapy session. Dogs may become fearful because the therapy situation is unfamiliar, because it has been associated with pain, discomfort or fear in the past, or because you or others are giving signals that the dog interprets as threatening. Avoid standing over the dog or reaching for it, especially with sudden or quick movements. Avoid staring at the dog, getting face to face with it, or using low, gruff tones while talking to it.

The patient may also be less fearful if you let it become familiar with the therapy situation and specific devices or instruments that will be used. Taking a few minutes to expose the patient to these things in a nonthreatening manner before therapy begins may result in better cooperation and less discomfort for the dog, and greater safety for the therapist.

For dogs that come into the therapy situation in a fearful state or become fearful or threatening during therapy, behavior modification techniques may help reduce the fear or perceived threat. These techniques are known as desensitization and counterconditioning. Briefly, desensitization involves gradual exposures to the things that cause the fear, but in such a manner that it does not cause a fearful response.

Counter conditioning involves creating an emotional response in the animal that is incompatible with the fear and that blocks it. Giving the dog a treat, for example, often creates a happy state that is incompatible with fear. It is beyond the scope of this chapter to explain the details of these techniques, but they are described elsewhere.[4,5] If at all possible, do not continue therapy that creates more than just mild anxiety or fear or that creates any threat or aggression, because this will cause more anxiety, fear, or aggression and make it more difficult for you and the patient in future therapy sessions.

Using strong rewards for the dog in the therapy session is helpful not only in reducing fears and threats, but also in motivating the dog to cooperate. If you use treats, play, petting, or praise, the patient may work more enthusiastically during therapy. Operant conditioning techniques may also be used to teach the dog specific movements or postures. If done carefully, such training may take a matter of minutes or may be done over one or a few therapy sessions. For example, you may want to teach a dog to move in a particular manner to extend the range of motion of a particular limb. When using rewards to teach behavior, it is important to reward each small step in the process. The basics of operant conditioning are explained elsewhere,[4] with a more detailed introduction to learning and teaching dogs given in reference 6. A particularly fast and effective way to teach dogs is the use of clicker training, which is a form of operant conditioning that makes use of a recognizable cue, the sound of a metal clicker, to teach the dog. An introduction to clicker training has been published.[7]

Recognize that the stronger the reward, the quicker and the more reliable the learning will be. When used in counterconditioning, more powerful rewards are more effective in blocking fears and threats. For many dogs, food is a powerful reward. Play can be very rewarding for some dogs. For some dogs, petting, massage, or praise may be rewarding, but in general, these are not as powerful as food or play. When using food, the owners or others familiar with the dog should be asked what foods the dog prefers. Not all dogs like the same things. It is not necessary to use large amounts of food when providing rewards to dogs in these settings. Dogs find very small pieces, no bigger than the end of your little finger, very rewarding. This is especially important because many rehabilitation patients are already obese, and low-

---

■ ■ ■ **BOX 4-2** Behavioral Considerations When Performing Physical Rehabilitation

- Question owners or others familiar with the dog about its behavior *before* beginning treatment. Ask if the dog has ever shown threats or aggression when in pain or afraid. Ask whether the dog threatens, is aggressive, struggles, or tries to escape when handled or restrained.
- Ask what things the dog finds powerfully rewarding.
- Try to avoid places, things, or procedures that frighten the dog. Change the environment to make it more pleasant and less fearful.
- Let the animal acclimate to unfamiliar places and equipment before beginning any treatment.
- Constantly monitor the body language and sounds of the dog. Be particularly alert to signs of pain, discomfort, conflict, fear, and threat.
- Avoid behaviors the dog may perceive as threatening such as leaning over, reaching down to touch or pet, making sudden movements, staring, getting your face close to the dog's, or using loud speech or gruff tones of voice.
- When possible, avoid or stop procedures or treatments that cause pain, anxiety, or fear.
- When possible, avoid or stop procedures or treatments that cause threat or aggression. If it is not possible to avoid or stop these things, use restraints or a muzzle.
- Use strong positive rewards before, during, and after therapy sessions. Use food treats, play, petting, praise, or whatever the dog finds rewarding.
- Reward every small step in the therapy process. Reward as you go along and reward as soon as the dog displays the desired behavior. Reward consistently.
- Be proactive. Always assume that a fearful, uncomfortable, or painful dog will bite. Take steps to protect yourself, and other people and animals.

---

calorie treats and small amounts of food help prevent additional weight gain. In some cases, asking that the dog not eat a few hours before the therapy session can make the food more rewarding.

Your safety, the safety of those working with you, and the safety of the dog are of primary importance in the therapy session. By reading the body language and recognizing pain, fear, threats, and conflict behavior in canine patients, you may avoid most injuries to people and dogs. This requires constant and careful monitoring of the dog's behavior because motivations and emotions can change very quickly.

Box 4-2 lists some things to consider when planning or performing therapy sessions. The owners and others who have worked with the dog should be asked about aggressive tendencies. Also ask if there are certain manners of handling or care that the dog does not tolerate. These questions should be asked before beginning therapy with the dog. If the dog displays threatening behavior or if you think the dog may become threatening or aggressive, either

muzzle the dog or end the therapy session. A basket-style muzzle is more comfortable for most dogs and will allow them to pant and take treats while wearing it.

REFERENCES
1. Dewsbury DA: *Comparative animal behavior,* New York, 1978, McGraw-Hill.
2. Hart BL: *The behavior of domestic animals,* New York, 1985, WH Freeman.
3. Simpson BS: Canine communication. In Houpt KA, ed: *The veterinary clinics of North America: small animal practice, progress in companion animal behavior,* vol 27, no 3, pp 445-464, Philadelphia, 1997, WB Saunders.
4. Hens S: *Pet behavior protocols: what to say, what to do, when to refer,* Lakewood, Colo, 1999, American Animal Hospital Association Press.
5. Voith VL, Borchelt PL: Fears and phobias in companion animals. In Voith VL, Borchelt PL, eds: *Reading in companion animal behavior,* pp 140-152, Trenton, NJ, 1996, Veterinary Learning Systems.
6. Reid PJ: *Exel-erated learning: explaining in plain English how dogs learn and how best to teach them,* Oakland, Calif, 1996, James and Kenneth.
7. Tillman P: *Clicking with your dog,* Waltham, Mass, 2000, Sunshine Books.
8. Overall KL: *Clinical behavioral medicine for small animals,* St Louis, 1997, Mosby.

Chapter 5

Canine Anatomy

Cheryl Riegger-Krugh, Darryl L. Millis, and Joseph P. Weigel

This text is intended for people who already possess knowledge of either veterinary or human anatomy. To assist communication among human rehabilitation and veterinary colleagues, some anatomical terms used for dogs will appear in regular print with the analogous terminology for humans in parentheses following the canine term. These comparisons have been minimized, as this is a chapter about canine anatomy and not a chapter about comparative anatomy. Comparative anatomy between dogs and humans has been described in other sources.[1-3]

We have chosen to use some terms consistently throughout the chapter, rather than use equally acceptable synonyms. The canine forelimb is known also as the thoracic limb and the pectoral limb, but we will use the term *forelimb*. The canine hindlimb is known also as the pelvic limb or rear limb, but we will use the term *hindlimb*. Because the term *foot* can be interpreted as a front foot or a hind foot, the term *foot* will be clarified when used or specified as forepaw or manus or hindpaw or pes. The terms trunk, neck, and head refer to the same body segments in dogs and humans. The word *canine* is an adjective and the word *dog* is a noun; these terms will be used in this consistent grammatical form throughout the chapter.

Directional Terms and Anatomical Planes

Directional Terms From Normal Stance (Anatomical Position)

The dog stands upright on digits or phalanges of each forepaw or manus and each hindpaw or pes (Figure 5-1). This type of stance is termed a digitigrade stance. The human stands upright on the feet, with the plantar aspect of the feet contacting the floor and adjacent to each other. The upper limbs hang at the sides of the body, palms facing forward. This type of stance is called a plantigrade stance.

Directional terms from anatomical position in dogs are more directly compared to the directional terms in humans when the human is in a quadruped position or the dog is in an upright stance posture. Directional terms include cranial, caudal, rostral, dorsal, palmar, plantar, medial, and lateral. Other specific directional terms include (1) radial and ulnar to indicate toward the radius and ulna, respectively; (2) axial and abaxial to indicate toward or away from the axis of the digits, which is between the third and fourth digits of the forepaw, and the third and fourth digits of the hind paw, respectively; and (3) tibial and fibular to indicate toward the tibia and fibula, respectively.

Anatomical Planes

The main planes of motion for dogs are as follows (see Figure 5-1):

- *Sagittal plane:* The plane that divides the dog into right and left portions. If this plane were in the midline of the body, this is the median plane or median sagittal plane.
- *Dorsal plane:* The plane that divides the dog into ventral and dorsal portions.
- *Transverse plane:* The plane that divides the body into cranial and caudal portions.

Axes of Rotation

Motion may occur in any of three planes of motion or some combination. Joint motion

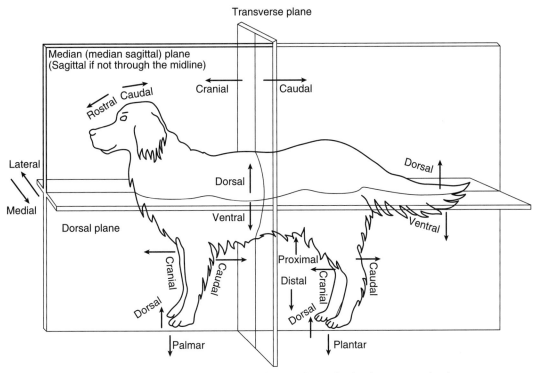

Figure 5-1   Orientation to planes of motion and directional terms for the dog. (Reprinted with permission from Riegger-Krugh C, Millis D: *Canine anatomy and biomechanics I (forelimb)*, LaCrosse, Wis, Jan 2000, Wis, Orthopaedic Section, Inc.)

within a plane usually occurs around an axis of rotation, which may be centered within the joint space or within the bone comprising the joint. Some joint motions are planar or gliding motions and do not occur around an axis of rotation.

An axis of rotation for a joint motion is a straight line or rod that is 90 degrees to the plane of motion. For each axis of rotation listed below, the plane of motion around which joint motion occurs can be viewed from Figure 5-1.

AXES OF ROTATIONAL JOINT MOTION

The axes of rotational joint motion are as follows:

- *Transverse axis:* Sagittal plane motion occurs around an axis of rotation that is directed mediolaterally.
- *Ventrodorsal axis:* Dorsal plane motion occurs around an axis of rotation that is directed ventrodorsally.
- *Craniocaudal axis:* Transverse plane motion, such as rotation of the trunk, occurs around an axis of rotation that is directed craniocaudally.

Most joints allow motion in more than one plane. Dogs and humans have the ability to selectively produce motion in one, some, or all of the planes of motion at one time. Dogs have much more limitation in motion in the dorsal and transverse planes.

Bones

The bones of the dog skeleton and limbs are illustrated in Figures 5-2, 5-3, and 5-4. Bony landmarks on the bones of the limbs are shown in Figures 5-5 through 5-11.

Forelimb

The forelimb skeleton consists of the thoracic or pectoral girdle and bones of the forelimb (Figures 5-5 and 5-6). Size of forelimb bones varies a great deal, because of the greater variation in size for breeds of dogs. The forelimbs bear 60% of the dog's weight.

The canine scapula is positioned close to the sagittal plane. Dogs have a very abbreviated clavicle that does not articulate with the

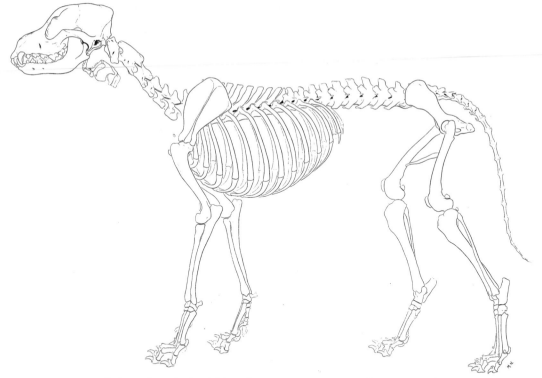

Figure 5-2   Skeleton of a male dog, left lateral view. (From Evans HE: *Miller's anatomy of the dog*, ed 3, Philadelphia, 1993, WB Saunders.)

rest of the skeleton. It is a small oval plate often 1 cm or less in length and ⅓ cm wide, located at the tendinous intersection of the brachiocephalicus muscle. The adult canine clavicle is mostly cartilage and is usually not visible on radiographs.

The canine humeral head is less rounded compared to the human head, to assist with weight bearing. Distally, there is an olecranon fossa and supratrochlear foramen for the secure positioning of the protruding anconeal process of the ulna for more stability in weight bearing.

The radius is the medial forearm bone and is the main weight-bearing bone of the antebrachium distally. The proximal surface of the radius articulates with the humeral capitulum, which is not as prominent as in the human. The canine distal radius has distinct facets for articulation with carpal bones, providing stability in weight-bearing.

The ulna is the lateral forearm bone and has a very prominent olecranon process, which allows secure attachment for the large triceps brachii muscle, needed as an antigravity muscle for weight bearing in dogs. The ulna is the longest bone of the canine body. It articulates distally with the ulnar carpal and accessory

carpal bones by two distal facets and does not have an articular disk. The dog has an anconeal process, which is near the attachment site of the anconeus muscle. The anconeal process is needed for stability in weight-bearing.

At the carpus or wrist (Figure 5-7), there are seven carpal bones. The radial carpal bone is analogous to the fused scaphoid and lunate. There are five metacarpal bones. The first metacarpal is very short and nonfunctional. Dogs have many sesamoid bones that are embedded in tendons or near them. Sesamoid bones occur when there are significant changes in directions of pull on tendons in addition to the tensile forces produced during muscle contractions. They allow for constant good alignment of angles of insertion of tendons at their attachment sites, which helps relieve stress on the tendinous insertions for animals that walk on their digits. Dogs are digitigrade animals and weight-bear on digits II to V, with the main weight-bearing occurring on digits III and IV. The sesamoid bones at the dorsal surface of each metacarpophalangeal joint align the extensor tendons for optimal muscle action. Those on the pad surface of the manus align the flexor tendons.

canine pelvis shape from a ventral view resembles a rectangle. The symphysis pelvis is relatively long and has two portions, the symphysis ischii and symphysis pubis, compared to the relatively shorter joining of the anterior aspect of the human innominates at the symphysis pubis. The distinction of the shape of the male and female pelvic inlet and outlet in humans is not made in dogs.

The canine femur is the heaviest[4] and largest[5] canine bone. In most dogs, it is slightly shorter than the tibia and the ulna and about one-fifth longer than the humerus. The average canine angle of inclination or cervicofemoral angle is 144.7 degrees.[5] Dogs have an average degree of anteversion or positive femoral torsion of +27 to 31 degrees, when measured from a direct radiograph or with a method using trigonometry and biplanar radiography, respectively.[5] The canine femur has a relatively thick and short femoral neck, a caudomedially located lesser trochanter, a prominent lateral greater trochanter, and a relatively short and wide shaft with a narrow isthmus in the middle. The greater trochanter has a craniolateral prominence called the cervical tubercle. Dogs have a third trochanter, which is the attachment site of the superficial gluteal muscle. Canine medial and lateral femoral condyles are equally prominent, but the articular surface of the medial femoral condyle projects more cranially than that of the lateral femoral condyle.

There are three sesamoid bones in the caudal stifle joint region. Two are located in the heads of the gastrocnemius muscle caudal to the stifle joint and are called fabellae. The sesamoid in the lateral head is the largest, is palpable, and articulates with the lateral femoral condyle, whereas the one in the medial head is smaller and may not have a distinct facet on the medial femoral condyle. The third is the smallest, is located in the proximal attachment of the popliteus muscle, and articulates with the lateral tibial condyle.

The canine patella or kneecap is the largest sesamoid bone in the body. It is an ossification in the quadriceps femoris muscle. The patella alters the pull, increases the moment arm, and protects the quadriceps tendon, as well as provides a greater contact surface for the tendon on the trochlea of the femur than would exist without the patella. The canine patellar articular surface is mildly convex.

The canine tibia is the major bone in the crus. The triangular proximal tibia is wider than the distal cylindrical tibia. Medial and

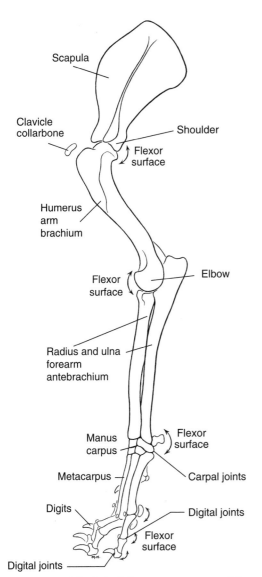

Figure 5-3 Left forelimb skeleton, noting joints and flexor surfaces. (From Evans HE, deLahunta A: *Miller's guide to the dissection of the dog*, ed 5, Philadelphia, 2000, WB Saunders.)

Hindlimb

The hindlimb skeleton includes the pelvic girdle, consisting of the fused ilium, ischium, and pubis, and the bones of the hindlimb (Figures 5-8 and 5-9). The size of hindlimb bones varies a great deal, because of the great variation in size for breeds of dogs. The hindlimbs bear 40% of the dog's weight.

The canine pelvis is positioned between the dorsal and transverse planes and closer to the dorsal plane. The canine pelvis is relatively small and narrow. The canine ischiatic or ischial tuberosities are wide and project caudally to form a broad ischiatic table. The

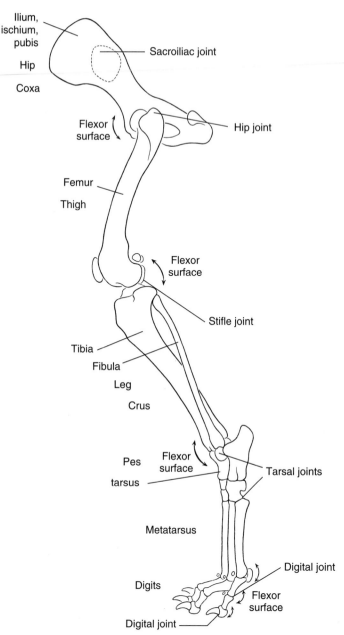

Figure 5-4   Left hindlimb skeleton, noting joints and flexor surfaces. (From Evans HE, deLahunta A: *Miller's guide to the dissection of the dog*, ed 5, Philadelphia, 2000, WB Saunders.)

lateral tibial condyles, an intercondylar eminence, and a tibial tuberosity are on the proximal tibia. The medial tibial plateau slopes distally on the most medial aspect. The extensor groove, on the cranial tibia and lateral to the tibial tuberosity, provides a pathway for the long digital extensor muscle. There is a popliteal notch on the caudal tibia in the midline, where the popliteal vessels course. The tibia articulates with the fibula proximally, along the interosseous crest, and distally. The

tibial cochlea articulate with the trochlea of the talus to form the talocrural joint.

The canine fibula is a long, slender bone, which articulates with the tibia and also serves as a site for muscle attachment. There is a distinctive groove in the lateral malleolus, the sulcus malleolaris lateralis, through which course the tendons of the lateral digital extensor and peroneus brevis muscles.

The tarsus, or hock, consists of the talus, calcaneus, a central tarsal bone, and tarsal

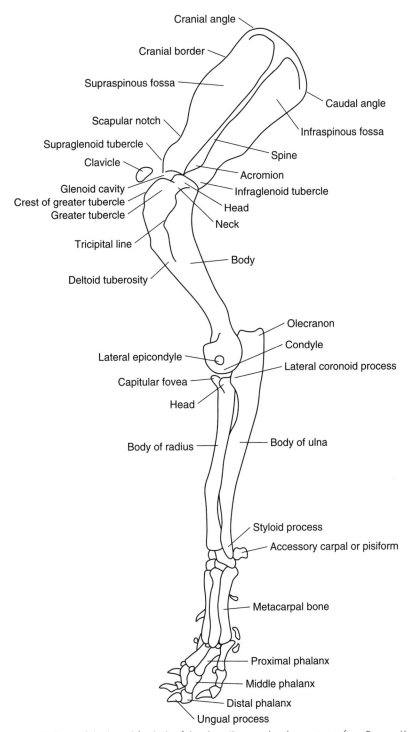

Figure 5-5   Skeleton of the lateral forelimb of the dog. (Reprinted with permission from Riegger-Krugh C, Millis D: *Canine anatomy and biomechanics I (forelimb)*, LaCrosse, Wis, Jan 2000, Orthopaedic Section, APTA, Inc.)

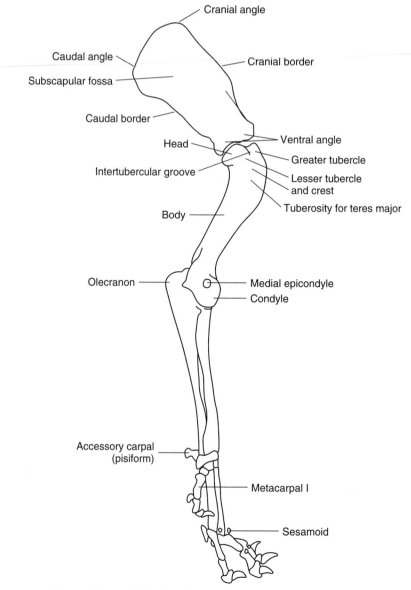

Figure 5-6   Skeleton of the medial forelimb of the dog. (Reprinted with permission from Riegger-Krugh C, Millis D: *Canine anatomy and biomechanics I (forelimb)*, LaCrosse, Wis, Jan 2000, Orthopaedic Section, APTA, Inc.)

bones I to IV (Figure 5-10). The talus articulates with the distal tibia and has prominent ridges. At the talocrural joint, two convex ridges of the trochlea of the talus articulate with two reciprocal concave grooves of the cochlea of the tibia. The orientation of the grooves and ridges deviates laterally about 25 degrees from the sagittal plane. This deviation allows the hindpaws to pass lateral to the forepaws when dogs gallop.[4] The calcaneus is large and serves as the insertion of the common calcaneal tendon. The central tarsal bone lies between the talus and the numbered tarsal bones I to III. Tarsal IV is

large and articulates with the calcaneus and metatarsal bones, spanning this entire region.

The canine hindpaw has five metatarsal bones; however, the first metatarsal can be very short or absent. Dogs have many sesamoid bones that are embedded in tendons where there are significant compressive and tensile forces produced during muscle contractions. The sesamoid bones at the dorsal surface of each metatarsophalangeal joint align the extensor tendons for optimal joint action. The sesamoid bones on the plantar surface of the hindpaw align flexor tendons.

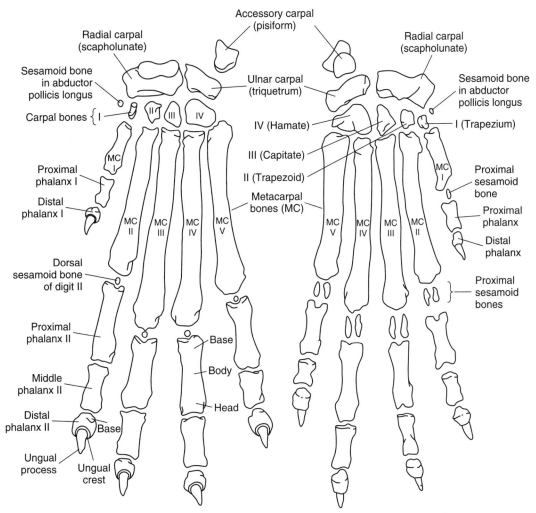

Figure 5-7   Skeleton of the left dorsal (A) and left palmar (B) forepaw of the dog. (Reprinted with permission from Riegger-Krugh C, Millis D: *Canine anatomy and biomechanics I (forelimb)*, LaCrosse, Wis, Jan 2000, Orthopaedic Section, APTA, Inc.)

Spine

The spine consists of five areas of the vertebral column: the cervical vertebrae and its articulation with the head, thoracic vertebrae, lumbar vertebrae, sacral vertebrae, and the coccygeal vertebrae (Figures 5-11 to 5-14). The number of vertebrae is listed in Box 5-1.

All vertebrae, except the sacral vertebrae, remain separate and form individual joints. Four sites exist within the canine spine which have limited motion.[6] These sites occur at areas where the cranial and caudal articular surfaces are inclined in a nonparallel manner and in different directions. The nonparallel alignment of the articular surfaces markedly restricts joint accessory motions, such as glides. The restricted joint motions and areas resulting from these joint alignments include atlantoaxial

motion other than rotation, the C7-T1 junction, the caudal thoracic region, and the sacrum.

Individual vertebral bone size and shape vary among breeds. For any one breed, canine cervical through lumbar vertebrae are fairly consistent in size. The consistent size in dogs reflects the relatively equivalent cranial-to-caudal compressive loading. Because dogs are quadruped, there is weight bearing on all four limbs. There is cervical spine compression as a result of the positioning of the dog's head as a cantilever, which requires cervical extensor muscle activity to maintain head posture. The massive cervical extensor muscle activity requires relatively large and strong cervical vertebrae to support the muscle mass. Canine intervertebral disks likewise change little in size from the cervical through the lumbar vertebrae. The cervical (C) C5-C6 area is a site

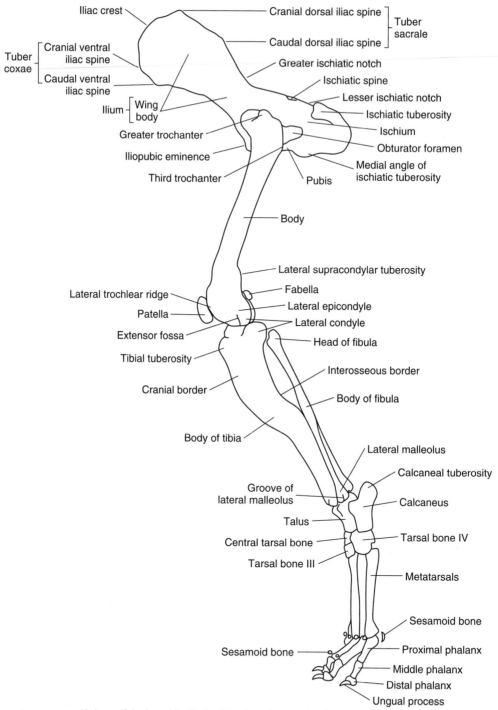

Figure 5-8   Skeleton of the lateral hindlimb of the dog. (Reprinted with permission from Riegger-Krugh C, Weigel J: *Canine anatomy and biomechanics II (hindlimb)*. LaCrosse, Wis, Feb, 2000, Orthopaedic Section, APTA, Inc.)

of relative hypermobility in large dogs. The spinal cord ends at L6-L7.

The canine atlas or C1 vertebra (Figure 5-12) has a transverse foramen in each transverse process, a craniodorsal arch, and right and left lateral vertebral foramina for the passage of cervical spinal nerve 1. The atlas has correspondingly shaped condyles for articulation with the occiput. The canine lateral wings or transverse processes are prominent and

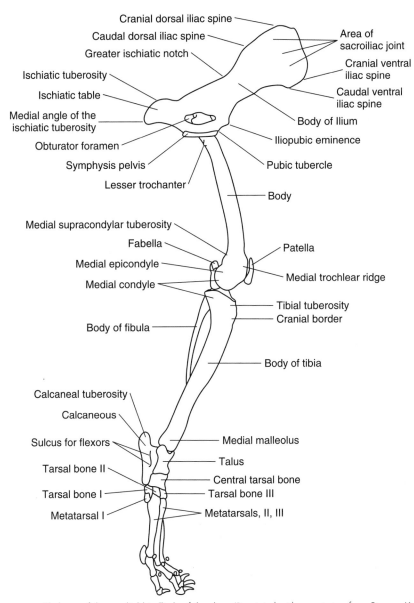

Cranial dorsal iliac spine
Caudal dorsal iliac spine
Greater ischiatic notch
Ischiatic tuberosity
Ischiatic table
Medial angle of the ischiatic tuberosity
Obturator foramen
Symphysis pelvis
Lesser trochanter

Area of sacroiliac joint
Cranial ventral iliac spine
Caudal ventral iliac spine
Body of Ilium
Iliopubic eminence
Pubic tubercle
Body

Medial supracondylar tuberosity
Fabella
Medial epicondyle
Medial condyle

Patella
Medial trochlear ridge

Body of fibula

Tibial tuberosity
Cranial border

Body of tibia

Calcaneal tuberosity
Calcaneous
Sulcus for flexors
Tarsal bone II
Tarsal bone I
Metatarsal I

Medial malleolus
Talus
Central tarsal bone
Tarsal bone III
Metatarsals, II, III

Figure 5-9   Skeleton of the medial hindlimb of the dog. (Reprinted with permission from Riegger-Krugh C, Weigel J: *Canine anatomy and biomechanics II (hindlimb).* LaCrosse, Wis, Feb, 2000, Orthopaedic Section, APTA, Inc.)

easily palpable from the skin surface. The canine axis or C2 has a large spinous process with an expanded arch, a wide body, and large transverse processes (see Figure 5). The spinous process is nonbifid. The canine axis is very large relative to the size of other canine cervical vertebrae. The axis has a dens, which projects cranially to allow pivotal motion between the atlas and axis. The condyles are oriented near the transverse plane to allow cervical spine rotation. The C3-C6 vertebrae have nonbifid spinous processes, large and flat spinous processes, caudal and cranial articular surface facets that are narrower than the transverse processes, large transverse processes, and transverse foramina for the passage of vertebral arteries. Caudal and cranial articular surfaces are oriented between the dorsal and transverse planes to facilitate cranial and caudal glides needed for cervical spine flexion and extension. The C7 vertebra has a similar shape, a large prominent nonbifid spinous process,

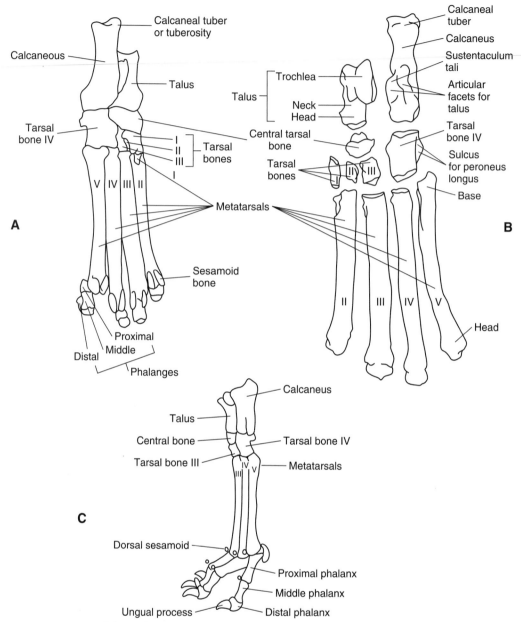

Figure 5-10 Skeleton of the left plantar **(A)**, left lateral **(B)**, and left dorsal **(C)** hindpaw of the dog. (Reprinted with permission from Riegger-Krugh C, Weigel J: *Canine anatomy and biomechanics II (hindlimb)*. LaCrosse, Wis, Feb, 2000, Orthopaedic Section, APTA, Inc.)

and caudal and cranial articular surfaces, which are oriented nearly craniocaudally.

Thoracic vertebrae (Figure 5-13) have small bodies relative to the size of the entire vertebrae. Canine spinous processes are relatively long. The spinous processes block excessive extension of the thoracic spine. At T10, the size of the body begins to increase and the length of spinous process decreases. The spinous processes are oriented close to the transverse plane. Cranial to T11, the spinous processes project caudally, but caudal to T11, they project cranially. Caudal and cranial articular surfaces are oriented close to the dorsal plane.

Lumbar (L) vertebrae (see Figure 5-13) have bodies that are larger than thoracic vertebral bodies. Canine lumbar transverse processes are long and thin, and they project lateroven-

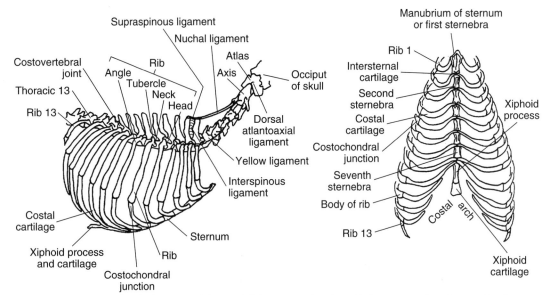

Figure 5-11   Identified portions of the axial skeleton cranial to the 13th thoracic vertebra. (Reprinted with permission from Riegger-Krugh C, Millis D: *Canine anatomy and biomechanics III (spine)*. LaCrosse, Wis, March, 2000, Orthopaedic Section, APTA, Inc.)

trocranially. In the cranial lumbar spine, cranial and caudal articular surfaces are oriented between the transverse and sagittal planes, which facilitate lumbar spine flexion and extension. The L7-S1 joint appears to orient between the sagittal and frontal planes to allow more rotation at this intervertebral level. The canine sacrum is relatively narrow and is linked to the pelvis with sacroiliac joints (Figure 5-14).

Caudal (Cd) vertebrae (Figure 5-14) have distinct bodies and transverse processes. The cranial articular surfaces are similar to those in more cranial vertebrae in shape and location; however, the caudal articular processes are bifid and are more centrally located, whereas articular processes in more cranial vertebrae are located more laterally. Hemal arches are separate bones that articulate with the ventral surfaces of the caudal ends of the bodies of Cd4-Cd6. The hemal arches provide protection for the median coccygeal artery, which is enclosed by the arches. In vertebrae caudal to Cd6 and in relatively the same position as the hemal arches are the paired hemal processes, which extend from Cd7-Cd17 or Cd18.

The ribs have vertebral attachments (see Figure 5-11). There are nine pairs of vertebrosternal or true ribs and four pairs of vertebrocostal or false ribs. The sternum is relatively long and has a manubrium and xiphoid process, with a prominent xiphoid cartilage.

The ribs limit overall thoracic spine motion and protect internal organs.

Joint Motion

The body segments of the forelimb and hindlimb are illustrated in Figures 5-3 and 5-4, respectively, with the major joints and their flexor and extensor surfaces. Body segments are listed and defined in Box 5-1. Types of joints are listed in Box 5-2.

Joint Motion and Shape of Articular Surfaces

The shape of articular surfaces of bones helps define the motions available for a joint. Articular surfaces of two bones forming a joint are usually concave on one bone and convex on the other bone. Some articular surfaces are flat. Occasionally adjacent bones are convex on both joint surfaces. Intraarticular structures, such as the medial and lateral menisci in the stifle joint, may modify adjacent surfaces. Understanding the concave-convex relationships as a guiding principle in determining joint motion allows prediction of possible joint motions based on articular surface shape. Ligamentous and other soft tissue around the joint guide and restrict the motion that would be possible based on articular surface shape alone.

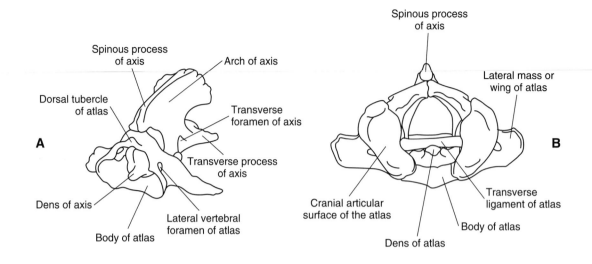

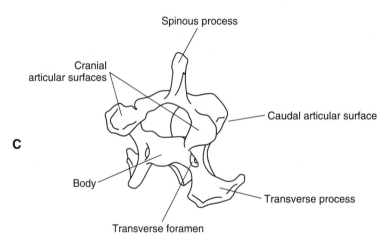

Figure 5-12   Detailed skeletal anatomy of the atlas and axis from a craniolateral view **(A)**, atlas and axis from a cranial view **(B)**, and C5 vertebra from a craniolateral view **(C)**. (Reprinted with permission from Riegger-Krugh C, Millis D: *Canine anatomy and biomechanics III (spine).* LaCrosse, Wis, March, 2000, Orthopaedic Section, APTA, Inc.)

Joint motions are named, most commonly, by movement of the distal bone relative to the proximal bone. For example, cranial movement of the tibia on a stable femur is named stifle joint extension. The major direction of motion, such as flexion of the stifle, is physiologic or osteokinematic motion.

Accessory or arthrokinematic motion is smaller in magnitude and less observable. Examples of accessory motions are glide or slide, rotary motion, distraction or traction, and compression or approximation. A normal amount of glide occurs in normal functioning joints. Glides are shear type or sliding motions of opposing articular surfaces. Rolls involve one bone rolling on another. Gliding motion in

combination with rolling is needed for normal physiologic joint motion. Spins are joint surface motions that result in continual contact of articular cartilage areas on opposite sides of a joint. Distraction or traction accessory motions are tensile or pulling-apart movements between bones. Compressive or approximation accessory motions are compressive or pushing-together movements between bones.

Normal joint motion involves both physiologic motion and accessory motion. Physiologic motion in joints with opposing concave and convex articular surfaces involves both roll and glide. Roll occurs in the same direction as the movement of the moving segment of the bone, but glide directions differ

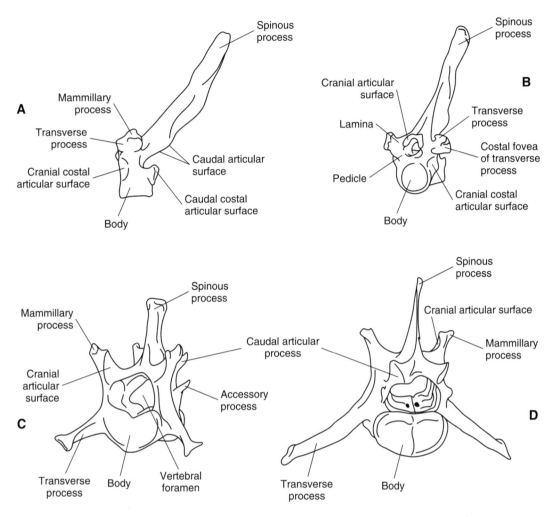

Figure 5-13   Detailed skeletal anatomy of T6 vertebra from a lateral view **(A)** and craniolateral view **(B)**, L1 vertebra from a craniolateral view **(C)**, and L5 vertebra from a caudolateral view **(D)**. (Reprinted with permission from Riegger-Krugh C, Millis D: *Canine anatomy and biomechanics III (spine)*. LaCrosse, Wis, March, 2000, Orthopaedic Section, APTA, Inc.)

based on whether the moving articular surface is concave or convex. A glide is described by identifying the joint motion, the direction of the glide, and which bone is moving. For example, stifle flexion involving the tibia and femur is termed caudal glide of the tibia on the femur.

Joint Motion in the Limbs and Spine

Joint motions are named by one body segment approaching or moving away from another body segment or movement of some referenced body landmark. Joint motions are named below and described (Figures 5-3 and 5-4) as they refer to the limbs, starting from

normal stance. Limb motion is usually described by motion of the joint rather than a body segment. For example, elbow flexion is recommended rather than forearm flexion. Occasionally, body segment motion is used to describe limb motion when motion does not involve axial motion with a joint as a pivot point. For example, rotation of the forelimb might be observable when pronation at the radioulnar joint would be difficult to observe clinically.

FLEXION

During flexion, a limb is retracted or folded, a digit is bent, and the back or neck is arched dorsally (i.e., the convex portion of the arch is

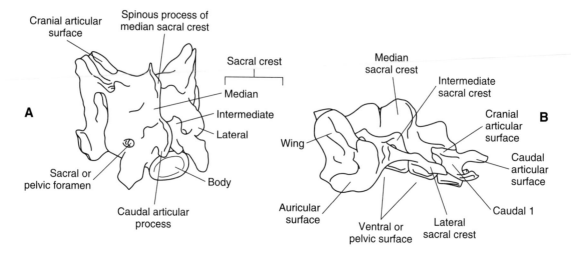

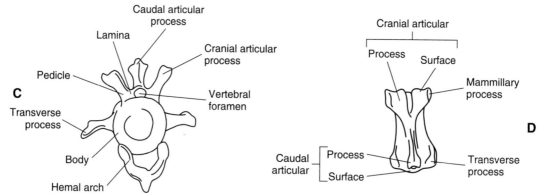

Figure 5-14   Detailed skeletal anatomy of the sacrum from a caudolateral view **(A)**, sacrum and caudal 1 or Cd1 vertebra from a lateral view **(B)**, Cd4 vertebra from a cranial view **(C)**, and Cd6 vertebra from a dorsal view **(D)**. (Reprinted with permission from Riegger-Krugh C, Millis D: *Canine anatomy and biomechanics III (spine)*. LaCrosse, Wis, March, 2000, Orthopaedic Section, APTA, Inc.)

directed dorsally). In the limbs, flexion motion occurs as the bones on either side of a joint move closer together and the joint angle becomes more acute. Flexion may also be referenced to limb motions involving closing angles during the swing phase of gait. Flexion motions of the limb joints are noted in Figures 5-3 and 5-4. In the spine, flexion occurs as the back or neck arches dorsally (i.e., the convex portion of the arch is directed dorsally).

A notable difference between dogs and humans is the meaning of shoulder flexion. In dogs, caudal retraction of the humerus in relation to the scapula is shoulder flexion, whereas cranial motion of the humerus in relation to the scapula is shoulder extension. The direction of shoulder flexion motion is opposite to this in humans. The terminology used in dogs is consistent with naming flexion as described above.

In normal stance, as shown in Figure 5-2, a dog's spine is flexed at the atlantooccipital and atlantoaxial joints, straight (neither flexed nor extended) in the remainder of the cervical spine, extended at the cervicothoracic junction, slightly lordotic in the thoracic spine, and flexed or normally kyphotic in the lumbar spine. There is either a slightly flexed or extended sacrum on the lumbar spine, depending on the tail posture. The flexed canine lumbar spine is beneficial to running speed. During running, the lumbar spine moves through varying degrees of flexion as running speed changes.

EXTENSION

During extension, the limb reaches out, the digit is extended, and the back or neck is less arched dorsally or arched ventrally. Extension is motion in the sagittal plane in the direction

■ ■ ■ BOX 5-1 Body Segments

Forelimb
- Forelimb: Arm, forearm, and forepaw
- Thoracic or pectoral girdle
  Scapula, clavicle
- Arm or brachium: Shoulder to elbow
- Forearm or antebrachium: Elbow to carpal joint
- Forepaw or manus
  Carpus or carpals
  Metacarpus or metacarpals
  Phalanges or digits
- Sesamoid bones or cartilages
  Dorsal on MCP joints in common digital extensor tendons of digits II to V; one per digit; small
  Pad surface on MCP joints in interosseous tendons of digits II to V; two per digit; smaller
  Dorsal and palmar on DIP joints of digits I to V; cartilage; small
- One sesamoid bone in the tendon of the abductor pollicis longus
- Digits or phalanges I to V, numbered medial to lateral
  No common names for digits
  Anatomical name: pollex for digit I
- Dewclaw or pollex or digit I with 2 phalanges
- Pads on the paws or digital pads: Weight-bearing pads
  Carpal pad: Small pad palmar to the carpus
  Metacarpal pad: Largest pad palmar to the MCP joints; triangular in shape
  Digital pads: Palmar to the DIP joints; ovoid and flat
- Ungual process: Extension of the phalanx into the claw
- Nails or claws

Hindlimb
- Hindlimb pelvic limb, or rear limb
  Thigh, leg, hindpaw
- Hip bone or os coxae
  Ilium, ischium, pubis
- Pelvic girdle
  Right and left hip bones and sacrum
- Thigh: Hip to stifle or knee
- Leg or crus: Stifle to talocrural joint
- Hindpaw or hind foot or pes
  Tarsus or tarsals (hock area)
  Metatarsus or metatarsals
  Phalanges or digits or toes
- Sesamoid bones or cartilages
  Dorsal on MTP joints in long digital extensor tendons of digits II to V; one per digit; small
  Plantar surface on MTP joints in interosseous tendons of digits II to V; two per digit; large
  Digit I: One per digit, smaller

- Dorsal and plantar on DIP joints—cartilaginous; one per digit I to V; small
- Digits or phalanges or toes
  I to V
- Dewclaw or digit I or hallux—may be absent, fully developed and articulating with a metatarsal, or may be a vestigial, that is, a trace or rudimentary structure, with a terminal phalanx and no proximal phalanx or metatarsal bone
- Digital pads or pads on the hindpaws—weight-bearing pads
  Tarsal pad: Small pad plantar to the talocrural joint
  Metatarsal pad: Largest pad plantar to the MTP joints; triangular in shape
  Digital pads: Plantar to the DIP joints; ovoid and flat
- Ungual process: Extension of the distal phalanx into the nail
- Nails or claws

Spine
- Trunk
  Borders: Inguinal ligament to C7-T1 disk
- Neck or cervical spine
- Head
- Tail
- Spinal regions
  Cervical: C1 through C7
  Thoracic: T1 through T13
  Lumbar: L1 through L7
  Sacral: S1 through S3
  Caudal or coccygeal: Cd1-Cd20; some dogs have more or fewer
- Ribs: 13
- Bones in the dog skeleton (excludes auditory ossicles)
  Vertebral column: 50
  Skull: 49
  Hyoid bone: 1
  Ribs: 26
  Sternum: 8 fused bones—manubrium or first sternebra, 6 additional sternebrae, and the xiphoid process
  Forelimbs: 90
  Hindlimbs: 96
  Total: 320
  Other: os penis in males—1
- Hip bone or os coxae
  Ilium, ischium, pubis
- Sacrum
- Pelvic girdle: Right and left hip bones and sacrum
- Pelvic complex: Hip bones, lumbar spine, sacral spine, caudal spine, sacroiliac joints, and hip joints

C, Cervical; *Cd*, caudal; *Cx*, coccygeal; *DIP*, distal interphalangeal; *L*, lumbar; *MCP*, metacarpophalangeal; *MTP*, metatarsophalangeal; *S*, sacral; *T*, thoracic.

opposite to that of flexion motion. In the limbs, extension motion occurs as the bones that are already close together and already form an acute angle move farther apart, such that the angle formed at the joint is increased

or straightened. Extension beyond 180 degrees is sometimes termed hyperextension. In the spine, extension occurs as the back or neck is arched ventrally (i.e., the convex portion of the arch is directed ventrally).

■ ■ ■ **BOX 5-2**   Types of Joints

Forelimb
- Artificial joint: Not described as a joint
- Ball and socket: Shoulder
- Hinge: Elbow, metacarpophalangeal I
- Pivot: Proximal, and distal radioulnar
- Syndesmosis: Middle radioulnar
- Hinge with lateral motion: Carpal
- Ellipsoid: Antebrachiocarpal, radiocarpal
- Plane: Middle carpal or midcarpal, intercarpal, inter-metacarpal
- Saddle plane: First carpal with MC I,
- Plane: Second carpal with MC II, third carpal with MC III, fourth carpal with MC IV and V intermetacarpal
- Hinge: Metacarpophalangeal I
- Condylar or condyloid: MC II to V with the same numbered phalanx
- Saddle/condylar
  Proximal interphalangeal II to V
  Distal interphalangeal II to V
  Interphalangeal of thumb

Hindlimb
- Synovial and fibrous: Sacroiliac
- Symphysis: Symphysis pelvis
- Ball and Socket: Hip or coxofemoral
- Complex condylar: Stifle, the term *knee* is used commonly with an animal's owner
- Plane
  Patellofemoral
  Tarsal joints or hock joints (this joint is referred to as the hock joint in common usage)
    Talocalcaneal
    Talocancaneocentral and calcanoeoquartal joints combined
    Proximal intertarsal or talocentral
    Calcaneoquartal
    Calcaneocentral
    Centroquartal

Centrodistal
Distal intertarsal: Central bone with tarsal III
Tarsal I with II, II with III
Tarsal III with IV
Tarsometatarsal
  Tarsal I with metatarsal I
  Tarsal II with metatarsal II
  Tarsal III with metatarsal III
  Tarsal IV with metatarsals IV and V
Intermetatarsal
- Tibiofibular
Synovial: Proximal and distal tibiofibular
Syndesmosis: Middle tibiofibular
- Hinge: Talocrural, tarsocrural, tibiotarsal or ankle joint; the term *ankle* is commonly used with an animal's owner (the tarsocrural has been referred to as the talocrural and the talocalcaneal joints combined)
Metatarsophalangeal I—metatarsal I with digit I
- Condylar: Metatarsal II to V with the same numbered digit
- Saddle
Proximal interphalangeal II to V
Distal interphalangeal II to V
Interphalangeal of hallux

Spine
- Part synovial and part fibrous: Sacroiliac
- Symphysis: Symphysis pelvis
- Condyloid: Atlantooccipital
- Pivot: Atlantoaxial—dens of C2 and atlas
- Plane
Atlantoaxial—articular surfaces
Between cranial and caudal articular surfaces
Costovertebral
Sternocostal: Sternum and true ribs
- Synchondrosis: Costochondral—ribs with cartilage

ABDUCTION

Limb joint abduction is movement in the transverse plane such that the distal aspect moves away from the midline of the body. Abduction of the digits is not routinely measured in dogs. Separation of the toes may be noted as splayed toes or abducted toes. The reference line for abduction of the digits passes between digits III and IV. Digit I, or the dewclaw, in dogs is nonfunctional and is not considered in a discussion of skeletal motion.

ADDUCTION

Limb joint adduction is movement in the transverse plane such that the distal aspect moves toward the midline of the body. Adduction of the digits is not routinely measured in dogs. The reference line for adduction is the same as for abduction.

SIDE BEND

In the trunk and head, side-to-side movement occurs in the dorsal plane such that lateral aspects of adjacent areas of the spine approximate or move away from each other. For example, side bend to the right involves the right side of adjacent spinal areas approximating each other.

CIRCUMDUCTION

Circumduction is movement at a joint, during which a bone or body segment outlines the surface of a cone or circle. This motion does not require rotation at the joint, but rotation at the joint may occur. Forelimb circumduction occurs primarily at the shoulder. Hindlimb circumduction occurs at the hips. While circumduction at individual limb joints is possible in dogs, veterinarians commonly observe and document circumduction of the entire limb, without distinction of the joints that contribute to the overall motion.

ROTATION

Internal rotation of a limb occurs with reference to the cranial aspect of the limb rotating toward the midline of the body or median plane and continuing in that direction. External rotation of a limb occurs with reference to the cranial aspect of the limb rotating away from the midline of the body and continuing in that direction. Limb rotational motions occur in the dorsal plane. With reference to the ventral aspect of a vertebral body, rotation to the right or left is called rotation to the right or left, respectively. Spinal rotations occur in the transverse plane.

SUPINATION

In the limbs, supination is external rotation of the limb, such that the pad surface of the paw faces medially. Supination motion, therefore, could involve forelimb carpal and forepaw supination, as well as other motions such as shoulder external rotation, or hindlimb talocrural and hindpaw supination, as well other motions such as hip joint external rotation. Scapular motion and glenohumeral external rotation occurring as part of supination occur in the dorsal plane. However, dorsal plane scapular motion is blocked by contact of the scapula with the trunk.

PRONATION

In the limbs, pronation is internal rotation of the limb, such that the pad surface of the paw faces laterally. Pronation motion, therefore, could involve forelimb carpal and forepaw pronation, as well as other motions, opposite to those of supination.

OTHER SHOULDER GIRDLE MOTIONS

Other shoulder girdle motions that are defined for humans exist in dogs, but have not been defined and measured in dogs. They include the human motions of scapular protraction, retraction, upward rotation, downward rotation, elevation, depression, anterior tilt and return from anterior tilt of the scapula, and glenohumeral horizontal abduction and horizontal adduction. Human scapulohumeral rhythm has not been defined in dogs, but may exist.

PELVIC AND SACROILIAC MOTIONS

Pelvic and sacroiliac motions and postures are less well defined in dogs than in humans. Human pelvic and sacroiliac motions and postures are described in depth, although terminology is not consistent among authors and clinicians. When pelvic and sacroiliac motions and postures are analyzed and described in dogs, the terminology listed below could be useful for correct identification and for accurate communication. Pelvofemoral rhythm, the human lower limb counterpart to human scapulohumeral rhythm, has not been defined in dogs, but may exist.

Pelvic Motion
VENTRAL AND DORSAL PELVIC TILT

Orientation of the pelvis with respect to the sagittal plane describes tilt of the pelvis. Ventral tilt would involve approximation of the ventral pelvis and cranial femur, and dorsal tilt would involve the ventral pelvis moving away from the cranial femur. These motions occur with the hip joints as the axes of rotation. Relative to a longitudinal axis through the entire spine, the canine pelvis appears tilted dorsally on the canine longitudinal axis.

LATERAL TILT OF THE PELVIS

Lateral tilt is dorsal plane movement such that the lateral aspect of the pelvis approximates the lateral aspect of the thigh or the trunk. Lateral pelvic tilt to the right, for example, would occur as the cranial border of the pelvis tilts to the right, approximating the right lateral side of the pelvis toward the right thigh.

PELVIC ROTATION

With reference to the movement of the ventral aspect of a pelvis, rotation toward the right or left is called rotation to the right or left, respectively. This motion occurs in the transverse plane. Pelvic rotation can be referenced to the floor and one lower limb. If this convention were used, internal rotation with reference to the right hindlimb would occur as the ventral pelvis rotates to the left. Internal rotation motion of the right hindlimb would occur in the same direction, that is, with the cranial aspect of the thigh or femur rotating to the left and the ventral aspect of the leg or tibia and fibula rotating to the left.

SACROILIAC MOTION

The suggested but as yet undefined terminology uses application of human terminology, with movements of the canine cranial and caudal aspects of the sacrum correlated to movement of the human superior and inferior aspects of the sacrum, respectively.

SACROILIAC FLEXION OR NUTATION

Sacroiliac flexion involves the cranial aspect of the sacrum tilting ventrally.

SACROILIAC EXTENSION
OR COUNTERNUTATION

Sacroiliac extension involves the cranial aspect of the sacrum tilting dorsally.

SACROILIAC SIDE BEND OR LATERAL FLEXION

Sacroiliac lateral flexion involves the cranial aspect of the sacrum tilting to the side. Right side bend or lateral flexion occurs as the cranial aspect of the sacrum tilts to the right.

SACROILIAC ROTATION

Sacroiliac rotation involves rotation around a longitudinal axis through the sacrum. Rotation of the sacrum would be named by the motion of the ventral sacrum to be consistent with terminology for humans. For example, rotation of the ventral sacrum to the left would be called sacral rotation to the left.

Overall spinal motion is determined and affected by many things. Among them are the orientation of the articular surfaces (facets); disk shape and size; structural blockages, such as ribs and orientation of spinous processes; ligament fiber direction, strength, and tightness; and muscle-tendon unit strength and tightness.

Normal Joint Motions and Ranges of Motion

Appendix 1 summarizes normal joint motions and ranges of motion for the peripheral joints.[5,7,8] Joint ranges of motion for the spine have not been documented in dogs.

Distinction of Maintained Joint Postures Versus Joint Motion

Motion is described by either referencing the joint or referencing a body segment. Terms to describe motion include flexion, flexing, abduction, abducting, etc. Motion occurs in a consistent direction, independent of the starting point of the motion. For example, the movement of the carpal joint from neutral to flexion is carpal joint flexion. Movement of the carpal joint from full extension to neutral is carpal joint flexion. Postures are maintained positions. Terms to describe postures include *flexed* or *abducted*, *maintained flexion*, or *abduction*.

Skeletal Alignment

Limbs

Skeletal alignment is important, because it is closely linked to mobility, function, and pathology. A functional example of the importance of skeletal alignment is seen at the talocrural joint. Alignment at this joint influences angulation of the hindlimbs in relation to speed during the gallop. Figures 5-5, 5-6, 5-8, and 5-9 show the normal alignment of the limbs.

Skeletal alignment is the alignment between bones at joint surfaces or the alignment of one portion of a bone in relation to another portion of the same bone. Skeletal malalignment would be abnormal alignment of either of these two relationships.[9] Skeletal alignment at any one joint affects the alignment at other joints, especially at joints functioning in weight-bearing closed-chain activities rather than non–weight-bearing or open-chain activities. Skeletal malalignment can lead to arthritis of a malaligned joint or of a compensating joint.

Normal skeletal alignment results in normal correlated motions and postures, which occur naturally and are normally related to the motion or posture imposed at the joint. Correlated motions and postures may not occur at all but can occur at any or several joints along the chain. This concept is well defined in human physical therapy, although clinicians use different terms to describe it. These concepts have been discussed in relation to dogs, mostly in the context of canine gait and related to correlated motion as a result of a limb with pain or dysfunction, rather than from skeletal malalignment alone.[10] An example of correlated posture or motion is the lateral rotation of the proximal forelimb or hindlimb that occurs when the dog supinates at the paw. Another example is the excessive shoulder or hip adduction and medial positioning of the elbow or stifle joints, which occur when the digits angle or point laterally in the forepaw or hindpaw, respectively.

For any skeletal malalignment or associated abnormal correlated motion or posture, compensatory motions or postures can occur. They occur to normalize mobility, improve cosmetic appearance of the limb, or improve foot contact with the ground. The term *compensation* is used to describe abnormal motion and posture in dogs.[10] An example would be excessive weight bearing on one limb when dysfunction exists in the other limb. Another example of a compensatory motion would be limb circumduction while advancing that limb during gait, as a result of inability to flex the joints of a limb during swing.

Spine

Complex correlated and compensatory postures and motions occur within the spine and pelvic complex. The pelvic complex for dogs and humans is defined in Box 5-1. Human correlated and compensatory postures and motions related to the spine and pelvis are described in great detail in the physical therapy literature[11-14]; however, there is controversy and even contradiction related to which motions and postures are correlated or compensatory for other motions and postures. This concept has been applied in less detail to spinal and pelvic postures and motions in dogs; however, development and use of terminology is encouraged for analysis of spinal motion and posture.

Fascia (Fasciae)

Fascia (fasciae), formed by flat, enveloping connective tissue, weaves throughout the body and provides structural connection. With damage, it can become adhered to adjacent structures. Physical therapists and other clinicians intervene in such circumstances with treatments such as stretching, transverse friction massage, and soft tissue mobilization to reduce this adherence.

Forelimb

The superficial and deep fascia of the shoulder and brachium are continuous with the superficial and deep fascia of the cervical spine and thorax. The superficial fascia in the region of the sternum is continuous with the medial brachium, and it covers the cephalic vein during its course. Distal to the elbow, the superficial fascia is more adhered to the deep structures. The cutaneous nerves and vessels of the forelimb travel long distances deep to the superficial fascia before entering the skin.

The deep fascia of the lateral shoulder and brachium, called the fascia omobrachialis lateralis, covers the muscles' superficial surfaces and adheres to the spine of the scapula. The deep antebrachial fascia forms a single dense sleeve around the muscles in the caudal antebrachium and is thickest medially. Intermuscular septa extend to the radius and ulna to separate the flexor and extensor carpal muscle groups.

The deep fascia is closely joined with the connective tissue around the tendons of the carpal joint. A thick and strong extension, the flexor retinaculum, bridges the flexor tendons to the carpal joint and digits. On the palmar surface of the metacarpophalangeal joints, thick extensions attach to the sesamoid bones and are called transverse ligaments.

Hindlimb

The hindlimb also has superficial and deep layers of fascia. At times the fascial layers are separable, especially with a layer of fat in obese dogs, and at times they are not. In general, the deep fascia is stronger than the superficial.

The superficial fascia on the dorsal trunk is continuous with the superficial gluteal fascia of the hip area, whereas the superficial fascia on the ventrolateral abdomen is continuous as the superficial lateral fascia of the lateral thigh and gluteal region. The superficial fascia encompasses the thigh almost to the patella and is closely connected to the deep fascia of the biceps femoris muscle. The superficial and deep fascia are also closely associated near the proximal sartorius muscle, the femoral canal, and the gracilis muscle. The superficial fascia of the crus, tarsus, and hindpaw is similar to that in the forelimb.

The strong lateral femoral fascia, or fascia lata (iliotibial band in humans), is formed on the lateral thigh from the gluteal fascia and the fascia of the tensor fasciae latae muscle and attaches to the lateral femur by an intermuscular septum between the biceps femoris and vastus lateralis muscles. The more loosely adhered medial femoral fascia joins the lateral femoral fascia to envelop the thigh and attach to the medial femur by a septum caudal to the vastus medialis. Both lateral and medial fascial layers attach to the patella and femoral condyles. The fascia extends around both the medial and lateral aspects of the stifle, but it thins as it merges with the patellar ligament and patella. The deep fascia continues in the crus as the crural fascia. The crural fascia has a superficial layer, which extends to the metatarsus, and a deep layer. The superficial and deep leaves are united near the distal tendons of the biceps femoris and semitendinosus, where they contribute to the common calcaneal tendon. The layers are also united to the distal tendons of the semimembranosus and cranial tibial muscles. The deep crural fascia thickens to form the crural extensor retinaculum, which envelops the long digital extensor and cranial tibial tendons, and the tarsal extensor retinaculum, which envelops the long digital extensor muscle. These retinacula ensheath all tendons and superficial muscles of the hindpaw and secure them to the bones in the hindpaw.

Trunk and Neck

The superficial and deep fascial layers of the neck and head are continuous. Although the deep fascia is stronger than the superficial fascia, it is deeper and more difficult to palpate; therefore the superficial fascia will be emphasized here. The superficial fascia of the neck ensheathes the entire neck, is continuous toward the forelimb as the superficial brachial fascia, and is continuous ventrally with the superficial fascia of the trunk in the sternal region. Caudally, the superficial external fascia of the trunk is continuous with the superficial gluteal fascia. At the dorsal midline in dogs, there is no attachment of the superficial fascia to deep structures, allowing the superficial fascia to be lifted in a big fold when the skin is gently lifted. Large quantities of subfascial fat are deposited in areas where the superficial fascia and skin move freely on deeper structures.

The deep external fascia is attached to the supraspinous ligament on the spinous processes of thoracic and lumbar vertebrae and ends cranially on the transverse processes of C7 and T1. In the trunk, it is continuous with the lateral abdominal muscles. The deep fascia attaches to the sternum and costal cartilages cranially and the ilium caudally. The dorsally located thoracolumbar fascia has two layers and lies deep to large amounts of fat in well-nourished dogs. The main layer serves as an attachment site for the serratus dorsalis cranialis and the internal and external abdominal oblique muscles. The deep fascia is continuous with the deep gluteal fascia and other deep fascia of the thigh.

Compartments

Fascial layers and the bones they attach to can form well-defined volumetric spaces called compartments. Compartments are described in the limbs and contain muscles and their associated neurovascular supply. Compartments become important when interstitial fluid hydrostatic pressure within the compartment exceeds physiologic levels, causing ischemia, disruption of membrane integrity, edema, and loss of viable muscle tissue.

Four distinct compartments have been described in the dog: (1) craniolateral compartment of the crus; (2) caudal compartment of the crus; (3) caudal compartment of the antebrachium; and (4) femoral compartment.[15] Unlike the others, the femoral compartment is not a single space but consists of three fascial envelopes; one contains the quadriceps muscles, another the hamstring group, and the final one surrounds the adductor muscle.

Muscles

Muscles are characterized as primary movers (i.e., critical in performing joint actions) and secondary movers (less important in performing joint actions). Primary movers are the muscles that produce the necessary moments for normal (physiologic) joint motion and have the best combination of characteristics: large physiologic cross section, large moment arm, and a good line of action based on the desired joint motions. Primary movers usually cross the joint with the desired motion at the last joint crossed.

Muscle strength depends on the multiplied product of the muscle force applied in the direction of the desired joint motion(s) and the moment arm of the muscle force. The size of the muscle and the direction of its line of action force vector determine its ability to produce specific motion. Muscle force is related to the physiologic cross-sectional areas of muscle fibers. The line of action determines the length of the moment arm, which determines the moment arm's contribution to the muscle moment that can be produced.

Interestingly, some canine muscles have been named according to the number of heads in analogous human muscles, but the actual number of heads making up the muscle may be different. For example, the biceps brachii in dogs has one head and the human biceps brachii has two heads, but both muscles are called biceps brachii.

Forelimb

Muscle number, size, and location are related closely to forelimb function as a weight-bearing limb (Figures 5-15 to 5-21). In addition, the need to suspend the head and neck increases the need for muscle mass and strong ligaments that extend between the head, neck, and forelimb. The canine head and neck function mechanically like a cantilever beam. The weight of the head at the end of the "beam" produces a large neck flexion moment, which must be balanced by spinal ligaments and neck extensor muscles.

Dogs have a large muscle mass in shoulder adductors and elbow extensors because of the weight-bearing function of the forelimb. These antigravity muscles support the dog in weight bearing. Antigravity muscle groups for the forelimb include the following (see Figures 5-15 to 5-21):

- Shoulder extensors in closed chain and end-range open chain, and shoulder flexors in open chain from normal stance posture
- Shoulder adductors and abductors, depending on the weight-bearing posture

- Elbow extensors in closed chain, and flexors in open chain from stance
- Carpal and digit flexors in closed chain and end-range open chain, and extensors in open chain from normal stance

Prime movers for forelimb muscle groups are as follows:

- Shoulder flexors—latissimus dorsi, deltoideus, long head of the triceps brachii, teres major, teres minor
- Shoulder extensors—cleidobrachialis, biceps brachii, supraspinatus, brachiocephalicus
- Elbow flexors—biceps brachii and brachialis
- Elbow extensors—triceps brachii
- Carpal flexors—flexor carpi radialis, ulnaris lateralis, flexor carpi ulnaris
- Carpal extensors—extensor carpi radialis; carpal flexor and extensor muscles have flexor and extensor retinacula to keep tendons to the digits in proper alignment
- Digit flexors—superficial and deep digital flexors
- Digit extensors—common and lateral digital extensor muscles

Appendix 2 contains information on muscles, attachment sites, joint actions, analogous human muscles (muscle that performs a similar function in humans), and innervation for prime movers of joint actions of the forelimb, hindlimb, and trunk and neck.

Hindlimb

The antigravity muscles of the hindlimb support the dog in weight bearing or closed chain (Figures 5-22 to 5-30). In normal stance, the angle of the hip and stifle are both about 110 to 150 degrees, with perhaps more flexion in the stifle joint. This posture creates a constant requirement for large hip extensor and stifle extensor moments. The main antigravity muscle groups for closed-chain function in the hindlimb are as follows:

- Hip extensors in the sagittal plane
- Hip adductors in the frontal plane
- Stifle extensors
- Talocrural extensors
- Digit flexors

Prime movers for hindlimb muscles include the following:

- Hip flexors—iliopsoas, sartorius, tensor fasciae latae
- Hip extensors—gluteal muscles, biceps femoris, semitendinosus, semimembranosus
- Hip abductors—middle gluteal

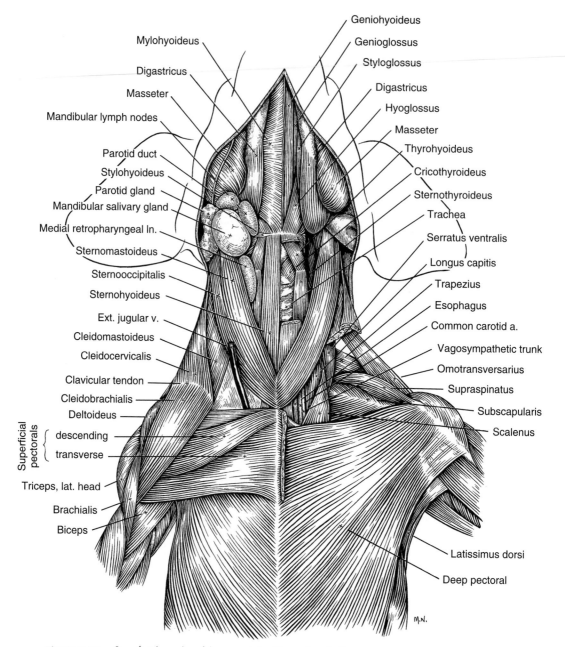

Figure 5-15 Superficial muscles of the ventral shoulder and neck. (From Evans HE: *Miller's anatomy of the dog*, ed 3, Philadelphia, 1993, WB Saunders.)

- Hip adductors—adductor magnus et brevis, pectineus
- Hip lateral rotators—internal and external obturator, gemelli
- Hip medial rotators—deep gluteal, semitendinosus
- Stifle extensors—quadriceps femoris: rectus femoris, vastus lateralis, vastus medialis, vastus intermedius
- Stifle flexors—biceps femoris, semitendinosus, semimembranosus
- Talocrural flexors—cranial tibial
- Talocrural extensors—gastrocnemius, superficial digital flexor
- Digit flexors—superficial and deep flexor
- Digit extensors—long digital extensor

Whereas the front limbs bear the majority of the static weight of the dog, the rear limbs

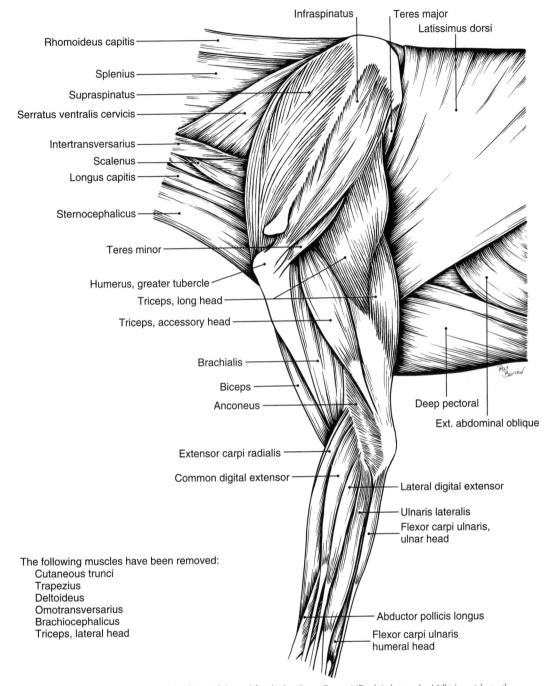

Figure 5-16   Deep muscles of the left lateral forelimb. (From Evans HE, deLahunta A: *Miller's guide to the dissection of the dog*, ed 5, Philadelphia, 2000, WB Saunders.)

provide the necessary propulsion for dynamic activity such as running and jumping. As a result, the hamstring muscles are large and therefore have a large force capacity. When compared to the human, the dog's ischial tuberosity is farther from the hip joint. Therefore the origin of the hamstrings on the

ischial tuberosity provides a longer moment arm and therefore a relatively larger extensor moment about the hip joint. At the region of the femorotibial joint, the entire biceps femoris muscle courses superficial to the vastus lateralis muscle and, as an aponeurosis, joins the fascia lata and the fascia cruris. Based on these

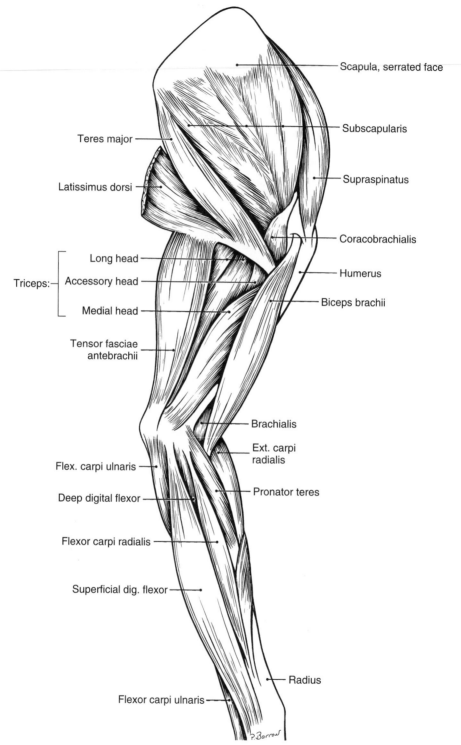

Figure 5-17   Muscles of the left medial forelimb. (From Evans HE, deLahunta A: *Miller's guide to the dissection of the dog*, ed 5, Philadelphia, 2000, WB Saunders.)

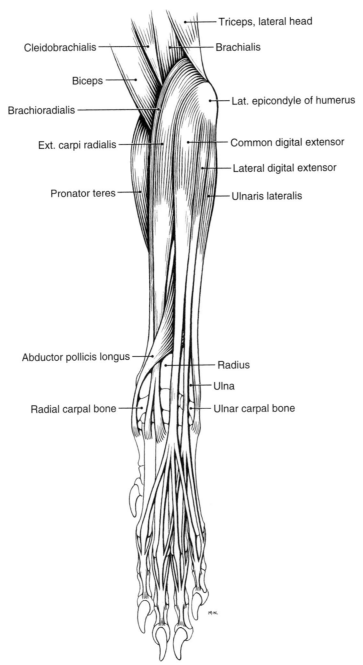

Triceps, lateral head

Cleidobrachialis

Brachialis

Biceps

Brachioradialis

Lat. epicondyle of humerus

Ext. carpi radialis

Common digital extensor

Lateral digital extensor

Pronator teres

Ulnaris lateralis

Abductor pollicis longus

Radius

Ulna

Radial carpal bone

Ulnar carpal bone

Figure 5-18   Muscles of the left antebrachium and forepaw, cranial view. (From Evans HE, deLahunta A: *Miller's guide to the dissection of the dog*, ed 5, Philadelphia, 2000, WB Saunders.)

attachments, the biceps femoris is very effective in producing hip extension and stifle flexion, making this muscle an effective source of propulsion. The middle gluteal and adductor muscles are large, thick muscles. The superficial gluteal is small and located more on the lateral hip than the caudal hip.

The quadriceps femoris muscles are large. This is consistent with the constant and large external stifle flexion moment due to the stifle position in normal stance.

At the talocrural joint, the canine gastrocnemius muscle is relatively large, and usually there is no soleus muscle. The long digital

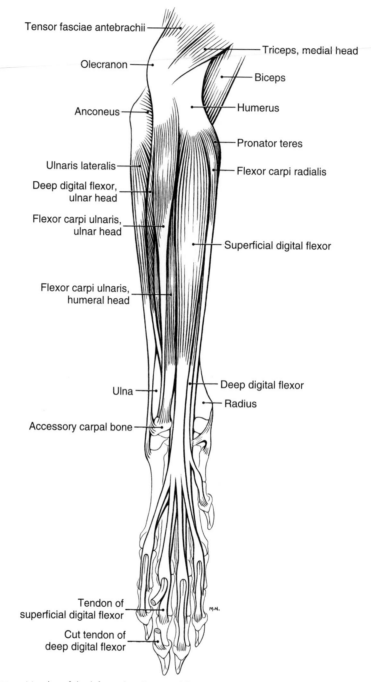

Figure 5-19 Muscles of the left antebrachium and forepaw, caudal view. (From Evans HE, deLahunta A: *Miller's guide to the dissection of the dog,* ed 5, Philadelphia, 2000, WB Saunders.)

extensor muscle crosses the stifle joint on the cranial surface. The tendons of the lateral digital extensor and peroneus brevis muscles travel in a distinctive groove, the sulcus malleolaris lateralis, on the lateral malleolus.

Trunk and Neck

Figures 5-31 to 5-36 display visual information about trunk and neck musculature. Canine muscles of the trunk and neck are characterized by nerve supply and embryological development into hypaxial and epaxial muscles. The

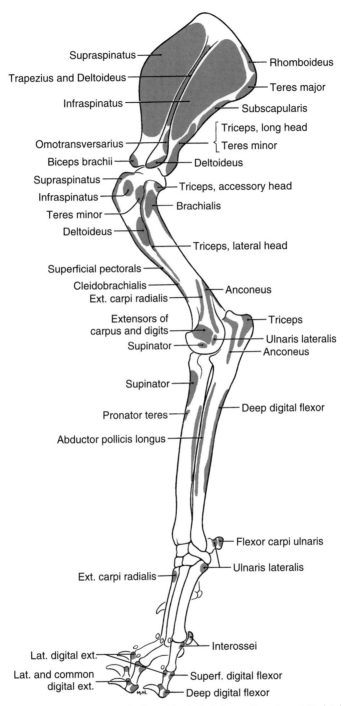

Supraspinatus
Trapezius and Deltoideus
Infraspinatus

Rhomboideus
Teres major
Subscapularis

Triceps, long head
Teres minor

Omotransversarius
Biceps brachii
Supraspinatus
Infraspinatus
Teres minor
Deltoideus

Deltoideus
Triceps, accessory head
Brachialis

Triceps, lateral head

Superficial pectorals
Cleidobrachialis
Ext. carpi radialis

Anconeus

Extensors of
carpus and digits
Supinator

Triceps
Ulnaris lateralis
Anconeus

Supinator

Pronator teres

Deep digital flexor

Abductor pollicis longus

Flexor carpi ulnaris

Ulnaris lateralis

Ext. carpi radialis

Interossei
Lat. digital ext.
Lat. and common
digital ext.

Superf. digital flexor
Deep digital flexor

Figure 5-20 Muscle attachment sites on the lateral forelimb skeleton. (From Evans HE, deLahunta A: *Miller's guide to the dissection of the dog*, ed 5, Philadelphia, 2000, WB Saunders.)

epaxial muscles develop locally in the trunk and are innervated by the dorsal rami of the spinal nerves. They include muscles that lie dorsal to the transverse processes of the vertebrae and have a main action of extension of the spine. The hypaxial muscles lie ventral to the transverse processes, are innervated by the ventral rami, and have a main action of flexion of the spine. The hypaxial group also includes the muscles of the abdominal and thoracic walls. The superficial dorsal trunk muscles act on the forelimb as well as the

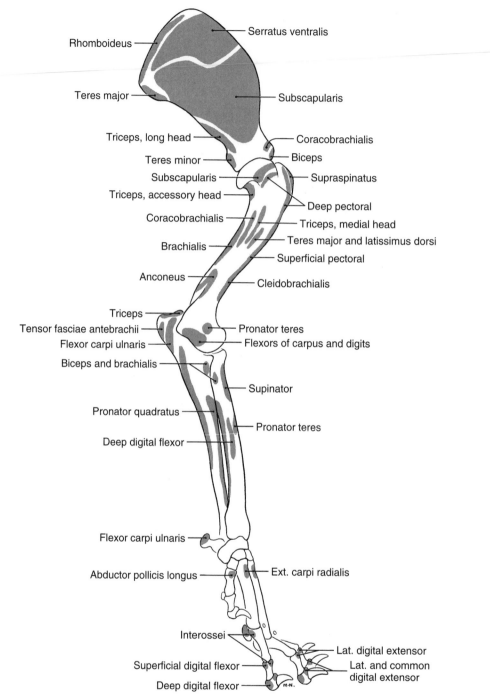

Figure 5-21 Muscle attachment sites on the medial forelimb skeleton. (From Evans HE, deLahunta A: *Miller's guide to the dissection of the dog*, ed 5, Philadelphia, 2000, WB Saunders.)

cervical spine and are innervated by the ventral rami.

Antigravity muscle groups for the spine are the trunk and neck extensors. Prime mover muscles for spine motion include the following:

- Cervical spine flexion of C1-C2—longus capitis and longus colli
- Cervical spine flexion caudal to C2—sternomastoideus, longus capitis, and longus colli
- Cervical spine extension—splenius
- Cervical spine side bend—scalenus

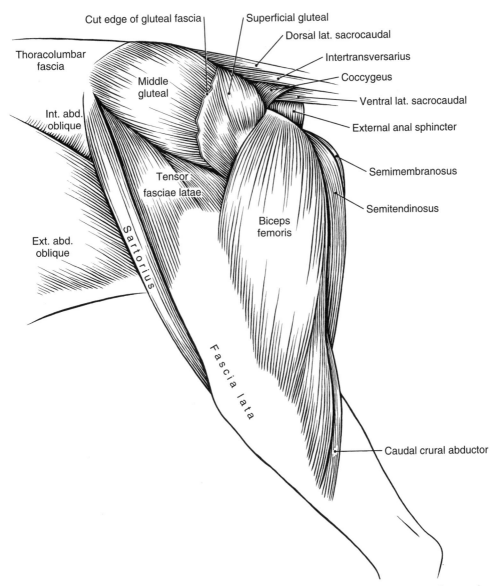

Cut edge of gluteal fascia

Superficial gluteal

Dorsal lat. sacrocaudal

Intertransversarius

Coccygeus

Ventral lat. sacrocaudal

External anal sphincter

Semimembranosus

Semitendinosus

Thoracolumbar fascia

Middle gluteal

Int. abd. oblique

Tensor fasciae latae

Ext. abd. oblique

Sartorius

Biceps femoris

Fascia lata

Caudal crural abductor

Figure 5-22   Superficial muscles of the left lateral hindlimb. (From Evans HE, deLahunta A: *Miller's guide to the dissection of the dog,* ed 5, Philadelphia, 2000, VVB Saunders.)

- Rotation of the cervical spine—splenius and sternomastoideus
- Flexion of the trunk (thoracic and lumbar spine)—rectus abdominis muscle
- Extension of the trunk—sacrospinalis or erector spinae muscles
- Side bend of the trunk—pars lumbalis of the external abdominal oblique
- Rotation of the trunk—longissimus and pars costalis of the external abdominal oblique

The posturing of the dog's head and neck as a cantilever beam produces a large amount of external or resisting neck flexion moment on the cervical spine. This posture creates a constant requirement for large neck extensor muscle activity. In response, there is a large amount of neck extensor muscle mass. Trunk flexor and extensor muscle masses are both large, reflecting a large requirement for trunk extensor and flexor muscle activity. The abdominal muscles have a big role in supporting the weight of the internal organs.

The deep dorsal trunk musculature, the extensor muscle groups, consists of three longitudinal muscle masses, each having many overlapping fascicles. The three masses are the

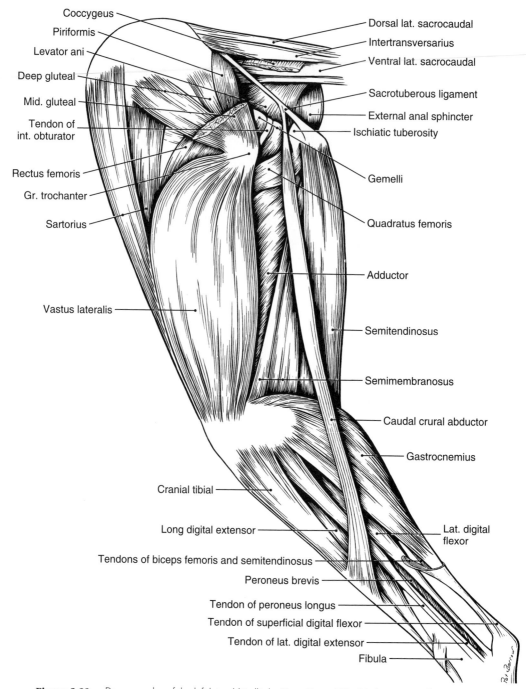

Figure 5-23   Deep muscles of the left lateral hindlimb. (From Evans HE, deLahunta A: *Miller's guide to the dissection of the dog*, ed 5, Philadelphia, 2000, WB Saunders.)

iliocostalis muscle system laterally, the longissimus muscle system intermediately, and the transversospinalis muscle system medially. Different arrangements of fused portions of these three primary segmental muscle masses exist, based on the running abilities of the breed. Dogs that run fast may have longer fascicles, which allow muscles to attach to the spine for increased leverage. These breeds have fused caudal portions of the iliocostalis muscle with the longissimus muscle to form the erector spinae or sacrospinalis muscle group.

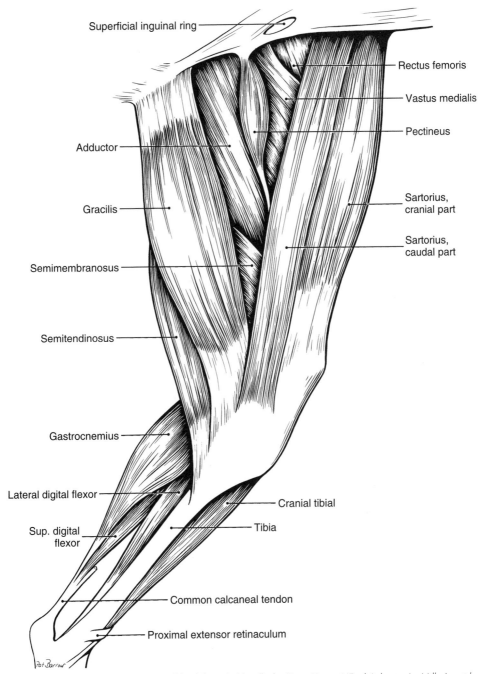

Figure 5-24 Superficial muscles of the left medial hindlimb. (From Evans HE, deLahunta A: *Miller's guide to the dissection of the dog*, ed 5, Philadelphia, 2000, WB Saunders.)

Lymph Node Anatomy

Forelimb

Superficial cervical lymph nodes are located just cranial to the shoulder joint. They are deep to the cleidocephalicus and omotransversarius muscles and are on the lymph drainage path from the cutaneous area of the head, neck, and forelimb. The superficial cervical lymph nodes are almost always palpable. Axillary lymph nodes are located dorsal to the deep pectoral muscle and generally are not palpable unless they are abnormally enlarged. The deep structures of the forelimb, as well as

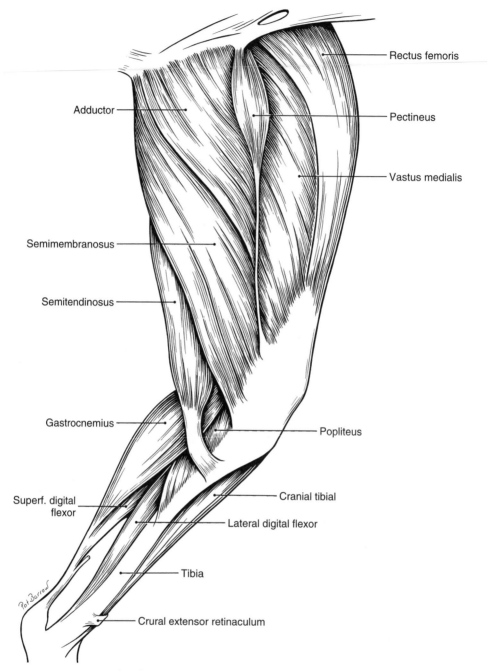

Figure 5-25   Deep muscles of the left medial hindlimb. (From Evans He, deLahunta A: *Miller's guide to the dissection of the dog*, ed 5, Philadelphia, 2000, WB Saunders.)

lymph vessels from the thoracic wall, drain into these nodes.

Hindlimb

The popliteal lymph node lies in the fat just caudal to the stifle joint and at the caudal border of the biceps femoris muscle. This is the largest lymph node in the hindlimb. The hindlimb structures distal to the stifle joint drain into this lymph node. The femoral lymph node is not consistently present and is small when present. It lies in the fat deep to the deep medial femoral fascia at the distal part of the femoral triangle. The femoral vessels lie cranial to the femoral lymph node.

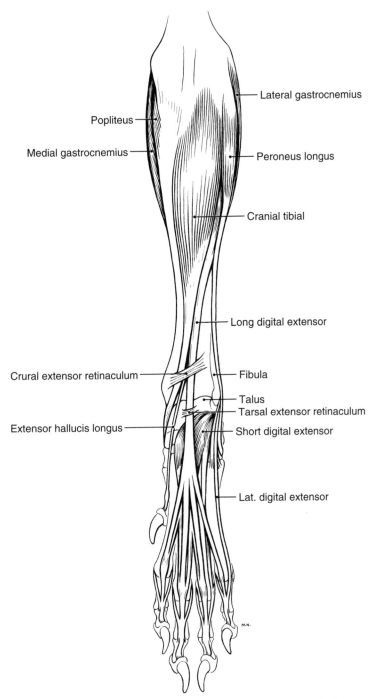

Figure 5-26 Muscles of the left leg and hindpaw, cranial view. (From Evans HE, deLahunta A: *Miller's guide to the dissection of the dog*, ed 5, Philadelphia, 2000, WB Saunders.)

Trunk and Neck

The superficial inguinal lymph nodes are important lymph nodes in the trunk. In addition to the lymph nodes, trunk internal organ anatomy that is particularly relevant for rehabilitation includes the lung lobes, the anatomy of which is critical when administering postural drainage of individual lobes for dogs with respiratory insufficiency.[16]

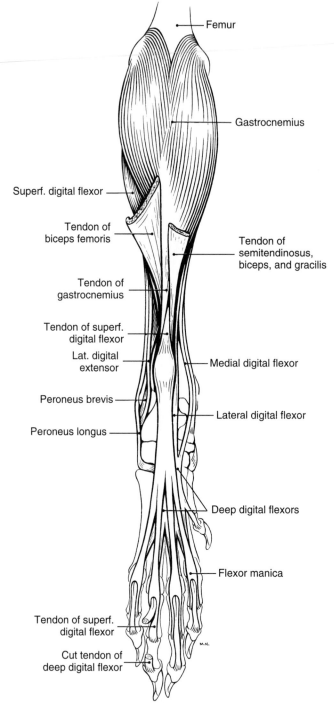

Figure 5-27 Muscles of the left leg and hindpaw, caudal view. (From Evans HE, deLahunta A: *Miller's guide to the dissection of the dog*, ed 5, Philadelphia, 2000, WB Saunders.)

Ligaments

Information about attachment, fiber direction, and motion restricted by the major forelimb, hindlimb, and spinal ligaments is noted in Appendix 3.[4,17] Listed order of the fiber direction in three planes is noted by the main orientation of the fibers first and follows in sequence for the second orientation of importance and then the third.

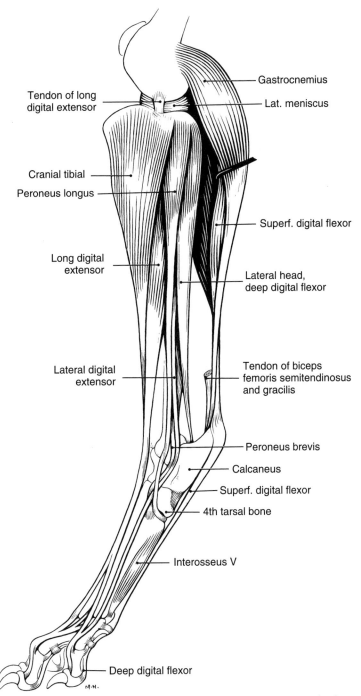

Figure 5-28 Muscles of the left leg and hindpaw, lateral view. (From Evans HE, deLahunta A: *Miller's guide to the dissection of the dog*, ed 5, Philadelphia, 2000, WB Saunders.)

Forelimb

Figures 5-37 and 5-38 display ligament attachment site, location, and line of direction for the major ligaments of the forelimb. The canine shoulder joints have medial and lateral gleno-

humeral ligaments, which are mildly thickened regions of fibrous joint capsule. The transverse humeral retinaculum holds the tendon of the biceps brachii securely in place. The annular ligament holds the proximal radius securely to

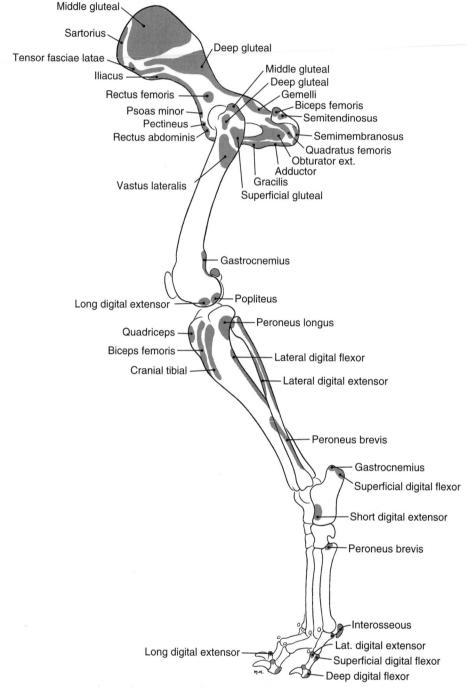

Figure 5-29 Muscle attachment sites on the lateral hindlimb skeleton. (From Evans HE, deLahunta A: *Miller's guide to the dissection of the dog*, ed 5, Philadelphia, 2000, WB Saunders.)

the ulna. The medial and lateral collateral ligaments of the elbow are substantial structures and contribute to elbow stability. Although there are no carpal collateral ligaments that span all the joints of the carpus, there are individual collateral ligaments at the various levels that are critical to carpal stability. Palmar liga-

ment and fibrocartilaginous support of the carpus are vital for normal weight-bearing.

Hindlimb

Figures 5-39 to 5-41 display hindlimb ligament attachment site, location, and line of direction

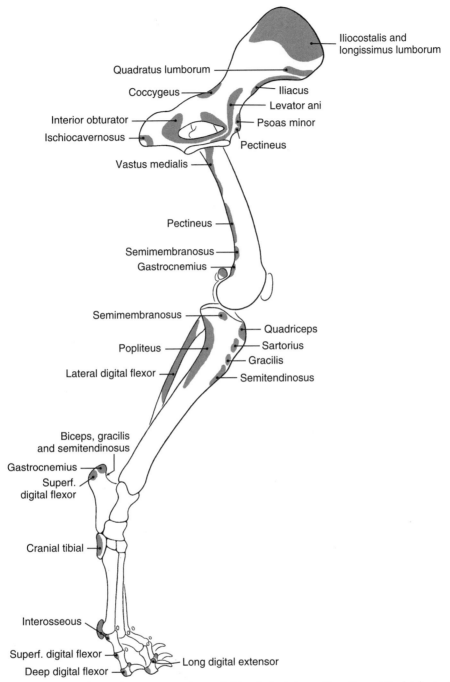

Figure 5-30   Muscle attachment sites on the medial hindlimb skeleton. (From Evans HE, deLahunta A: *Miller's guide to the dissection of the dog*, ed 5, Philadelphia, 2000, WB Saunders.)

for the major ligaments of the hindlimb. The iliofemoral, pubofemoral, and ischiofemoral ligaments are not present in the dog. The ligament of the femoral head does not contribute to hip stability as much as the capsule, but is important in the development of the hip.

The transverse acetabular ligament traverses the acetabular notch and thereby completes the rim of the acetabulum. Without the transverse acetabular ligament, the hip may luxate ventrally. Although the sacrotuberous ligament is a pelvic ligament, rather than a

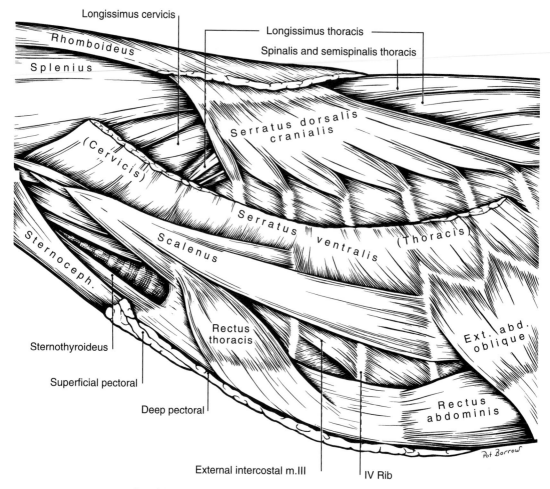

Figure 5-31 Muscles of the left lateral neck and thorax. (From Evans HE, deLahunta A: *Miller's guide to the dissection of the dog*, ed 5, Philadelphia, 2000, WB Saunders.)

hip-joint ligament, it is mentioned here because of its importance as one of the origins of the biceps femoris muscle.

The cranial (anterior) and caudal (posterior) cruciate ligaments are critical stabilizing ligaments that restrain stifle motion within physiologic limits. The cruciate ligaments are named by their cranial or caudal attachment to the tibia. Injury to the cranial cruciate ligament is common. The cranial cruciate ligament has different fiber bundles, the craniomedial and caudolateral bands. Throughout the normal range of motion, these bands accept varying stress loads depending on the stage of motion. With the stifle in moderate flexion, excessive stifle internal rotation stretches the cranial cruciate ligament under the weight of the medial femoral condyle, causing disruption of the ligament.

The medial and lateral collateral ligaments of the stifle joint are substantial and important to joint stability. The medial meniscus is attached to the tibia cranially and caudally, and to the medial collateral ligament. The lateral meniscus is attached to the tibia cranially and the femur caudally (through the meniscofemoral ligament) and is separated from the lateral collateral ligament. Although the menisci move with flexion and extension, the more fixed medial meniscus is less accommodating than the lateral if subluxation occurs with loss of the cranial cruciate ligament. Therefore the medial meniscus is often damaged in cases of cranial cruciate rupture.

The fibrous extensor retinaculum secures the patella. The contribution from the fascia lata to the extensor retinaculum is particularly important in holding the patella in the trochlea.

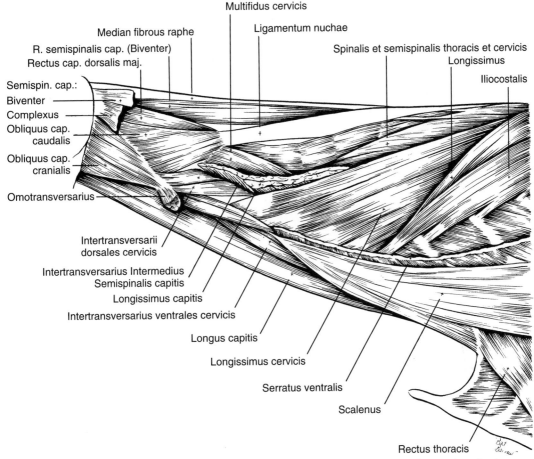

Multifidus cervicis

Ligamentum nuchae

Median fibrous raphe

Spinalis et semispinalis thoracis et cervicis

R. semispinalis cap. (Biventer)

Longissimus

Rectus cap. dorsalis maj.

Iliocostalis

Semispin. cap.:

Biventer

Complexus

Obliquus cap.
caudalis

Obliquus cap.
cranialis

Omotransversarius

Intertransversarii
dorsales cervicis

Intertransversarius Intermedius
Semispinalis capitis

Longissimus capitis

Intertransversarius ventrales cervicis

Longus capitis

Longissimus cervicis

Serratus ventralis

Scalenus

Rectus thoracis

Figure 5-32   Deep muscles of the left lateral neck. (From Evans HE, deLahunta A: *Miller's guide to the dissection of the dog*, ed 5, Philadelphia, 2000, WB Saunders.)

Femoropatellar ligaments are mildly thickened regions of the fibrous capsule and are observed only in large dogs. The tendon of the popliteus muscle separates the lateral collateral ligament from the lateral meniscus. The patellar ligament is a strong support between the patella and tibial tuberosity. There is no tendon from the quadriceps muscle to the patella. The quadriceps is attached to parapatellar fibrocartilage.

There are three joint or synovial pouches in the stifle, two femorotibial joint pouches and one retropatellar joint pouch. The femorotibial joint pouches incorporate the articulations of the sesamoids of the gastrocnemius muscle, but exclude the cruciate ligaments. The lateral femorotibial pouch continues distally through the extensor groove as the tendon sheath for the tendon of the proximal long digital extensor muscle and also surrounds the tendon of

the proximal attachment of the popliteus muscle. The tibiofibular joint has ligamentous support from the ligament of the fibular head, the interosseous membrane, and the cranial tibiofibular ligament.

Medial and lateral collateral ligaments of the tarsocrural joint provide stability to the tarsus. There are long and short portions of the collateral ligaments. Plantar ligaments are more developed and substantial in the dog than in the human because of the upright weight-bearing stance in humans. Ligaments in the hindpaw maintain what is described as a rigid tarsocrural area in dogs. The tendons coursing into the hindpaw are secured by the fascia pedis, which forms retinacula to stabilize tendons and superficial muscles of the hindpaw and secure them to all the projecting bones in the hindpaw.

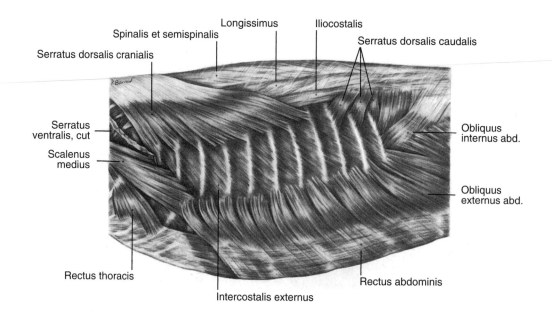

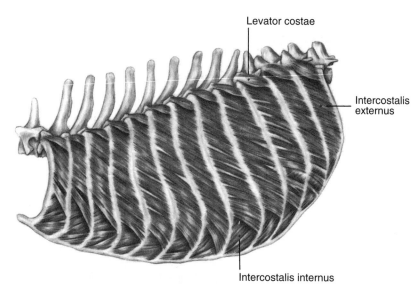

Figure 5-33   Superficial muscles of the left lateral thoracic cage. (From Evans HE, deLahunta A: *Miller's guide to the dissection of the dog*, ed 5, Philadelphia, 2000, WB Saunders.)

Spine

Figures 5-11, 5-12, 5-32, and 5-42 display ligament attachment sites, locations, and lines of direction for some ligaments of the spine. Spinal ligaments are extensive. Strong ligamentous support in the spine is thought to decrease the risk of disk herniation. The liga-

mentum nuchae or nuchal ligament is attached at the cranial and caudal extents of the cervical spine. This strong ligament acts as a tension band to oppose flexion of the head and neck and helps to hold the dog's head up with passive force, sparing muscle activity. This allows the dog relief from muscle fatigue.

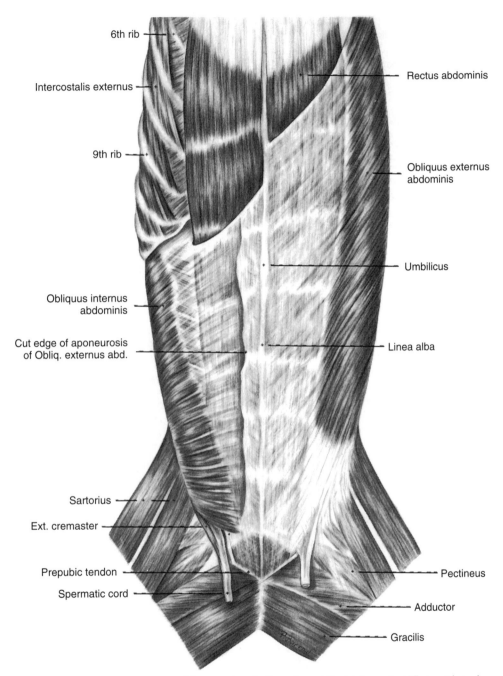

6th rib

Intercostalis externus

9th rib

Obliquus internus abdominis

Cut edge of aponeurosis of Obliq. externus abd.

Sartorius

Ext. cremaster

Prepubic tendon

Spermatic cord

Rectus abdominis

Obliquus externus abdominis

Umbilicus

Linea alba

Pectineus

Adductor

Gracilis

Figure 5-34 Superficial muscles of the ventral trunk. (From Evans HE, deLahunta A: *Miller's guide to the dissection of the dog*, ed 5, Philadelphia, 2000, WB Saunders.)

General Nerve Supply

Forelimb

Figures 5-43 to 5-45 show the main nerves of the forelimb. The brachial plexus innervates the forelimb. It is formed by ventral rami cervical 6 or C6 through thoracic 2 or T2.

Sometimes C5 contributes to the brachial plexus. The nerves appear along the ventral border of the scalenus and enter the forelimb through the axillary space. The nerves of the canine brachial plexus include the suprascapular (C6-C7), subscapular (C6-C7), thoracodorsal (C6-C8), brachiocephalic (C6-C7),

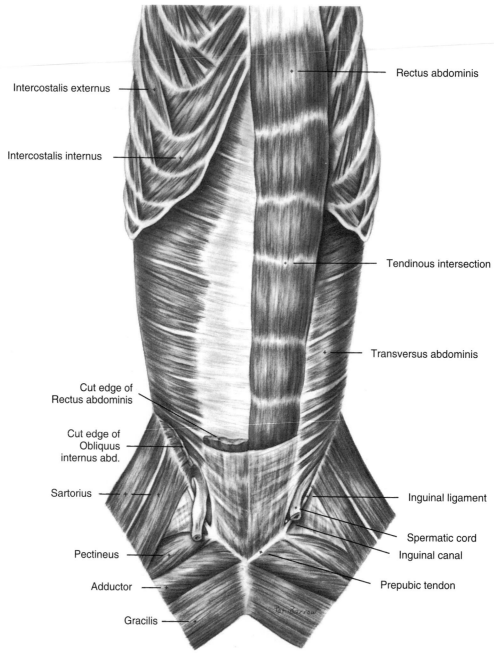

Intercostalis externus

Intercostalis internus

Rectus abdominis

Tendinous intersection

Transversus abdominis

Cut edge of
Rectus abdominis

Cut edge of
Obliquus
internus abd.

Sartorius

Pectineus

Adductor

Gracilis

Inguinal ligament

Spermatic cord

Inguinal canal

Prepubic tendon

Figure 5-35   Deep muscles of the ventral trunk. (From Evans HE, deLahunta A: *Miller's guide to the dissection of the dog*, ed 5, Philadelphia, 2000, WB Saunders.)

lateral thoracic (C8-T1), caudal pectoral (C6-C8), musculocutaneous (C6-C8), axillary (C6-C8), radial (C6-T2), median (C7-T1), and ulnar (C8-T2) nerves. Innervations of muscles of the forelimb are included in Appendix 2.

Autonomous zones are areas of skin or cutaneous sensation that are innervated by only one peripheral nerve. Main front-limb autonomous zones of the brachial plexus are the regions of

the axillary, musculocutaneous, radial, median, and ulnar nerves. Autonomous zones of the front limb and cranial trunk are displayed in Figure 5-46.

Hindlimb

Figures 5-47 to 5-49 show the main nerves of the hindlimb. The lumbosacral plexus inner-

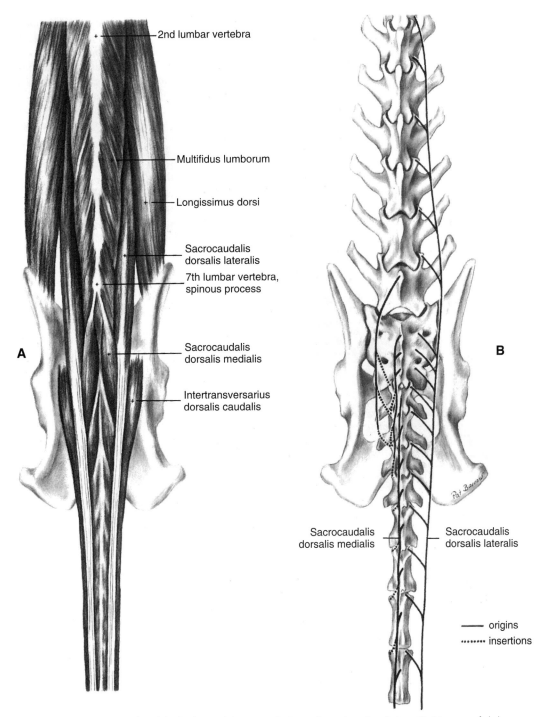

2nd lumbar vertebra

Multifidus lumborum

Longissimus dorsi

Sacrocaudalis
dorsalis lateralis

7th lumbar vertebra,
spinous process

Sacrocaudalis
dorsalis medialis

Intertransversarius
dorsalis caudalis

A

B

Sacrocaudalis
dorsalis medialis

Sacrocaudalis
dorsalis lateralis

——— origins
·········· insertions

Figure 5-36   Muscles of the lumbocaudal region. **A,** Epaxial muscles, dorsal view. **B,** Diagram of skeleton and sacrocaudal muscle attachments, dorsal view. (From Evans HE, deLahunta A: *Miller's guide to the dissection of the dog,* ed 5, Philadelphia, 2000, WB Saunders.)

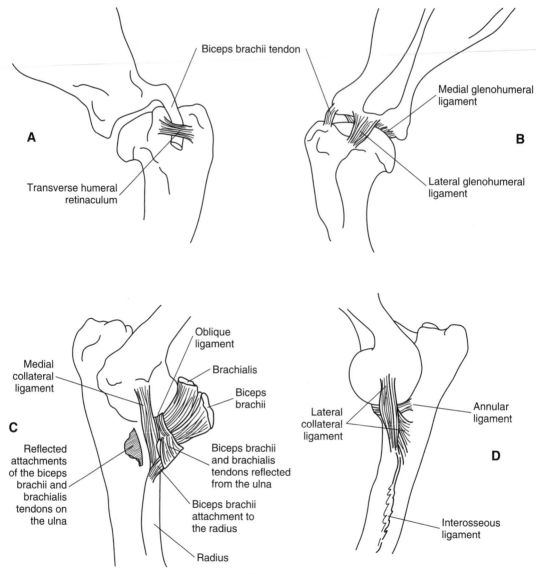

Figure 5-37   Ligaments of the medial (**A**) and lateral (**B**) left shoulder and medial (**C**) and lateral (**D**) left elbow in the dog. (Reprinted with permission from Riegger-Krugh C, Millis D: *Canine anatomy and biomechanics I (forelimb)*, LaCrosse, Wis, Jan 2000, Orthopaedic Section, APTA, Inc.)

vates the hindlimb. This plexus can be divided into lumbar and sacral plexuses; however, there are always communications between the two plexuses. The plexus consists of ventral rami from the caudal five lumbar, or L, nerves and the three sacral, or S, nerves. There are seven lumbar nerves and three sacral nerves. The lumbosacral trunk is the largest and most important part of the lumbosacral plexus and becomes the sciatic nerve outside the pelvis.

The lumbar plexus is generally formed by ventral rami from L3-L5, sometimes L2-L6. The nerves of the lumbar plexus include the

ilioinguinal from L3, genitofemoral from L3 and L4, lateral cutaneous femoral from L3 and L4, femoral from L4-L6, saphenous from L4-L6, and obturator from L4-L6 nerves. Innervations of the rear limb muscles are included in Appendix 2.

The sacral plexus is formed by ventral rami from L6-S3. The nerves of the sacral plexus that relate to the hindlimb include the cranial gluteal from L6-S1, caudal gluteal from L7 (S1), caudal cutaneous femoral from S1-S2,[18] sciatic from L6-S1, common, superficial, and deep peroneal from L6-L7, tibial from L6-S1,

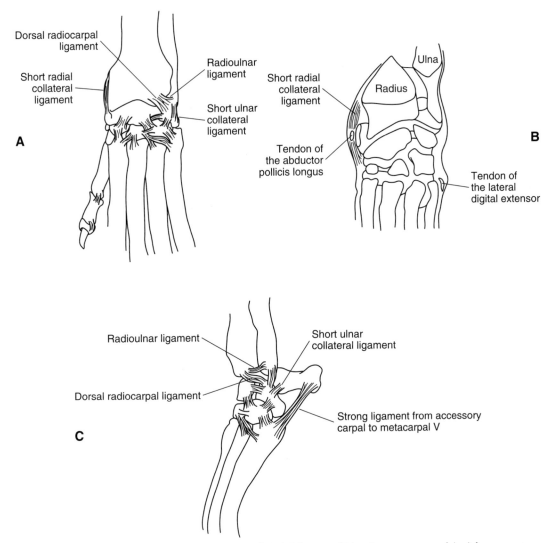

Figure 5-38   Ligaments of the dorsal aspect of the left forepaw **(A)**, schematic section of the left carpus **(B)**, and lateral aspect of the left forepaw **(C)** in the dog. (Reprinted with permission from Riegger-Krugh C, Millis D: *Canine anatomy and biomechanics I (forelimb)*, LaCrosse, Wis, Jan 2000, Orthopaedic Section, APTA, Inc.)

proximal caudal cutaneous sural from L6-S1, and lateral cutaneous sural from L6-L7. In the hindpaw the dorsal metatarsal nerves are continuations of the deep peroneal nerve, and the medial plantar and lateral plantar nerves are the distal continuations of the tibial nerve. Innervations of muscles of the hindlimb are included in Appendix 2.

Main hindlimb autonomous zones are the regions of distribution of the genitofemoral, femoral, lateral femoral cutaneous, saphenous, caudal cutaneous femoral, sciatic, tibial, and peroneal nerves. Autonomous zones of the hindlimb and caudal trunk are displayed in Figure 5-50.

Trunk and Neck

The superficial muscles of the dorsal and lateral neck and trunk are innervated by the brachial plexus for muscles near the forelimb and by the lumbosacral plexus for muscles near the hindlimb. Most of the deep musculature of the neck and trunk is innervated segmentally by dorsal rami of spinal nerves (see Appendix 2). These deep muscles on the dorsal neck and trunk are epaxial muscles, that is, they developed in the dorsal neck or trunk area and received muscular innervation locally from the dorsal rami. The advantage of the segmental innervation from many nerves

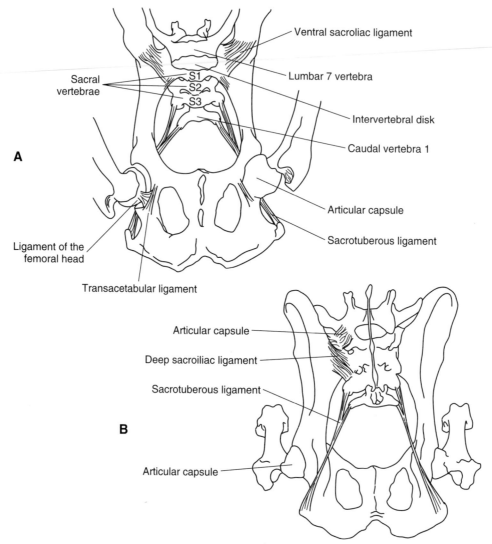

Figure 5-39   Ligaments of the hip and pelvis from a ventral **(A)** and dorsal **(B)** view. (Reprinted with permission from Riegger-Krugh C, Weigel J: *Canine anatomy and biomechanics II (hindlimb)*. LaCrosse, Wis, Feb, 2000, Orthopaedic Section, APTA, Inc.)

is that there is less chance of a strength deficit from damage to any one nerve.

The hypaxial muscles of the lateral and ventral abdominal wall developed in the lateral and ventral abdomen and received innervation from the ventral rami (i.e., the branch of the spinal nerve that traveled laterally and ventrally and innervated the local structures).

The spinal nerves exit between the vertebrae through the intervertebral foramina. All of the spinal nerves, except the cervical nerves, exit the intervertebral foramen caudal to the vertebra of the same number. In the cervical region, there are eight cervical nerves and seven cervical vertebrae. C2-C7 exit the intervertebral foramen cranial to the vertebra of the same number. C1 emerges through the lateral vertebral foramen of the arch of the atlas. C8 exits the intervertebral foramen caudal to C7.

Neck and trunk autonomous zones are circumferential strips of skin sensation around the dorsal neck and trunk. Because of extensive overlap in cutaneous sensation, a sensory deficit does not often occur unless a minimum of two consecutive spinal nerves are damaged.

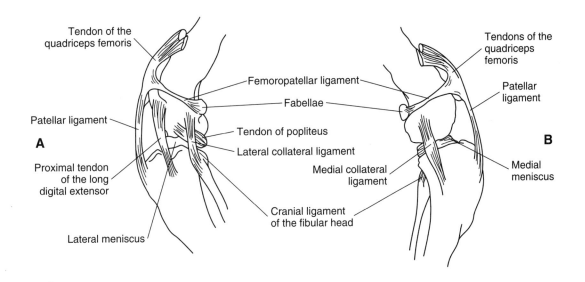

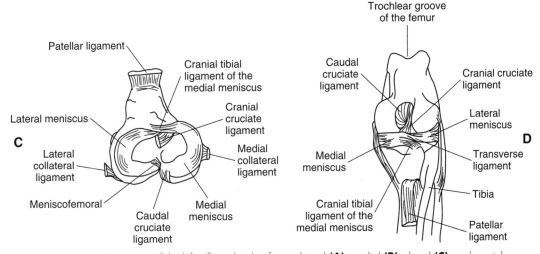

Figure 5-40 Ligaments of the left stifle in the dog from a lateral **(A)**, medial **(B)**, dorsal **(C)**, and cranial **(D)** view. (Reprinted with permission from Riegger-Krugh C, Weigel J: *Canine anatomy and biomechanics II (hindlimb)*. LaCrosse, Wis, Feb, 2000, Orthopaedic Section, APTA, Inc.)

General Blood Supply

Forelimb

Primary blood vessels to the dog's forelimb are the subclavian, axillary, brachial, common interosseous, and median arteries (Figure 5-51). The axillary artery and branches, the external thoracic, lateral thoracic, subscapular, and cranial and caudal circumflex humeral, supply the scapular and shoulder area. The brachial artery and branches, deep brachial, bicipital, collateral ulnar, superficial brachial, and common interosseous, supply the arm and forearm. Common interosseous branches

are the ulnar, cranial, and caudal interosseous arteries, which supply the deep forearm. The median artery, a continuation of the brachial artery, has two branches, the superficial palmar arch, which is the distal continuation of the median artery, and the radial artery. Arterial pulses are not easily palpable in the front limb and are not commonly used to assess cardiovascular function.

Hindlimb

The abdominal aorta divides into the common iliac arteries. The two branches of the

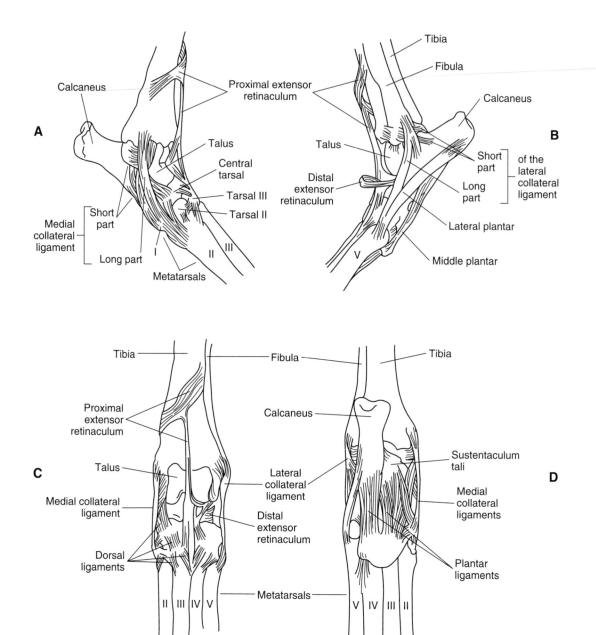

Figure 5-41   Ligaments of the left hindpaw in the dog from a medial **(A)**, lateral **(B)**, dorsal **(C)**, and plantar **(D)** view. (Reprinted with permission from Riegger-Krugh C, Weigel J: *Canine anatomy and biomechanics II (hindlimb)*. LaCrosse, Wis, Feb, 2000, Orthopaedic Section, APTA, Inc.)

common iliac arteries are the internal iliac artery, supplying the pelvic area, and the external iliac, which supplies the lower limb (Figure 5-52). The internal iliac artery supplies the caudal thigh via the caudal gluteal artery. The external iliac branches to the deep femoral, which gives rise to the medial circumflex femoral and the femoral arteries. The femoral artery gives rise to the lateral circum-

flex femoral, saphenous, descending genicular, distal caudal femoral, and popliteal arteries. Arterial pulses are palpable in the femoral artery in the inguinal region. From the caudal stifle area, the femoral artery becomes the popliteal, which divides into the cranial tibial, which continues as the dorsal pedal and arcuate arteries supplying the dorsal hindpaw, and the caudal tibial or posterior tibial arteries.

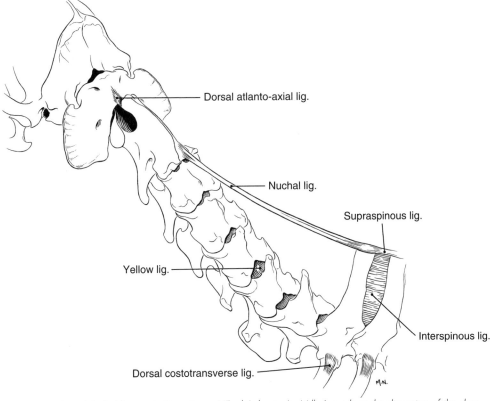

Dorsal atlanto-axial lig.

Nuchal lig.

Supraspinous lig.

Yellow lig.

Interspinous lig.

Dorsal costotransverse lig.

Figure 5-42 Nuchal ligament. (From Evans HE, deLahunta A: *Miller's guide to the dissection of the dog,* ed 5, Philadelphia, 2000, WB Saunders.)

The dorsal pedal artery is the principal blood supply to the hindpaw. The saphenous artery from the femoral sends genicular branches to the stifle before dividing into a superficial and caudal branch. The superficial branch anastomoses with the superficial branch of the cranial tibial artery to form a series of dorsal metatarsal, common digital, and axial and abaxial proper dorsal digital arteries coursing between the toes. The caudal branch of the saphenous artery forms the larger medial and a smaller lateral plantar arteries, and from these are formed a series of plantar common digital arteries. A perforating branch of dorsal metatarsal artery II, which is a branch of the arcuate artery, forms the deep plantar arch, from which form the plantar metatarsal arteries. The plantar metatarsal arteries join the plantar common digital arteries to form axial plantar digital arteries, which travel on the axial sides of the toes.

The cranial branch of the lateral saphenous vein is commonly a site for venipuncture. It is located on the dorsal tarsus and courses proximocaudally along the lateral surface of the leg.

Palpation of the Dog

Structures that are sufficiently superficial may be palpated. Palpation of structures, linked with knowledge of location of structures and the variation of feel with pathology, is an important skill in accurate palpation. Palpation is more difficult in some dogs, depending on the type and thickness of hair, skin, and subcutaneous fat. Structures that can be palpated in dogs are numerous. Almost all figures in this chapter illustrate some palpable structures.

Forelimb
BONY AREAS

The bony areas that are easily palpated include the following:
- *Scapula:* Borders, spine, acromion.
- *Humerus:* Greater tubercle, intertubercular groove, deltoid tuberosity, medial and lateral epicondyles.
- *Radius:* Head, styloid process.

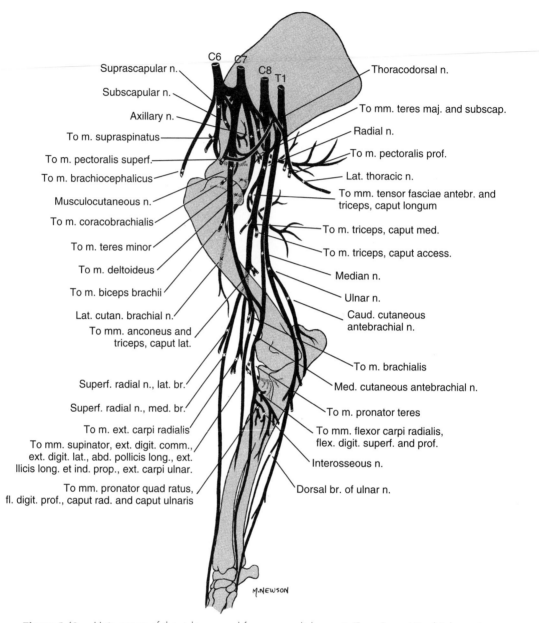

Figure 5-43   *Main nerves of the right arm and forearm, medial aspect. (From Evans HE, deLahunta A: Miller's guide to the dissection of the dog, ed 5, Philadelphia, 2000, WB Saunders.)*

- *Ulna:* Olecranon, styloid process. The medial coronoid process is usually covered by too much soft tissue to be palpable, but the location can be painful on palpation if the coronoid is fragmented.
- *Carpus and digits:* Accessory carpal bone, metacarpals, phalanges, metacarpophalangeal and interphalangeal joints, metacarpal pad in relation to the metacarpophalangeal joints, digital pad in relation to the distal interphalangeal joints.

JOINTS

Joint motion can be palpated and observed with flexion and extension of the shoulder, elbow, carpus, and the metacarpophalangeal and interphalangeal joints.

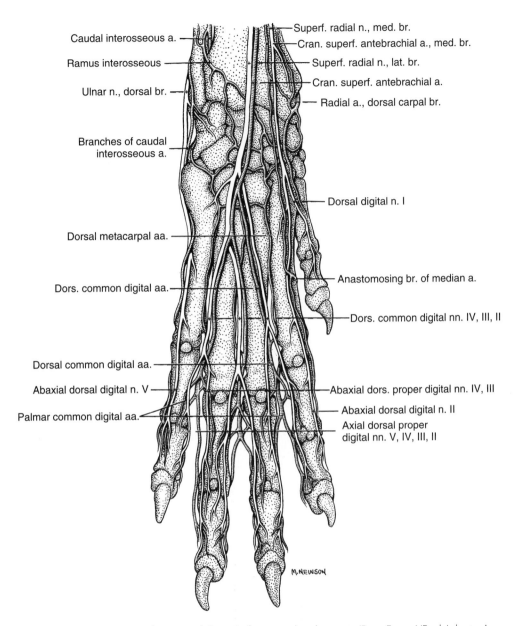

Caudal interosseous a.

Ramus interosseous

Ulnar n., dorsal br.

Branches of caudal interosseous a.

Dorsal metacarpal aa.

Dors. common digital aa.

Dorsal common digital aa.

Abaxial dorsal digital n. V

Palmar common digital aa.

Superf. radial n., med. br.

Cran. superf. antebrachial a., med. br.

Superf. radial n., lat. br.

Cran. superf. antebrachial a.

Radial a., dorsal carpal br.

Dorsal digital n. I

Anastomosing br. of median a.

Dors. common digital nn. IV, III, II

Abaxial dors. proper digital nn. IV, III

Abaxial dorsal digital n. II

Axial dorsal proper digital nn. V, IV, III, II

M.NEWSON

Figure 5-44   Nerves and arteries of the right forepaw, dorsal aspect. (From Evans HE, deLahunta A: *Miller's guide to the dissection of the dog*, ed 5, Philadelphia, 2000, WB Saunders.)

MUSCLES

The forelimb muscles to be palpated include the following:

- *Scapulothoracic:* Rhomboideus, trapezius
- *Glenohumeral:* Superficial pectoral, deep pectoral, brachiocephalicus, latissimus dorsi, supraspinatus, infraspinatus, deltoideus, long head of triceps, biceps brachii tendon in the intertubercular groove, biceps brachii

medially and brachialis laterally on the distal cranial humerus.

- *Elbow:* Triceps brachii and tendon of insertion.
- *Forepaw:* Flexor muscles on the medial humeral epicondyle, distal attachments of the flexor carpi ulnaris and ulnaris lateralis on the accessory carpal, flexor carpi radialis as it tightens with carpal extension, extensor muscles, tendons of the extensor carpi radialis and the common digital extensor.

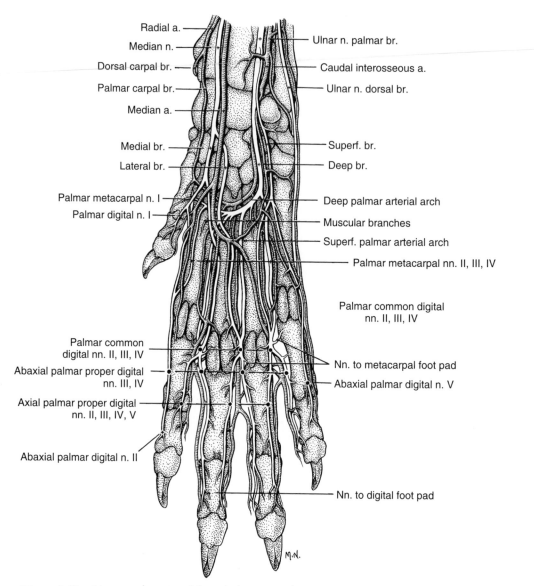

Figure 5-45   Nerves and arteries of the right forepaw, palmar aspect. (From Evans HE, deLahunta A: *Miller's guide to the dissection of the dog*, ed 5, Philadelphia, 2000, WB Saunders.)

- *Digit:* Tendons of the superficial digital flexors at the carpal canal, and digital flexor tendons and extensor tendons as groups.
- *Soft tissue:* Although the medial and lateral collateral ligaments of the elbow, annular ligament, short radial collateral, and short ulnar collateral ligaments of the carpal joint are not palpable, their integrity can be evaluated by applying controlled stresses to the joints.

NERVES

The ulnar nerve may be palpable caudal to the medial epicondyle. The median nerve is located just cranial to the humeral medial epicondyle where it is accessible for nerve stimulation but is not distinctly palpable.

ARTERIES

The brachial artery is located just cranial to the humeral medial epicondyle but may not be

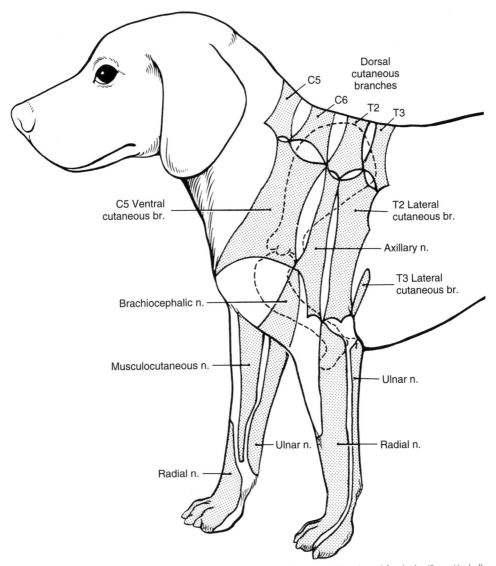

Figure 5-46   Autonomous zones of cutaneous innervation of the cranial trunk and forelimb. (From Kitchell RL et al: Electrophysiologic studies of cutaneous nerves of the thoracic limbs of the dog. *Am J Vet Res* 41: 61-76,1980.

palpable. The median artery passes deep to the flexor carpi radialis at the carpal joint, where the pulse may be palpable

VEINS

The cephalic vein becomes prominent for palpation with compression of the cranial aspect of the proximal antebrachium.

LYMPH NODES

The superficial cervical lymph nodes can be palpated cranial to the shoulder.

Hindlimb

BONY AREAS

The bony areas to be palpated include the following:

- *Pelvis:* Iliac crests, sacrum, cranial dorsal and ventral iliac spines, ischiatic tuberosities, ischiatic arch.
- *Femur:* Greater trochanter, trochlea of the femur and patella that articulates with the trochlea, femoral condyles.
- *Tibia:* Tibial condyles, tibial tuberosity, cranial border, medial side of the body of the tibia, medial malleolus.

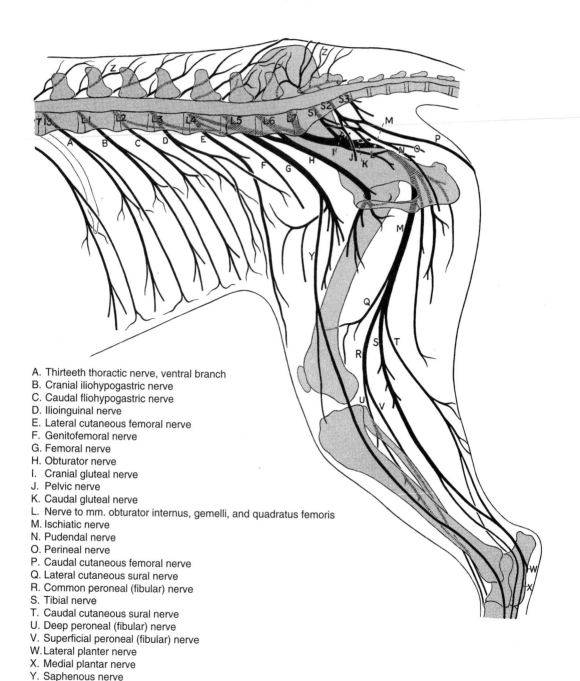

A. Thirteeth thoractic nerve, ventral branch
B. Cranial iliohypogastric nerve
C. Caudal fliohypogastric nerve
D. Ilioinguinal nerve
E. Lateral cutaneous femoral nerve
F. Genitofemoral nerve
G. Femoral nerve
H. Obturator nerve
I. Cranial gluteal nerve
J. Pelvic nerve
K. Caudal gluteal nerve
L. Nerve to mm. obturator internus, gemelli, and quadratus femoris
M. Ischiatic nerve
N. Pudendal nerve
O. Perineal nerve
P. Caudal cutaneous femoral nerve
Q. Lateral cutaneous sural nerve
R. Common peroneal (fibular) nerve
S. Tibial nerve
T. Caudal cutaneous sural nerve
U. Deep peroneal (fibular) nerve
V. Superficial peroneal (fibular) nerve
W. Lateral planter nerve
X. Medial plantar nerve
Y. Saphenous nerve
Z. Dorsal branches of lumbar and sacral nerves

Figure 5-47 Main nerves of the left caudal trunk, thigh, and leg, lateral aspect. (From Evans HE: *Miller's anatomy of the dog*, ed 3, Philadelphia, 2000, WB Saunders.)

- *Fibula:* Head of the fibula, lateral malleolus.
- *Tarsus:* Trochlea of the talus and lateral ridge, tuber calcanei, phalanges, metatarsal pad in relation to the metatarsophalangeal joints, digital pad in relation to the distal interphalangeal joints.

CARTILAGE

The parapatellar fibrocartilages sometimes can be palpated.

JOINTS

Joint motion can be palpated and observed in the hip, stifle, tarsocrural, metatarsophalangeal, and interphalangeal joints.

MUSCLES

The hindlimb muscles to be palpated include the following:
- *Hip:* Superficial gluteal, middle gluteal, sartorius, biceps femoris, semitendinosus,

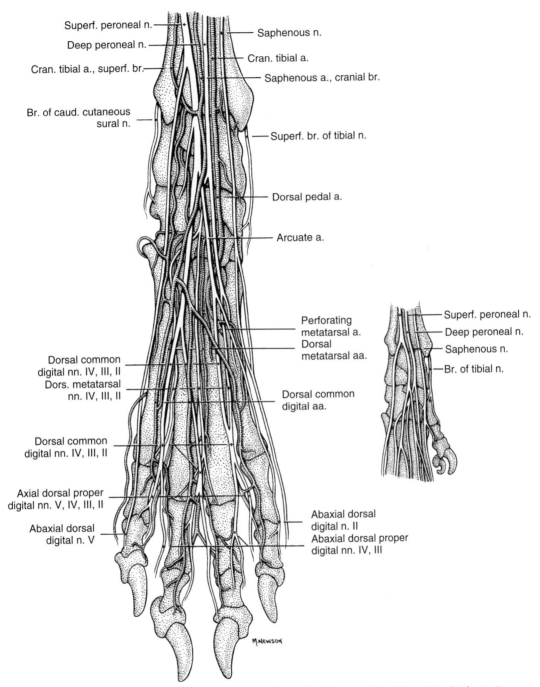

Superf. peroneal n.

Deep peroneal n.

Cran. tibial a., superf. br.

Br. of caud. cutaneous sural n.

Saphenous n.

Cran. tibial a.

Saphenous a., cranial br.

Superf. br. of tibial n.

Dorsal pedal a.

Arcuate a.

Perforating metatarsal a.

Dorsal metatarsal aa.

Dorsal common digital nn. IV, III, II

Dors. metatarsal nn. IV, III, II

Dorsal common digital aa.

Dorsal common digital nn. IV, III, II

Axial dorsal proper digital nn. V, IV, III, II

Abaxial dorsal digital n. V

Superf. peroneal n.

Deep peroneal n.

Saphenous n.

Br. of tibial n.

Abaxial dorsal digital n. II

Abaxial dorsal proper digital nn. IV, III

M. NEWSON

Figure 5-48 Nerves and arteries of the right hindpaw, dorsal aspect. (From Evans HE, deLahunta A: *Miller's guide to the dissection of the dog,* ed 5, Philadelphia, 2000, WB Saunders.)

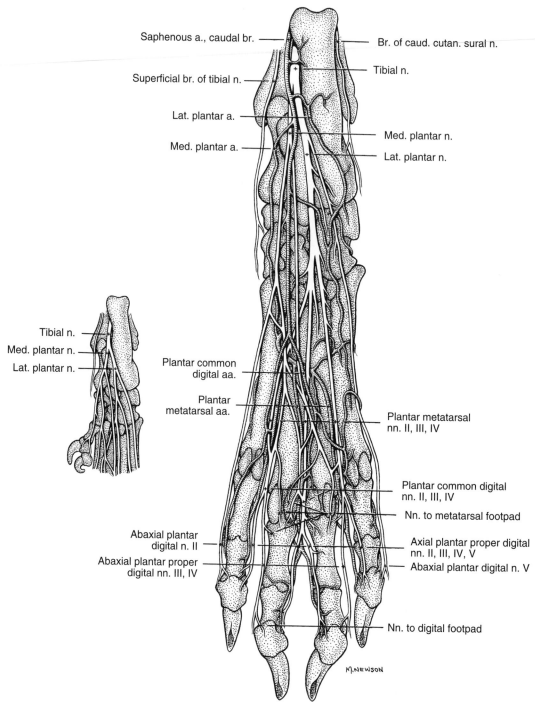

Figure 5-49   Nerves and arteries of the right hindpaw, plantar aspect. Inset is the nerve and blood supply to a double dew claw. (From Evans HE, deLahunta A: *Miller's guide to the dissection of the dog,* ed 5, Philadelphia, 2000, WB Saunders.)

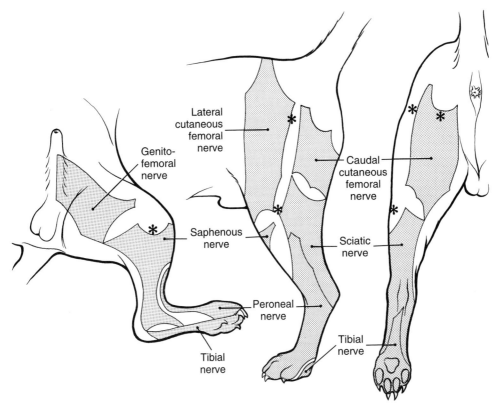

Figure 5-50 Autonomous zones of cutaneous innervation of the caudal trunk and hindlimb. Asterisks indicate palpable bony landmarks (medial and lateral tibial condyles, greater trochanter and lateral end of the ischiatic or ischial tuberosity). The sciatic nerve autonomous zone is for lesions proximal to the greater trochanter and includes the zones for the peroneal and tibial nerves. For sciatic nerve lesions caudal to the femur, the autonomous zone varies, depending on how many of its cutaneous branches are affected. (From Kitchell RL et al: Electrophysiologic studies of cutaneous nerves of the thoracic limbs of the dog, *Am J Vet Res* 41:61-76,1980)

semimembranosus, gracilis, and pectineus. In the caudal thigh, the biceps femoris, semitendinosus, semimembranosus, and gracilis are palpated in sequence from lateral to medial.

- *Stifle:* Vastus medialis, rectus femoris, vastus lateralis, biceps femoris, semitendinosus, semimembranosus, medial and lateral gastrocnemius and their associated sesamoid bones (fabellae), gracilis.
- *Tarsus:* Craniolateral muscle group that forms the tarsocrural flexors and digital extensors, gastrocnemius muscles, common calcaneal tendon, superficial digital flexor tendon, and portions of the biceps femoris, semitendinosus, and gracilis tendons.
- *Digits:* Digital flexors and extensors as groups, digital flexors in the caudal leg and plantar tarsus.

SOFT TISSUE

The medial collateral and lateral collateral ligaments of the stifle and tarsocrural joints, and the patellar ligament, are palpable. The extensor retinaculum may be palpable.

NERVES

The common peroneal nerve is palpable on the lateral surface of the proximal fibula. The tibial nerve is palpable cranial to the commoncalcaneal tendon and proximal to the tarsus.

ARTERIES

The femoral artery is palpated in the area of the medial femoral triangle and just cranial to the pectineus muscle. A pulse is palpable where the cranial branch of the saphenous

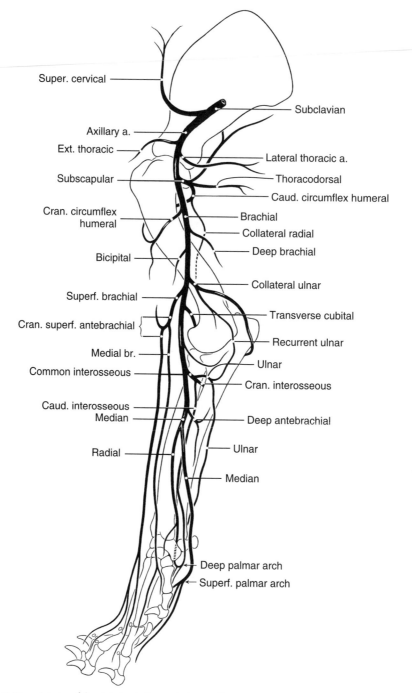

Figure 5-51 Arteries of the right forelimb, medial view. (From Evans HE, deLahunta A: *Miller's guide to the dissection of the dog,* ed 5, Philadelphia, 2000, WB Saunders.)

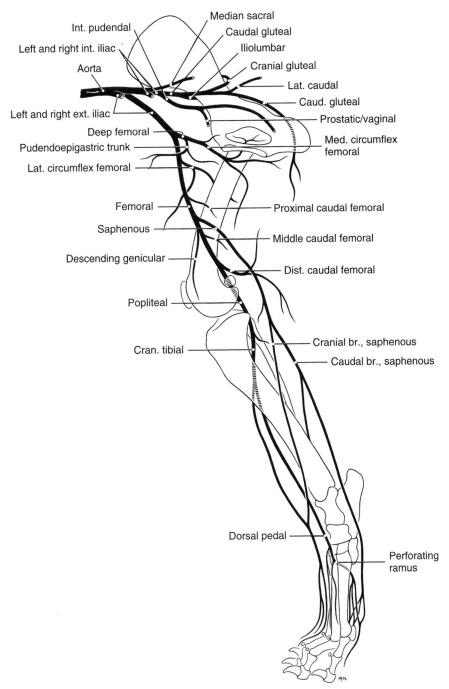

Figure 5-52   Arteries of the right hindlimb, medial view. (From Evans HE, deLahunta A: *Miller's guide to the dissection of the dog*, ed 5, Philadelphia, 2000, WB Saunders.)

artery typically crosses the medial side of the middle third of the tibia. The dorsal pedal artery can be palpated on the dorsal tarsus, often between the proximal ends of the second and third metatarsal bones.

VEINS

The lateral saphenous vein is palpable and is a common site for venipuncture.

LYMPH NODES

The popliteal lymph node, between the distal ends of the biceps femoris and the semitendinosus, is palpable.

Trunk

BONY AREAS

Palpable bony areas of the trunk include spinous processes of thoracic and lumbar vertebrae, transverse processes of the lumbar vertebrae, wings or lateral masses of atlas, spine of the axis, transverse processes of C3-C6, T13 spinous process from location of rib 13, cranial dorsal iliac spine, rib expansion with breathing, iliac crests and L7 spinous process between the iliac crests, sternum from manubrium to the xiphoid process, ribs.

JOINTS

Joint motion may be palpated and observed during intervertebral joint motion.

MUSCLES

The cervical and trunk extensor muscle mass and the rectus abdominis muscle are palpable.

SOFT TISSUE

The lumbosacral space caudal to the last lumbar spinous process is palpable.

NERVES

No nerves are readily palpable in the neck and trunk.

ARTERIES

The heartbeat can be felt over the left ventral thorax, carotid artery. No veins are palpable in the neck and trunk, but with compression at the thoracic inlet, the external jugular vein is palpable.

LYMPH NODES

The inguinal lymph nodes are palpable.

Summary

This chapter presents canine anatomy in the context of association learning and the relevant anatomy for movement rehabilitation. Some of the relevant biomechanics that enhance association learning have been included. Knowledge of relevant anatomy and biomechanics is important in understanding movement function and dysfunction in animals.

REFERENCES

1. Riegger-Krugh C, Millis D: *Canine anatomy and biomechanics I (forelimb)*, LaCrosse, Wis, Jan 2000, Orthopedic Section of the APTA, home study course.
2. Riegger-Krugh C, Weigel J: *Canine anatomy and biomechanics II (hindlimb)*. LaCrosse, Wis, Feb 2000, Orthopedic Section of the APTA, home study course.
3. Riegger-Krugh C, Millis D: *Canine anatomy and biomechanics III (spine)*. LaCrosse, Wis, March 2000, Orthopedic Section of the APTA, home study course.
4. Evans HE: *Miller's Anatomy of the dog*, ed 3, Philadelphia, 1993, WB Saunders.
5. Mann FA, Wagner-Mann C, Tangner CH: Manual goniometric measurement of the canine pelvic limb, *J Am Anim Hosp Assoc* 24:189-194, 1988.
6. Komarek V: Vertebrae inflexae, *Folia Vet* 29:103-125, 1985.
7. Millis DL: *Laboratory manual for canine physical therapy I*, LaCrosse, Wis, 1999, Orthopedic Section, American Physical Therapy Association.
8. Newton CD: Normal joint range of motion in the dog and cat. Appendix B. In *Textbook of small animal orthopedics*, Philadelphia, 1985, JB Lippincott.
9. Riegger-Krugh C, Keysor JJ: Skeletal malalignments of the lower quarter: correlated and compensatory motions and postures, *J Orthop Sport Phys Ther* 23:164-170, 1996.
10. Gillette RL, Gannon JR: Physical examination of the athletic dog: biomechanics in rehabilitation. Papers presented at First International Symposium on Rehabilitation and Physical Therapy in Veterinary Medicine, Aug 7-11, 1999, Corvallis, Ore.
11. Kapandji IA: *Physiology of the joints*, vol III, New York, 1974, Churchill Livingstone.
12. Twomey LT, Taylor JR: Lumbar posture, movement and mechanics. In Twomey LT, Taylor JR, eds: *Physical therapy of the low back*, New York, 1987, Churchill Livingstone.
13. Lee D: *The pelvic girdle*, New York, 1989, Churchill Livingstone.

14. Norkin CC, Levangie PK: *Joint structure and function: a comprehensive analysis*, ed 2, Philadelphia, 1992, FA Davis.
15. Basinger RR et al: Osteofascial compartment syndrome in the dog, *Vet Surg* 126:427-434, 1987.
16. McGonagle L: Respiratory physical therapy for animals. *Orthopaed Phys Ther Pract* 11:47-48, 1999.
17. Evans HE, deLahunta A: *Miller's guide to the dissection of the dog*, ed 4,. Philadelphia, 1996, WB Saunders.
18. Piermattei DL, Flo GL: *Brinker, Piermattei, and Flo's handbook of small animal orthopedics and fracture repair*, ed 3, Philadelphia, 1997, WB Saunders.

Suggested Reading

General Canine Anatomy Texts and References

Bloomberg MS, Dee JF, Taylor RA: *Canine sports medicine and surgery*, Philadelphia, 1998, WB Saunders.

Boyd JS: *Clinical anatomy*, Boston, 1995, Mosby-Wolfe.
deLahunta A, Habel RE: *Applied veterinary anatomy*, Philadelphia, 1986, WB Saunders.
Douglas SW, Williamson HD: *Veterinary radiological interpretation*, Philadelphia, 1970, Lea & Febiger.

Canine Anatomy Atlases

Boyd JS, Paterson D, Msay AH: *A color atlas of clinical anatomy of the dog and cat*. Bucks, UK, 1991, Mosby-Wolfe.
Popesko P: *Atlas of topographical anatomy of the domestic animals: I, II, III*, ed 3,. Philadelphia, 1979, WB Saunders.

Wound Healing: Tendons, Ligaments, Bone, Muscles, and Cartilage

James (Ned) Williams

Injury to tissue initiates a complex series of events involving many cellular and biochemical responses that ultimately result in wound healing. The series of events depends on the severity of the injury and the tissues involved. The goal is regeneration or repair of the injured or traumatized tissue. Bone generally restores tissue architecture by regeneration of the normal cell population while other connective tissues respond by repair of the injured area.[1] The wound repair response is generally described by three major phases: inflammation, reparative (proliferative or fibroblastic), and remodeling (maturation).[1-3] These phases of healing overlap, and their sequence and timing vary with the tissue involved and the severity of the injury. The focus of this chapter will be the basic wound healing response as well as the specific healing patterns of bone, muscle, tendon, ligament, and cartilage.

General Wound Healing

Inflammatory Phase

Most tissues undergo an initial inflammatory phase that involves an acute vascular response followed by cellular infiltration.[1,3] The immediate vascular component of the response is centered around hemostasis in the wound. Blood vessel disruption within the wound allows extravascular movement of blood elements and exposure of subendothelial collagen to platelets causing activation of the coagulation cascade.[1,3-5] The result is formation of a fibrin network to support the hemostatic plug and act as a scaffold for cellular infiltration.

The cellular aspect of the inflammatory phase follows the initial vascular response.

The release of cytokines associated with the hemostatic plug and increased vascular permeability incites the chemotaxis of cells into the wound environment (Figure 6-1). Neutrophils are the first cells migrating into the area, appearing by 6 hours after injury and peaking over a 2- to 3-day period.[1,3,5] The roles of the neutrophil are initial debridement and phagocytosis of microorganisms, thereby minimizing the potential for infection. The extent of neutrophil action within the wound depends on the severity of the wound and degree of contamination. The contribution by neutrophils in a noncontaminated wound is not essential for normal wound healing to occur.[1,5]

Macrophages appear within the wound approximately 24 to 48 hours after neutrophil migration.[1] The influx of macrophages into the wound appears key to the transition from the inflammatory phase to the reparative phase and appropriate wound repair.[1,3] They are central to five major functions including phagocytosis, wound debridement, matrix synthesis regulation, cell recruitment and activation, and angiogenesis.[3] Phagocytosis and wound debridement occur with the release of oxygen radicals, nitric oxide, and collagenases.[3] Working in conjunction with the neutrophil, the macrophage creates an optimal environment for entering into the reparative (fibroblastic) phase of wound healing. This activity is at a maximum in the first 3 to 4 days after injury. In addition, the macrophage releases a host of cytokines, growth factors, prostaglandins, and enzymes that subsequently activate and mediate angiogenesis and fibroplasia.[3] The macrophage appears to be the central figure in control of cellular and biochemical events in general wound healing.

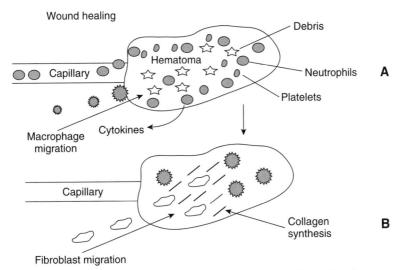

Figure 6-1   Inflammatory **(A)** and reparative **(B)** phases of wound healing.

The presence of macrophages also attracts and activates lymphocytes, whose function remains controversial.[1,3] Lymphocytes secrete lymphokines such as interferons and interleukins that stimulate fibroblast migration and collagen synthesis.[1,3,6] Their activity appears to peak approximately 6 days after injury.[1,5]

Reparative Phase

The reparative (proliferative or fibroblastic) phase of wound healing is characterized by the cellular response of endothelial cells and fibroblasts.[1,3] Fibroblast proliferation and migration predominate and are followed by matrix synthesis of collagen, elastin, and proteoglycans. The fibroblasts begin appearing in the wound within 3 days of the injury; however, there is a lag phase of 2 to 3 days before collagen production with maximal proteoglycan synthesis not occurring until 2 weeks after injury.[5] Matrix synthesis increases over the following few weeks with concurrent increases in tensile strength.[1]

In addition, endothelial cells adjacent to the wound begin to proliferate and form new capillaries that gradually migrate into the wound. The newly developing capillaries follow immediately behind the migrating fibroblast and collagen scaffold and continue until normal oxygen tension in the wound is restored.[5] This dense network of macrophages, fibroblasts, and neovascularization during the proliferative phase is generally recognized as granulation tissue.

Remodeling (Maturation) Phase

The remodeling phase is the final aspect of wound healing during which collagen fibers reorient parallel to lines of stress and strain and the fibers cross link in a stable formation.[7,8] This is the most important aspect of wound healing for connective tissues, because appropriate collagen deposition and alignment is critical to adequate tensile strength development in the repaired tissue. Although collagen deposition reaches a maximal point 2 to 3 weeks after injury, tensile strength continues to progressively increase over the course of approximately 1 year (Table 6-1). This period allows for removal of biomechanically inferior collagen fibers (type 3) and replacement with the fibers suitable for the specific tissue involved (generally type 1 collagen). In addition, decreasing proteoglycan concentration leads to a decrease in water content, resulting in compression of the collagen fibers. As fibers become closer in proximity because of realignment and compression, increased surface area is available for cross linking, subsequently increasing tensile strength.[5] Thus a proper equilibrium between collagenolysis and matrix accumulation becomes essential.

Bone Healing

Bone Structure

Bone is a dynamic tissue composed of 35% organic material and 65% mineral.[2,9-11] The organic portion comprises cellular constituents (osteocytes, osteoblasts, and osteoclasts) and matrix components. The osteocytes are cells of mature bone that remain within spaces (lacunae) surrounded by lamellar bone and are responsible for normal mineral homeostasis. Osteoblasts are responsible for osteoid production while osteoclasts function in bone resorption.[11,12] A fine balance of bone resorption and deposition is maintained for mineral homeostasis as well as continuous remodeling secondary to mechanical stresses placed on the bone in accordance with Wolff's law.[12,13]

Bone matrix is composed of predominately type 1 collagen and ground substance containing glycosaminoglycans.[8,11,12] Calcium and phosphorus deposit in association with the collagen fibrils and serve as the primary reservoir for overall calcium homeostasis. Hydroxyapatite crystals of calcium and phosphorus are aligned with the collagen fibrils and provide the structural rigidity to bone.[11,12] This unique arrangement between collagen and mineral creates the viscoelastic property of bone with the crystal supplying resistance to compressive forces and the collagen providing tensile support.[12]

Blood supply to bone is based primarily on the nutrient artery that bifurcates into ascending and descending branches within the medullary cavity (Figure 6-2). In addition, there is vascular support from metaphyseal arteries and periosteal arterioles.[11] The metaphyseal vessels anastomose with the nutrient artery branches within the medullary canal to provide complete collateral circulation. The vascular flow is centrifugal, with elevated pressure in the medullary cavity driving blood toward the periosteum. The efferent system is a venous drainage system using

■ ■ ■ **Table 6-1** Tissue Healing Rates	
Tissue	**Maximal Strength**
Skin	Collagen stabilizes (at approximately 21 days) with 20% of normal strength, 70% at 1 yr.
Muscle	Normal collagen ratio takes >6 wk. Decreases in muscle contraction strength are directly related to the degree of strain injury and the ingrowth of fibrous tissue.
Tendon	56% of normal tensile strength at 6 wk, 79% at 1 yr.
Ligament	50%-70% of normal tensile strength at 1 yr.

Above rates are generalizations of individual tissue healing. Each injury will vary depending on the severity, chronicity, and age of the individual.

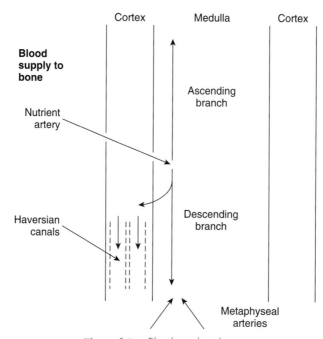

Figure 6-2 Blood supply to bone.

periosteal venules and the medullary venous sinus. Cortical vessels flow through Haversian canals in which small vascular channels are surrounded by layers of lamellar bone.[9-11] These channels in the cortical bone provide perfusion to the osteocytes within their lacunae.[12] The periosteal arterioles are the least important contributors of the vascular supply in healthy intact bone and are primarily of concern in areas of soft tissue attachment. Injury to the bone results in disruption of the vascular supply to varying degrees and is dependent on the severity of the fracture. If the endosteal supply remains intact, it will predominate during healing. However, if the endosteal supply is disrupted, as in most fractures, the periosteal support becomes extremely important, thus making careful maintenance and handling of soft tissue attachments crucial to healing.[14]

Primary Bone Healing

As discussed previously, bone is one of the few tissues that can undergo direct cellular regeneration to restore 100% of the original biomechanical properties. This can occur through two major types of healing, primary or secondary. Primary, or direct, bone healing occurs when there is a minimal fracture gap with rigid stability, and it proceeds by either contact or gap healing. Contact healing involves the direct formation of bone across a

fracture line less than 0.1 mm wide by creating resorption cavities, or "cutting cones," through the Haversian canals parallel to the long axis of the bone (Figure 6-3).[9,10,15,16] Osteoclasts lead the front edge of the resorption cavity across the fracture line and remove bone and calcified matrix in preparation for osteoblastic activity immediately following. Finally, nutritional support is supplied by capillary loops following the advancing osteoblasts.[9,15,16] This progressive Haversian remodeling continues across the fracture line until the surrounding bone has been remodeled into new Haversian systems.

When the fracture line is greater than 0.1 mm but less than 0.5 mm, primary bone union can still occur through gap healing.[10,16] This distance cannot be directly crossed by a resorption cavity. As a result, lamellar bone produced from cells lining the medullary cavity and periosteum first fills the void in a transverse direction. Subsequently, resorption cavities cross the newly formed lamellar bone and again create new Haversian systems in the proper longitudinal direction.[10,16] In fracture repair, both gap and contact healing will occur in different aspects of the same fracture line.[16] With primary bone healing, there is little radiographic callous formation, and the fracture line gradually disappears. Although direct healing entails direct formation of lamellar bone and remodeling of Haversian systems without intermediate

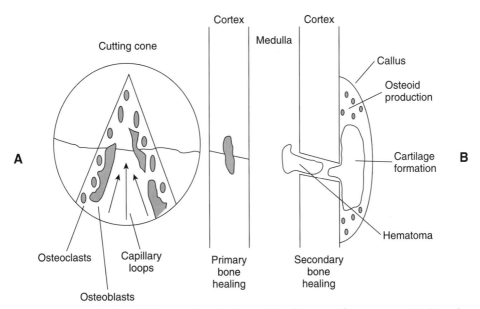

Figure 6-3   Bone healing. **A,** Primary bone healing with the formation of cutting cones. **B,** Secondary bone healing.

fibrous or cartilaginous tissue, it does not reduce the time for fracture healing, and weeks to months may still be required before complete union.[15] Radiographic evaluation is generally pursued at 4- to 6-week intervals until the fracture line has resolved. The goal is to achieve recovery of function and early weight-bearing with implants employing interfragmentary compression so rehabilitation can begin at an early stage.

Secondary Bone Healing

Secondary, or indirect, bone healing occurs when there is a lack of rigidity or absence of anatomic reduction such that the fracture gap is greater than 0.5 mm and is characterized by the formation of callus (see Figure 6-3).[16,17] The degree of callus formation is related to the amount of instability at the fracture site. In general, secondary bone healing proceeds through the same phases as basic wound healing.[9,10,18]

Similar to basic wound healing, hemostasis is the initial response during the inflammatory phase. Immediate hemorrhage and hematoma formation occur within the fracture gap in addition to injury to the surrounding soft tissues. Destruction of the Haversian canals at the site of injury causes osteocyte death and necrosis of bone. The process proceeds with the migration of neutrophils followed by macrophages into the injured site for necrotic debris removal. In addition, biochemical mediators such as bone morphogenetic proteins, platelet-derived growth factor, osteonectin, prostaglandins, and osteocalcin enter the fracture site to contribute to bone healing.[10] As the inflammatory response previously described subsides (24 to 72 hours), the repair process begins.[9,10,18]

The reparative phase begins with the surrounding tissue providing mesenchymal cells which enter the fracture site to form osteoblasts, chondroblasts, and fibroblasts. During the initial 3 weeks, a fibrous and cartilaginous "soft" callus is formed by the deposition of types I, II, III, V, IX, and X collagen synthesized by mesenchymal cells. Types III and V collagen initially appear during the inflammatory phase, whereas types II and IX collagen peak during the cartilaginous aspect of the reparative phase 1 to 2 weeks after injury. Collagen type I is initially present at low levels in the first 2 weeks but becomes the predominant type by day 14.[8,13] The function of the soft callus is to unite the fracture ends

and decrease interfragmentary motion and strain.[16] The fibrocartilage deposited is gradually transformed to bone by the process of endochondral ossification similar to that which occurs during physeal growth.[8,18] Chondrocytes progress to a hypertrophied stage followed by mineralization of the surrounding matrix. Invasion by capillaries brings cells that resorb the mineralized matrix, produce osteoid, and deposit bone. This transition from soft callus to hard callus is directly related to the blood supply available and the interfragmentary strain at the fracture gap. With high interfragmentary strain or poor blood supply, activity of osteoblasts and osteoid production is limited, and the callus remains as fibrocartilage.[10,16]

The remodeling or maturation phase proceeds following transition from soft to hard callus. The fracture gap is bridged and stabilized with endosteal and periosteal callus consisting primarily of woven bone that must be remodeled to lamellar bone according to weight-bearing forces as directed by Wolff's law. In addition, the normal blood supply is reestablished. As the endosteal callus is gradually remodeled, the medullary cavity and its blood supply are restored. Similarly, as cortical bone is restored, the Haversian system is recreated and the normal centrifugal vascular pattern can return with concurrent resorption of the temporary extraosseous supply.[17,18]

Factors Affecting Healing

Biomechanical factors at the fracture site are important to healing. As discussed previously, Wolff's law has a tremendous impact on bone deposition and resorption. The stress placed on the bone is beneficial to stimulating healing as long as the micromotion created does not exceed the acceptable interfragmentary strain for osteoid deposition.[17] If the mechanical load exceeds the strength of the reparative tissues, inhibition of bone healing occurs. Thus, it is important that no or minimal motion between fracture fragments occur early in the healing phase to allow adequate establishment of the extraosseous blood supply. Once the vascular supply is established and callus formation has occurred, then controlled axial micromotion can stimulate appropriate bone remodeling. As such, destabilization of rigidity in external fixator frames has been recommended at approximately 4 to 6 weeks following frame application to "dynamize" the fracture line.[19,20]

Electrical fields have been demonstrated in normal and injured bone and are related to either mechanical forces or bioelectric potentials.[21] Strain-related potentials occur secondary to mechanical loading of the bone and are related to piezoelectric activity resulting from collagen deformation and fluid flowing through space in the extracellular matrix.[10] Bioelectric potentials are generated by cellular functions associated with metabolic processes in the cell.[21] These electrical fields can be stimulated exogenously and have been demonstrated to favorably affect bone remodeling. Electrical stimulation can be provided by invasive or noninvasive methods. Invasive stimulation includes direct surgical implantation of a cathode at the site of stimulation and the anode placed in the surrounding soft tissue. Noninvasive stimulation can be accomplished by capacitive or inductive coupling of current to the appropriate site. With capacitive coupling, the electrodes are placed on the skin on opposite sides of the stimulation site, and electrical fields between 1 and 10 mV/cm are generated. Inductive coupling utilizes external electromagnetic coils to establish an electromagnetic field of time-varying or pulsed nature to create a secondary electrical field in the bone.[21] Currently, the mechanism of electrical stimulation of bone healing is not completely understood, but its use has been advocated with nonunion fractures.[22,23]

Alterations in endocrine balance can influence bone healing as well. Hormones such as parathormone, calcitonin, vitamin D, and thyroid can have effects on bone resorption and deposition.[10] Corticosteroids and diabetes mellitus can have inhibitory effects on bone healing.[10,24] In addition, there are numerous other miscellaneous factors that need to be considered with respect to fracture healing, including patient age, fracture configuration, fracture location, and whether the site was grafted.[10,16] Young patients heal faster than geriatric individuals. The fracture configuration is also important because highly comminuted fractures or those with significant bone loss require more time to achieve bony union. Furthermore, fractures closer to the metaphysis in locations of high cancellous bone, or those that have been grafted, may have more rapid healing potential.

Efforts to develop enhanced in fracture healing continue along many pathways. The ability to stimulate bone healing with the use of growth factors is a future possibility, and research continues in the field of electrical stimulation. In addition, research has demonstrated potential advantages to using ultrasound technology for the enhancement of fracture healing.[23,25]

Muscle Healing

Muscle Structure

Skeletal muscle is composed of aggregations of muscle cells termed fibers (myofibers) consisting of multiple nuclei within each fiber (Figure 6-4). Each individual muscle belly is composed of numerous fibers bound together by connective tissue into multiple diffuse bundles (fascicles). A dense fibrous connective tissue sheath termed the epimysium surrounds the entire muscle. The perimysium is the connective tissue support surrounding each fiber bundle within the muscle belly and the endomysium represents sheets of connective tissue surrounding each independent muscle fiber.[26,27] Capillaries, nerves, and lymphatics traverse to the muscle fibers through the surrounding connective tissue sheaths, eventually reaching the endomysium, where a rich capillary network highly sensitive to sympathetic vasomotor tone is established around the individual myofibers.[28]

Each muscle fiber has an extensive subcellular structure. Myofibrils within the muscle fiber are composed of both thick (myosin) and thin (actin) filaments, troponin, and tropomyosin, which function to provide the contractile properties of the muscle fiber.[26,28] The myofibrils are surrounded closely by the sarcoplasmic reticulum, which plays a role in storage and release of calcium for muscular function.[28] Profound variations in the composition of the myofibers and sarcoplasmic reticulum result in different types of fibers (slow or fast twitch) for varying muscular functions and fatigue resistance.

Muscle Injury and Healing

Injury to muscle occurs as a result of lacerations, contusions, ruptures, ischemia, and strains. A strain is described as an injury to the muscle/tendon unit having a tendency to occur near the myotendinous junction. Strains are described as grade 1 through 4, with grade 1 strains being disruption of a few muscle fibers and grade 4 being complete rupture of the muscle belly.[29] Often the cause of nonpenetrating injuries is forceful contraction of the muscle belly with concurrent passive extension.[27]

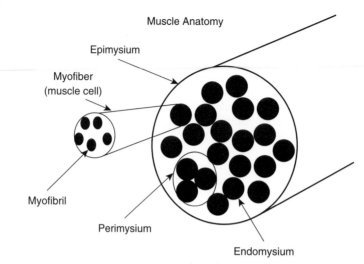

Figure 6-4   Anatomy of muscle connective tissue.

Damage to the muscle results in tearing of the muscle fibers and disruption of the vascular or connective tissue support. The problem may be acute or chronic, and the severity may vary from mild injury to complete rupture.

Muscle healing progresses in the same basic pattern as general wound healing. An initial period of hemostasis and inflammation precedes repair. Following hematoma formation, the edema and ischemia can result in necrosis of adjacent ruptured muscle fibers.[30] The initial inflammatory phase continues with neutrophil and macrophage removal of necrotic debris during the first 24 to 72 hours.[27,29] A distinct relationship between macrophage penetration and myofiber regeneration has been suspected; however, the essential component is reestablishment of the vascular supply to the injured fibers.[28] The repair phase follows and is a competitive process involving either regeneration of functional myofibers or production of fibrous scar tissue, depending on the severity of the injury and size of muscle gap.[29] The repair by means of scar tissue production is not as desirable because of the higher chance of recurrent injury and the decrease in muscle contractile strength of approximately 50%.[29,31]

As in general wound healing, the repair phase continues with production of extracellular matrix by fibroblasts including proteoglycans, fibronectin, and collagen. Type III collagen appears within the injured site in the first 3 days and generally precedes the thicker type I collagen fiber production.[32] This extracellular matrix provides a scaffold for myofiber regeneration across the injury site.[29] Myoblastic stem cells from the surrounding wound environment (satellite cells and mononuclear leukocytes) migrate to the viable ends of myofibers and align across the gap providing a route for myotubules to cross the injured site and repair the myofiber.[29] The alternative form of healing occurs when there is an inadequate source of myoblasts, inadequate vascularization, inadequate innervation, or stress across the injured site creating a significant gap.[27,29] In this situation, excessive collagen deposition and fibroblastic activity lead to formation of fibrous tissue within the injured site. The result is a barrier to myofibers crossing the injury site and inadequate return to normal muscle function.

Timing of appropriate stress and motion at the injury site is important to the type of healing that occurs. For optimal muscle fiber healing and return to maximal function, mobility across the injury site should not begin until late in the reparative or early in the remodeling phases. During the reparative and remodeling phases, the muscle fibers can be aligned parallel to the line of action if appropriate stresses are allowed.[29] If motion is excessive, gap widening occurs and the muscle heals with more fibrous tissue.

Prolonged immobilization allows penetration of regenerating myofibers and decreased fibrous tissue activity; however, the muscle fibers tend to orient inappropriately to lines of stress and tension. This decreases the tensile strength of the muscle fibers, and if the fibrous tissue elongates during the remodeling phase, significant loss of muscle power can occur.[27,29] An initial immobilization period of 5 days followed by controlled mobilization accelerates the appearance of type I collagen fiber production and subsequently increases tensile strength.[32] Considering the normal timing associated with wound healing, recommendations have been made for 4 to 6 weeks of protected activity before increased activity.[27] Adequate approximation of the myofiber ends and controlled mobilization are extremely important to good long-term muscle healing and function.

Tendon Healing

Tendon Structure

Tendons, similar to ligaments, are composed primarily of type I collagen (>95%) organized into parallel bundles with surrounding extracellular matrix. Fibroblasts or tenocytes are the predominant cellular component of the tissue and function in repair and maintenance of the structure. The individual collagen bundles are surrounded by a loose connective tissue termed endotenon. The epitenon covers the entire group of bundles while the paratenon covers and separates different tendon bellies, providing the potential for smooth gliding function.[27,33] Tendons are classified as either vascular (lacking synovial sheaths) or avascular (encased within a synovial lining). Tendons within synovial sheaths lack the typical paratenon. The blood supply to the tendon arises from three primary sources: the musculotendinous junction, the osseous point of insertion, and adjacent muscle and paratenon.[27]

Tendon Healing

The process of tendon healing follows the general course of wound healing as previously discussed with initial fibroplasia and collagen deposition followed by maturation and reorientation of the collagen fibrils. The primary variable in tendon healing is whether the tendon is a vascular paratenon-covered tendon or a synovial sheathed tendon. Paratenon-covered tendons rely less heavily on the intrinsic blood supply, as fibroblasts and capillaries invade the injured tendon ends from the surrounding tissue. This establishes the "one wound–one scar" theory.[33] With synovial lined tendons, a longer period is required to achieve adequate tensile strength and healing because healing depends on the tendon's intrinsic blood supply or inflammatory repair tissue infiltration. Thus immobilization is extremely important in the initial period to resist gap formation at the repair site and allow adequate healing.[29,34,35]

Early descriptions of tendon healing involved an extrinsic process in which an influx of cells from the synovial sheath, paratenon, or epitenon allowed phagocytosis, fibroplasia, and subsequent collagen deposition.[27,36,37] The inflammatory stage is seen within the first 3 days and is quickly followed by randomly oriented collagen deposition by the fifth day. The reparative phase follows with progressively increasing collagen content through the first 4 weeks. Similar to muscle healing, the initial collagen is generally type III, which is replaced with the biomechanically superior type I collagen as repair and remodeling progress.[8,38] Research has demonstrated that healing of tendon ends by collagen deposition requires a minimum of 28 days for fibers to align parallel to lines of stress. In addition, collagen bundles are distinguishable from normal tendons until 112 days after injury.[36] Evaluation of healing of canine triceps tenotomies (a vascular tendon lacking a synovial sheath) demonstrated only 56% of breaking strength at 6 weeks and only 79% tensile strength 1 year following injury.[34]

More recently, evidence has been presented of the potential for intrinsic repair controlled predominately by the epitenon and endotenon.[39-42] This repair mechanism occurs primarily in synovial sheathed tendons with minimal damage to the synovial lining. If there is severe damage to the synovial sheath, the extrinsic mechanism overwhelms the capacity for intrinsic healing. The intrinsic pattern of cellular proliferation and sequencing is similar to extrinsic healing; however, there is a balance between epitenon and endotenon contributions and there is minimal adhesion formation.[38] The intrinsic healing process can be stimulated by early controlled mobilization, decreasing the risk of adhesion formation and providing greater tensile strength due to proper alignment of collagen fibers along the lines of stress.[39-44] Early controlled passive motion beginning within 21 days of repair appears to be ideal; however, the duration and magnitude of motion for optimal healing remains unknown. In addition, patient compliance in veterinary medicine is a problem and must be considered to ensure a good outcome.[29,40,44]

Tendon Repair

The goal of treatment is to minimize adhesion formation and return to maximum function. The appropriate treatment is surgical apposition of the transected or injured tendon ends. Numerous suture patterns have been designed to maximize tensile strength and attempt to minimize gap formation at the injury site. Commonly used techniques include the locking-loop and three-loop pulley patterns.[33,45-50] Adherence to several fundamental concepts is required. Meticulous hemostasis is necessary to minimize hematoma formation within the injury site and minimize adhesion formation. In addition, atraumatic technique and minimal handling of the tendon ends is important. Suture materials should be monofilament to minimize reactivity and nonabsorbable to allow time for the return of adequate tensile strength. Monofilament suture also allows efficient gliding through the tissue and even distribution of weight-bearing forces and tendon tension.[27,33]

Ligament Healing

Ligament Structure

Ligaments are dense connective tissue structures consisting of fibroblasts, water, collagen, proteoglycans, fibronectin, and elastin that connect two or more bones.[11,51] They tend to widen at insertion points to blend with the periosteum and generally provide support to the articulating surfaces. Ligaments are primarily composed of long parallel or spiral collagenous fibers that are strategically arranged in multiple directions to restrain the joint from excessive excursions secondary to both normal and abnormal motions.[8,11] Histologically, the fibroblasts have elongated basophilic nuclei lying between collagen bundles.[51] The cellular and collagenous density vary with each ligament. Collagen makes up 70% to 80% of ligament dry weight composition with the majority being type I fibers, and approximately 10% being type III fibers.[51] The collagen fibers are generally crimped or buckled and can be stretched out with stress to provide elasticity and the potential to withstand rapid load application.[51]

Ligament Healing

Currently, a great deal of information remains unanswered regarding timing of ligamentous healing, especially with respect to postoperative mobilization techniques. This is because ligaments heal differently depending on the location. For example, the healing potential of the medial collateral ligament of the stifle is very good, but the cranial cruciate ligament, which has received the most investigation, demonstrates virtually no healing response following injury.[51] However, it appears that ligaments generally heal according to the same basic pattern of inflammation, repair, and remodeling.[51,52]

Within hours of injury, the defect is filled with an organized hematoma and the surrounding tissue becomes edematous from perivascular leakage of fluid. This inflammatory stage is characterized by an influx of inflammatory cells as in general wound healing. Monocytes and macrophages are found in the wound by 24 hours and respond by cleaning up the site and transitioning to the next phase. This stage lasts for approximately 48 to 72 hours.[51]

The reparative phase begins 2 to 3 days after injury and persists approximately 6 weeks.[51] Both cellular and matrix production predominate, with granulation tissue and vascular ingrowth filling the defect between friable ligament ends. The scar in the first few weeks is highly cellular with fibroblasts actively synthesizing primarily types I and III collagen and other extracellular matrix components.[51] During this aspect of ligament healing, the scar cross section reaches a maximum.[29] Type I collagen predominates and tensile strength of the ligamentous repair tissue increases as time progresses.

The final stage of remodeling and maturation progresses as with normal wound healing and may take more than 12 months to complete. At that point, ligament strength is only 50% to 70% of the original tensile strength.[51] Fibroblast and macrophage numbers decrease, and the collagen fibers become more densely packed and appropriately aligned. Factors that are important to appropriate repair of tissue include ligament end apposition, nutritional status, endocrine imbalances, severity of injury, blood supply, and mechanical stresses placed across the healing tissue.[29,51] As with muscle healing, allowing the ligament to heal across a large gap results in excessive scar tissue formation obstructing histologically normal ligament from bridging the defect.[29]

Articular Cartilage Healing

Articular Cartilage Structure and Function

Diarthrodial (synovial) joints consist of two or more hyaline cartilage surfaces that are tightly adherent to the underlying cortical end plates of apposing bones. Hyaline cartilage is designed to provide a smooth, low-friction, gliding surface for joint movement and to transmit weight-bearing forces to the underlying bone structure.[11,53-56] Cartilage is primarily avascular and without lymphatics. It is approximately 70% to 80% water by weight with the remainder composed of chondrocytes, type II collagen (90% to 95% of the total cartilage collagen), and proteoglycan aggregates.[11,53-57] Collagen provides tensile strength to the joint surface, which is divided into three zones. The most superficial layer, the tangential zone, has collagen fibers aligned parallel to the joint surface creating primary resistance to shear and tensile stresses placed on the cartilage surface. Deeper within the cartilage, the collagen fibers become oriented in a more oblique fashion and form the intermediate zone. The final, and largest, zone is the radial zone in which the collagen fibers are oriented in a perpendicular columnar arrangement and become embedded into the subchondral bone.[53-57]

Chondrocytes comprise less than 10% of the total cartilage volume.[57] The chondrocytes are oriented similar to collagen except for an additional zone of calcification present deep within the cartilage to provide transition to the subchondral bone. Surrounding each chondrocyte is the cartilage matrix separated into three regions classified as pericellular, territorial, and interterritorial. The function of the chondrocyte early in life is primarily cell proliferation and matrix synthesis. As maturation proceeds, these processes slow, with cellular density decreasing and interterritorial matrix size increasing.[53-57]

Proteoglycan aggregates provide the compressive strength to cartilage and progressively increase in quantity from the intermediate to the radial zones of the cartilage.[54] The primary constituents of the proteoglycan aggregate are a series of glycosaminoglycans attached to a core protein, which in turn are linked to a backbone chain of hyaluronic acid. The glycosaminoglycans are composed of chondroitin-6 sulfate, keratan sulfate, and some chondroitin-4 sulfate. These highly sulfated and carboxylated structures carry negative charges that strongly repel each other, resulting in stiffly extended aggregates. In addition, they are highly hydrophilic. The resulting osmotic swelling pressure, along with the fixed anionic charges, produces dramatic compressive resistance. These products are synthesized by chondrocytes and provide supportive structure to the collagen fiber network.[53-57]

A capsule surrounds the joint and is created by an outer fibrous layer and an inner synovial membrane. The outer fibrous layer, continuous with the periosteum, is composed primarily of collagen and helps to provide mechanical support. The inner synovial membrane is a thin layer of synovial cells closely associated with a subsynovial vascular plexus.[11,53-55] The cellular component of the synovial membrane is divided into type A synoviocytes, which are primarily responsible for phagocytic activity, and type B synoviocytes, which are responsible for hyaluronic acid production.[53,54] Synovial fluid is a plasma ultrafiltrate from the subsynovial plexus, which allows molecules less than 12,000 daltons to permeate into the joint. To this ultrafiltrate, the type B synoviocytes add hyaluronic acid.[53,54] Synovial fluid provides joint lubrication and cartilage nutrition, which occur through two separate processes.[11,53,54] Boundary lubrication is associated with the synovial membrane, the periphery of the cartilage surface, and hyaluronic acid. Hydrostatic lubrication is a process created by the weight-bearing force on the cartilage surface, which pushes water to the surface during weight bearing. Weight bearing and joint motion also improve the diffusion of nutrients to the chondrocytes and the removal of waste metabolites.

Cartilage Healing

Injury to articular cartilage and the subsequent healing response are directly related to the type of trauma incurred. Similar to the basic pattern of general wound healing, the ideal response includes initial necrosis and inflammation, followed by vascular ingrowth and the reparative phase. The limiting factor for the repair of articular cartilage is its avascular nature. As a result, injury to the articular surface results in two separate responses based on whether the injury is limited to the cartilage surface or extends into the subchondral bone.[58,59]

Injury limited to the cartilage surface results in a number of secondary responses. A traumatic laceration perpendicular to the joint surface (without invasion below the calcified cartilage layer) results in localized death of the chondrocytes and subsequent loss of matrix support. Consequently, a matrix defect occurs that is characterized by a lack of vascular infiltration and no inflammatory response. As a result, there is no fibroblastic response, and the local chondrocytes must proliferate and fill the defect with new matrix.[58,59] The chondrocytes respond with an initial increase in mitotic activity adjacent to the defect.[60] However, the chondrocytes may not completely fill the defect and a lesion often remains. With a lesion parallel to the cartilage surface, a similar response ensues with initial limited cellular proliferation and increased proteoglycan and matrix synthesis to fill the injured site. The primary problem is the limited durability of the repair process and the failure to completely replace the cartilage matrix. If the defect is large, then degenerative joint disease may ensue. It appears that if the defect is small, such as in a surgical laceration, it will generally be limited in progression and not proceed to significant degenerative change within the joint.[58,59,61]

Full-thickness injury to the level of the subchondral bone allows access of marrow stem cells and vascular capillaries to the cartilage defect. As a result, the injury can respond similar to general wound repair with an initial debridement and inflammatory phase. Within 48 hours a fibrin clot forms, providing a scaffold for migration of fibroblasts.[59,61] Fibroblasts and collagen replace the clot in 5 to 7 days and metaplasia to fibrocartilage begins. Matrix formation occurs with a proteoglycan-rich environment, and defect repair takes approximately 2 months to complete.[59,61] Wound healing continues with remodeling and maturation. At 6 months, the glycosaminoglycan concentration decreases significantly and tends to be rich in dermatan sulfate, which is smaller and less wear resistant than other glycosaminoglycans. Type I collagen predominates in the early stages but slowly decreases with time (40% at 8 weeks, 20% at 1 year).[59] The repair tissue remains more fibrous and is biomechanically inferior to the normal surrounding hyaline cartilage with a gross distinction permanently remaining.[58,59,61]

Because of the poor repair potential of articular cartilage, research has focused on methods of facilitating repair of hyaline cartilage. Surgical debridement continues to play an important role in treatment of articular surface defects. Arthroscopic shaving of partial-thickness defects essentially relieves clinical signs associated with defects; however, it does not appear to dramatically alter healing potential.[58,59] Recent advances have lead to the concept of perforation or abrasion of the calcified cartilage layer and invasion to the subchondral region to elicit vascular invasion and a local repair response.[59,62] Another important approach to repair of articular defects is the concept of early continuous passive motion postoperatively, because prolonged immobilization impairs the biomechanical and biochemical healing capacity of articular cartilage.[58,59,63] Additional research includes the potential for electrical stimulation, cartilage grafting, and the effects of growth factors on cartilage healing.[59]

Advances for the Future

Wound healing remains an area with tremendous research potential. An exciting area of interest includes the potential for modulation of wound healing with the use of various growth factors. Growth factors are low-molecular-weight polypeptide molecules that are located throughout the body and have a powerful influence on cellular activity. Factors such as transforming growth factor alpha and beta, platelet-derived growth factor, fibroblast growth factor, epidermal growth factor, and insulin-like growth factor modulate cellular activity by binding to receptors on appropriate target cells, resulting in stimulation of specific cellular activities. These substances may have various effects, including chemotaxis, mitogenesis, cellular activation, and stimulation of all aspects of wound healing, with their exogenous use intended to expedite the repair of injured tissues.[64-66]

Summary

Wound healing in most tissues involves an initial process of hemostasis followed by inflammation. This allows for debridement of the injured region followed by chemotaxis of the appropriate pleuripotential cells for production of repair tissue. In general, the repair process involves production of collagen, bone, or myofibrils. Maturation occurs over time allowing for appropriate alignment of collagen and tissue for resistance of tensile forces. The initiation of physical therapy in the postoperative period is important for rehabilitation purposes, and the techniques should be used to augment the maturation phase to maximize early return of tensile strength and function. The time of initiation of various therapeutic modalities is important, and knowledge of the basic patterns of wound healing is imperative.

REFERENCES

1. Fowler D: Principles of wound healing. In Harari J, editor: *Surgical complications and wound healing in the small animal practice*, Philadelphia, 1993, WB Saunders.
2. Mast B: Healing in other tissues, *Surg Clin North Am* 77:529-547, 1997.
3. Witte M, Barbul A: General principles of wound healing, *Surg Clin North Am* 77:509-528, 1997.
4. Gentry P, Downie H: Blood coagulation. In Swenson MJ, editor: *Duke's physiology of domestic animals*, ed 10, Ithaca, NY, 1984, Cornell University Press.
5. Kanzler M, Gorsulowsky D, Swanson N: Basic mechanisms in the healing cutaneous wound, *J Dermatol Surg Oncol* 12:1156-1164, 1986.
6. Barbul A et al: The effect of in vivo T helper and T suppressor lymphocyte depletion on wound healing, *Ann Surg* 209:479-483, 1989.
7. Bailey A, Bazin S, Delaunay A: Changes in the nature of the collagen during development and resorption of granulation tissue, *Biochim Biophys Acta* 328:383-390, 1978.
8. Liu S et al: Collagen in tendon, ligament, and bone healing, *Clin Orthop* 318:265-278, 1995.
9. Kraus K: Healing of bone fractures. In Harari J, editor: *Surgical complications and wound healing in the small animal practice*, Philadelphia, 1993, WB Saunders.
10. Mann F, Payne J: Bone healing, *Sem Vet Med Surg* 4:312-321, 1989.
11. Evans H, Christensen G: *Miller's anatomy of the dog*, ed 2, Philadelphia, 1979, WB Saunders.
12. Wasserman R: Bones. In Swenson MJ, editor: *Duke's physiology of domestic animals*, ed 10, Ithaca, NY, 1984, Cornell University Press.
13. Styles S, Einhorn T: Fracture healing and responses to skeletal injury. In Dee R, Hurst LC, Gruber MA, Kottmeier SA, editors: *Principles of orthopaedic practice*, New York, 1997, McGraw-Hill.
14. Motoki D, Mulliken J: The healing of bone and cartilage, *Clin Plast Surg* 17:527-543, 1990.
15. Perren S: Primary bone healing. In Bojrab MJ, editor: *Disease mechanisms in small animal surgery*, Philadelphia, 1993, Lea and Febiger.
16. Hulse D, Hyman B: Fracture biology and biomechanics. In Slatter B, editor: *Textbook of small animal surgery*, ed 2, Philadelphia, 1993, WB Saunders.
17. Brown S, Kramers P: Indirect (secondary) bone healing, In Bojrab MJ, editor: *Disease mechanisms in small animal surgery*, Philadelphia, 1993, Lea and Febiger.
18. McKibbin B: The biology of fracture healing in long bones, *J Bone Joint Surg* 60B:150-162, 1978.
19. Foxworthy M, Pringle R: Dynamization timing and its effect on bone healing when using the Orthofix dynamic axial fixator, *Injury* 26:117-119, 1995.
20. Noordeen M et al: Cyclical movement and fracture healing, *J Bone Joint Surg* 77B:645-648, 1995.
21. Aaron R, Coimbor D: Electrical stimulation of bone induction and grafting. In Habal MB, Reddi AH, editors: *Bone grafts and bone substitutes*, Philadelphia, 1992, WB Saunders.
22. Lavine L, Grodzinsky A: Current concepts review: electrical stimulation of repair of bone, *J Bone Joint Surg* 69A:626-630, 1987.
23. Einhorn T: Enhancement of fracture healing, *Instruct Course Lect* 45:401-416, 1996.
24. Loder R: The influence of diabetes mellitus on the healing of closed fractures, *Clin Orthop* 232:210-216, 1988.
25. Kristiansen T et al: Accelerated healing of distal radial fractures with the use of specific, low intensity ultrasound: a multicenter, prospective, randomized, double blind, placebo controlled study, *J Bone Joint Surg* 79A:961-973, 1997.
26. Goll D, Robson R, Stromer M: Skeletal muscle. In Swenson MJ, editor: *Duke's physiology of domestic animals*, ed 10, Ithaca, NY, 1984, Cornell University Press.
27. Killingsworth C: Repair of injured peripheral nerves, tendons, and muscles. In Harari J, editor: *Surgical complications and wound healing in the small animal practice*, Philadelphia, 1993, WB Saunders.
28. Caplan A et al: Skeletal muscle. In Woo S, Buckwalter J, editors: *Injury and repair of the musculoskeletal soft tissues*, Park Ridge, Illinois, 1991, American Academy of Orthopedic Surgeons Symposium.
29. Montgomery R: Healing of muscle, ligaments, and tendons, *Semin Vet Med Surg* 4:304-311, 1989.
30. Nikolaou P et al: Biomechanical and histological evaluation of muscle after controlled strain injury, *Am J Sports Med* 15:9-14, 1987.
31. Garrett W et al: Recovery of skeletal muscle after laceration and repair, *J Hand Surg* 9A:683-692, 1984.
32. Lehto M, Duance, V, Restall D: Collagen and fibronectin in a healing skeletal muscle injury, *J Bone Joint Surg* 67B:820-828, 1985.
33. Bloomberg M: Muscles and tendons. In Slatter, editor: *Textbook of small animal surgery*, ed 2, Philadelphia, 1993, WB Saunders.
34. Dueland R, Quenin J: Triceps tenotomy: biomechanical assessment of healing strength, *JAAHA* 16:507-512, 1980.
35. Chaplin D: The vascular anatomy within normal tendons, divided tendons, free tendon grafts, and pedicle tendon grafts in rabbits, *J Bone Joint Surg* 55B:369-389, 1973.
36. Potenza A: Tendon healing within the flexor digital sheath in the dog, *J Bone Joint Surg* 44A:49-64, 1962.
37. Spurlock G: Management of traumatic tendon lacerations, *Vet Clin North Am Equine Pract* 5:575-590, 1989.
38. Gelberman R et al: Tendon. In Woo S, Buckwalter J, editors: *Injury and repair of the musculoskeletal soft tissues*, Park Ridge, Illinois, 1991, American Academy of Orthopedic Surgeons Symposium.
39. Gelberman R Flexor tendon healing and restoration of the gliding surface, *J Bone Joint Surg* 65A:70-80, 1983.
40. Gelberman R et al: The effects of mobilization on the vascularization of healing flexor tendons in dogs, *Clin Orthop Rel Res* 153:283-289, 1980.
41. Matthews P, Richards H: The repair potential of digital flexor tendons, *J Bone Joint Surg* 56B:618-625, 1974.
42. Manske P et al: Intrinsic flexor tendon repair, *J Bone Joint Surg* 66A:385-396, 1984.
43. Steinberg D: Acute flexor tendon injuries, *Orthop Clin North Am* 23:125-140, 1992.
44. Lister G et al: Primary flexor tendon repair followed by immediate controlled mobilization, *J Hand Surg* 2:441-451, 1977.
45. Aron D: Tendons. In Bojrab MJ, editor: *Current techniques in small animal surgery*, Philadelphia, 1990, Lea and Febiger.
46. Berg J, Egger E: In vitro comparison of the three loop pulley and locking loop suture patterns for repair of

canine weight bearing tendons and collateral ligaments, *Vet Surg* 15:107-110, 1986.

47. Tomlinson J, Moore R: Locking loop tendon suture use in repair of five calcanean tendons, *Vet Surg* 11:105-109, 1982.

48. Jann H, Stein L, Good J: Strength characteristics and failure modes of locking loop and three loop pulley suture patterns in equine tendons, *Vet Surg* 19:28-33, 1990.

49. Easley K et al: Mechanical properties of four suture patterns for transected equine tendon repair, *Vet Surg* 19:102-106, 1990.

50. Pennington D: The locking loop tendon suture, *Plast Reconstr Surg* 63:648-652, 1979.

51. Frank C et al: Normal ligament: structure, function, and composition. In Woo S, Buckwalter J, editors: *Injury and repair of the musculoskeletal soft tissues,* Park Ridge, Illinois, 1991, American Academy of Orthopedic Surgeons Symposium.

52. Frank C et al: Medial collateral ligament healing: a multidisciplinary assessment in rabbits, *Am J Sports Med* 11:1983, 379-389.

53. Beale B, Goring R: Degenerative joint disease. In Bojrab MJ, editor: *Disease mechanisms in small animal surgery,* Philadelphia, 1993, Lea and Febiger.

54. Clyne M: Pathogenesis of degenerative joint disease, *Equine Vet J* 19:15-18, 1987.

55. Clark D: The biochemistry of degenerative joint disease and its treatment, *Comp Contin Educ Pract Vet* 13:275-284, 1991.

56. McIlwraith CW: Current concepts in equine degenerative joint disease, *JAVMA* 180:239-250, 1982.

57. Buckwalter J et al: Articular cartilage: composition and structure. In Woo S, Buckwalter J, editors: *Injury and repair of the musculoskeletal soft tissues,* Park Ridge, Illinois, 1991, American Academy of Orthopedic Surgeons Symposium.

58. Trippel S, Mankin H: Articular cartilage healing, In Bojrab MJ, editor: *Disease mechanisms in small animal surgery,* Philadelphia, 1993, Lea and Febiger.

59. Buckwalter J et al: Articular cartilage: injury and repair. In Woo S, Buckwalter J, editors: *Injury and repair of the musculoskeletal soft tissues,* Park Ridge, Illinois, 1991, American Academy of Orthopedic Surgeons Symposium.

60. Mankin H: Localization of tritiated thymidine in articular cartilage of rabbits: repair in immature cartilage, *J Bone J Surg* 44:688, 1962.

61. Manjin H: The reaction of articular cartilage to injury and osteoarthritis, *New Engl J Med* 24:1285-1292, 1974.

62. Frisbie D et al: Arthroscopic subchondral bone plate microfracture technique augments healing of large chondral defects in the radial carpal bone and medial femoral condyle of horses, *Vet Surg* 28:242-255, 1999.

63. Salter R et al: The effect of continuous passive motion on the healing of articular cartilage defects, *J Bone Joint Surg* 57A:570, 1975.

64. Steed D: The role of growth factors in wound healing, *Surg Clin North Am* 77:575-586, 1997.

65. Inoue H et al: Stimulation of cartilage matrix proteoglycan synthesis by morphologically transformed chondrocytes grown in the presence of fibroblast growth factor and transforming growth factor beta, *J Cell Physiol* 138:329-337, 1989.

66. Cook J et al: Effects of EGF, FGF, and PDGF on canine chondrocytes in three dimensional culture, *Vet Orth Comp Traum* 10:210-213, 1997.

Chapter 7

Responses of Musculoskeletal Tissues to Disuse and Remobilization

Darryl L. Millis

Rehabilitation of patients with acute or chronic neurologic or orthopedic conditions involves the application of controlled challenges to tissues to improve strength, condition, and function. The tissues most affected by immobilization are cartilage, muscle, ligament, tendon, and bone. Knowledge of how and in what time frame these tissues respond to disuse and immobilization is important in understanding the need for physical rehabilitation and the types of deleterious tissue changes that occur. For example, stress deprivation of joints results in proliferation of connective tissue within the joint space, adhesions between synovial folds, adherence of connective tissue to cartilage surfaces, atrophy of cartilage, reduced proteoglycan (PG) content, ulceration at points of cartilage-to-cartilage contact, disorganization of cellular and fibrillar ligament alignment, reduced collagen mass, increased ligament compliance, weakened ligament insertion sites, reduced load-to-failure and energy-absorbing capacity of the bone-ligament-bone complex, and osteoporosis of the involved extremity.[1]

Perhaps more important is understanding how to safely remobilize tissues after injury and a period of immobilization. Rehabilitation must sufficiently challenge tissues to enhance and positively influence their recovery and healing. However, if tissues are overchallenged, they may be damaged, ultimately delaying recovery. There must be a balance between the simultaneous demands for protection against undue stress to facilitate healing, and the need for stress to attenuate atrophy of musculoskeletal tissues.[2] A review of these concepts forms the basis for a rational approach to developing rehabilitation programs.

Cartilage

Disorders of articular cartilage and joints represent some of the most common and debilitating diseases encountered in veterinary practice. Understanding the normal structure and function of articular cartilage is a prerequisite to understanding the pathologic processes. The mechanical properties of articular cartilage arise from the complex structure and interactions of its biochemical constituents. The viscoelastic properties of cartilage, due primarily to fluid flow through the solid matrix, can explain much of the deformational response observed during loading. For example, cartilage that is loaded rapidly is stiffer than the same cartilage that is loaded slowly. Degenerative processes can often be explained by a breakdown of the normal constituents of cartilage, especially the collagen network and PGs, which affects the mechanics of fluid flow through the cartilage. Factors contributing to such a breakdown include direct trauma, obesity, immobilization, and excessive repetitive loading of the cartilage. Training activities, without traumatic injury, do not appear to be a risk factor for developing osteoarthritis (OA) in a normal joint, but such activity may be harmful to an abnormal joint.[3]

Normal Articular Cartilage

Articular cartilage covers the ends of long bones and is composed of chondrocytes, extracellular matrix, and water. Articular cartilage is avascular, aneural, and alymphatic. Synovial fluid is present on joint surfaces and provides a near frictionless, wear-resistant, weight-bearing surface. Articular cartilage

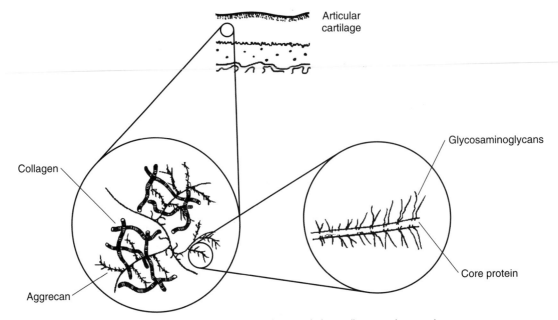

Figure 7-1   Diagram of articular cartilage, including collagen and proteoglycans.

dissipates contact stresses during loading, distributing compressive and shearing forces, which are transmitted through subchondral bone to the stiffer cortical bone.

Chondrocytes are metabolically active and make up less than 5% of the tissue volume. Metabolism of the cells is modulated by their location within the cartilage, aging, and biomechanical stresses. The chondrocytes produce and maintain the extracellular matrix and pericellular environment. The substrates for these processes come mainly from the synovial fluid. Weight-bearing results in pumping of synovial fluid, which facilitates the transfer of nutrients and waste exchange by diffusion from the cartilage surface.

The extracellular matrix is composed of collagen, PGs, and water (Figure 7-1). The orientation of the collagen and PGs functions to distribute forces over the subchondral bone and provide a smooth surface that allows movement of joints.[3] Collagen provides tensile strength for the cartilage and structural support for the extracellular matrix. Type II collagen is the primary form in articular cartilage and is unique to cartilage. Type IX collagen is also unique to articular cartilage and links type II fibrils together, limits the separation of collagen fibrils, limits fibril diameter, and binds PGs to collagen. Processes resulting in loss of articular cartilage cause collagen degradation enzymatically, mechanically, or both together. Type IX

collagen is especially susceptible to enzymatic degradation.

PGs make up most of the extracellular matrix that is not collagen and comprise 22% to 38% of the dry weight of articular cartilage. PGs are highly hydrophilic, which results in water retention, creating swelling pressure and turgidity that is essential to articular cartilage function. A PG monomer consists of a core protein with one or more types of glycosaminoglycan (GAG) chains attached (Figure 7-2). The core protein has a hyaluronan binding region, a GAG binding region, and a carboxy-terminal end. A link protein binds the PG chain to hyaluronan. Hyaluronan is a nonsulfated GAG located in the extracellular matrix, and forms a chain, to which the PG monomers are covalently bound. Aggrecan refers to a PG monomer that combines with hyaluronan.

GAGs are chains with varying lengths of repeating disaccharides. Chondroitin sulfate and keratan sulfate are the major GAGs, making up almost 90% of total articular cartilage GAGs. GAGs are negatively charged, causing them to repel one another when attached to a core protein and to occupy a large area.

Water comprises 65% to 80% of total cartilage weight. Although PGs are highly hydrophilic, enclosure in the collagen meshwork limits their ability to expand. This keeps cartilage turgid, resisting deformation. Water moves slowly within the cartilage matrix

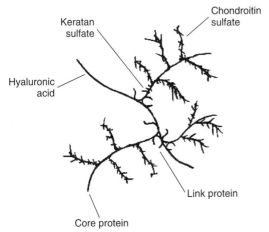

Figure 7-2 Proteoglycan molecule consisting of a core protein, the glycosaminoglycans chondroitin sulfate and keratan sulfate, hyaluronan backbone, and link protein.

during loading because of resistance of flow through the collagen meshwork and the hydrophilic nature of the PGs. Water is forced out of articular cartilage during loading, and some water weeps onto the articular surface, allowing hydrostatic lubrication. When the load ceases, water is reabsorbed. With rapid loading, cartilage is stiffer because water distributes more slowly. Cartilage is more compliant with slow loading.

Histologically, cartilage may be divided into various zones based on their depth within the cartilage and their characteristics. These zones include a relatively thin superficial layer; a middle layer with the cells arranged in vertical columns; and a tidemark, which is the upper limit of the zone of calcified cartilage, which in turn interdigitates with the subchondral bone plate.

The subchondral bone is the thin layer of bone beneath the calcified cartilage layer. It is 10 times more deformable than cortical bone and is important in distributing forces during loading. Its relatively high compliance helps to diminish the peak load placed on the cartilage, decreasing damage to the articular surface. The subchondral bone becomes stiffer with OA. As the bone becomes more sclerotic and denser, the cartilage does not deform normally, and the chondrocytes and matrix are more likely to be damaged with loading.

Response of Cartilage to Disuse and Immobilization

The effects of immobilization on articular cartilage should be understood by clinicians who

attempt to restore joint motion. Disuse of cartilage may result in atrophic or degenerative changes, and these changes are more marked and appear sooner in areas of weight-bearing.[4] Immobilization leads to a decrease in matrix and cellular components, disorganization of cartilage, and potential irreversible damage if immobilization is prolonged.[5] In addition to a reduction in synovial fluid production with immobilization, nutrition to cartilage is diminished as a result of reduced synovial pumping and nutrient diffusion. Several models of joint immobilization and disuse have been studied, including casting with the limb in flexion or extension, external skeletal fixation, and non–weight-bearing models. Immobilization of a joint in extension results in increased muscle contraction against the immobilization device and changes in articular cartilage similar to those seen in OA. Immobilization with a joint in flexion does not generally lead to arthritic changes in the short term, but cartilage atrophy occurs.

The cartilage of limbs casted in flexion for 3 to 11 weeks is grossly normal with no osteophytes.[6,7] However, there is a 13% to 60% early and progressive reduction of PG content following immobilization, with the depletion being most severe in the superficial zones.[4,7-9] Immobilization for as little as 6 days may result in a 40% reduction in cartilage PG synthesis and up to 60% for joints immobilized for 8 weeks.[4] In addition, there is a 10-20% increase in water content. The accelerated PG turnover appears to be caused by a combination of decreased synthesis and increased proteolysis of PGs.[10] The loss of PGs is somewhat selective, with preferential loss of chondroitin 6-sulfate.[8] The levels of synovial fluid PG components, including link protein, keratan sulfate, and total sulfated GAG, were determined in dogs after a 3-week recovery period following either 4 or 8 weeks of immobilization with the stifle in flexion.[9,11,12] The concentrations of keratan sulfate and sulfated GAG in the synovial fluid lavages were increased after disuse and after disuse with recovery compared with controls, but the levels of link protein remained low. This pattern of catabolism differs from that found in osteoarthritis, in which link protein is elevated in synovial fluid lavages, along with keratan sulfate and sulfated GAG.

After 3 weeks of immobilization, PG aggregation is poor. These changes are reversible, however, because PG aggregates were normal 2 weeks after removal of a cast that had been worn for 6 weeks.[4] The interaction of PGs with hyaluronic acid (HA) may be reduced in older dogs because of an abnormality in the HA binding region of the PG core protein,[4] but others have shown no abnormality in aggregation in young dogs.[8,10]

Young immature dogs subjected to 11 weeks of immobilization by splinting had a significant reduction in hyaluronan concentration in the tibial and femoral condyles, and the patellar surface of the femur, with a concurrent decrease in aggrecan, but the ratio of hyaluronan to aggrecan was unchanged.[13] Young dogs may respond differently, because there was no change in hyaluronan content in skeletally mature dogs following 4 to 8 weeks of immobilization, as compared to an 80% decrease during early osteoarthritis.[9] This difference supports the concept that the mechanism of cartilage degradation in disuse and osteoarthritis is different, and immature dogs may respond differently than older dogs to immobilization. It may also help explain why the changes in cartilage following immobilization may be reversible, whereas the changes in osteoarthritic cartilage are not reversible.

Cartilage thickness may be reduced 30% to 50% with immobilization, but the location of thinning within the cartilage is not consistent. In mature dogs, thinning occurs primarily in the uncalcified cartilage, whereas in young dogs it tends to occur in the calcified cartilage under the tidemark.[4,7] Immobilization may result in 30% fewer chondrocytes per unit area in cartilage.[4] The subchondral bone also atrophies.

Sling immobilization of the stifle for 4 weeks results in elevation of gelatinase (MMP-2 or neutral metalloproteinase) and almost complete suppression of tissue inhibitor of metalloproteinases (TIMP), especially in the superficial zone, as well as reduced protein synthesis by chondrocytes.[14] In contrast, collagenase activity is normal. The return of MMP-2 and TIMP levels to normal was observed with a 2-week remobilization period or treatment with insulin-like growth factor-1 and pentosan polysulfate. This suggests that cartilage is remodeling, similar to bone remodeling in disuse atrophy, but the material properties of the articular surface remain relatively intact following a period of immobilization with a sling.

Contact forces between articulating surfaces appear to be necessary to maintain normal PG content of articular cartilage.[8] The greatest depletion of GAGs (64%) occurred at the cranial and caudal extremes of the femoral condyles in the stifle joint cartilage of young Beagle dogs following cast immobilization for 11 weeks in 90 degrees of flexion. These were locations where the immobilized cartilage lost contact with the opposing cartilage.[8]

The biochemical changes that occur with immobilization also affect the biomechanical properties of articular cartilage. Splint immobilization of stifle joints of young dogs for 11 weeks caused significant softening of femoral and tibial cartilage with no visible changes of the cartilage surface.[15] The rate of deformation during loading increased 42% and the average thickness of the cartilage decreased 9% as compared with controls. Loading of cartilage may be necessary to maintain cartilage stiffness, because stiffness was maintained in the contact area between the patella and patellar surface of the femur as a result of sustained loading between the femur and the patella produced by the flexion of the knee joint, whereas cartilage softening was greatest in nonloaded areas. There is correlation between cartilage stiffness and PG concentration. Therefore loss of PGs during immobilization may also affect biomechanical properties. Immobilization of stifles with a cast caused significant softening of up to 30% in the lateral femoral and tibial cartilages.[16] The GAG content of the cartilage was slightly decreased after immobilization, especially in the superficial zone of cartilage. The changes in stiffness correlated with alterations in GAG content of the superficial and deep zones. This confirms the key role of PGs in the regulation of cartilage stiffness. There may also be changes in the compressive and shear stiffness of cartilage from nonimmobilized contralateral limbs, possibly due to increased loading.[17]

The changes that occur to articular cartilage during immobilization are probably due to a combination of decreased joint motion and reduced loading. Although both are important in maintaining cartilage integrity, normal loading is particularly important with contraction of muscles that span the joint and stabilize the limb during weight-bearing.[6] In a non–weight-bearing model that allowed joint motion of the stifle joint, cartilage thickness, PG content, and PG synthesis were reduced, while water content was increased.[18] These changes were similar to those that occur with immobilization in a flexed position and suggest that weight-bearing is necessary to prevent the bulk of changes. Nevertheless, some motion of the joint during immobilization is beneficial. Stifles immobilized for 6 weeks with a cast, allowing 8 to 15 degrees of motion, had less PG loss and a smaller decrease in PG synthesis than occurred with more rigid fixation. The limited motion provided by casting was protective.[10]

The age of the dog, as well as the form of immobilization used, may affect results. The changes in mechanical behavior and biochemical composition of articular cartilage appear to be less dramatic in limbs immobilized in a sling than in limbs immobilized in a cast. Adult Greyhound dogs had stifles placed in a sling at 90 degrees of flexion for 4 or 8 weeks, which allowed some limited motion of the stifle, and had no changes in the compressive properties of cartilage, PG content, collagen content, or cartilage thickness.[19] This suggests that immobilization with a sling may be less deleterious to articular cartilage compared with other models of joint disuse in which cartilage changes are both progressive and degenerative.[19]

The elimination of motion by rigid fixation induces even more pronounced atrophic changes to articular cartilage. To study the effects of immobilization on the ultrastructure and surface contour of articular cartilage, knee joints of adult dogs were immobilized with circular external fixation for 2 to 4 weeks.[20] The degree of cartilage changes increased with the length of immobilization and consisted of destruction of the superficial cartilage layer, cleft formation in the surface, and erosion of the articular cartilage. In another study, knees of mature dogs were immobilized for 6 weeks with external fixators. There was a 7% increase in water content compared with normal knee cartilage and a 28% decrease in GAG content, which was greater than if some motion was allowed.[10] More importantly, GAG content did not return to normal after a 1-week remobilization period as it did in dogs which were not rigidly immobilized.

Immobilization of the stifle in flexion may be beneficial when joint instability exists, such as occurs with a ruptured cranial cruciate ligament (CCL), because bearing weight on an unstable stifle results in osteoarthritis. Dogs that underwent transection of the CCL either had their stifle joints maintained in flexion or were permitted ad libitum ambulation in a pen for 12 weeks.[21] Dogs allowed to bear weight had osteophytes, fibrillation, and decreased cartilage PG content, although cartilage thickness was normal. PG synthesis was 80% greater than that in cartilage from the

contralateral knee. In contrast, osteophytes were not seen when the leg was immobilized in flexion immediately after transection of the ligament, and the articular surface remained intact. The cartilage became atrophic, however, and PG content and PG synthesis were decreased compared with cartilage from the contralateral knee. Knee cartilage from immobilized limbs after cruciate ligament transection therefore resembled that from dogs whose limbs were immobilized without ligament transection.

The effect of position of the limb during immobilization on blood flow to the joint must also be considered. For example, forced abduction of experimentally induced hip dysplasia with secondary osteoarthritis results in significant reduction of blood flow, whereas immobilization in flexion results in the highest blood flow to the femoral head.[22]

The Effects of Remobilization on Cartilage

The response of cartilage to remobilization depends on the biomechanical demand to which the joint is exposed, the condition of the cartilage, and the length of the immobilization and remobilization period. If the joint is subjected to high stresses and repeated loading immediately after immobilization, cartilage may not be able to resist the stresses and may become damaged because of injury to the softened matrix. The duration and the degree of load-bearing after immobilization are factors that determine the cartilage response (Figure 7-3). Also, the ability to restore biomechanical properties may depend on an intact collagen network.

The atrophic changes of cartilage that occur with a limb casted in flexion are somewhat reversible. Remobilization of a normal limb casted in flexion for 6 weeks by allowing

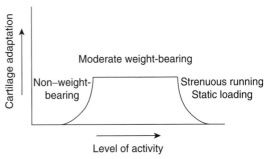

Figure 7-3 Adaptive responses of articular cartilage to activity (based on a diagram from Hallett and Andrish[43]).

ambulation for 3 weeks after cast removal resulted in the cartilage becoming normal.[4]

Longer periods of immobilization in young dogs may result in more long-standing effects, even with a gentle remobilization period. Skeletally immature female Beagle dogs were immobilized in a cast for 11 weeks in 90 degrees of flexion followed by remobilization for 15 weeks.[8] Following remobilization, PG content remained an average 18% lower than controls, with content at the minimum contact sites 33% lower. GAG concentration was restored in the more loaded regions of the patellofemoral region and tibial condyles, but remained lower than the control values in the less loaded peripheral regions of the femoral condyles.[23] Uncalcified cartilage thickness of the femoral condyles was 15% less than in the controls, and the thickness of the calcified zone was reduced in most regions of the remobilized stifles. The thinness of the calcified zone may be due to advanced bone growth from the subchondral bone during remobilization. Softening of the articular cartilage during immobilization may expose the calcified zone to increased mechanical loading and result in mineralization and thickening of subchondral bone. The changes induced by unloading are reversible to a great extent, but full restoration of articular cartilage may not occur at all sites following 15 weeks of remobilization. Immobilization of the skeletally immature joint therefore may affect the development of articular cartilage in such a way that very slow recovery or permanent alterations are induced.

Longer periods of remobilization may be more beneficial. Hindlimbs of immature dogs were immobilized for 11 weeks and then remobilized for 50 weeks.[16,24,25] After the immobilization period, cartilage GAG concentration was reduced similar to that found in other studies. The amount of collagen cross-links was also reduced during immobilization. After 50 weeks of remobilization, GAG concentration was restored at most sites, but remained 9% to 28% lower than controls in the patella, medial femoral condyle, tibial condyles, and the proximal femoropatellar surface. Collagen cross-links were restored to control levels, indicating that collagen is resistant to reduced joint loading and slow remobilization. Although the articular cartilage of immobilized limbs became similar to control cartilage following long periods of remobilization, full restoration of articular cartilage GAG concentration was not obtained in all sites, even after remobilization for 50 weeks. This suggests that joint

immobilization of young dogs can cause long-lasting articular cartilage PG alterations.

Because GAGs exert strong influence on the biomechanical properties of cartilage, the biochemical changes that occur in cartilage during remobilization may also affect the biomechanical properties. The restoration of the biomechanical properties of articular cartilage was studied after 15 weeks of remobilization of the knee joint in mature Beagles previously immobilized with a cast for 11 weeks.[26] Remobilization improved the decreased stiffness and cartilage thickness in femoral, tibial, and patellar cartilage created by immobilization and approached values of nonimmobilized controls. However, stiffness of the femoral condylar cartilage remained lower and cartilage permeability was higher compared with the controls. A study with the same period of immobilization but with a remobilization period of 50 weeks resulted in restoration of the biomechanical properties of cartilage in the lateral condyle of tibia, but not in the lateral condyle of femur, where stiffness remained 15% below the control level following remobilization.[16] Similar to biochemical changes, articular cartilage biomechanical properties return toward normal during remobilization, although the recovery is not complete in all parts of the knee even after 50 weeks of remobilization. Immobilization of joints of young dogs may cause long-term, if not permanent, alterations of cartilage biomechanical properties, similar to changes observed in biochemical components of articular cartilage. This may predispose joints to degenerative changes later in life.

The atrophic changes seen in cartilage following immobilization are less reversible following immobilization with a rigid external fixator. However, in one study, 2 to 4 weeks of remobilization following 2 to 4 weeks of immobilization with an Ilizarov external fixator demonstrated that the longer the period of remobilization, the greater the reparative processes.[20]

In contrast to the improvements seen with mild remobilization strategies, vigorous exercise after a period of immobilization may have deleterious effects on cartilage.[27] Dogs that ran daily (9.5 km/day) on a treadmill for 3 weeks after cast removal had continued decreases in cartilage thickness (20%) and PG content (35%), even though net PG synthesis was 16% greater than in cartilage from contralateral nonimmobilized stifles. Therefore vigorous loading of the joint following a period of immobilization may prevent reversal of cartilage damage and ultimately be detrimental to cartilage. It appears that the atrophic changes are more reversible with gentle spontaneous reloading.

Meniscal Cartilage Changes

Various experimental models for producing atrophy of meniscal tissue have yielded contradictory results. These models have included denervation of the stifle, immobilization (both internal and external), and disarticulation. Active motion of the stifle may play a more important role than weight-bearing in preventing meniscal atrophy. In one study, internal skeletal fixation, which did not allow motion of the stifle joint, was applied for 12 weeks. There was significant atrophy of the lateral meniscus, despite the opportunity for weight-bearing.[28] Another study evaluated the effect of active joint motion on the maintenance of meniscus mass in a unilateral ankle disarticulation non–weight-bearing model of disuse. This model maintained active knee motion without weight bearing. Despite the loss of collagen and calcium mass in the femur and tibia because of decreased weight-bearing, there was no loss of meniscal mass.[29]

Although meniscal mass may be maintained when motion is allowed in stifles with limited weight-bearing, there may be profound changes in biomechanical and biochemical properties. Meniscal cartilage stiffness decreased by 30% 8 weeks after transection of the CCL and immediate stabilization of the stifle in one study, despite the normal appearance of the meniscus.[30] Although weight-bearing and joint motion were not restricted following surgery, limb use was reduced, and it is possible that a combination of inflammation and decreased limb use after surgery resulted in decreased stiffness. Chronic stifle instability may result in further deterioration of the meniscus, because clinical cases undergoing partial meniscectomy had a 60% decrease in meniscal stiffness.

The effect of early motion on healing meniscal repairs has been evaluated in humans at the time of anterior cruciate ligament (ACL) reconstruction. In one study, 80% of patients undergoing immediate postoperative range of motion and early partial weight-bearing had complete meniscal healing with no deleterious effects of immediate knee motion on meniscal repairs.[31] Although meniscal repair is not generally performed in dogs,

studies of healing medial meniscal incisions demonstrated that dogs with immediate limb mobilization had greater collagen content in the healing meniscus than those that were immobilized in a cast.[32] There were no significant differences in collagen between the repaired menisci with mobilization and the control menisci. Prolonged immobilization resulted in decreased collagen formation in healing tissue. The vascular response during meniscal healing is also affected by immobilization.[33] In a study of rabbits with meniscal injury, meniscal blood flow was increased fivefold in animals in which the stifle was allowed motion, but this increase was prevented by immobilization 4 weeks after injury. Furthermore, healing was diminished in immobilized knees.

Partial or complete meniscectomy is more commonly used to treat meniscal damage in dogs. In general, meniscal removal results in degeneration of articular cartilage, and biomechanical properties of cartilage, including cartilage stiffness, are affected.[34] Less severe changes occur with partial meniscal resection, but the changes are greater on the tibial surface.[35,36] Early joint motion may be beneficial to these patients. In studies of bilateral medial meniscectomy in dogs, one group was allowed immediate joint movement, while another group underwent knee joint immobilization with an external skeletal fixator for 5 weeks immediately following meniscectomy. After removal of the fixation, the animals were allowed free movement for 21 weeks.[37,38] The menisci (regrown and normal) were examined for collagen content, collagen assembly, and GAG distribution. Although the collagen content of regrown tissues was not different from normal menisci, fiber development and GAGs were not normal. Movement following meniscectomy is likely beneficial to matrix formation in the regenerating tissue. Regarding articular cartilage, twice as much PG was present in femoral condyles of meniscectomized animals encouraged to bear weight on joints immediately after surgery compared to controls or joints immobilized after surgery.

Adaptations of Cartilage to Increased Stress

Many reports have suggested an association between the biochemical and biomechanical properties of cartilage and the mechanical stress to which it is subjected. For example, the increased weight-bearing in the limb opposite a limb casted in flexion caused a 19% increase in uncalcified cartilage thickness and a 25% to 35% increase in GAG concentration in the intermediate, deep, and calcified zones of the femoral condyles.[7] It appears that increased weight-bearing augments local PG content of the articular cartilage matrix. In fact, PG content and cartilage thickness are generally greater in central weight-bearing areas than in peripheral areas, and contact forces help maintain normal cartilage matrix.[7] In general, chondroitin sulfate predominates in pressure-bearing regions, whereas dermatan sulfate predominates in tension-transmitting regions of connective tissues.[39]

The influence of static and intermittent stress on articular cartilage metabolism was examined in vitro using full-thickness plugs of cartilage from femoral condyles of normal adult dogs.[39] When cartilage was exposed to a static stress equivalent to 3 times body weight, or to cyclic stresses at a duty cycle of 60 seconds on/60 seconds off, net GAG synthesis was suppressed to 30% to 60% of that in controls. Protein synthesis also decreased, and water content increased. In contrast, when a duty cycle of 4 seconds on/11 seconds off was used, GAG synthesis was increased by 34%, but protein synthesis and water content were not affected. The changes in GAG synthesis do not appear to be due to changes in diffusion of nutrients during loading. These results suggest that regular, intermittent stresses, such as those obtained with walking, are important to maintain normal articular cartilage.

Continuous strong compression or heavy impact loading to joints may cause deterioration of articular cartilage (see Figure 7-3).[40] Blunt trauma applied to cartilage results in changes in the zone of calcified cartilage, with an increase in cellular clones, bony bar formation in the calcified cartilage, vascular invasion, and decreased PG content, thickness of the calcified cartilage, and number of chondrocytes.[41,42] Blunt trauma to articular cartilage causes significant alterations in the deeper layers of cartilage, without disruption of the articular surface.

EFFECTS OF TRAINING ON CARTILAGE

The adaptation that occurs in functioning joints is known as Leed's hypothesis, which states that cartilage becomes conditioned to transmit, without sustaining damage, the stresses to which it is most regularly subjected.[26] Exercise places biomechanical and physiologic demands on articular cartilage.[43] Mild to moderate levels of running in dogs may stimulate adaptation, but strenuous levels can cause detrimental articular cartilage changes. There may be activity thresholds below and above which articular cartilage is maintained or destroyed. Between these thresholds, cartilage seems to adapt to the loads placed upon it.

Intermittent compression tends to stimulate chondrocyte biosynthesis. Joint motion without compression results in articular cartilage thinning, and static loading causes decreased chondrocyte biosynthesis.[43] Cartilage subjected to high stress has higher PG content and is stiffer than cartilage exposed to low stress levels. Most studies of moderate running indicate no injury to articular cartilage, assuming there are no abnormal biomechanical stresses acting on the joints.

Mild to Moderate Training

Young Beagle dogs running 4 km/day at a 15-degree incline on a treadmill for 15 weeks had no macroscopic damage to the cartilage surface and a 6% increase in mean cartilage stiffness, with most of the increase occurring on the patellar surface of the femur and the tibial condyles.[44] In general, most of the increase in stiffness occurred in areas that were heavily loaded during exercise. Cartilage thickness also increased by a mean of 11%, with increases of 19% to 23% in the lateral condyle and patella surface of the femur. In addition, there was a 28% increase in GAG content of the femoral condyles, located mainly in the intermediate and deep zones.[45] This degree of exercise had a mildly anabolic effect on properties of cartilage. Running 20 km/day on a treadmill for 15 weeks did not further improve mechanical properties.[46]

Severe Training

Skeletally immature dogs were subjected to 15 weeks of running exercise at a rate of 40 km/day. There was no change in cartilage total hyaluronan or PGs after long-term exercise.[13] However, running 20 km/day for nearly 1 year resulted in a 6% reduction in thickness of the uncalcified cartilage of the medial femoral condyle, with an 11% reduction in GAG content.[47] Although tibial cartilage was stiffer, femoral condyle stiffness was unchanged with this degree of training.[46]

In similar studies of running 40 km/day, the effects on young canine articular cartilage of training for 1 year were investigated. The cartilage response to running training was found to be site-dependent.[48,49] Cartilage stiffness decreased 12% to 14% in the lateral, but not in the medial, condyles of the femur and tibia, perhaps because of excessive impact loading and damage to the lateral region.[48] GAG content was depleted in the superficial weight-bearing areas of the joint, including the lateral femoral condyle.[49] There were slight increases in the thickness of the uncalcified and calcified cartilage, and the subchondral bone.[50] There also appears to be reorientation of the superficial zone collagen network.[51] Although no overt cartilage damage was seen, softening of the cartilage may jeopardize the ability of cartilage to maintain its normal structural and functional properties over time. The response to long-term exercise may be different in other joints. Although there was a decrease in GAG content and cartilage thickness in the head of the humerus following training, cartilage stiffness was not affected.[48,49] The articular cartilage of the femoral head appears to adapt very well to long-term distance training.[52]

Strenuous training protocols in older dogs may result in deleterious changes to cartilage. Running aged dogs on a treadmill at 9.6 to 12.8 km/hr for 1 hr/day, 6 days/week for 8 months led to matrix degradation in the femoral head. PG content was decreased and there was irreversible destruction of collagen fibrils, with erosion and fibrillation of the cartilage surface. Older dogs may be more vulnerable to mechanical stress changes than younger animals.[53]

Lifelong Training

One study evaluated the effect of lifelong low-impact exercise on articular cartilage.[54] Dogs were exercised on a treadmill at 3 km/hr for 75 min, 5 days/week for 527 weeks while wearing jackets so that the total weight carried was 130% of body weight. There was no ligament, meniscal, or cartilage injury or osteophytes. Biochemical, cartilage thickness, and biomechanical properties were not affected by training. These results suggest that a lifetime of relatively low impact weight-bearing exercise in dogs with normal joints does not cause alterations in the structure and mechanical properties of articular cartilage that might lead to joint degeneration.[54]

EFFECTS OF EXERCISE ON CARTILAGE DURING ACUTE INFLAMMATION

Excessive exercise during periods of acute joint inflammation may be detrimental to articular cartilage. Passively exercising the stifle joints of dogs in a model of acute inflammation for 5 seconds resulted in a twofold increase in the synovial fluid leukocyte count, whereas exercise for 5 minutes produced a ninefold increase in inflamed joints.[55] Forms of acute inflammatory arthritis may require periods of physical inactivity for recovery. Observations of humans with rheumatoid arthritis suggest that excessive activity may increase the severity of the disease.[56] Immobilization was chondroprotective to guinea pig stifles following an intraarticular injection of iodoacetate. Animals that were not immobilized had decreased GAG content and a 10% to 20% reduction in the number of chondrocytes 1 week after injection. Three weeks after injection, cell death and loss of GAG progressed, and surface fibrillation and osteophytes developed. Although the loss of GAGs was not altered by immobilization after iodoacetate injection, the depletion of chondrocytes was reduced. Furthermore, neither osteophytes nor fibrillation developed.[57] Therefore immobilization may be protective during acute bouts of inflammatory joint disease.

ABNORMAL BIOMECHANICAL STRESSES

Whereas moderate training programs appear to have no detrimental effects on articular cartilage in animals with normal joints, training programs may be deleterious to articular cartilage in dogs with abnormal biomechanical stresses acting on joints. Transection of the CCL is a common model to produce OA. OA occurs as a result of joint instability during weight-bearing. Joint immobilization may be somewhat protective against OA development. In a CCL transection model, the stifle joint of one group was immobilized in a cast for 12 weeks, and the other group had no immobilization for 12 weeks.[21] Stifles of dogs with CCL transection without immobilization had changes typical of OA, including increased water content and PG synthesis, and decreased PG content, but the cartilage thickness was normal. Osteophytes were not seen with CCL transection and immobilization, but the cartilage was atrophic (40% thinner), water content was increased, and PG content and synthesis were diminished. These data suggest that OA develops with cruciate ligament transection as a result of mechanical instability. If the knee is immobilized after cruciate transection so that loading is reduced, OA does not develop in the short term.

Effects of Medications on Immobilized Cartilage

Medications are commonly prescribed for dogs with joint injuries. Many of these drugs may have deleterious effects on articular cartilage metabolism, especially if the joint is immobilized. For example, fluoroquinolones, such as enrofloxacin and ciprofloxacin, may be toxic to chondrocytes, resulting in cellular changes which alter cell adhesion.[58] Knowledge of these effects may result in more effective rehabilitation strategies to minimize damage to cartilage. Alternatively, some drugs may provide beneficial effects to immobilized cartilage.

Nonsteroidal antiinflammatory drugs, such as aspirin, are commonly used in the management of OA. Aspirin suppresses PG synthesis in normal canine knee cartilage, as well as in early OA cartilage, such as that following CCL transection.[59,60] Aspirin may affect GAG synthesis by inhibiting uridine diphosphate-glucose dehydrogenase, an enzyme important in the synthesis of chondroitin sulfate.[60] Uptake of acetylsalicylic acid increases by 35% in osteoarthritic cartilage, suggesting that the drug permeates it more readily than in normal cartilage. The lower PG content of OA cartilage may be more important than fibrillation or surface disruption in rendering it vulnerable to aspirin.[61] In addition, aspirin suppresses GAG synthesis in unloaded cartilage to a much greater extent in vitro than it does in loaded cartilage.[62,63] Aspirin also markedly reduces prostaglandin E_2 synthesis by the cartilage, and drug concentrations in cartilage from loaded zones are lower than those in cartilage from unloaded sites.

Aspirin administration aggravates the changes that occur in cartilage during limb immobilization. In one study, a high dose of aspirin (40 mg/kg tid) was administered daily for 6 weeks while one hindlimb was immobilized in a cast.[64] While the cartilage of contralateral nonimmobilized limbs in dogs receiving aspirin had normal GAG content, the decreases in GAG content and net PG synthesis were significantly greater in immobilized stifles receiving aspirin as compared with immobilized stifles alone. Aspirin also apparently causes synthesis of type I rather than type II collagen by atrophic articular cartilage during immobilization.[65] Although these results indicate that aspirin has an adverse effect on articular cartilage of immobilized joints, aspirin administration did not preclude reversal of the above changes if the dog was allowed to walk freely for 3 weeks after cast removal.[64] However, if dogs ran daily on a treadmill for 3 weeks after cast removal, the decrease in GAG content of immobilized knees persisted and actually worsened in dogs receiving aspirin.

Treatment with corticosteroids may also have detrimental effects on normal cartilage and cartilage of immobilized limbs. Prednisone given to normal dogs with immobilized stifle joints results in a 58% loss of GAG content.[66] In nonimmobilized joints of dogs receiving prednisone, GAG content decreased 11% to 31%, compared with controls.

The use of HA in dogs may have some benefit to articular cartilage following immobilization. In one study, stifles were immobilized for 4 weeks using transarticular external skeletal fixation.[67] Treated dogs received HA. The PG content was reduced after immobilization in all dogs. Remobilization of the stifles was associated with damage to the surface and tangential layers of cartilage. However, remobilization with HA improved PG content and reduced structural damage. In another study, casts were placed on the hindlimbs of dogs for 92 days. Beginning on day 56, dogs received intraarticular injections of HA. Injections were repeated at 4-day intervals until the end of the study. Although femoral condylar articular cartilage had decreased PG content in all cast groups, the decrease was less in the HA-treated group. HA may inhibit inflammatory mediators, such as tumor necrosis factor-alpha and stromelysin.[68] Treatment with HA may not be as beneficial for treatment of OA, however. HA treatment of dogs in which a CCL was transected failed to prevent the progression of OA, and GAG content was 10% to 30% lower than in the contralateral stifle, compared with dogs receiving intraarticular injections of saline that had a 30% to 60% greater GAG content.[69]

Joint Capsule Changes

The functional and structural consequences of remobilization of the glenohumeral joint after 12 weeks of immobilization were studied in 10

Beagle dogs.[70] One forelimb was immobilized in a cast. The cast was removed and remobilization was allowed for 4, 8, and 12 weeks. After 12 weeks of immobilization, the passive range of motion was markedly impaired, intraarticular pressure was raised during movements, and the filling volume of the joint cavity was reduced. There was synovial lining hyperplasia and vascular proliferation in the wall of the joint capsule, but there was no increase of fibrous collagen in the capsular wall. Both the functional and structural changes were unaltered after 4 weeks of remobilization, but after 8 weeks they began to reverse, and they returned to normal levels after 12 weeks. Both functional and structural changes after 12 weeks of immobilization of the glenohumeral joint are reversible by remobilization. The collagen composition of the capsule seems unrelated to the degree of capsular contraction that occurs during 12 weeks of immobilization.

Similar changes were observed in the carpus and elbow in dogs in which the forelimb was immobilized for 16 weeks.[71] All dogs had a 20% to 30% decrease in range of motion in the elbow and carpal joints, which returned to normal within 6 weeks after remobilization. In addition, all dogs were significantly lame immediately following immobilization, but returned to soundness within 6 weeks after remobilization began.

Limbs casted for 32 weeks had severe joint stiffness and muscle atrophy, and recovery of normal limb use was delayed by several weeks.[72] Deficits were also present after only 12 weeks of immobilization, but full function resumed much sooner.

Muscle

Canine Muscle Fiber Types

Several types of muscle fibers exist, which perform somewhat specialized functions. Traditionally, they have been classified as two general types: type I (slow twitch) and type II (fast twitch) fibers. Type I fibers are more adapted for oxidative metabolism and functions, such as maintaining posture, whereas type II fibers are associated with glycolytic metabolism and the generation of power and speed during muscle contraction. Fiber types identified in immature and mature canine skeletal muscles include types I, IIA, and IIC, with the last representing less than 10% of the total fiber population.[73-75] Type IIC fibers

likely represent a transitional fiber between types I and II and are precursors to type IIA and IIB fibers in neonatal animals. Type IIA fibers have more oxidative capacity, but they still function in the generation of speed and power. Type IIB fibers have less oxidative capacity. The presence of true type IIB fibers has been debated in the dog, and type IIDog fibers, which are peculiar to the dog, have been suggested as a fiber type that is similar to, but does not correspond exactly with, classical type IIB fibers of other species.[75,76] The interpretation of fiber type composition depends on the staining and incubation methods used.[75] Type IIB or type IIDog fibers are not found in all muscles and were biologically significant only in the semitendinosus muscle in one study.[74] The metabolic potential of these fibers is fairly similar to that of IIA fibers, but significantly different from that of IIB fibers in other mammals, suggesting that they may be designed to play a different role during locomotion. All canine muscle fibers have an abundant capillary supply and moderate to high oxidative capacity, which may be related to the extraordinary athletic capability of dogs.

One study of the semitendinosus muscle found that hound-type dogs had the largest muscle fibers, but the fiber-type percentages were similar compared with mixed-breed and Beagle dogs with similar activity levels.[77] In general, there are no differences between the left and right limb muscles, but there may be significant differences in the percentages of muscle fiber types between individuals of the same breed for the same muscle.[78] Other studies have shown that Greyhounds have greater fiber size and a higher percentage of type II fibers than mixed-breed dogs, presumably because of the demand for intense physical activity.[79] However, there were no differences in fiber types in trained versus untrained Greyhounds, indicating that the distribution of fiber types may be more dependent on breed and genetics than level of training for this breed.

Different muscle groups have variable muscle-fiber type patterns that may be due to function and use.[74,80] In fact, muscle fiber type may change if muscle function is altered by transposing muscles. In one study, the fibularis longus tendon was severed and surgically transferred to the tendon of the cranial tibial muscle, a functionally different muscle. Later muscle biopsies demonstrated an increase in type I and type IIB fibers, which was similar to the fiber composition of the cranial tibial muscle. These findings indicate that muscle-fiber changes may occur and suggests that changes in muscle-fiber type are manifestations of functional adaptation.

Muscle biopsy technique may affect the results of muscle fiber typing.[78,81] For example, the percentage of type I fibers in the cranial tibial and semitendinosus muscles progressively increases from the superficial and middle regions to the deepest portion. Although the distance of the section from the origin of the muscle does not significantly affect the mean percentage of fiber types, the variation in fiber types varies less deeper within the muscle, so a needle biopsy taken from deep within muscle should provide a more consistent and reliable estimate of fiber type proportion than a superficial specimen.

Factors Affecting Muscle Contraction

SKELETAL MUSCLE BLOOD FLOW

The ability of muscles to contract is dependent on blood flow to the muscle. Small decreases in blood flow are associated with reduced contraction strength. When muscles contract, muscle blood flow typically increases, depending on the metabolic rate that is established by the contraction pattern and frequency. The ability of canine oxidative skeletal muscle to maintain developed isometric force is limited by blood flow.[82] This limitation implies a mismatching of blood flow and the metabolic rate. The blood flow past a muscle cell is determined by the number of capillaries per fiber, the vascular conductance, the capillaries perfused, and vascular autoregulation. The resulting mismatching of flow and metabolism accelerates the fatigue process.

The frequency of muscle contraction and tension development affect blood flow during muscle contractions.[83] The magnitude of the blood flow response to maximal exercise in different muscles is extremely varied. For example, in one study skeletal muscle blood flow increased progressively up to maximal oxygen uptake in the gracilis, semitendinosus, and semimembranosus muscles of dogs.[84] However, the blood flow response to maximal exercise leveled off during submaximal exercise in the gastrocnemius muscle. In addition, there are species differences in skeletal muscle blood flow.[85] Muscle blood flow can reach 300 to 400 ml/100 g of tissue/min in dogs, ponies, and rats, whereas it only reaches 75 ml/100 g

of tissue/min in a 75-kg man. The role of the diffusion gradient of oxygen from the blood to muscle cells is also important in exercising muscle.[86]

Muscle capillarity decreases in aged dogs.[87] Endurance training, however, enhances capillarity, and old rats and humans can attain levels of capillarity comparable to their active young counterparts, even when performing considerably less exercise.[88] In addition, there were no age-related effects on blood flow to the triceps, deltoideus, flexor carpi ulnaris, superficial digital flexor, gastrocnemius, gracilis, semimembranosus, and semitendinosus muscles of dogs during maximal exercise on a treadmill.[87]

SKELETAL MUSCLE OXIDATIVE CAPACITY

Oxygen uptake by the gastrocnemius muscle group of dogs appears to be linearly related to external work rate and to the load against which the muscles shorten.[89] The major contribution to oxygen uptake during contraction appears to be the number of contracting muscle fibers. Oxygen uptake of muscle also increases with stimulation frequency, reaching a peak at 5 twitches/second.[90] Further increases in stimulation frequency result in lower oxygen uptake, perhaps secondary to mechanical restraints imposed by contraction duty cycle and vascular compression. However, muscle contractions may have only a small direct effect on muscle blood flow. Their main effect may be to reduce venous pressures.[91] The limiting factors for skeletal muscle oxygen uptake vary according to the intensity of muscle contractions.[92] During transitions from rest to contractions of dog gastrocnemius muscles with 70% of peak oxygen uptake, oxygen delivery to muscle, intramuscular blood flow, and peripheral oxygen diffusion are not limiting factors for skeletal muscle oxygen uptake kinetics. Oxygen uptake may be mainly determined by intrinsic skeletal muscle oxidative metabolism.

Maximum oxygen uptake is limited by oxygen delivery as a result of a limited and uneven distribution of muscle blood flow. When oxygen delivery is reduced, hypoxia results in reduction of muscle performance. Endurance training results in an increased number of capillaries in muscle over time. Hypoxia enhances angiogenesis in canine skeletal muscle after endurance exercise, while lactic acid appears to inhibit vascular endothelial cells.[93] Increased oxygen delivery to muscle may decrease fatigue. Metabolic rates can be increased by increasing oxygen supply.[86] During high metabolic rate isotonic tetanic contractions, muscle fatigue was diminished by polycythemia, but the effect appears to be transient.[94] Norepinephrine can produce large increases in muscle recovery oxygen consumption, whereas beta-blockers, such as propranolol, reduce the rate of oxygen uptake during exercise and postexercise recovery.[95] Catecholamines may make a significant contribution to postexercise recovery oxygen consumption.

Oxidative capacity may decline in many muscles of sedentary individuals. Endurance training can greatly improve endurance in old age with an increase in muscle oxidative capacity.[88] With endurance training, old individuals may attain levels of muscle oxidative capacity similar to those in identically training young individuals.

SKELETAL MUSCLE CARBOHYDRATE METABOLISM

Muscle fatigue may be the result of several factors, with the relative contribution of each dependent on the condition and nature of the exercise, including the intensity, duration, muscle mass, and energy substrate. Fatigue may occur as the result of accumulation of hydrogen ions, inorganic phosphate, substrate depletion, and alterations in calcium ion function.[96] Adequate cellular oxygen content and maintenance of ATP levels are critical to avoid fatigue.

An increase in muscle oxidative capacity contributes to reduced glycogen depletion. Muscle glucose transport is enhanced after a bout of exercise, regardless of age.[88] Muscle glycogen depletion, creatine phosphate depletion, and lactate accumulation during contractile activity are exaggerated in older animals, apparently secondary to reduced muscle oxidative capacity and blood flow. Resting muscle glycogen concentration is diminished in older humans, probably in part because of a more sedentary lifestyle. Although several months of endurance training raises muscle glycogen concentration in older people, levels still remain below those of younger individuals.

Studies of the role of intracellular oxygen on the efflux of lactate from skeletal muscle during graded exercise from submaximal to maximal effort indicate that a constant intracellular oxygen content is unrelated to increasing lactate efflux.[86] Furthermore, muscle tension development is reduced by lactate.[96] This effect of the lactate ion appears to be independent of pH.

AGING

Muscle mass typically declines in old age, secondary to muscle fiber loss and atrophy.[88] The loss of strength in old age is predominantly accounted for by reduced muscle mass. Although there are no apparent effects of aging on muscle fiber type percentages in dogs, there is a 25% reduction of cross-sectional area of type II fibers in aged dogs.[87] The cross-sectional area of type I fibers is relatively unchanged, however, and may actually increase in some muscles. The mechanism for age-related atrophy is unknown, but may be related to a loss in the number of alpha motoneurons.[88]

HEART DISEASE AND SKELETAL MUSCLE

Patients with chronic heart failure may be limited by exertional fatigue. Changes in skeletal muscle may contribute to this fatigue, because biochemical and histologic abnormalities of skeletal muscle may develop in patients with chronic heart failure. Dogs with chronic heart failure have changes in skeletal muscle fiber type, fiber size, and fiber ultrastructural properties.[97,98] Skeletal muscle weights, muscle fiber area, and the percentage of skeletal muscle type I fibers may be reduced, whereas the percentage of skeletal muscle type II fibers may be increased with heart failure. There are apparently no differences in developed tension per gram muscle during stimulation, maximal developed tension, muscle fatigability, or preferential atrophy or hypertrophy of either muscle fiber type in skeletal muscle of dogs with heart failure. Although skeletal muscle atrophy occurs with heart failure, the remaining muscle appears to exhibit normal performance and metabolism. These changes may be the result of adaptations of skeletal muscle to anaerobic metabolism.

Response of Muscle to Disuse and Immobilization

The muscles that are most vulnerable to disuse atrophy are the postural muscles that contain a relatively large proportion of type I (slow twitch) muscle fibers and cross a single joint. Conversely, those that are least susceptible to atrophy are those that are not used as postural muscles (antagonist muscles), that cross multiple joints, and that are predominantly composed of type II (fast twitch) muscle fibers.[56,99] Immobilization reduces the chronic load on these muscles, which results in decreased cross-sectional diameter of the muscle and muscle fibers (Figure 7-4). Muscle strength decreases rapidly during the first week of immobilization, with further losses occurring more gradually over time.[100] Loss of muscle force production is not entirely explained by muscle atrophy. There may be up to a 50% reduction in peak force, even when the muscle mass has been normalized to constant muscle mass. This suggests that a cellular component may be involved, such as an alteration in sarcoplasmic reticulum function. In addition, there is decreased mitochondrial function and reduced protein synthesis. Interestingly, there is often an increase in capillary density and sometimes blood flow to muscles undergoing atrophy.[101,102]

Removal of weight-bearing activity has less impact on type II muscle fibers because these do not perform a major function in maintaining posture. In fact, with reduced stress, there may be an increase in type II muscle fibers.

This results in increased maximum muscle velocity, not only in type II muscle fibers, but also in type I muscle fibers. These changes help to attenuate a decline in power output as a result of atrophy. The length at which the muscle is immobilized also affects the degree of atrophy, with muscles immobilized in a shortened position atrophying to a greater degree, with reduced force-generating capacity and oxidative activity. When a muscle is immobilized in a shortened position, the number of sarcomeres decreases, leading to a reduced length of muscle fibers. If the muscle is immobilized in a stretched position, the fibers become lengthened because of addition of sarcomeres.[101] Connective tissue is increased in atrophic muscles, which may result in increased muscle stiffness.

Models of reduced limb usage include hindlimb immobilization (HI), hindlimb suspension (HS), denervation, and spaceflight. There is greater muscle atrophy with HS than with HI because HI muscles are able to contract against the immobilizing material. In contrast, HS muscles contract, but there is no load to contract against.

The change in muscle fiber size and fiber percentage was studied in three heads of the

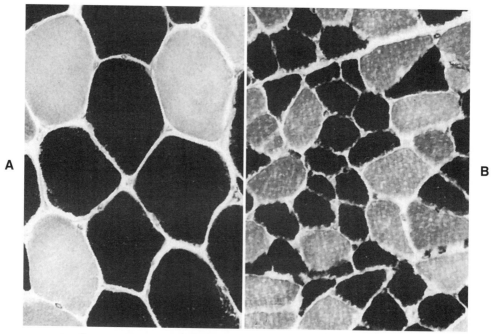

Figure 7-4   Photomicrographs of biceps femoris muscle. **A,** Normal muscle. **B,** Same muscle following 60 days of disuse. There is general atrophy of both types I (light stained) and II (dark stained) muscle fibers. (Figure 9-9 from Carlton WW, McGavin MD, *Thompson's special veterinary pathology*. St. Louis, 1995, Mosby.)

dog quadriceps following 10 weeks of rigid immobilization with an external skeletal fixator.[99] Muscle fiber atrophy was greatest in the vastus medialis and least in the rectus femoris. The atrophic response for type I fibers was, in order from most to least atrophied, vastus medialis, vastus lateralis, and rectus femoris; for type II fibers, atrophy of the vastus medialis was equal to vastus lateralis, and both atrophied more than the rectus femoris. In fact, vastus medialis type I and II muscle fiber areas were only about one-third normal following immobilization. Tetanic torque also declined by about 60%, and muscle fiber diameter correlated strongly with torque.[103] The rectus femoris acts as a knee extensor and hip flexor and crosses two joints, which makes it less susceptible to atrophic changes because the hip joint was not immobilized in this model. The changes in the vastus medialis suggest that this muscle performs a greater postural function than the vastus lateralis. A similar study with 10 weeks of immobilization indicated that there was a significant decrease in both type I and type II fiber area, and muscle fiber areas recovered to only about 70% of control values following 4 weeks of remobilization.[104] Tetanic torque improves during remobilization, but remains below preimmobilized levels.[103]

In general the muscles most vulnerable to immobilization-induced atrophy are those that cross a single joint and have a large proportion of type I muscle fibers, such as the vastus medialis and vastus intermedius.[99] The next most susceptible muscles are antigravity muscles that cross multiple joints and have primarily type I muscle fibers. Examples of these muscles are the gastrocnemius and rectus femoris muscles. Muscles least susceptible to atrophy following immobilization are those that are intermittently activated and have predominantly type II muscle fibers, including the cranial tibial, long digital extensor, and biceps femoris muscles.

Biochemical changes also occur in muscles with immobilization. The effect of immobilization on muscle carbohydrate metabolism was investigated in dogs.[105] Total carbohydrate and glycogen content of skeletal muscle fell during immobilization. The glycogen-degrading enzyme phosphorylase was activated 1 week after immobilization. Thereafter, enzyme activity decreased and remained significantly lower. In contrast, muscle glucose and lactate concentrations were unchanged. Oxidative and glycolytic enzyme activities

may be reduced and are associated with reduced capacity for energy production. Immobilization may also result in reduced glutathione content.[106] Reduced muscle activity may reduce the responsiveness of muscle to insulin, which affects the ability of muscle to take up glucose. There is also increased total muscle calcium concentration, decreased sarcoplasmic reticulum calcium uptake, and reduced Ca-ATPase activity following immobilization.

Protein and RNA synthesis also decrease with immobilization.[102] Quadriceps muscle protein turnover was assessed in men immediately after the end of 37 days of leg immobilization in a plaster cast after tibial fracture.[107] Quadriceps muscle protein synthetic rate was 0.046%/hr in the contralateral leg, but was only 0.034%/hr in the immobilized leg. Muscle RNA activity in the immobilized leg was 50% that of the nonimmobilized leg. Immobilization was associated with significant atrophy of type I muscle fibers, but no significant change occurred in type II fiber diameter. Mean quadriceps fiber volume was smaller in the injured leg by 10.6%, and the difference in muscle thigh volume was 8.3%.

Although it is believed that muscle atrophy occurs as a result of an imbalance of protein formation and degradation with the balance shifted to degradation, the exact mechanism is unknown. Recently, attention has focused on the role of the ubiquitin-proteasome pathway of intracellular protein degradation. It is believed that this system accounts for the majority of nonlysosomal protein degradation and is a complex multicomponent system that selectively targets proteins for destruction.[108] The pathway uses ubiquitin, a protein, which covalently binds to targeted proteins and acts as a destruction signal for the proteins. A number of conjugating enzymes are involved in this process. The ubiquitin-tagged proteins are then degraded by a large protease complex, the 26S proteosome. Studies of rats in a hindlimb suspension model have shown increased function of the ubiquitin-proteasome pathway, with increased ubiquitin mRNA levels, conjugating enzymes, and proteasome subunits, indicating the potential importance of this pathway of muscle degradation. Manipulation of this system of muscle degradation may alter the process of muscle atrophy and preserve muscle mass during periods of immobilization.

Muscle use and disuse apparently govern the number of acetylcholine receptors which are regulated through a feedback mechanism. Immobilization of skeletal muscle results in disuse atrophy and resistance to nondepolarizing muscle relaxants. Dogs undergoing cast immobilization of a hindlimb for 3 weeks had resistance to metocurine, a muscle relaxant, by the fourth day of casting.[109] This resistance persisted for 2 weeks after cast removal, but was normal 6 weeks after cast removal. These responses suggest that there may be up-regulation of muscle acetylcholine receptors as a result of immobilization.[110] These changes may also occur in patients in the intensive care unit that have muscle weakness. A canine intensive care model that involved 3 weeks of anesthesia with pentobarbital and positive-pressure ventilation indicated that the absence of muscle tone and reflex responsiveness for 3 weeks was also associated with exaggerated resistance to neuromuscular blockade.[111]

The blood supply to the myotendinous junction is also affected by immobilization. In one study of rats, the vascular density of the myotendinous junction was decreased by 30% after 3 weeks of immobilization.[112] Vascular density returned to normal after 8 weeks of cage remobilization. Progressively increasing running resulted in greater vascular density. The effects of immobilization on peak oxygen uptake and effective oxygen diffusive conductance in skeletal muscle were studied.[113] Dogs were cage confined for 8 weeks, with immobilization of a hindlimb for the last 3 weeks. Gastrocnemius muscles were electrically stimulated to elicit peak oxygen uptake at three levels of arterial oxygenation. Immobilization was sufficient to reduce muscle mass by 31% and citrate synthase activity by 68%; however, it had no effect on peak oxygen uptake or oxygen diffusive conductance.

Other species have similar changes in muscle with immobilization. Immobilization of a hindlimb of sheep for 9 weeks resulted in an 8% reduction in thigh circumference and a slight decrease in the area of type I fibers.[114] In addition, Na^+-K^+ pump concentration and citrate synthase activity were reduced, which may contribute to fatigue during activity. A modified rat tail suspension model, which allows the rear limbs to remain mobile without any weight-bearing, was used to determine the atrophic response of muscle with unloading.[115] Maximal muscle atrophy occurred within 14 to 30 days. The gastrocnemius was less severely affected by suspension than by other immobilization techniques, suggesting that muscle atrophy in the suspension model

is different from immobilization atrophy. One significant response was decreased blood flow, which may indicate that hypodynamic nonimmobilized muscle has altered functional demands. Similar changes occur in humans. Patients immobilized with a long leg cast after tibial fractures or ligamentous injuries had decreased limb circumference immediately after removal of the cast.[116] These differences persisted even after 81 days of remobilization.

Prolonged bedrest in people causes changes in muscle mass.[117] A period of 4 to 5 weeks of bedrest results in a 10% loss of muscle mass in the lower limbs of humans. Four months of bedrest results in 20% to 30% loss of muscle mass. Ten minutes of standing per day during bed rest attenuates muscle atrophy by 25% in people. If some resistance exercise is added, such as pulling a weight uphill, muscle atrophy is attenuated by up to 50%.

Spaceflight may also result in significant loss of muscle mass because of the loss of weight-bearing and loading.[117] MRI was used to obtain the muscle volumes of the calf, thigh, and lower back before and after an 8-day Space Shuttle mission. The soleus-gastrocnemius (−6.3%), anterior calf (−3.9%), hamstrings (−8.3%), quadriceps (−6.0%), and intrinsic back (−10.3%) muscles were decreased 24 hours after landing compared to baseline. After 2 weeks, the hamstrings and intrinsic lower back muscles were still below baseline.

Reflex inhibition of muscles, a situation in which sensory stimuli impede the voluntary activation of muscle, may occur with joint injury and result in muscle atrophy and in loss of strength and activation of the muscle. Reflex inhibition may be measured directly by electromyography, or the sequelae of reflex inhibition may be measured, such as thigh circumference measurement and muscle biopsy.[118] The most frequently cited causes of muscle reflex inhibition in joint injury are pain, joint effusion, and joint immobilization. Finally, there may be selectivity of affected muscles and muscle fibers with reflex inhibition following joint injury. In light of these findings, several suggestions have been offered for preventing reflex inhibition and that can be applied to rehabilitate the most affected muscle group, the quadriceps femoris. These include cryotherapy, transcutaneous electrical nerve stimulation, electromyo stimulation, traditional exercise training, joint mobilization, rest, and proper positioning of the limb in rest and exercise.

Neurogenic Muscle Atrophy

Muscles undergo denervation atrophy with damage to the spinal motoneurons or to the motor nerves in the ventral roots.[119] It has been well documented that there is an early rapid loss, followed by stabilization, of muscle mass with neurogenic muscle atrophy (Figure 7-5).[119,120] On the other hand, disuse atrophy occurs with damage to the central nervous system. Neural activity is generally reduced with spinal cord lesions, but varies with the type of lesion and the level of spasticity.

Structural and biochemical changes occur with neurogenic atrophy, including changes in glycolytic and oxidative metabolic enzymes. Functional recovery following nerve injury and repair is directly related to the degree of muscle atrophy that takes place during the period of nerve regeneration and the ability of surviving motoneurons to sprout and reinnervate the denervated muscle fibers.[119,121] For injuries with more than 15% of the motor supply to a partially denervated muscle intact, denervated muscle fibers are reinnervated and the partially denervated muscle recovers. Conversely, lesions with injury to more than 85% of the motoneurons result in inadequate sprouting and incomplete recovery. Motoneurons may increase the number of

muscle fibers that they normally supply by fivefold with sprouting. However, the distance over which sprouting occurs is limited, and with extensive denervation nerve sprouts may not grow far enough to reinnervate muscle. The extent of muscle atrophy is related to a number of factors including the distance through which the nerve must regenerate, the age of the patient, and the type of nerve injury and other associated tendon, soft tissue, and bony damage. In animals with spinal cord injuries, the capacity of paralyzed muscles to sustain contractions is reduced, therefore reducing muscle endurance. Adequate nursing care of paraplegic or tetraplegic animals is necessary to prevent muscle atrophy from disuse.[122] Secondary conditions, such as disuse osteoporosis of bones and contracture of joints, must also be considered in dealing with patients having neurogenic muscle atrophy.

Computed tomography was used to evaluate neurogenic muscle atrophy in dogs with induced sciatic nerve injury.[123] The cross-sectional area of muscles decreased 1 to 2 weeks after denervation, and the differences were significant after 3 weeks. Additional decreases were minimal after 28 days, after which time there was significant infiltration of adipose tissue into the muscle. The cross-sectional areas

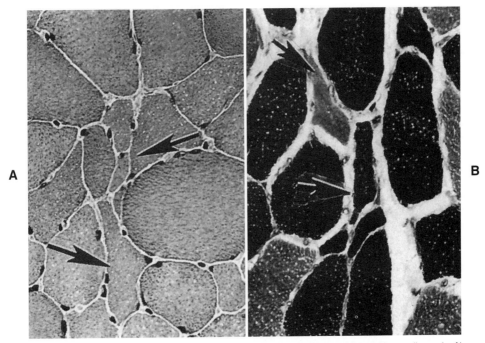

Figure 7-5 Neurogenic muscle atrophy. **A,** Early denervation atrophy, as indicated by small angular fibers (arrows). **B,** Atrophic angular fibers of both type I (light) and type II (dark) muscle fibers. (Figure 9-8 from Carlton WW, McGavin MD, *Thompson's special veterinary pathology.* St. Louis, 1995, Mosby.)

of the biceps femoris, semimembranosus, and semitendinosus muscles decreased by approximately 30% by 60 days, with most of the changes occurring in the first 2 to 3 weeks. In a study of denervated latissimus dorsi muscle, there was a 20% loss of lean muscle mass after 6 weeks, 45% loss at 6 months, and 55% loss at 9 months.[120] Histologically, there was atrophy of individual muscle fibers. With denervation atrophy, there is preferential atrophy of type II muscle fibers.[102]

Denervated dog gastrocnemius muscle has a progressive decrease in total protein content, alanine aminotransferase, aspartate aminotransferase, and glutamate dehydrogenase activity levels and elevation in free amino acid, ammonia, urea, glutamine contents, and AMP deaminase activity levels following neurectomy.[124] Total protein content decreased 50% by 4 weeks after muscle denervation. Catabolism of muscle protein may result in increased metabolites, including ammonia, urea, and glutamine.

Serum carbohydrate metabolism was evaluated in denervation atrophied and denervation electrical-stimulated dogs.[125] Neuromuscular electrical stimulation was applied to the gastrocnemius muscles of the latter group for 30 min/day for 15 days, using biphasic pulses of 10 V, 100 ms duration, and 2 Hz. Denervation atrophy may result in hyperglycemia possibly as a result of the lack of uptake by the muscle. Electrical stimulation applied to denervated muscle may reverse the hyperglycemia, indicating that muscular work may be important in modulating serum carbohydrate metabolism.

Continuous electrical stimulation of denervated muscles during the period of nerve regeneration appears to help maintain the integrity of the muscle fibers and their potential functional capacity.[121] In addition, electrical stimulation may be applied for extended periods with little evidence of discomfort. This modality may be useful in patients with the potential for partial or complete recovery from nerve injury.

Muscle Changes With Selected Orthopedic Conditions

HIP CONDITIONS

Hip conditions are common in dogs and may affect muscle mass. In some conditions, such as hip dysplasia, lameness and reluctance to exercise may result in pelvic limb muscle atrophy with compensatory shoulder muscle hypertrophy.[126] Excision of the femoral head and neck is sometimes performed as a treatment for severe hip dysplasia or fractures of the acetabulum. Although fewer dogs show lameness or pain in the operated hip after recovery from surgery, muscle atrophy is noted in approximately 50% of dogs following femoral head and neck excision, even after 8 years.[127] Moderate or marked muscle atrophy is most common in larger breeds of dogs. Difficulty in jumping and in climbing stairs may be noted postoperatively in larger breeds of dogs and may be related to the loss of power needed for jumping and hip extension following femoral head and neck excision. Legg-Calvé-Perthes disease, or aseptic necrosis of the femoral head, is a condition affecting small breeds of dogs that is also treated with a femoral head and neck excision. In a clinical study of dogs with avascular necrosis of the femoral head, muscle atrophy was present in 25 of 35 dogs at the time of diagnosis as a result of pain and lameness.[128]

CRANIAL CRUCIATE LIGAMENT INJURY

Changes in muscle mass are common in dogs with CCL rupture and following surgical treatment of the injury. In one study, dogs with CCL deficiency were examined before surgical treatment and 1.5, 7, and 13 months after surgery.[129] The degree of quadriceps muscle atrophy present before surgery correlated significantly with the degree of cartilage fibrillation, indicating a relationship with the severity of the condition. Although there was slightly greater muscle atrophy 6 weeks after surgery, muscle mass improved 7 and 13 months after surgery, but significant residual muscle atrophy remained in many dogs even after 1 year. A measure of quadriceps atrophy may be a useful tool for assessing long-term outcome.

Information regarding changes in specific muscles following CCL rupture and stifle stabilization surgery may be useful to target specific muscles for rehabilitation. Muscle atrophy was studied in a group of dogs undergoing surgical transection of a CCL and immediate stifle stabilization using a modified retinacular imbrication technique.[130] Thigh circumference and body composition measured by dual-energy X-ray analysis (DEXA) were used to estimate muscle mass before surgery, and 2, 5, and 10 weeks after surgery. Actual mass of rear limb muscles was determined at

10 weeks. Muscle mass decreased with transection of the CCL, despite immediate stifle stabilization (Figure 7-6). The changes were evident by 2 weeks and continued until 5 weeks, followed by a slight recovery at 10 weeks. The muscles most affected at 10 weeks were the quadriceps, biceps femoris, and semimembranosus, and these muscles weighed only 60% as much as the intact contralateral side (Figure 7-7). Similar changes were also seen in the muscles of the crus (Figure 7-8). Changes in thigh girth and DEXA lean tissue mass were similar over time and indicated significant muscle atrophy following cruciate transection and repair. The quadriceps and biceps femoris muscles are important in supporting weight during stance and should be targeted during rehabilitation to improve muscle mass and strength. The time course of changes suggests that postoperative physical rehabilitation should continue for at least 5 weeks after surgery.

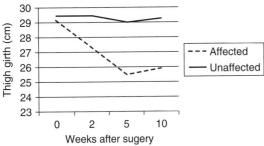

Figure 7-6 Rate of muscle atrophy in a limb with following cranial cruciate ligament transection and immediate stifle stabilization with no postoperative rehabilitation.

Girth measures are also commonly used in people to assess muscle atrophy following surgery for torn ACLs. Thigh and calf girth measurements of involved and noninvolved extremities were determined before and following knee surgery for acute and chronic knee injuries.[131] Although thigh and calf girth measurement differences existed between the involved and noninvolved extremities before and after surgery, the bulk of the girth measurement differences existed before surgery for both groups. The differences between involved and noninvolved limbs were in the 2% to 6% range, which were similar to differences observed in another study.[132] They concluded that altered gait and reflex inhibition contributed to muscle atrophy following injury and surgery. Muscular changes more than 5 years following ACL injury were evaluated to determine whether there were differences between patients with ACL reconstruction and conservative treatment.[133] Thigh circumference was measured, and the relationship of strength to electrical activity and muscle size was analyzed. Only minimal differences in thigh circumference were found between the uninjured and injured limb of both groups; however, isokinetic torque and EMG values showed significant differences. These changes may be due to modified use of muscle fibers and altered joint receptor afferent signaling following injury.

Normal quadriceps femoris strength may not be achieved in humans following ACL surgery despite aggressive rehabilitation. One study evaluated the correlation of thigh muscle size and strength with thigh circumference,

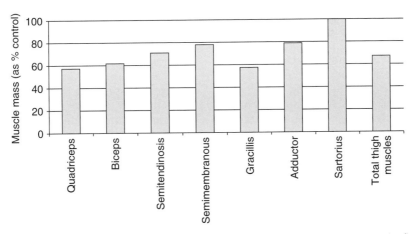

Figure 7-7 Mass of thigh muscles 10 weeks after cranial cruciate ligament transection and stifle stabilization with no rehabilitation. Values are percentage of the mass of the unaffected contralateral limb.

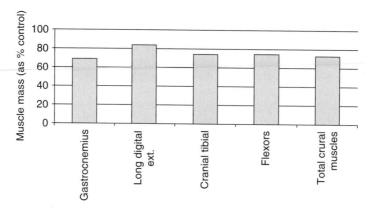

Figure 7-8   Mass of crus muscles 10 weeks after cranial cruciate ligament transection and stifle stabilization with no rehabilitation. Values are percentage of the mass of the unaffected contralateral limb.

muscle cross-sectional area by MRI, and isokinetic strength.[134] Patients were evaluated 48 months after surgery. There was a significant 1.8% decrease in thigh circumference, a 10% decrease in average quadriceps torque, and an 8.6% decrease in quadriceps cross-sectional area by MRI in the involved extremities compared with the uninvolved extremities. Persistent quadriceps weakness and decreased cross-sectional area 48 months after surgery and rehabilitation suggest that some patients may not completely recover from surgery, despite aggressive therapy. Strength deficits may persist for long periods, even with less severe injuries, such as partial tears of the medial collateral ligament (MCL).[135] Muscle atrophy that occurs following cruciate injury and surgery may result in early muscle fatigue, which also affects EMG patterns of quadriceps and hamstring muscles.[136] As little as 10 minutes walking may affect the gait pattern, particularly the activity of the hamstring muscles. This suggests that endurance training, in addition to strength and stabilization training, should be emphasized during rehabilitation.

Various specific techniques can be used for strengthening of the hamstring and quadriceps muscles in people following surgery for ACL repair, with or without resistive equipment.[137] In addition, electrical stimulation may help prevent muscle wasting due to immobilization. People are generally able to return to full activity and competitive sports after 6 to 12 months.

FRACTURES

Muscle atrophy may occur following fractures, particularly those with severe com-

minution. A stable repair with anatomic reduction is vital to encourage early weight-bearing, joint motion and use of the limb. Distal femoral fractures treated with limb immobilization in extension for 3 to 7 weeks resulted in limb hyperextension, generalized muscle atrophy, abducted gait, and limited range of joint motion.[138] Lesions found in muscle biopsies included fiber size variability, increased fibrosis, and focal necrosis. Histochemical and morphometric studies showed significant type I fiber atrophy in the vastus lateralis muscle, with a reduction of the number of type I fibers. Atrophic changes in the gastrocnemius and biceps femoris muscles were not significant. The atrophy seen in the vastus lateralis muscle may be a result of immobilizing the limb in extension, which results in shortening of this muscle group. Immobilization of a muscle in a shortened position results in preferential atrophy because of a reduced number of sarcomeres in series and reduced protein synthesis. In contrast, passive stretch of muscles in a lengthened state promotes muscle growth and may explain the relative sparing to the biceps femoris and gastrocnemius muscles.

A follow-up experimental study evaluated the effect of splinting in extension for 2 weeks after trauma to the distal portion of the quadriceps femoris muscle in dogs.[139] Flexion of the stifle joint was limited after splinting. A reversible type I fiber atrophy of the vastus lateralis, biceps femoris, and gastrocnemius muscles occurred. Early type II fiber atrophy was seen in a few muscles. Multifocal fiber necrosis was the only irreversible change seen. Relative fiber percentages did not change appreciably during splinting or recovery.[139]

ARTHRITIS

The relationship between arthritis and muscle mass is unknown in dogs, but we suspect that muscle mass and strength decline with the progression of osteoarthritis and the subsequent reduction in activity. In humans, the ratio of quadriceps to hamstrings muscle strength is important for knee stability and for protection from excessive stress.[140] People with knee OA have weak knee flexor and extensor strength, with relatively greater weakness in the quadriceps muscles. The mean quadriceps to hamstring strength ratio of 1.4 is below ratios reported for young healthy adults of 2.0. The low ratio might be explained by reflex inhibition due to pain associated with disease, because the quadriceps muscle can be selectively inhibited by pain and effusion in the joint leading to decreased production of muscle tension. In fact, joint enlargement had a negative correlation with the ratio of quadriceps to hamstring muscle strength in one study.[141]

The severity of the arthritis may also affect muscle mass. The strength and bulk of the quadriceps muscle of children with juvenile chronic arthritis was studied over a 2-year period.[142] Children with high OA severity scores had the least strength and muscle bulk. As the arthritis progressed and the severity score worsened, there was a corresponding reduction in muscle strength and bulk. The presence and intensity of local arthritis may be one important factor affecting muscle function in dogs with chronic arthritis.

Effects of Remobilization on Muscle

Fortunately, most of the changes that occur in skeletal muscle during immobilization are reversible. One rule of thumb regarding humans states that a remobilization period of twice the duration of the immobilization period is necessary for a return of limb circumference to normal values.[116] The effect of remobilization following splinting the stifle joint of young dogs with and without muscle injury was studied.[139] A rear limb was splinted in extension for 3 weeks and the biceps femoris, vastus lateralis, and gastrocnemius muscles were studied after splint removal and following 6 weeks of free activity. Despite a stifle range of motion of only 40 degrees immediately following splinting, after remobilization, range of motion and flexion were similar in all groups. A reversible type I fiber

atrophy occurred in most splinted muscles. Relative fiber percentages did not change appreciably during splinting or recovery. Beagle dogs undergoing HI by external fixation for 10 weeks had a 60% decline in tetanic torque, which improved somewhat during a 5-week remobilization period.[103] The diameters of type I and type II fibers measured from the vastus lateralis muscle followed the same trend.

Similar improvements occur with remobilization in humans and other animals. Changes in limb circumference and passive resistance of the human knee caused by immobilization were studied during remobilization.[116] Patients immobilized with a long leg cast after tibial fractures or ligamentous injuries were evaluated immediately after cast removal and after 18, 36, and 81 days of remobilization. Although improved, differences in mid-thigh circumference were still present after 81 days of remobilization. During remobilization, the increased resistance to flexion found immediately after removal of the cast resolved. This may indicate a rapid readaptation of muscle length (shortened due to immobilization in a shortened position) to almost normal values. After cast immobilization for 3 weeks, rat limbs were remobilized by free cage activity or treadmill running.[143] Typical changes of muscle atrophy occurred during the immobilization period. Remobilization, especially treadmill running, resulted in return of muscle toward normal, particularly the fiber size, capillary number, and fiber type distribution. Another study of the same model that compared low- and high-intensity treadmill training after immobilization found that high-intensity activity was more effective in restoring muscles to normal than was low-intensity exercise.[144] Sheep hindlimbs were immobilized in a plaster splint for 9 weeks, followed by remobilization for 9 weeks.[114] There was a slight decrease in type I fiber area at 9 weeks, and a slight increase at 18 weeks. The Na^+-K^+ pump density and citrate synthase activity were reduced by 39% and 30%, respectively, after 9 weeks of immobilization. During remobilization both increased to the same level as in the control animals.

Adaptations of Muscle to Increased Mechanical Stress

Mechanical stress may be induced by endurance training or strength training. Endurance training consists of repetitive, low-intensity contractions that result in changes in oxidative metabolism. Strength training is characterized by a limited number of contractions that occur against a high (often maximal) mechanical load.

ENDURANCE TRAINING

Endurance training does not affect muscle fiber number or cross-sectional area, but it alters metabolic responses. There is a twofold increase in oxidative capacity of all muscle fiber types with endurance training. There is an increase in muscle mitochondrial density, oxidative enzyme activity, muscle glycogen, and intracellular lipids.[145] Fatty acid use increases while reliance on carbohydrate metabolism is reduced. Muscles become more fatigue-resistant with training. Endurance training also elevates the antioxidant and detoxicant status of muscle.[106] For example, total glutathione, glutathione peroxidase, glutathione reductase, and gamma-glutamyl transpeptidase increased in the leg muscles of Beagle dogs treadmill trained for 40 km/day at 5.5 to 6.8 km/hr, 15% upgrade, 5 days/wk for 55 weeks.

Training also results in augmentation of muscle capillarity by new capillary formation, which may increase the available surface area for oxygen diffusion and decrease the distance over which oxygen must diffuse to reach cells.[113] Training also appears to improve the functional blood-tissue gas exchange properties of muscle. The effects of exercise training on peak oxygen uptake and effective oxygen diffusive conductance in skeletal muscle were investigated in dogs exercised on a treadmill 1 hr/day, 5 days/wk for 8 weeks.[113] Peak oxygen uptake by gastrocnemius muscles was 38%, 33%, and 19% greater and oxygen diffusive conductance was 71%, 75%, and 68% greater during normoxia, moderate hypoxia, and severe hypoxia, respectively, in exercised dogs as compared to controls.

Endurance training can induce changes in muscle fiber types. The alterations of muscle fiber type distribution initiated by long-distance running were studied in young dogs run on a treadmill for 55 weeks, 5 days/wk.[146] The daily running distance was gradually increased to 40 km and maintained at that level for the final 15 weeks. In the triceps brachii muscle, there was a shift from type II to type I fibers, which was also observed in the thoracic and cervical spinal muscles. In addition, there was also a shift toward a higher oxidative capacity of type II fibers. However, in the lumbar muscles, the percentage of type II muscle fibers increased significantly in the running group. Training can induce changes in fiber type composition not only in limb muscles but also in the stabilizing spinal muscles.

Although endurance training brings about changes in muscle metabolic properties, muscle mass may not be affected.[147] Young Beagle dogs trained on a treadmill for 1 year, gradually increasing running to 40 km/day at a speed of 5.5 to 6.8 km/hr with a 15-degree inclination during the last 15 weeks, while control dogs were kept in their cages. There was no difference in mass of cranial tibial and semitendinosus muscles between trained and control dogs.

STRENGTH TRAINING

Strength training uses brief, maximal contractions and requires a relatively high rate of anaerobic energy production. In addition to increased enzyme activity for glycolysis and glycogenolysis, there is an increase in muscle strength and size. Muscle fiber cross-sectional area is directly related to the tension the muscle is capable of exerting.[148] Strength training by overloading muscle increases the cross-sectional area of all fiber types, especially the fast-twitch fibers. New myofibrils are synthesized, and there may also be hyperplasia of muscle fibers. There is also improved synchronization of motor units.[145] This may help explain why the changes in muscle cross-sectional area are smaller than the changes in maximal voluntary force production.[149] Resistance training may especially result in increased cross-sectional area of type II fibers.[88]

The contraction time is increased with muscle hypertrophy because of the greater distance that must be traveled in the sarcoplasmic reticulum during contraction.[148] The increases in strength may not become apparent until the training program is well under way.[149] There is little effect on oxidative metabolism by muscle cells compared with endurance training. In fact, mitochondrial density may decline with strength training because of a dilutional effect by the larger quantity of myofibrils, although the absolute volume of mitochondria is unchanged.[149] In some instances, there may be a mild increase in oxidative capacity, suggested by the increase in type IIa muscle fibers with strength training seen in some studies.[150] In models of muscle hypertrophy, collagen content increases, with changes in collagen metabolism beginning as early as 3 days after increased loading.[56] Muscle fiber damage may also occur during vigorous strength training. Lactate accumulation in overworked muscles may contribute to increased collagen synthesis by stimulating proline hydroxylase. The increased collagen content may prevent skeletal muscles from contracting against excessive loads.

Compensatory hypertrophy of muscles may be induced by removal of one or more muscles of a synergistic group of muscles.[148] This results in overloading of the remaining muscle(s), with increased muscle weight and enlargement of remaining muscle fibers. In addition, there may be an increase in the number of fibers as a result of muscle fiber splitting. Weight training results in muscle fiber splitting of cats trained to lift weights.[148] The degree of fiber splitting is related to the intensity of exercise, and all muscle fiber types are affected.

Unfortunately, there is relatively little information regarding the effect of strength training on muscles in dogs, perhaps because of the difficulty in having them perform strength training activities. A study of cats trained to move a bar and lift weights for a food reward resulted in muscle hypertrophy of 7% to 34% after 40 weeks.[151] A variety of studies have evaluated strength training in humans. Men participating in an exercise program designed to strengthen the quadriceps muscles had increased thigh girth, and muscle strength increased 40% with training.[152] In addition, endurance and time to exhaustion while cycling and running increased, indicating some benefit to endurance exercise. The impact of adding heavy-resistance training to increase leg-muscle strength was further studied in humans undergoing endurance training.[153] After 10 weeks, leg strength increased an average of 30%, but thigh girth, muscle fiber areas, and oxidative activities were unchanged. Short-term endurance was increased by 12%. Exercise to exhaustion also increased after strength training, indicating that certain types of endurance performance, particularly those requiring fast-twitch fiber recruitment, can be improved by strength-training supplementation.

Muscle strengthening may occur, even in older individuals. For example, one study of geriatric men compared the training effects of voluntary isometric contraction on the quadriceps femoris to determine whether exercise changes age-related muscle weakness.[154] Maximal voluntary isometric contraction torque increased with even low training loads during 12 training sessions over 4 weeks. Altering dietary intake to achieve carbohydrate loading has been used to enhance muscle mass before competitions in humans, but one study indicated there was no advantage to carbohydrate loading to enhance muscle girth over weight-lifting alone.[155]

Although gender differences associated with strength training are unknown in dogs, female cats had greater muscle hypertrophy following weight training than male cats.[156] Gender differences also exist regarding skeletal muscle hypertrophy subsequent to heavy-resistance training in humans. Absolute changes in muscle mass are generally greater in males than females, but the percentage changes may not be significantly different.[157] For example, women completing a 20-week heavy-resistance weight training program for the lower extremity consisting of squats, vertical leg presses, leg extensions, and leg curls twice a week had a significant increase in maximal isotonic strength and hypertrophy of muscle fiber types I (15%), IIA (45%), and IIA + IIB (57%).[150] These data are similar to those in men and suggest that considerable hypertrophy of muscle fiber types occurs in women if exercise intensity and duration are sufficient.[155]

The Effects of Medications on Immobilized Muscles

STEROIDS

Naturally occurring or iatrogenic hyperadrenocorticism has been associated with myopathy in dogs.[158] Most dogs have muscle stiffness, proximal appendicular muscle enlargement, and myotonic discharges on electromyography. Muscle weakness and muscle atrophy may be present in some dogs. Histologic changes are characteristic of noninflammatory degenerative myopathy. Clinical signs of the myopathy may improve to varying degrees following treatment of hyperadrenocorticism. Steroids have a catabolic effect on muscle proteins, reduce protein synthesis, and alter the insulin responsiveness of muscle that is immobilized.[102] During treatment with corticosteroids or during catabolic conditions, glutamine synthetase increases and glutamine, the most abundant amino acid in muscle, is released at a high rate. On the other hand, endurance exercise reduces basal levels of glutamine synthetase.[159] In addition, treatment with cortico steroids results in increased susceptibility of type II fibers to atrophy, and type IIb fibers are more susceptible to atrophy than type IIa fibers.

Resistance exercise training may help attenuate the muscle loss associated with glucocorticoid administration by up to 40%.[159] Endurance training may also prevent glucocorticoid-induced muscle atrophy. Running attenuated muscle loss by 25% to 50% in rats receiving corticosteroids concurrently with the start of training. Prior endurance training does not appear to offer any advantage in preventing atrophy associated with corticosteroid administration compared with beginning training at the same time of steroid administration. Initiation of endurance exercise shortly after the onset of steroid treatment helps to prevent further muscle atrophy from that time on, but does not prevent the atrophy that has already occurred. Atrophy sparing seems to occur to a greater extent in muscle types that are highly recruited during endurance training.

Androgens and synthetic anabolic steroids have been recommended to help attenuate loss of muscle mass because of their ability to increase protein synthesis and promote muscle growth.[159] Although the effects of anabolic steroids on athletes and athletic performance are controversial, they do not appear to enhance aerobic metabolism. Anabolic steroids do seem to be beneficial in patients in negative nitrogen balance, such as those that are undernourished. The influence of oral anabolic steroids on body mass index (BMI), lean body mass, anthropometric measures, and functional exercise capacity among humans with chronic obstructive pulmonary disease was evaluated.[160] A group receiving testosterone and daily oral stanozol for 27 weeks had increased weight, whereas the control group lost weight. Lean body mass, BMI, arm muscle circumference, and thigh circumference increased in the treated group, but there were no changes in endurance exercise capacity. Anecdotally, there may be some benefit to administration of anabolic steroids to dogs with chronic medical conditions that may result in muscle atrophy.

ANTIINFLAMMATORY DRUGS

The exact role of nonsteroidal antiinflammatory drugs (NSAIDs) in the treatment of acute muscle injuries is unknown, but it has been suggested that these agents may be contraindicated, perhaps because NSAIDs delay muscle regeneration following injury. The effects of two different NSAIDs and physiotherapy modalities on the healing of acute hamstring muscle tears of humans were studied.[161] Patients received meclofenamate, diclofenac, or a placebo. All patients received the same intensive physical therapy, including rest, ice, compression, elevation, therapeutic ultrasound, deep transverse friction massage, stretching, and exercise over a 7-day treatment period. Pain, swelling at the site of the muscle tear, and isokinetic muscle strength were improved in all groups, but there was no difference among groups. In fact, the pain score of the more severe injuries was significantly lower in the physiotherapy group than in those receiving NSAIDs and physiotherapy at day 7. Therefore there may not be an additive effect on the healing of acute muscle injuries when NSAIDs are added to standard physiotherapeutic modalities.

GROWTH HORMONE

Growth hormone (GH) may attenuate muscle atrophy as a result of immobilization or denervation.[102] The actions of GH are mediated by complex interactions among several hormones, receptors, and binding proteins.[162] One of the primary effects of GH is the production of insulin-like growth factor-I (IGF-I) by the liver, which in turn also affects muscle tissue. GH results in stimulation of protein synthesis. In addition, amino acid and glucose uptake are increased, and lipolysis is increased. Treatment with GH results in an increase in lean body mass in humans and rats, although strength is probably not improved. IGF-I may be a mediator of the response of GH because it also results in increased amino acid uptake and protein synthesis.[163] IGF-I stimulates muscle satellite cells to enter the cell cycle and proliferate, with some differentiating and fusing with myofibers. However, most studies indicate that IGF-I has minimal effect on the adaptation of muscle to changes in loading. The GH response to acute aerobic exercise may be augmented with repeated bouts of exercise.[164] During prolonged administration, resistance to the anabolic effects of GH may occur.

Administration of GH during periods of non–weight-bearing activity may not result in maintenance of muscle mass.[130,162] However, treatment during recovery may be beneficial. Beagle dogs receiving a GH secretagogue during a 10-week immobilization and 5-week remobilization period had a 60% decrease in tetanic torque during immobilization, which was similar to that in untreated dogs, but had a threefold increase in tetanic torque in the treated group compared to controls during remobilization.[103] The diameters of type I and type II fibers measured from the vastus lateralis muscle followed the same trend. These data suggest that the GH secretagogue increased the size and strength of the quadriceps muscle during remobilization. GH may also attenuate the catabolic effects of corticosteroid treatment on muscle mass.[162]

Ligaments and Tendons

Ligament and Tendon Structure and Biomechanics

Ligaments and tendons consist primarily of type I collagen that forms parallel fibers. Ligaments extend between bones to stabilize joints, while tendons permit movement of bones by connecting muscles to bones.[56] Both are relatively pliant and flexible to allow natural movements of bone to which they attach. They are also strong and relatively inextensible to offer resistance to applied forces, especially tensile forces. Ligament and tendon structure and chemical composition are very similar in humans and many animal species, including rats, rabbits, dogs, and monkeys. They are composed of dense connective tissue with primarily parallel fibers of collagen, with a small number of collagen fibers that run perpendicular to the predominant direction of stress. Cross-links that form between collagen chains are important to collagen tensile strength and resistance to proteases.[165] Reducible cross-links are found in newly formed collagen, whereas nonreducible cross-links are found in mature collagen and account for stronger and stiffer collagen. The concentration of cross-links and their ratio varies between species and location. For example, the rabbit CCL has 3 to 5 times more nonreducible cross-links than the patellar tendon.[165] Ligaments also have more cells per mass than tendons.

Most ligaments do not function as a unit structure because at a particular joint position, one portion of a ligament may be taut while another part is relaxed.[166] This is relevant because certain joint positions may need to be avoided to reduce stress on healing ligaments. Ligament insertions may be direct or indi-

rect.[166] With a direct insertion, collagen fibrils course directly into the bone, with some fibers blending with the periosteum. In contrast, indirect insertions have a zone of fibrocartilage and mineralized fibrocartilage between the ligament and cortical bone. These zones are important when considering ligament insertions and their responses to stress and rehabilitation from injury.

The biomechanical responses of ligaments and tendons are nonlinear because of progressive fiber recruitment and viscoelastic properties. The structural properties of the entire bone-ligament-bone complex that must be considered are dependent on the mechanical properties of the ligament, macroscopic and microscopic ligament geometry, the cross-sectional area and length of the ligament, and the material properties of the fibrous and ground substance constituents.

When initially loaded, ligaments and tendons stretch with a slight increase in load. Histologically, the fibers change from a relaxed wavy appearance to a parallel alignment as the fibers become oriented in the direction of loading. This region on a load-deformation curve is known as the toe region (Figure 7-9). As the load is increased, the curve becomes more linear, corresponding to full orientation of the fibers. The linear portion of the curve also indicates elastic deformation, with return to normal structure when the load is released. If loading continues, the load-deformation curve exits the linear region and

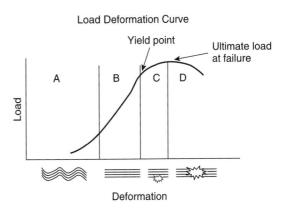

Figure 7-9 Load-deformation curve of ligament biomechanical testing. *A,* Toe region. Note the bottom portion of the diagram indicating the wavy appearance of the collagen fibers. *B,* Linear physiologic loading and zone of elastic deformation. The collagen fibers become taut. *C,* Early permanent damage and zone of plastic deformation. There is damage to some of the fibers. *D,* Ultimate load at failure. There is gross disruption of the ligament.

enters the region of plastic deformation. This point is termed the yield point. Histologically, some microfailure may occur even before the yield point is reached, resulting in damage to the ligament or tendon. After the yield point is reached, gross failure of the ligament occurs, and permanent structural damage takes place and remains even if the load is released. When the ligament or tendon fails and can support only a negligible load, the ultimate failure point has been reached. It is important to note that the ligament may retain continuity despite micro- and macro-failure.

The mechanical properties of ligaments and tendons are a reflection of their material characteristics and allow for uniform comparison between other ligaments and tendons. They also reflect the orientation and organization of the collagen fibers. High strain-rate techniques for studying knee ligament failure in people have replaced the previous low strain-rate methods and distinguish the failure mechanism of ligaments from that of bone. For example, anterior cruciate bone-ligament-bone preparations of primates failed at a higher load and absorbed more energy at a faster rate of deformation than at a slower rate.[167] Specimens failed by ligament disruption at faster rates, and by tibial avulsion fractures at slower rates. Ligament function is further defined by measuring the restraining force provided by specific ligaments. Advances in analytical techniques and models permit precise analysis of joint position, motion, and laxity.[167] Recent studies have indicated that, in addition to tendon and ligament support, neuromuscular reflexes may play a large role in joint stability.[166] Impulses from mechanoreceptors in the joint capsule, menisci, and ligaments transmitted to the spinal cord result in instantaneous reflex regulation of muscles acting on a joint to provide coordinated joint function and stability. Canine lateral collateral ligaments have nerve fibers and Golgi-Mazzoni and Ruffini corpuscles, some of which resemble Golgi tendon organs.[169] Mechanoreceptors are more numerous at the ends than in the middle of ligaments; they are present in both the subsynovial and the interfascicular connective tissue and are surrounded by vessel networks. The number of corpuscles may be related to the type of stress to which a ligament is subjected. ACL-deficient humans have disruption of an ACL-hamstring rapid reflex arc that normally helps to limit anterior motion of the tibia.[166] Instead, a slower reflex originating from the knee joint

capsule limits anterior tibial motion. Rehabilitation techniques to help restore ligament-muscle reflexes should be considered.

Knowledge of the blood supply to ligaments and tendons is necessary to understand how healing and the rehabilitation program may be affected. Blood flow to the proximal, middle, and distal parts of the CCL were 3.0, 2.2, and 3.5 ml per 100 g of tissue per minute, respectively, in one study.[170] The respective values in the caudal cruciate ligament were 2.8, 2.8, and 3.2 ml per 100 g of tissue per minute. The cruciate ligaments are relatively hypovascular, with blood flow only 50% of that of the synovium of the suprapatellar pouch.[171] Application of a cranial stress diminishes the blood flow to the ligament to one fifth of the baseline value, an effect that is reversible. Division of the infrapatellar fat pad causes a twofold decrease in perfusion to the ligament, whereas dissection of the enveloping synovium results in a complete cessation of blood flow.

Many factors affect the ligament-bone unit response. Increasing age weakens the tissue-bone preparation.[172] Tendons also respond biochemically to the stresses placed on them.[39] In compression regions of rabbit tendons, the GAG content is 15 times greater than in tension-transmitting regions. Dermatan sulfate predominates in regions of tension, whereas chondroitin sulfate is the major GAG in regions of compression. The relative GAG content changes with alterations in the stresses placed on tendons induced by transposing the tendon, and the content reverts back to normal when the tendon is replaced to its original position. Other factors affecting tendons and ligaments include the amount of activity the animal undergoes and medications the patient may receive.

Response of Ligaments and Tendons to Disuse and Immobilization

Immobilization is commonly used to treat injuries to ligaments and tendons. There are many models of ligament and tendon disuse, including internal and external fixation methods, casts and slings, denervation, disarticulation, and bed rest. These models have allowed the study of histologic, biochemical, and biomechanical changes that occur with disuse. There is an adverse decline in structural and material properties of ligaments and tendons with immobilization of the joints that they cross. The bone-tendon/bone-ligament complex is especially affected by immobilization. The effects of stress deprivation appear to be time and dose dependent, and differences may exist in the responses of various ligaments and tendons within the same animal because of differences in cellular, structural, and biochemical properties. For example, the CCL may be more resistant to stress deprivation than the MCL.[173,174] Typically, there is reduction of cross-sectional area, disorganization of the parallel structure of fibrils and cells, increased collagen turnover with increased collagen synthesis and degradation, a net decrease in collagen mass, and reduced GAG, HA, chondroitin sulfate, dermatan sulfate, and water content.[173] Remobilization returns the mechanical properties to nearly normal over time, but the recovery of the bony insertion sites is prolonged compared with the ligament/tendon midsubstance. Knowledge of the detrimental effects of immobilization may influence the management of ligament and tendon injuries.

It is well recognized that a reduction of activity, such as confinement to a cage, may affect ligament and tendon properties.[174] A study of related rhesus monkeys showed a 0.2% loss in CCL strength and energy to failure per week of captivity.[175] More profound effects may be expected with complete immobilization of a limb. In a classic study, the effect of body cast immobilization on the biomechanical properties of bone-CCL-bone units of rhesus monkeys was studied.[176] After 8 weeks of total-body plaster immobilization, there were significant decreases in maximum failure load and energy absorbed to failure (39% and 32%, respectively). There was also a 69% decrease in ligament stiffness. These changes likely indicate an alteration in the functional capacity of the ligament to resist loading and elongation, factors that relate to the ligament's ability to provide joint stability. The immobilized ligament units frequently failed by avulsion fractures of the bone, which correlated with bone resorption in the cortex immediately beneath the ligament insertion site. The effect of immobility on ligaments of the knee depends, in part, on the histologic characteristics of the ligament-bone attachment. The ligament-bone junctions with zones of fibrocartilage were little affected. In contrast, the MCL, which inserts directly into the tibia and periosteum without well-defined zones of cartilage, showed marked interruption after immobility due to bone resorption in the sub-

periosteal and outer cortical regions. In some places the ligament was attached only to the overlying periosteum. After 5 months of remobilization following total body immobilization, there was only partial recovery in ligament strength, although ligament stiffness and compliance parameters returned to control values. As much as 12 months was required for nearly complete recovery of ligament strength.

Similar effects of immobilization have been noted on canine ligaments. The effect of immobilization on the CCL of dogs was studied using a model of internal skeletal fixation for 12 weeks.[28] Failure of the femur-ligament-tibia complex occurred through the tibial insertion of the ligament for both experimental and control limbs. The load at failure and stiffness were 45% and 73%, respectively, of the nonimmobilized CCLs. Even though there was a 13% reduction in soft tissue mass, the loss of collagen was greater in the tibia and femur than in the CCL and correlated with mechanical failure at the bony insertion. Bone atrophy was the result of increased resorption of bone rather than decreased bone formation. This study demonstrated that there was significant atrophy of the CCL and bone in immobilized joints of dogs.

Other studies have confirmed the importance of bone resorption and the reduction of bone collagen due to disuse and its relationship to strength of the medial collateral and CCL complexes.[174,177] In canine stifles immobilized in a cast for up to 12 weeks, changes in the tibial insertion of the ligament were apparent, including the presence of many osteoclasts, numerous large fibroblasts, replacement of bone by loosely arranged fibrous tissue, and attachment of the ligament to periosteum only.[174] Interestingly, in this study the femoral attachments of the medial and lateral collateral ligaments and the origin and insertion sites of the CCLs showed little bone resorption, indicating that the response to immobilization may be site-specific. Even so, MCL strength decreased 40% following 6 weeks of immobilization.[178] Restriction of activity to cage confinement also causes significant bone atrophy of the tibial insertion sites of the collateral ligaments if adequate activity is not allowed. Additionally, there is decreased thickness of ligament and tendon fiber bundles, greater extensibility per unit load, and unchanged collagen content after immobilization.

Whereas stress deprivation with immobilization appears to reduce the mechanical properties of ligaments and tendons in a time- and dose-dependent manner, stress deprivation with continued mobility may have different effects. Maintaining joint motion and reducing the period of immobilization may help preserve ligament properties. The effects of stress deprivation with joint motion on the CCL were studied in dogs by freeing the tibial insertion of the ligament, moving it caudally, and securing it with a screw.[179] Stifle joints were allowed complete mobility. The cross-sectional area of the ligament was 115% larger than controls at 6 weeks. The tensile strength was unchanged at 6 weeks, but was only 67% of control values at 12 weeks. This model of stress deprivation with continued joint motion on the CCL suggests that there may be an increase in ligament cross-sectional area and a concurrent decrease in biomechanical properties after a period of time.[173] Other models of stress deprivation with joint motion for relatively short periods have shown different results. The effect of active joint motion on ligament and meniscus mass in a non–weight-bearing model of disuse was studied. A unilateral ankle disarticulation model of disuse that maintained active knee motion without weight-bearing for 8 weeks was studied in dogs.[29] A large and similar loss of collagen and calcium mass occurred in the femur and tibia, indicating bone resorption and little replacement with new bone. No loss of tissue mass occurred for the collateral and cruciate ligaments or menisci. The strength of the femur-CCL-tibia complex was not qualitatively or quantitatively different between control and experimental limbs. So although immobilization for greater than 8 weeks results in atrophy of bone, ligament, tendon, and meniscus in some canine studies, the absence of weight bearing for 6 to 8 weeks with maintenance of joint motion appears to help preserve femur-ligament-tibia complex mechanical strength, despite the occurrence of bone atrophy.

The effects of immobilization on the biomechanical and morphological properties of the femur-MCL-tibia (FMT) complex and its components have also been investigated in rabbits.[180] After 9 weeks of immobilization, stiffness was significantly reduced, the ultimate load to failure and energy-absorbing capacity were reduced by 69% and 82%, respectively, and an increased number of failures occurred by tibial avulsion. Histologically, the femoral and tibial insertion sites showed increased osteoclastic activity, resorption of bone, and disruption of the normal attachment of the bone to the ligament. The cross-sectional area of the CCL also decreased with immobilization of the stifle joint.[181] Diminished stress also results in increased collagen turnover, with formation of immature collagen.[166]

There is a dose-dependent effect of stress shielding on the mechanical properties of rabbit patellar tendons.[173] In addition to decreased ultimate stress of tendons with stress shielding, there is a significant increase in the cross-sectional area of tendons, despite fewer numbers of collagen fibrils per unit area. Although there is significant loss of ultimate stress on tendons after 1 to 3 weeks, applying tension for 3 to 12 weeks results in significant gains in biomechanical properties, but they are not completely recovered by this time.[173]

As the above studies have indicated, ligaments and tendons are not metabolically inert structures, although their oxygen consumption is approximately 10 times lower than liver tissue and 7.5 times less than skeletal muscles. Immobilization of rat limbs causes an additional 36% reduction in oxygen consumption and decreased aerobic enzyme activity, suggesting that the metabolic activity of ligaments and tendons is lowered with decreased levels of physical activity.[182]

Effects of Remobilization on Ligaments and Tendons

Although the mechanical properties of immobilized ligaments return to normal relatively quickly,[173] the load to failure of the bone-ligament-bone complex lags behind, indicating that there is asynchronous healing of the bone-ligament-bone complex. After 6 weeks of immobilization of the lower limbs of dogs, 18 weeks of remobilization was necessary for return of the normal structural properties of the FMT complex.[174] In fact, as much as 1 year of remobilization may be required for normalization of the ligament-tibia complex in some instances, while the mechanical properties of the ligament return to normal in a relatively short period of time, as newly synthesized collagen fibers gradually mature and strengthen with subsequent stress resumption.

In the study of immobilized stifles of rhesus monkeys, 5 or 12 months of remobilization was allowed after casting for 8 weeks.[176] Following 5 months of rehabilitation, there was still a 20% deficit in load to failure and energy stored at failure, but only a 7% deficit in stiffness. After 12 months of rehabilitation, there was only a 9% deficit in load to failure and an 8% deficit in energy stored to failure.

The effects of remobilization following 9 weeks of immobilization were studied in the rabbit FMT complex.[180] With 9 weeks of remobilization, the ultimate load and energy-absorbing capabilities of the bone-ligament complex improved to about 80% of normal. One year was required to recover the functional properties following 12 weeks of immobilization. Failure by tibial avulsion became less frequent, and the stress-strain characteristics of the MCL returned to normal. Histologically, the sites of insertion of the ligament also showed evidence of recovery.

Postoperative Healing of Tendons and Ligaments With Motion

The function of tendons and ligaments is to transmit tensile forces. Early studies suggested that healing ligaments should be immobilized for proper healing. Immobilization of surgically repaired tendons or ligaments for 6 weeks results in a wound with approximately 50% the normal tensile strength for tendons and ligaments.[183] Recently, it has been suggested that early, controlled mobilization of healing tendon and ligament repairs may be beneficial. Earlier tension across a ligament or tendon wound orients the healing fibers and results in stronger healing. For example, MCLs of canine stifles sutured with polyester suture in a locking loop pattern and immobilized for 3 weeks, followed by active motion, resulted in valgus-varus laxity of 150% and ultimate strength of 92% compared with intact controls. In comparison, 6 weeks of immobilization resulted in valgus-varus laxity of 300% and only 14% of the ultimate strength of controls. Repaired canine tendons immobilized for 3 to 6 weeks after surgery also apparently have sufficient strength to allow protected active motion. Current knowledge of healing tendons and ligaments suggests that postoperative immobilization for 3 weeks will allow acceptable return to function while minimizing the risk of damage if appropriate suturing techniques are used. The immobilization splint should be designed to allow some active motion of the joints, but should limit the amount of weight-bearing.[184] After immobilization devices are removed, the amount and type of exercise allowed should be severely limited and increased gradually

over time. By 6 weeks after repair, tendons have approximately 50% of tensile strength as compared to normal. It is believed that tendons need only 25% to 33% of their strength to withstand the forces of normal physiologic muscle contractions, indicating that some light activity should not be detrimental to healing.[183]

MEDIAL COLLATERAL LIGAMENT

Several studies have evaluated early mobilization following injury to the MCL. Injury to the MCL was induced by making incisions through the superficial and deep portions of the ligament, and then repair was performed by suturing the incision.[178] Ligaments that were not immobilized during the 6-week healing period were stronger than those that were immobilized with a cast, suggesting that ligament strength is sensitive to physical activity. The effects of early mobilization and exercise on healing of injured MCL were further studied.[185-187] Transected canine MCLs were subjected to one of the following: no surgical repair with 6 weeks of mobilization; surgical repair with 3 weeks immobilization at 90 degrees followed by 3 weeks remobilization; or surgical repair with 6 weeks of immobilization. Knees were tested in tension to determine the structural properties of the FMT complex and the mechanical properties of the healing MCL. Laxity increased in all knees, but early mobilization resulted in the best joint stability. The structural properties of the FMT complex and the MCL substance were also improved in the early mobilization groups. Stiffness of the MCL in early mobilization groups was about 60% of controls, whereas stiffness of prolonged immobilization stifles was only 36% of that of control stifles. The load at failure of the FMT complex was approximately 40% and 20% of normal stifles in early mobilized versus immobilized stifles, respectively. Similarly, the tensile strength of the MCL was approximately four times greater in stifles that underwent early mobilization, but values of immobilized limbs were only 20% of normal stifles. These studies indicate that early mobilization (less than 3 weeks of immobilization) is the treatment of choice in cases with isolated MCL injuries. It is important to realize that an intact CCL provides significant stability to the stifle joint and allows the MCL to heal. If the CCL is intact, implementation of early motion is recommended.

Injuries to multiple stifle ligaments, however, may affect healing of the MCL. Although the previous studies have suggested that with normal stifle motion, the functional deficit of the MCL in valgus rotation is compensated for by the remaining structures, especially the CCL, MCL strength was just 14% of normal after 14 weeks of healing when both ligaments were transected, compared to transection of the MCL alone, which were 52% of controls.[188] There were also marked arthritic changes in the joint when both ligaments were transected.

Lateral collateral ligament healing is similar to healing of the MCL.[166] Repaired ligaments heal faster with more organized tissue than nonrepaired ligaments, but both are still weaker than control ligaments after 10 weeks of healing.[189]

CRANIAL CRUCIATE LIGAMENT

Transected ends of the CCL retract and do not join together, as other ligaments may do. Repair of transected ligaments results in resorption of 40% of the ligament 24 months after repair, and weakness persists after 4 years of healing.[190] The CCL is not normally in contact with synovial fluid because of an overlying synovial membrane. However, when the ligament is damaged, synovial fluid may bathe the damaged ligament, which may inhibit healing because of the inhibitory effects of synovial fluid on fibroblast proliferation.[166] In addition, there are increased levels of collagenase with cruciate ligament and meniscal injuries. A study of experimentally created CCL and MCL transection indicated that postoperative immobilization for 6 weeks resulted in greater arthritic changes in articular cartilage than in dogs undergoing early stifle mobilization.[191]

Human patients undergoing rehabilitation consisting of immediate knee motion and early weight-bearing do not have an increased incidence of abnormal knee displacement in the early phases after undergoing bone–patellar tendon–bone allograft or iliotibial band extraarticular stabilization of ACL injuries.[192] Although similar studies have not been conducted in dogs, our clinical impression is that there is not an increased incidence of stifle instability in dogs undergoing rehabilitation, and in fact, there may be less displacement because of the additional stability afforded by greater muscle mass of patients undergoing rehabilitation.

FLEXOR TENDONS

Immediate immobilization of flexor tendons following repair results in diminished ultimate tensile strength in the early postoperative period. Using an early passive motion protocol, ultimate tensile strength and ultimate load are increased two to three times more than if the limb is immobilized.[193] In addition, joint motion is significantly greater than if the joints are immobilized. Early protected passive motion augments biomechanical properties and excursion of healing flexor tendons. These results were confirmed in another study that compared different suturing techniques in dogs undergoing early mobilization following repair of lacerated deep digital flexor tendons. The mechanical and histologic healing of tendon repairs using early active motion was evaluated with three flexor tendon repair techniques.[184] Healing tendons were evaluated 5, 10, and 21 days after surgery. Adhesions occurred in 15% of the dorsal tendon splint repairs. Smooth tendon gliding was obtained in the other specimens in which repair was successful. Histologically, there was evidence of progressive healing without surrounding adhesions in repaired tendons. Improved suture techniques have the potential to withstand the stress produced by active digital motion protocols. Immobilization may also result in adhesion formation, reducing the excursion of healing tendons and reduced range of motion. In one study, 10 minutes of daily passive motion, with 1.5 to 1.7 mm of tendon excursion, prevented adhesions in a sharp transection model of the deep digital flexor tendon.[194,195] Doubling the excursion resulted in no additional improvement. Therefore, less aggressive passive motion exercises may be sufficient to prevent adhesion formation. In fact, overly aggressive range-of-motion rehabilitation may be deleterious. Tendons undergoing excessive motion with formation of a large gap between tendon ends are at risk for rupture during early healing.[196] Increased frequency of passive motion also has beneficial effects. In one study of healing canine digital flexor tendons, passive motion at a rate of 12 cycles/min for 5 min daily resulted in similar gliding function with significantly greater tensile properties than dogs receiving 1 cycle/min for 60 min.[197] Repair of tendons should occur within 7 days for optimum restoration of gliding function.[198] Although repair of tendons as long as 21 days after injury results in strength and stiffness similar to those of tendons undergoing immediate repair, there is significant loss of gliding function with delayed repair.

Rehabilitation of partial flexor tendon lacerations may be different than for complete lacerations. In one study of partial lacerations of the deep digital flexor tendon, dogs not undergoing surgical repair had higher ultimate loads and stiffness than repair groups.[199] In addition, passive rehabilitation of nonrepaired tendons resulted in less gap formation than unrestricted active mobilization of repaired tendons.

Retaining vascularity does not seem to prevent significant reduction in tendon properties that occurs postoperatively, nor does it accelerate the return in strength and stiffness.[200] The medial half of the patellar tendon was placed as a vascularized graft to replace the ACL on one side and as a nonvascularized graft on the other in monkeys. Grafts had only 57% of control ACL stiffness and 39% of control maximum force by 1 year. Elastic modulus and maximum stress also increased over time, but at 1 year were only 34% and 26% of normal values, respectively.

Adaptations of Ligaments and Tendons to Increased Stress

Much like Wolff's law for bone, ligaments also adapt to applied stress and motion. Ligaments are morphologically, biomechanically, and biochemically sensitive to stress deprivation as well as stress enhancement. Although testing procedures vary among studies, most have consistently demonstrated that training increases the strength of ligaments and tendons. Compared to other tissues, such as muscle, the metabolic activity of ligaments and tendons is lower, probably because of poorer vascularity and circulation.[201] The responses of ligaments and tendons to increased training stresses are therefore slower than in muscles. It is also important to consider the conditions under which laboratory animals are housed when interpreting the results of experimental studies because ligaments and tendons are very sensitive to stress deprivation, and limiting normal activity with cage confinement may affect strength of these tissues.[202]

Ligaments retain 80% to 90% of their baseline mechanical properties with minimal stimulation. The effects of exercise on ligaments and tendons are less profound than the effects of immobilization. In a healthy ligament, exercise is not likely to increase the strength and

stiffness by more than about 10% to 15%. Sprint training results in increases in ligament weight but not ligament-bone junction strength.[202] However, endurance activity with regular mechanical loads results in increases in junction strength ligament stiffness. Low duration (30 minutes) and high frequency (6 days/week) endurance exercise appears to have the most benefit to ligament strength. A program of low-intensity exercise combined with short bouts of high-intensity exercise in young horses resulted in thicker and stronger superficial digital flexor tendons as compared with horses that were stall rested or were stall rested with a single daily bout of high-intensity exercise.[203]

The effects of exercise on morphology and mechanical properties of the canine stifle MCL have been investigated.[178,204] Dogs undergoing treadmill exercise for 6 weeks had a 12% increase in failure load of the MCL and a 15% increase in hydroxyproline content of the lateral collateral ligament compared to control dogs. In addition, collagen fiber diameter was greater following training, although GAG content, water content, collagen concentration/dry weight, and collagen concentration per weight/length unit were unchanged.

Another study evaluated the effect of exercise on the structural properties of swine FMT complex. Animals were trained on a treadmill daily for 12 months. Exercised pigs had a significant increase in the ultimate load to failure of their ligaments when normalized for body weight, but there were no significant changes in ultimate load, deformation, or energy absorbed of ligaments. Results found in young rabbits that were trained on running wheels indicated that training increased the breaking strength of many ligaments and tendons, including the tibia-CCL-femur complex.[204] Studies in rats and mice have shown similar results and have suggested a possible additive role for testosterone in enhancing ligament and tendon strength with training.[56]

Studies in other species have not always demonstrated a corresponding increase in breaking strength, fiber diameter, and collagen content. For example, there was no increase in hydroxyproline content despite an increase in breaking strength in rats undergoing training.[56] In addition, there was an increase in collagen turnover with training. More of the newly formed collagen may be in the soluble form because of fewer cross-links. Metabolic changes have been noted in tendons and ligaments of rodents undergoing training, including increased tendon nitrogen content, malate dehydrogenase, NADH-oxidase, lactate dehydrogenase, isocitrate dehydrogenase, and succinate dehydrogenase early in the training period.[56] The water content does not change with training, but the number of cell nuclei per unit volume of tendon is greater in trained rats. Training results in an increase in oxygen consumption of less than 10% in ligaments and tendons, while there is a 58% elevation in muscle tissue. It is unclear why chronic exercise does not produce a greater effect.[182] Changes in the content of an elastic extracellular matrix protein, tenascin-C, have also been noted with immobilization and remobilization of ligaments and tendons.[205] Although rat tenascin-C was present at the normal rat bone–patellar tendon junction, it was almost completely absent after 3 weeks of cast immobilization. Remobilization in the form of cage activity for 8 weeks resulted in some increase, but not to normal levels. Tenascin-C activity was normal following remobilization with 8 weeks of treadmill training, however, especially around the chondrocytes and fibroblasts of the bone-tendon junction and the collagen fibers of the tendon belly.

Stretching is frequently recommended in dogs in training or during rehabilitation to help improve joint range of motion. In a study of rat tail tendons, stretching to 108% of the original length resulted in return to 104% of the original length when the stretch was released.[206] A second stretch resulted in more stretch per unit load (less stiffness). Histologically, there was evidence of damage to some strands of collagen. Despite the changes in stiffness, the maximum breaking load was not significantly altered after the second stretch.

Effects of Medications on Ligaments and Tendons

Drugs are sometimes administered locally or systemically in the treatment of musculoskeletal conditions. In particular, corticosteroids may be administered intraarticularly and have effects on ligaments and tendons. The effect of intraarticular corticosteroid injections on the mechanical properties of anterior cruciate bone-ligament-bone units was determined in rhesus monkeys.[207] Alterations in ligament strength and elongation properties were dependent on corticosteroid dosage and time after injection. Fifteen weeks after three weekly

injections of large doses of methylprednisolone acetate (6 mg/kg) there were significant decreases in the maximum failure load (20%), energy absorption before failure (11%), and stiffness (11%) of the ligament unit. In contrast, only minimal alterations occurred after 6 weeks. A third group of animals received intraarticular injections (0.6 mg/kg) spaced 2 weeks apart. Although decreases occurred in maximum failure load (9%) and energy absorption (8%) by 15 weeks, the magnitude of changes was less. There was microscopic evidence of collagen fiber failure at multiple levels throughout the ligament. Although high and frequent doses of intraarticular corticosteroids produce the greatest alterations in ligament strength and function, even low doses given infrequently affected ligament properties. A single intraarticular injection or injections repeated at intervals of several months is recommended to minimize ligament damage. Furthermore, direct injection of corticosteroid into the ligament should be avoided because fibrocyte death and alterations in ligament strength and stiffness may occur for up to 1 year.[207]

Injection of corticosteroid inside a tendon has deleterious effects, with collagen necrosis and decreases in tensile strength occurring.[208] Peritendinous injections are generally safer, and with proper indications, there may be fewer complications. Systemic administration of corticosteroids also has fewer adverse effects on tendons than intratendinous injection. However, administration of very high doses (10 mg/kg) may result in reduced breaking strength of sutured canine tendons.[208] In rabbits receiving corticosteroids, bony insertion sites became osteoporotic and failure tended to occur by fracture.[209] Tissues with shorter turnover times, such as bone, tend to weaken faster than tissues with longer turnover times, such as tendons and ligaments, when corticosteroids are administered. In fact, tendons may initially become slightly stiffer early in the course of steroid administration because fibroblast proliferation and collagen production are reduced, resulting in decreased insoluble collagen. Long-term steroid use eventually results in weakening of ligaments and tendons because of the continued inhibition of collagen synthesis.

Treatment with topical dimethyl sulfoxide (DMSO) has been recommended for the rehabilitation of local inflammatory conditions, including injuries to tendons and muscles. However, topical treatment with DMSO of the

Achilles tendons of mice indicated that the tensile strength of the tendon was related to the length of time the mice were treated with DMSO.[210] The maximum decrease of 20% was seen 7 days after treatment began. These data suggest that vigorous muscle activity should be avoided during treatment with DMSO.

Fluoroquinolone antibiotics may contribute to tendinopathies. The incidence of tendinitis and tendon rupture in human patients treated with ciprofloxacin suggests that these antibiotics alter tendon fibroblast metabolism. There was a 67% decrease in cell proliferation compared with control cells, and a 36% to 48% decrease in collagen synthesis of canine Achilles tendon, paratenon, and shoulder capsule fibroblasts incubated with serum levels of ciprofloxacin in cell culture.[211] Ciprofloxacin also caused a 14% to 60% decrease in PG synthesis and significant increases in matrix-degrading proteolytic activity. These changes suggest that ciprofloxacin stimulates matrix-degrading protease activity from fibroblasts and inhibits fibroblast metabolism, which may contribute to the clinically described tendinopathies associated with ciprofloxacin therapy.

Certain pharmacological agents may positively affect ligaments and tendons. For example, treatment with bone morphogenetic protein-2 results in more extensive bone formation around tendons placed through bone tunnels with closer apposition of new bone to the tendon in treated limbs, resulting in higher tendon pull-out strength.[212] Bone morphogenetic protein can accelerate the healing process when a tendon graft is transplanted into a bone tunnel.

Bone

Normal Bone

Bone consists of organic and inorganic components. The organic component consists of collagen fibers embedded in a matrix of GAGs, among other components of ground substance. The inorganic component consists primarily of calcium and phosphorus in the form of hydroxyapatite crystals. These crystals are embedded within the organized collagen fibers. Bone provides the musculoskeletal tissues with compressive strength during weight-bearing. Long bones have a compact portion of lamellar bone found in the outer cortex, and loosely woven trabecular bone found in the inner medulla. The inner medullary bone is typically more metabolically active because of the relatively large surface area, but it is also relatively weaker as compared with the more dense outer cortical bone.

Response of Bone to Disuse and Immobilization

Many models exist to study the effects of immobilization on the skeleton, including local or systemic immobilization. Local immobilization involves casting, splinting, denervation, paralysis, disarticulation, and limb suspension, whereas systemic immobilization is accomplished with body casting, bedrest, or spaceflight. Reduced stress on bones may also result from stress shielding following application of implants for repair of fractures. Care must be taken in employing the various models. They have similar patterns of bone loss, but they respond slightly differently in the location and the amount of bone loss, depending upon the degree of unloading.

Models of forelimb and hindlimb immobilization that prevent weight-bearing on the limb induce a reduction in cortical and cancellous bone mass, reduce cortical bone density and stiffness, and increase turnover in cancellous bone.[213,214] The changes that occur following immobilization vary depending on the length of immobilization and remobilization, the age of the animal, and the bone involved. The effects appear to be more profound in younger dogs (Figure 7-10). In fact, immobilization during growth may result in permanent changes in bone mass and the relation of bone mineral content (BMC) to body weight.[215] Older animals may have less preexisting bone mass as a result of senile osteoporosis, and these dogs may lose less bone following immobilization than those with higher initial bone mass.[72,216] Trabecular bone is affected to a greater degree than cortical bone, and the effects of immobilization are more extensive in the more distal weight-bearing bones (Figures 7-11 to 7-13).[216,217] Diaphyseal bone loss during immobilization affects the cranial and caudal cortices to a greater extent than the medial and lateral cortices.[218] These changes are consistent with those seen in other species, including rats.[218]

The response to cast immobilization of bone in young adult dogs may be divided into three stages of histologic response.[219] In stage I, there is rapid initial loss of bone, reaching its maximum rate of loss at 6 weeks, with

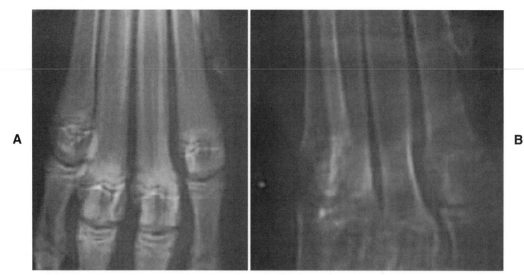

Figure 7-10   Radiographs of the metacarpal bones of a 10-month-old dog with fractures of the distal radius and ulna. **A,** At the time of fracture. **B,** Four weeks after cast placement. Note thinning of the cortices and generalized bone atrophy.

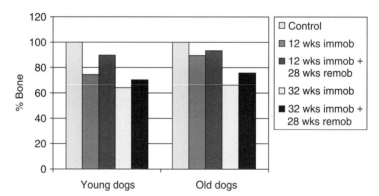

Figure 7-11   Trabecular bone volume of the radius following varying periods of immobilization and remobilization. Note the relatively greater loss of bone volume in trabecular bone compared to the diaphyseal bone in Figure 7-12.

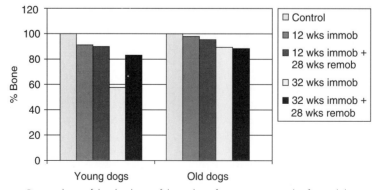

Figure 7-12   Bone volume of the diaphysis of the radius after varying periods of immobilization and remobilization. Bone loss is greater in young dogs immobilized for long periods of time.

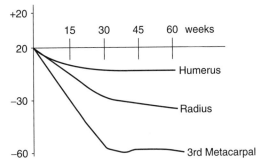

Figure 7-13   Effects of immobilization on density of various bones.

relatively equal contributions of the periosteal, Haversian, and endosteal regions to the loss. The rate of bone loss slows during stage II, which consists of 24 to 32 weeks of immobilization. The majority of the bone loss during this stage comes from the periosteal envelope. Stage III, characterized by greater than 32 weeks of immobilization, results in bone mass that has been reduced by 30% to 50% of original values. This pattern is qualitatively similar in all bones of the forelimb, but the distal bones are affected to a greater degree. Another study of immature dogs demonstrated a 55% decrease in bone mass of the distal tibial metaphysis following 4 weeks of unilateral hindlimb cast immobilization.[220]

The extent of resorption surface and the increase in the total histologically "active" periosteal envelope parallel the phases of bone loss. The type of metabolic bone activity also varies depending on the length of immobilization. In cast-immobilized young adult Beagle dogs, the total active metacarpal bone surface (resorption and formation) was reduced 60% below control values during the first 2 to 4 weeks, increased 50% above controls at 6 weeks, and subsequently returned to control values at 8 to 12 weeks.[219] The response of bone to immobilization differs in mature dogs and is related to the length of immobilization.[72] In one study, bone volume was estimated in the third metacarpus, radius, ulna, and humerus at the mid-diaphysis and the distal metaphysis of dogs with forelimb immobilization for up to 32 weeks. In both young and mature dogs, bone volume decreased with the duration of immobilization, and the types of changes were similar in the metaphysis and diaphysis. The old dogs, which began the study with 10% less bone

than the younger dogs, showed smaller proportional losses than younger dogs, most evident in the diaphysis. In both age-groups, the distal, weight-bearing bones tended to show greater losses. Following 32 weeks of immobilization, young dogs had 54% less bone volume in the third metacarpal diaphysis, while older dogs had 38% less. Metacarpal trabecular bone decreased 50% in young dogs and 47% in older dogs. Adult dogs had a 45% decrease in bone mass of the distal radial metaphysis following 16 weeks of cast immobilization in another study.[221]

The amount of bone loss associated with the length of immobilization apparently has limits. Although immobilization studies have demonstrated bone loss of up to 60% of the trabecular bone mass, there appears to be a maintenance bone turnover level that occurs with continued immobilization.[216] The remaining maintenance level suggests a physiological threshold where basal hormonal and cellular activity is reached in the absence of mechanical stimuli. During the acute phase of immobilization, bone loss occurs in bone adjacent to marrow and from an increase in bone resorption and a decrease in bone formation.[217] There may be more erosion of the inner cortical surface in older dogs. Young growing dogs also have an interruption of periosteal bone deposition, resulting in smaller bone diameter. Immobilization also results in increased regional blood flow and bone marrow pressure. The flow of the entire long bone is approximately four times greater than that of cortical bone, indicating that cancellous bone receives much of the blood flow. There is no significant difference in flow rate between the endosteal and periosteal cortices, however. There are variations of blood flow among long bones, which might be due to differences in their structure and function, and which may help to explain the differences in bone loss following immobilization.[222] Secondary factors such as low dietary calcium or fluctuating hormone levels may also be involved. At steady state, or chronic phase, bone mass plateaus to a maintenance level with cellular activities returning to normal levels.

Biomechanical properties of cortical and cancellous bone are also significantly affected by immobilization. Forelimbs of dogs immobilized for 16 weeks had decreases in cortical load, yield, and stiffness as well as cancellous bone failure stress, yield stress, and modulus, compared with control limbs.[71] In general, immobilized limb cancellous bone mechanical properties were 28% to 74% of control values, and cortical bone mechanical properties were 71% to 98% of control values. Similar to the differences in bone loss that occur in different bones, biomechanical properties of different bones in the same immobilized limb may also vary. Torsional stiffness of radiuses and metacarpal bones immobilized for 12 weeks decreased approximately 12% and 30%, respectively, as compared with controls.[213,223] Increasing the length of immobilization results in further deterioration of biomechanical properties. Metacarpal bone immobilized for 26 weeks retained only 50% of normal stiffness.

There is increased urinary and fecal excretion of calcium and phosphorus in people with cast immobilization of a limb, and similar findings may be expected in dogs.[56] Excretion of hydroxyproline, an indicator of collagen content, also increases with disuse. Relatively equal proportions of bone matrix and bone mineral are lost during bone atrophy, suggesting that the organic and mineral composition of bone is similar following a period of immobilization. Histologically, there is an increase in osteoclast activity and vascularization with disuse, suggesting an increase in bone resorption. Prostaglandin E (PGE) may also be involved in the development of immobilization osteoporosis.[220] Osteoporosis induced by fiberglass-cast immobilization of the hindlimb of immature dogs for 4 weeks resulted in significant loss of bone mass and a twofold increase in bone PGE, suggesting that PGE plays a role in immobilization osteoporosis.

Bone resorption also occurs at insertion sites of ligaments as a result of disuse, and there is decreased mechanical strength and bone collagen associated with disuse.[177] An internal skeletal fixation model applied for 12 weeks resulted in significant atrophy of bone and loss of collagen in the tibia and femur at the insertion and origin of the CCL.[28] When a fast rate of deformation was applied, failure of the femur-ligament-tibia complex occurred through the tibial insertion of the ligament. Bone atrophy was the result of increased resorption of bone rather than decreased bone formation. Preservation of active joint motion during immobilization may have a protective effect on the bone-ligament-bone complex.[29] A unilateral tarsal disarticulation model of disuse that maintained active knee motion without weight bearing for 8 weeks maintained the strength of the femur-CCL-tibia

complex despite loss of collagen and calcium mass in the femur and tibia, suggesting that active joint motion helps to preserve the mechanical strength of the femur-ligament-tibia complex.

Bone loss may be reduced in paraplegic human patients who are ambulatory as compared with those who are nonambulatory, who develop osteoporosis of the pelvis and limbs.[56] A relatively low degree of physical training may inhibit the development of osteoporosis. Slow oscillation of bedridden human patients with intact neuromuscular function from a horizontal position to a 20-degree footdown position every 2 minutes may help preserve bone mass. The contraction of antigravity muscles during the downward tilt may be partially responsible for maintenance of bone mass by adding stress to bones during muscle contraction. There also appears to be an association of bone mass with muscle mass, with similar degrees of bone and muscle loss with disuse. Non–weight-bearing exercise of bedridden patients is relatively ineffective in reducing calcium loss, but standing for 3 hours reduces urinary excretion, suggesting that weight-bearing rather than physical activity is primarily responsible for reducing bone atrophy during bed rest.

In summary, young dogs tend to lose bone more quickly following immobilization as compared with older animals, even though older dogs may have less bone mass to begin with. The degree of bone loss increases with the length of immobilization, with the rate of loss slowing as the time of immobilization increases. Bone loss is greater in the more distal weight-bearing bones as compared with proximal minimally weight-bearing bones.

Bone Changes Resulting From Disease Conditions

Bone changes may be detected after total hip replacement and complications of this procedure. In one study, dogs with unilateral primary cementless total hip arthroplasty had no right-left difference in tibial BMC or cortical bone cross-sectional geometry after 6 months, but after 2 years there was a 5% to 6% difference in BMC, perhaps because of subclinical disuse of the operated limb.[224] In dogs with failed cemented prostheses, tibial BMC may be more than 20% lower in the operated limb. Successful revision of the total hip replacement results in improved BMC, suggesting that improved limb function after revision surgery may result in gain of previously lost bone.

Bone loss may also occur following knee surgery as a result of relative disuse of the affected limb. One study of dogs with surgically created CCL transection demonstrated that there was a dramatic 22% to 34% decrease in bone mineral density of the affected distal femur 12 weeks after surgery.[225] Studies of humans indicate similar decreases in bone mineral density of approximately 20% in the distal femur, patella, and proximal tibia up to 1 year after surgery for ACL injury.[226,227] In addition, bone density may be decreased by 3% to 9% 10 to 11 years after surgery.[228] Bone density had significant correlation with functional scores of the knee, but not with knee stability.

In addition to bone changes following ligament injury, it is possible that dogs may experience decreased bone density following fracture. In humans, 2% to 7% decreases in bone density were found in the distal femur, patella, proximal tibia, and calcaneus 10 years after femur fracture.[229] Relative bone density had correlation with pain and functional scores of the affected limb, but not with fracture type, fracture location, or non–weight-bearing time after injury. Similar decreases in bone density were seen 9 years after tibial fractures in another study.[230]

Denervation of a limb of a growing dog results in decreased lengths of the humerus and radius.[231] Furthermore, loss of innervation to a region may result in decreased bone density.[232] However, active muscle contraction, through either reflex walking or electrical stimulation, helps attenuate loss of bone density.[232] A functional neuromuscular stimulation–induced knee extension exercise system was used in human patients with spinal cord injuries up to three times per week for 36 sessions using a progressive resistance load.[233] Maintenance of bone density in some subjects suggests that training may retard the rate of bone loss that typically occurs with spinal cord injuries.

Stress Protection

Stress shielding or stress protection occurs when metal implants, such as bone plates and screws, are used to repair fractures or in joint replacement surgery. Although rigid metal plates stabilize the fracture site, help maintain contact between bone fragments, and allow early weight-bearing and patient mobility, the higher stiffness of the implant results in bone loss as a result of decreased physiologic loading of the bone. Calculations were made of the alterations in cyclic bone stresses due to the application of bone plates on canine femurs.[226] The magnitude of the reduction in the loads borne by the bone and the degree of shift in the bone stress neutral axis during the stance phase of gait were influenced by plate geometry, plate stiffness, and plate location. Bone remodeling is very sensitive to small changes in cyclic bone stresses. Changes in cyclic bone stresses of less than 1% of the ultimate strength can cause measurable differences in bone remodeling after a period of a few months.

The pattern of cortical atrophy induced by plate fixation for 7 months on canine femurs was evaluated in another study.[234] A pronounced reduction of cortical bone (approximately 15% less cortical area) was observed in the diaphysis of the plated bone at the end of the study period. The loss of cortical bone was mainly caused by endosteal resorption with enlargement of the medullary cavity. Neither periosteal resorption nor formation of woven bone under the site of the plate were observed. Osteoporosis due to rigid plate fixation may occur by thinning of the cortex rather than by reduction of the mechanical properties of the osseous tissue.[235] In addition to enlargement of the medullary canal, there may also be decreased cortical thickness under the plate as a result of endosteal resorption. The stiffer the implant and the longer the implant is in place, the greater the bone loss and the lower the recovery potential of the bone. For example, 6 weeks after screw application, some resorption of bone is evident, and by 14 weeks, more significant resorption occurs.

Implants may also interfere with blood circulation, and the weakened bone can refracture after plate removal.[236-238] Disturbance of blood supply may be the main cause of osteopenia in the early stage, whereas disuse of the affected limb may be the most important factor in later stages of fracture healing. Osteopenia may be treated, in part, by active exercises and normal weight-bearing before plate removal.[238]

Stress shielding may also occur following total hip arthroplasty.[239] Stiffness of the femoral stem is a design variable that is partially responsible for femoral remodeling. The basic pattern of bone remodeling is characterized by proximal cortical atrophy and distal cortical and medullary bone hypertrophy. Low-stiffness stems may alter this pattern, leading to reduced proximal bone loss, increased proximal medullary bone hypertrophy, and no distal cortical hypertrophy, suggesting that stem stiffness has a profound effect on stress shielding.

Effects of Remobilization on Bone

The recovery of mechanical and morphologic properties of bone following a period of immobilization depends on the length and type of immobilization, the type and intensity of remobilization, and the age of the animal.[240]

The potential for recovery of bone lost during disuse, in both the diaphyseal cortical and metaphyseal cancellous bone, was evaluated in young adult and old Beagle dogs.[72] Following immobilization of a forelimb for up to 32 weeks, there was considerable recovery of the original bone loss during remobilization. In both age-groups, the residual deficits increased with the duration of immobilization and were similar in the metaphysis and in the diaphysis. In addition, the distal, weight-bearing bones tended to show greater losses and also greater recovery in both diaphyseal and metaphyseal bone. The older dogs had greater residual deficits, most evident in the diaphysis. Following 32 weeks of immobilization and 28 weeks of remobilization, a 50% loss in the third metacarpal diaphysis of younger dogs immediately following the immobilization period decreased to 15% (a 70% recovery), whereas older dogs had a 38% loss that decreased to 23% (a 40% recovery). In contrast, immobilization for 6 or 12 weeks resulted in complete recovery of bone after remobilization of 10 or 28 weeks, respectively. In fact, bone volume of third metacarpal trabecular bone exceeded the original control values in some dogs.

The stages of bone loss that young adult dogs undergo in response to cast immobilization have been discussed.[219] The response to remobilization may be similarly divided into stages. In stage I, in which there is a rapid initial loss of bone following 6 weeks of immobilization, there is near full recovery of bone mass within 8 to 12 weeks of cast removal. Radiographic evidence of periosteal stress reactions of the metacarpal bones, indicated by external bone formation in the distal metacarpal metaphysis, was present in 60% of younger dogs but none of the older dogs following 12 weeks of immobilization and up to 28 weeks of remobilization.[218] In stage II, bone

loss slows, but recovery is also slower following 24 to 32 weeks of immobilization. During the remobilization period, young and old dogs immobilized for 32 weeks may have periosteal stress reactions of the metacarpal bones, indicated by external bone formation in the distal metacarpal metaphysis.[218] Although there was no evidence of a break in bone continuity, microdamage (mechanical fatigue) may have occurred at these sites, and periosteal stress-induced reactions may occur at sites of increased stress in the absence of actual fractures. Continued stress to bones during the remobilization period may indeed lead to stress reactions. Immobilization for longer than 32 weeks characterizes stage III, in which the loss of bone mass remains at 30% to 50% of original values, despite remobilization.

Complete recovery of trabecular bone following immobilization may be limited by changes in bony architecture.[240] Following 18 weeks of immobilization, trabecular area of rat tibias increased by 42% and 51% following 10 and 20 weeks of remobilization, respectively. Remobilization resulted in increased bone area by decreasing porosity during the first 10 weeks of remobilization, but little further increase occurred between 10 and 20 weeks of remobilization. The recovery of bone loss was mainly due to an increase in trabecular width. In fact, there was no recovery of the number of trabeculae lost during immobilization. Remobilization added bone on existing surfaces but was not anabolic enough to reconnect trabeculae. This may explain why there may be a persistent loss of bone following long periods of immobilization, despite a long remobilization period.

Whereas it is clear that a simple period of free exercise during the remobilization period may not result in complete recovery of bone following immobilization, high-intensity training following immobilization may result in more complete recovery. One study of rats undergoing limb immobilization and subsequent remobilization indicated that high-intensity treadmill running resulted in restored BMC and bone density of the affected limb, whereas animals undergoing free remobilization had BMC and density values below those of controls.[241,242] The expression of osteocalcin, a marker of osteoblastic activity, corresponded to bone formation during the remobilization period.[243] When the training period ceased, however, the beneficial effects of training were lost. It appears that intensified remobilization is necessary to restore bone mineral after disuse, but the benefits may be lost if activity is terminated.

A period of mild treadmill activity following free remobilization may also be beneficial for dogs with immobilized limbs. Forelimb immobilization of 1- to 2-year-old dogs for 16 weeks, followed by a remobilization period of 16 weeks of kennel confinement and 16 weeks of treadmill exercise administered three times per week, resulted in the return of cortical and cancellous bone mineral density and mechanical properties to essentially normal levels.[71]

Adaptation of Bone to Increased Stress

The bone response to mechanical loading is proportional to an applied load of given magnitude and frequency of application. There are also proportional increases in second messengers, growth factors, bone matrix, and bone strength with loading.[244] Animal models using dogs, turkeys, mice, rats, chickens, and pigs have demonstrated a threshold response and dose-response relationship to mechanical loading of bone, by either mechanical means or exercise. In general, relatively low-intensity training may have no or only mild effects on bone density or bone growth, whereas higher intensity training results in greater bone density but may inhibit growth in bone length and girth in growing animals.[56]

Despite much knowledge regarding the influence of physical activity on bone, precise information regarding the type, intensity, frequency, and duration of exercise on bone remains elusive. The remodeling of bone is slow, taking several months to complete. The age at which training begins is important. Initiation of activity early in life appears to be the most beneficial.[245] Within limits, loading of growing bone leads to a better result than loading of adult bone. The production of prostaglandins and growth factors may modulate the process of bone modeling. Although the optimal pattern of bone loading is unknown, evidence suggests that bone should be loaded with high peak forces and strain rates (high impacts), create strain throughout the bony column, consist of relatively few repetitions, and be long-term and progressive. In humans, weightlifters have the greatest bone mass, followed by throwers, runners, soccer players, and swimmers. This suggests that weight and strength training appear to provide the greatest effects on bone and swimming the least, perhaps because the buoyancy of water alters the load placed on bone as compared to weight lifting on land.

Resistance exercise training may also affect bone of animals. Rats conditioned to press levers, facilitating full extension and full flexion of the hindlimbs while wearing a weighted vest, had an increase in cancellous bone area of the proximal tibia after 6 weeks.[246] In addition, osteocalcin, trabecular number, thickness, and osteoid covering cancellous bone were greater in trained animals, suggesting that resistance training increases cancellous bone area by stimulating bone formation. A study of rats undergoing exercise with or without sudden impact loading of the femur indicated that cortical wall thickness increased with any activity, and breaking strength of the bones was greater in bones undergoing impact loading as compared to sedentary controls.[247] In spite of the enhanced biomechanical properties of impact-loaded bones, there was little difference in BMC in the exercised groups, suggesting that significant improvements may occur in biomechanical properties with little change in bone mass with impact loading.

In dogs, mild increases in loading of bones have little effect on bone mass or bone density. Impact loading or chronic moderate increases in loading result in increased bone mass and bone density. A study of mature Beagle dogs with an ostectomy of a radius showed that there was little change in bone mass and density of the contralateral radius and ulna (Figure 7-14).[248] This model allows weight-bearing on the limb undergoing ostectomy of the radius because the intact ulna allows for weight-bearing. Because all of the weight is borne by the intact ulna following ostectomy, the load on that bone is significantly greater as compared with the load-sharing seen with the intact radius and ulna of the contralateral limb (Figure 7-15). The increased load results in significant increases in bone mass and density in the ipsilateral ulna within a relatively short period of time.

Increasing weight-bearing on bones by exercising dogs with lead-weighted jackets results in increased bone mass.[249] Increasing the load carried to 130% of body weight and exercising on a treadmill for 75 min at 3.3 km/hr over a 70-week period resulted in a mild increase in BMC of the tibia when adjusted for actual body weight. This form of activity may increase bone mass and help reduce bone loss during aging.

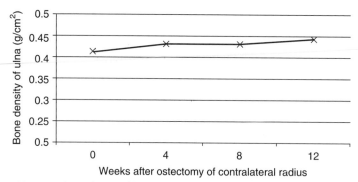

Figure 7-14 Change in bone density of the contralateral ulna following ostectomy of a radius. Compared with the situation in Figure 7-15, there is little change in bone density because both the intact radius and ulna continue to share loading.

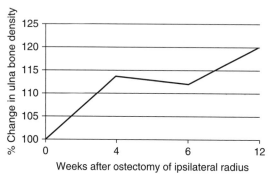

Figure 7-15 Relative change of the bone density of the ulna following ostectomy of the ipsilateral radius. Note the increased density as a result of the shift of weight-bearing from a paired two-bone system to the single remaining bone.

The effects of long-distance running training on bone growth have been studied in young growing dogs.[147] Young Beagle dogs trained on a treadmill for 1 year, gradually increasing running to 40 km/day at a speed of 5.5 to 6.8 km/hr with a 15-degree inclination during the last 15 weeks, while control dogs were kept in their cages. Ulna and radius bone mass as a ratio to body mass increased approximately 10% in trained dogs as compared with controls, while there was no change in mass of cranial tibial and semitendinosus muscles. Long-distance running apparently has a mild positive effect on bone mass in growing dogs.

In contrast, another study of immature dogs with a similar training regimen indicated that while intensive endurance training may increase bone mass of weight-bearing bones, the appendicular skeleton may have reduced bone density.[250] Trained dogs had larger and heavier radius, ulna, and hip bones, but reduced bone mineral density of thoracic vertebrae as compared with untrained controls. In addition, trained dogs developed more osteophytes in the spines but not in the extremities. Intense aerobic training of young dogs may alter bone mass, possibly because of altered biomechanical forces placed on the bones.

High-level activity, such as racing, may affect bone to a greater extent as compared with bone changes occurring with endurance training. One study of racing Greyhounds found that the cross-sectional and cortical areas of left metacarpals IV and V were greater than those of the right metacarpals.[251] In addition, osteonal density was greater on the dorsal surface of the bones than in the medial and lateral quadrants. These changes indicate site-specific adaptations to the bones as a result of asymmetrical loading from running in a counterclockwise fashion and greater loading of the inside limb.

A lifetime of weight-bearing physical exercise may decrease the amount of bone lost through the normal aging process in dogs.[252] Dogs in a trained group exercised for 90 min, 5 days/wk, for 527 weeks, running an average of 3.3 km/hr on a treadmill while carrying approximately 11.5 kg. The control group had normal cage activity in dog runs. Long-term exercise significantly reduced cortical porosity and marginally increased cortical area in aged dogs, because of a decrease in bone resorption rather than an increase in bone formation. The results of this study have implications for the role of exercise in delaying bone loss during aging. Training appears to alter mineral uptake and retention by bone. For example, in one study of geriatric dogs exercising 40 min/day at 2.4 km/hr on a 15-degree grade, dogs had less calcium excretion on exercise days.[253] Similar studies of humans support these findings and also indicate that bone deposition rate is increased with training.[56]

Although mechanical stimulation is important in promoting bone formation in normal dogs, fracture healing may also be enhanced with weight-bearing. Dogs with surgically created defects in the tibial cortex that were allowed to bear weight on the limb had significantly more woven bone in the defects as compared to dogs that were not permitted to bear weight.[254] This suggests that weight-bearing is a permissive factor for bone formation in bony defects. In addition, training may enhance healing if a fracture should occur after initiating training. A study of mice undergoing training before fracture had higher rates of collagen synthesis and higher concentrations of calcium in the healing fracture callus as compared with sedentary rats.[255]

Effects of Medications on Bone

A number of studies have evaluated the effects of various compounds on bone mass in dogs. Some of these substances are osteoprotective, whereas others, such as corticosteroids, may hasten bone loss in immobilized limbs.

Some drugs and hormones help protect against bone loss during immobilization. Dogs receiving 60 to 240 ng/kg of vitamin D_3 for 4 weeks had trabecular bone volume of the calcaneus in direct relation to the dosage of vitamin D_3 in a plaster cast disuse osteoporosis model for 4 weeks, with the highest dose resulting in bone volume equal to that of the control limb.[256] Unfortunately, this dose is considered to be toxic. Vitamin D_3 administered to Beagle dogs after ovariectomy was effective in maintaining normal urinary hydroxyproline excretion, suggesting that the treatment was effective in helping prevent the bone loss associated with ovariectomy.[257] In fact, bone mineral density of the lumbar vertebrae and femur of ovariectomized dogs receiving 2 or 10 µg/kg of vitamin D_3 were the same as those of nonovariectomized control animals 30 months after surgery, whereas density was 25% lower in untreated ovariectomized dogs.

Bone loss during disuse has been prevented with bisphosphonate compounds in humans following paralysis or bedrest. Using a forelimb immobilization model in dogs, pamidronate, a bisphosphonate compound, was administered

for 7 days followed by 3 weeks without treatment. This cycle was repeated three times for a total of 12 weeks. This treatment was effective in preventing cancellous bone loss and maintained cortical bone density and stiffness.[213] In addition, indices of bone formation and resorption were significantly reduced. Tamoxifen citrate administered to growing dogs with a hindlimb placed in a fiberglass cast for 28 days was moderately effective in sparing bone mass as compared to immobilized controls.[214] The calculated bone mass sparing effect of tamoxifen was 24.4%. This drug is a nonsteroidal antiestrogen compound, with some ability to inhibit prostaglandin synthesis, modulate signal transduction processes that control cell growth, and induce transforming growth factor-beta.

Aspirin may also be effective in diminishing bone loss during immobilization. Osteoporosis was induced in growing dogs using a cast immobilization model for 4 weeks.[220] Bone PGE concentrations doubled and bone mass was reduced in untreated immobilized dogs. Dogs receiving 25 mg/kg of buffered aspirin every 8 hours had a 13% bone mass sparing effect and a 65% reduction in bone PGE. Similar bone-sparing effects have been observed with other NSAIDs, such as ibuprofen, in the treatment of osteolytic conditions such as osteomyelitis and bone metastases.

REFERENCES

1. Akeson WH et al: Effects of immobilization on joints, *Clin Orthop* 219:28-37, 1987.
2. Paulos LE, Wnorowski DC, Beck CL: Rehabilitation following knee surgery: recommendations, *Sports Med* 11:257-275, 1991.
3. Cohen NP, Foster RJ, Mow VC: Composition and dynamics of articular cartilage: structure, function, and maintaining healthy state, *J Orthop Sports Phys Ther* 28:203-215, 1998.
4. Palmoski M, Perricone E, Brandt KD: Development and reversal of a proteoglycan aggregation defect in normal canine knee cartilage after immobilization, *Arthritis Rheum* 22:508-517, 1979.
5. McDonough AL: Effects of cortico steroids on articular cartilage: a review of literature, *Phys Ther* 62:835,1982.
6. Palmoski MJ, Bean JS: Cartilage atrophy induced by limb immobilization. In: Greenwald RA, Diamond HS, editors: *CRC handbook of animal models for the rheumatic diseases*. Boca Raton, FL, 1988, CRC Press.
7. Kiviranta I et al: Weight bearing controls glycosaminoglycan concentration and articular cartilage thickness in the knee joints of young beagle dogs, *Arthritis Rheum* 30:801-809, 1987.
8. Saamanen AM et al: Proteoglycan alterations following immobilization and remobilization in the articular cartilage of young canine knee (stifle) joint, *J Orthop Res* 8:863-873, 1990.

9. Muller FJ et al: Centrifugal and biochemical comparison of proteoglycan aggregates from articular cartilage in experimental joint disuse and joint instability, *J Orthop Res* 12:498-508, 1994.

10. Behrens F, Kraft EL, Oegema-TR J: Biochemical changes in articular cartilage after joint immobilization by casting or external fixation, *J Orthop Res* 7:335-343, 1989.

11. Ratcliffe A, Beauvais PJ, Saed NF: Differential levels of synovial fluid aggrecan aggregate components in experimental osteoarthritis and joint disuse, *J Orthop Res* 12:464-473, 1994.

12. Ratcliffe A et al: Synovial fluid analyses detect and differentiate proteoglycan metabolism in canine experimental models of osteoarthritis and disuse atrophy, *Agents Actions Suppl* 39:63-67, 1993.

13. Haapala J et al: Coordinated regulation of hyaluronan and aggrecan content in the articular cartilage of immobilized and exercised dogs, *J Rheumatol* 23:1586-1593, 1996.

14. Grumbles et al: Cartilage metalloproteases in disuse atrophy, *J Rheumatol Suppl* 43:146-148, 1995.

15. Jurvelin J et al: Softening of canine articular cartilage after immobilization of the knee joint, *Clin Orthop* 207:246-252, 1986.

16. Haapala J et al: Incomplete restoration of immobilization induced softening of young beagle knee articular cartilage after 50-week remobilization. *Int J Sports Med* 21:76-81, 2000.

17. Leroux MA et al: Altered mechanics and histomorphometry of canine tibial cartilage following joint immobilization. *Osteoarthr Cartilage* 9:633-640, 2001.

18. Palmoski MJ, Colyer RA, Brandt KD: Joint motion in the absence of normal loading does not maintain normal articular cartilage. *Arthritis Rheum* 23:325-334, 1980.

19. Setton LA et al: Mechanical behavior and biochemical composition of canine knee cartilage following periods of joint disuse and disuse with remobilization, *Osteoarthr Cartilage* 5:1-16, 1997.

20. Shevtsov VI, Asonova SN: Ultrastructural changes of articular cartilage following joint immobilization with the Ilizarov apparatus, *Bull Hosp Jt Dis* 54:69-75, 1995.

21. Palmoski MJ, Brandt KD: Immobilization of the knee prevents osteoarthritis after anterior cruciate ligament transection, *Arthritis Rheum* 25:1201-1208, 1982.

22. Schoenecker PL, Lesker PA, Ogata K: A dynamic canine model of experimental hip dysplasia. Gross and histological pathology, and the effect of position of immobilization on capital femoral epiphyseal blood flow, *J Bone Joint Surg* 66A:1281-1288, 1984.

23. Kiviranta I J, et al: Articular cartilage thickness and glycosaminoglycan distribution in the young canine knee joint after remobilization of the immobilized limb, *J Orthop Res* 12:161-167, 1994.

24. Haapala J et al: Remobilization does not fully restore immobilization induced articular cartilage atrophy, *Clin Orthop* 362:218-229, 1999.

25. Jortikka MO et al: Immobilisation causes longlasting matrix changes both in the immobilised and contralateral joint cartilage, *Ann Rheum Dis* 56:255-261, 1997.

26. Jurvelin J et al: Partial restoration of immobilization-induced softening of canine articular cartilage after remobilization of the knee (stifle) joint, *J Orthop Res* 7:352-358, 1989.

27. Palmoski MJ, Brandt KD: Running inhibits the reversal of atrophic changes in canine knee cartilage after removal of a leg cast, *Arthritis Rheum* 24:1329-1337, 1981.

28. Klein L et al: Isotopic evidence for resorption of soft tissues and bone in immobilized dogs, *J Bone Joint Surg* 64A:225-230, 1982.

29. Klein L et al: Prevention of ligament and meniscus atrophy by active joint motion in a non-weight-bearing model, *J Orthop Res* 7:80-85, 1989.

30. Noone TJ et al: Influence of canine recombinant somatotropin on biomechanical and biochemical properties of the medial meniscus in stifles with altered stability, *Am J Vet Res* 63:419-426, 2002.

31. Buseck MS, Noyes FR: Arthroscopic evaluation of meniscal repairs after anterior cruciate ligament reconstruction and immediate motion, *Am J Sports Med* 19:489-494, 1991.

32. Dowdy PA et al: The effect of cast immobilization on meniscal healing: an experimental study in the dog, *Am J Sports Med* 23:721-728, 1995.

33. Bray RC et al: Vascular response of the meniscus to injury: effects of immobilization, *J Orthop Res* 19:384-390, 2001.

34. Elliott DM et al: Tensile properties of articular cartilaage are altered by meniscectomy in a canine model of osteoarthritis, *J Orthop Res* 17:503-508, 1999.

35. Berjon JJ, Munuera L, Calvo M: Degenerative lesions in the articular cartilage after meniscectomy: a preliminary experimental study in dogs, *J Trauma* 31:342-350, 2001.

36. Cox JS et al: The degenerative effects of partial and total resection of the medial meniscus in dog's knees, *Clin Orthop* 109:178-183, 1975.

37. Ghosh P et al: Effect of postoperative immobilisation on the regrowth of the knee joint semilunar cartilage: an experimental study, *J Orthop Res* 1:153-164, 1983.

38. Ghosh P et al: The effects of postoperative joint immobilization on articular cartilage degeneration following meniscectomy, *J Surg Res* 35:461-473, 1983.

39. Palmoski MJ, Brandt KD: Effects of static and cyclic compressive loading on articular cartilage plugs in vitro, *Arthritis Rheum* 27:675-681, 1984.

40. Radin EL et al: Effects of mechanical loading on the tissues of the rabbit knee, *J Orthop Res* 2:221-234, 1984.

41. Donohue JM et al: The effects of indirect blunt trauma on adult articular cartilage, *J Bone Joint Surg* 65A:948-957, 1983.

42. Wang J: Response of calcified cartilage to blunt trauma, *Chinese J Sports Med* 9:65-66, 1990.

43. Hallett MB, Andrish JT: Effects of exercise on articular cartilage, *Sports Med Arthrosc Rev* 2:29-37, 1994.

44. Jurvelin J et al: Effect of physical exercise on indentation stiffness of articular cartilage in the canine knee, *Int J Sports Med* 7:106-110, 1986.

45. Kiviranta I et al: Moderate running exercise augments glycosaminoglycans and thickness of articular cartilage in the knee joint of young beagle dogs, *J Orthop Res* 6:188-195, 1988.

46. Jurvelin J et al: Indentation stiffness of young canine knee articular cartilage: influence of strenuous joint loading, *J Biomech* 23:1239-1246, 1990.

47. Kiviranta I et al: Articular cartilage thickness and glycosaminoglycan distribution in the anine knee joint after strenuous running exercise, *Clin Orthop* 283:302-308, 1992.

48. Arokoski J et al: Softening of the lateral condyle articular cartilage in the canine knee joint after long distance (up to 40 km/day) running training lasting one year, *Int J Sports Med* 15:254-260, 1994.

49. Arokoski J et al: Long-distance running causes site-dependent decrease of cartilage glycosaminoglycan content in the knee joints of beagle dogs, *Arthritis Rheum* 36:1451-1459, 1993.

50. Oettmeier R et al: Quantitative study of articular cartilage and subchondral bone remodeling in the knee joint of dogs after strenuous running training, *J Bone Miner Res* 7(suppl 2):S419-S424, 1992.

51. Arokoski JP et al: Decreased birefringence of the superficial zone collagen network in the canine knee (stifle) articular cartilage after long distance running training, detected by quantitative polarised light microscopy, *Ann Rheum Dis* 55:253-264, 1996.

52. Lammi M et al: Adaptation of canine femoral head articular cartilage to long distance running exercise in young beagles, *Ann Rheum Dis* 52:369-377, 1993.

53. Vasan N: Effects of physical stress on the synthesis and degradation of cartilage matrix, *Conn Tiss Res* 12:49-58, 1983.

54. Newton PM et al: The effect of lifelong exercise on canine articular cartilage, *Am J Sports Med* 25:282-287, 1997.

55. Agudelo CA, Schumacher HR, Phelps P: Effect of exercise on urate crystal-induced inflammation in canine joints, *Arthritis Rheum* 15:609-616, 1972.

56. Booth FW, Gould EW: Effects of training and disuse on connective tissue, *Exerc Sport Sci Rev* 3:83-112, 1975.

57. Williams JM, Brandt KD: Immobilization ameliorates chemically-induced articular cartilage damage, *Arthritis Rheum* 27:208-216, 1984.

58. Egerbacher M, Edinger J, Tschulenk W: Effects of enrofloxacin and ciprofloxacin hydrochloride on canine and equine chondrocytes in culture, *Am J Vet Res* 62:704-708, 2001.

59. Palmoski MJ, Colyer RA, Brandt KD: Marked suppression by salicylate of the augmented proteoglycan synthesis in osteoarthritic cartilage, *Arthritis Rheum* 23:83-91, 1980.

60. Brandt KD, Palmoski MJ: Effects of salicylates and other nonsteroidal anti-inflammatory drugs on articular cartilage, *Am J Med* 77:65-69, 1984.

61. Palmoski MJ, Brandt KD: Proteoglycan depletion, rather than fibrillation, determines the effects of salicylate and indomethacin on osteoarthritic cartilage, *Arthritis Rheum* 28:548-553, 1985.

62. Palmoski MJ, Brandt KD: Relationship between matrix proteoglycan content and the effects of salicylate and indomethacin on articular cartilage, *Arthritis Rheum* 26:528-531, 1983.

63. Palmoski MJ, Brandt KD: Effects of salicylate and indomethacin on glycosaminoglycan and prostaglandin E2 synthesis in intact canine knee cartilage ex vivo, *Arthritis Rheum* 27:398-403, 1984.

64. Palmoski MJ, Brandt KD: Aspirin aggravates the degeneration of canine joint cartilage caused by immobilization, *Arthritis Rheum* 25:1333-1342, 1982.

65. Gay RE et al: Aspirin causes in vivo synthesis of type I collagen by atrophic articular cartilage, *Arthritis Rheum* 26:1231-1236, 1983.

66. Olah EH, Kostenszky KS: Effect of loading and prednisolone treatment on the glycosaminoglycan content of articular cartilage in dogs, *Scand J Rheumatol* 5:49-52, 1976.

67. Keller WG et al: The effect of trans-stifle external skeletal fixation and hyaluronic acid therapy on articular cartilage in the dog, *Vet Surg* 23:119-128, 1994.

68. Comer JS et al: Immunolocalization of stromelysin, tumor necrosis factor (TNF) alpha, and TNF receptors in atrophied canine articular cartilage treated with hyaluronic acid and transforming growth factor beta, *Am J Vet Res* 57:1488-1496, 1996.

69. Smith GN et al: Effect of intraarticular hyaluronan injection in experimental canine osteoarthritis, *Arthritis Rheum* 41:976-985, 1998.

70. Schollmeier G et al: Structural and functional changes in the canine shoulder after cessation of immobilization, *Clin Orthop* 323:310-315, 1996.

71. Kaneps AJ, Stover SM, Lane NE: Changes in canine cortical and cancellous bone mechanical properties following immobilization and remobilization with exercise, *Bone* 21:419-423, 1997.

72. Jaworski ZF, Uhthoff HK: Reversibility of nontraumatic disuse osteoporosis during its active phase, *Bone* 7:431-439, 1986.

73. Braund KG, Hoff EJ, Richardson EY: Histochemical identification of fiber types in canine skeletal muscle, *Am J Vet Res* 39:561-565, 1978.

74. Rivero JL et al: Enzyme-histochemical profiles of fiber types in mature canine appendicular muscles, *Anat Histol Embryol* 23:330-336, 1994.

75. Latorre R et al: Skeletal muscle fibre types in the dog, *J Anat* 182:329-337, 1993.

76. Snow DH et al: No classical type IIB fibres in dog skeletal muscle, *Histochemistry* 75:53-65, 1982.

77. Rosenblatt JD et al: Fiber type, fiber size, and capillary geometric features of the semitendinosus muscle in three types of dogs, *Am J Vet Res* 49:1573-1576, 1988.

78. Newsholme SJ, Lexell J, Downham DY: Distribution of fibre types and fibre sizes in the tibialis cranialis muscle of beagle dogs, *J Anat* 160:1-8, 1988.

79. Guy PS, Snow DH: Skeletal muscle fibre composition in the dog and its relationship to athletic ability, *Res Vet Sci* 31:186:244-248, 1981.

80. Castle ME, Reyman TA: The effect of tenotomy and tendon transfers on muscle fiber types in the dog, *Clin Orthop* 186:302-310, 1984.

81. Gunn HM: Differences in the histochemical properties of skeletal muscles of different breeds of horses and dogs, *J Anat* 127:615-634, 1978.

82. Barclay JK: Hypothesis: local vascular regulation is a key to flow limited muscle function, *Can J Spt Sci* 15:9-13, 1990.

83. Dodd SL, Powers SK, Crawford MP: Tension development and duty cycle affect Q_{peak} and Vo_{2peak} in contracting muscle, *Med Sci Sports Exerc* 26:997-1002, 1994.

84. Musch TI: Skeletal muscle blood flow in exercising dogs, *Med Sci Sports Exerc* 20:(5 Suppl):S104-S108, 1988.

85. Rowell LB: Muscle blood flow in humans: how high can it go?, *Med Sci Sports Exerc* 20:S97-S103, 1988.

86. Richardson RS: What governs skeletal muscle Vo_{2max}? New evidence, *Med Sci Sports Exerc* 32:100-107, 2000.

87. Haidet GC, Parsons D: Reduced exercise capacity in senescent beagles: an evaluation of the periphery, *Am J Physiol* 260:H173-H182, 1991.

88. Cartee GD: Aging skeletal muscle: response to exercise, *Exerc Sport Sci Rev* 22:91-120, 1994.

89. Stainsby WN, Peterson CV, Barbee RW: O_2 uptake and work by in situ muscle performing contractions with constant shortening, *Med Sci Sports Exerc* 13:27-30, 1981.

90. Brechue WF et al: Blood flow and pressure relationships which determine Vo_{2max}, *Med Sci Sports Exerc* 27:37-42, 1995.

91. Naamani R, Hussain NA, Magder S: The mechanical effects of contractions on blood flow to the muscle, *Eur J Appl Physiol* 71:102-112, 1995.
92. Grassi B: Skeletal muscle Vo$_2$ on-kinetics: set by O$_2$ delivery or by O$_2$ utilization? New insights into an old issue, *Med Sci Sports Exerc* 32:108-116, 2000.
93. Burton HW, Barclay JK: Metabolic factors from exercising muscle and the proliferation of endothelial cells, *Med Sci Sports Exerc* 18:390-395, 1986.
94. Frisbee JC et al: Polycythemia decreases fatigue in tetanic contractions of canine skeletal muscle, *Med Sci Sports Exerc* 31:1293-1298, 1999.
95. Gladden LB, Stainsby WN, MacIntosh BR: Norepinephrine increases canine skeletal muscle Vo$_2$ during recovery, *Med Sci Sports Exerc* 14:471-476, 1982.
96. Hogan MC et al: Increased [lactate] in working dog muscle reduces tension development independent of pH, *Med Sci Sports Exerc* 27:371-377, 1995.
97. Sabbah HN et al: Decreased proportion of type I myofibers in skeletal muscle of dogs with chronic heart failure, *Circulation* 87:1729-1737, 1993.
98. Wilson JR, Coyle EF, Osbakken M: Effect of heart failure on skeletal muscle in dogs, *Am J Physiol* 262: H993-H998, 1992.
99. Lieber RL et al: Differential response of the dog quadriceps muscle to external skeletal fixation of the knee, *Muscle Nerve* 11:193-201, 1988.
100. Appell HJ: Muscular atrophy following immobilization: a review, *Sports Med* 10:42-58, 1990.
101. Appell HJ: Skeletal muscle atrophy during immobilization, *Int J Sports Med* 7:1-5, 1986.
102. Musacchia XJ, Steffen JM, Fell RD: Disuse atrophy of skeletal muscle: animal models, *Exerc Sport Sci Rev* 16:61-87, 1988.
103. Lieber RL et al: Growth hormone secretagogue increases muscle strength during remobilization after canine hindlimb immobilization, *J Orthop Res* 15:519-527, 1997.
104. Lieber RL, McKee WT, Gershuni DH: Recovery of the dog quadriceps after 10 weeks of immobilization followed by 4 weeks of remobilization, *J Orthop Res* 7:408-412, 1989.
105. Horl M et al: Carbohydrate metabolism of dog skeletal muscle during immobilization, *Res Exp Med* 187:81-85, 1987.
106. Sen CK et al: Skeletal muscle and liver glutathione homeostasis in response to training, exercise, and immobilization, *J Appl Physiol* 73:265-1272, 1992.
107. Gibson JN et al: Decrease in human quadriceps muscle protein turnover consequent upon leg immobilization, *Clin Sci* 72:503-509, 1987.
108. DeMartino GN, Ordway GA: Ubiquitin-proteasome pathway of intracellular protein degradation: implications for muscle atrophy during unloading, *Exerc Sport Sci Rev* 26:219-252.
109. Fung DL et al: The changing pharmacodynamics of metocurine identify the onset and offset of canine gastrocnemius disuse atrophy, *Anesthesiology* 83:134-140, 1995.
110. Fung DL et al: The onset of disuse-related potassium efflux to succinylcholine, *Anesthesiology* 75:650-653, 1991.
111. Gronert GA et al: Deep sedation and mechanical ventilation without paralysis for 3 weeks in normal beagles: exaggerated resistance to metocurine in gastrocnemius muscle, *Anesthesiology* 90:1741-1745, 1999.
112. Kvist M et al: Vascular density at the myotendinous junction of the rat gastrocnemius muscle after immobilization and remobilization. *Am J Sports Med* 23:359-364, 1995.
113. Bebout DE et al: Effects of training and immobilization on Vo$_2$ and Do$_2$ in dog gastrocnemius muscle in situ, *J Appl Physiol* 74:1697-1703, 1993.
114. Jebens E et al: Changes in Na$^+$,K($^+$)-adenosine-triphosphatase, citrate synthase and K$^+$ in sheep skeletal muscle during immobilization and remobilization, *Eur J Appl Physiol* 71:386-395, 1995.
115. LeBlanc A et al: Bone and muscle atrophy with suspension of the rat, *J Appl Physiol* 58:1669-1675, 1985.
116. Heerkens YF et al: Passive resistance of the human knee: the effect of remobilization, *J Biomed Eng* 9: 69-76, 1987.
117. LeBlanc A et al: Regional muscle loss after short duration spaceflight, *Aviat Space Environ Med* 66:1151-1154, 1995.
118. Morrissey MC: Reflex inhibition of thigh muscles in knee injury: causes and treatment, *Sports Med* 7:263-276, 1989.
119. Gordon T, Mao J: Muscle atrophy and procedures for training after spinal cord injury, *Phys Ther* 74:50-60, 1994.
120. Hagerty R, Bostwick J, Nahai F: Denervated muscle flaps: mass and thickness changes following denervation, *Ann Plast Surg* 12:171-176, 1984.
121. Williams HB: The value of continuous electrical muscle stimulation using a completely implantable system in the preservation of muscle function following motor nerve injury and repair: an experimental study, *Microsurgery* 17:589-596, 1996.
122. Braund KG, Shores A, Brawner WRJ: Recovering from spinal cord trauma: the rehabilitative steps, complications, and prognosis, *Vet Med* 85:740-744, 1990.
123. Orima H, Fujita M: Computed tomographic findings of experimentally induced neurogenic muscular atrophy in dogs, *J Vet Med Sci* 59:729-731, 1997.
124. Begum SJ et al: Skeletal muscle protein metabolism under denervation atrophy in dog, *Canis domesticus, Indian J Physiol Pharmacol* 30:341-346, 1986.
125. Reddy KV et al: Induced muscular work overload and disuse on the serum carbohydrate metabolism of dog, *Canis domesticus, Arch Int Physiol Biochim* 91:411-416, 1983.
126. Fry TR, Clark DM: Canine hip dysplasia: clinical signs and physical diagnosis, *Vet Clin North Am Small Anim Pract* 22:551-558, 1992.
127. Duff R, Campbell JR: Long term results of excision arthroplasty of the canine hip, *Vet Rec* 101:181-184, 1977.
128. Piek CJ et al: Long-term follow-up of avascular necrosis of the femoral head in the dog, *J Small Anim Pract* 37:12-18, 1996.
129. Innes JF, Barr AR: Clinical natural history of the postsurgical cruciate deficient canine stifle joint: year 1, *J Small Anim Pract* 39:325-332, 1998.
130. Millis DL et al: Changes in muscle mass following transection of the cranial cruciate ligament and immediate stifle stabilization, *Proc 27th Ann Conf Vet Orthop Soc* 2000, p 3.
131. Ross M, Worrell TW: Thigh and calf girth following knee injury and surgery, *J Orthop Sports Phys Ther* 27:9-15, 1998.
132. Soderberg GL, Ballantyne BT, Kestel LL: Reliability of lower extremity girth measurements after anterior cruciate ligament reconstruction, *Physiother Res Int* 1:7-16, 1996.
133. Fink C et al: Neuro-muscular changes following ACL-injury, *Hungarian Rev Sports Med* 34:89-98, 1993.

134. Arangio GA et al: Thigh muscle size and strength after anterior cruciate ligament reconstruction and rehabilitation, *J Orthop Sports Phys Ther* 26:238-243, 1997.

135. Kannus P, Jarvinen M: Thigh muscle function after partial tear of the medial ligament compartment of the knee, *Med Sci Sports Exerc* 23:4-9, 1991.

136. van Lent MET, Drost MR, Wildenberg FAJMvd: EMG profiles of ACL-deficient patients during walking: the influence of mild fatigue, *Int J Sports Med* 15: 508-514, 1994.

137. Kannus P, Jarvinen M: Nonoperative treatment of acute knee ligament injuries: a review with special reference to indications and methods, *Sports Med* 9:244-260, 1990.

138. Braund KG, Shires PK, Mikeal RL: Type I fiber atrophy in the vastus lateralis muscle in dogs with femoral fractures treated by hyperextension, *Vet Pathol* 17:164-176, 1980.

139. Shires PK, Braund KG, Milton JL, et al: Effect of localized trauma and temporary splinting on immature skeletal muscle and mobility of the femorotibial joint in the dog, *Am J Vet Res* 43: 454-460, 1982.

140. Hayes KW, Falconer J: Differential muscle strength decline in osteoarthritis of the knee: a developing hypothesis, *Arthritis Care Res* 5:24-28, 1992.

141. Hall KD, Hayes KW, Falconer J: Differential strength decline in patients with osteoarthritis of the knee: revision of a hypothesis, *Arthritis Care Res* 6:89-96, 1993.

142. Lindehammar H, Sandstedt P: Measurement of quadriceps muscle strength and bulk in juvenile chronic arthritis: a prospective, longitudinal, 2 year survey, *J Rheumatol* 25:2240-2248, 1998.

143. Kannus P et al: Effects of immobilization and subsequent low- and high-intensity exercise on morphology of rat calf muscles, *Scan J Med Sci Sports* 8:160-171, 1998.

144. Kannus P et al: Free mobilization and low- and high-intensity exercise in immobilization-induced muscle atrophy, *J Appl Physiol* 84:1418-1424, 1998.

145. Hoppeler H: Exercise-induced ultrastructural changes in skeletal muscle, *Int J Sports Med* 7:187-204, 1986.

146. Puustjarvi K et al: Running training alters fiber type composition in spinal muscles, *Eur Spine J* 3:17-21, 1994.

147. Arokoski J et al: Effects of aerobic long distance running training (up to 40 km.day^{-1}) of 1-year duration on blood and endocrine parameters of female beagle dogs, *Eur J Appl Physiol* 67:321-329, 1993.

148. Gonyea WJ: Muscle fiber splitting in trained and untrained animals, *Exerc Sport Sci Rev* 8:19-39, 1980.

149. Luthi JM et al: Structural changes in skeletal muscle tissue with heavy-resistance exercise, *Int J Sports Med* 7:123-127, 1986.

150. Staron RS et al: Muscle hypertrophy and fast fiber type conversions in heavy resistance-trained women, *Eur J Appl Physiol* 60:71-79, 1989.

151. Gonyea WJ, Ericson GC: An experimental model for the study of exercise-induced skeletal muscle hypertrophy, *J Appl Physiol* 40:630-633, 1976.

152. Hickson RC, Rosenkoetter MA, Brown MM: Strength training effects on aerobic power and short-term endurance, *Med Sci Sports Exerc* 12:336-339, 1980.

153. Hickson RC et al: Potential for strength and endurance training to amplify endurance performance, *J Appl Physiol* 65:2285-2290, 1988.

154. Caggiano E et al: Effects of electrical stimulation or voluntary contraction for strengthening the quadriceps femoris muscles in an aged male population, *J Orthop Sports Phys Ther* 20:22-28, 1994.

155. Balon TW, Horowitz JF, Fitzsimmons KM: Effects of carbohydrate loading and weight-lifting on muscle girth, *Int J Sports Nutr* 2:328-334, 1992.

156. Mikesky AE et al: Sexually dimorphic response in weight lifting cats, *Med Sci Sports Exerc* 18:566, 1986

157. Cureton KJ et al: Muscle hypertrophy in men and women, *Med Sci Sports Exerc* 20:338-344, 1988.

158. Greene CE et al: Myopathy associated with hyperadrenocorticism in the dog, *J Am Vet Med Assoc* 174:1310-1315, 1979.

159. Hickson RC, Marone JR: Exercise and inhibition of glucocorticoid-induced muscle atrophy, *Exerc Sport Sci Rev* 21:135-167, 1993.

160. Ferreira IM et al: The influence of 6 months of oral anabolic steroids on body mass and respiratory muscles in undernourished COPD patients, *Chest* 114:19-28, 1998.

161. Reynolds JF et al: Non-steroidal anti-inflammatory drugs fail to enhance healing of acute hamstring injuries treated with physiotherapy, *S Afr Med J* 85:517-522, 1995.

162. Yarasheski KE: Growth hormone effects on metabolism, body composition, muscle mass, and strength, *Exerc Sport Sci Rev* 22:285-312, 1994.

163. Adams GR: Role of insulin-like growth factor-I in the regulation of skeletal muscle adaptation to increased loading, *Exerc Sport Sci Rev* 26:31-60, 1998.

164. Kanaley JA et al: Human growth hormone response to repeated bouts of aerobic exercise, *J Appl Physiol* 83:1756-1761, 1997.

165. Eyre DR, Oguchi H: Collagens: their measurement, properties, and a proposed pathway of formation, *Biophys Res Commun* 92:403-407, 1980.

166. Loitz BJ, Frank CB: Biology and mechanics of ligament and ligament healing, *Exerc Sport Sci Rev* 21:33-64, 1993.

167. Noyes FR, DeLucas JL, Torvik PJ: Biomechanics of anterior cruciate ligament failure: an analysis of strain-rate sensitivity and mechanisms of failure in primates, *J Bone Joint Surg* 56A:236-253, 1974.

168. Noyes FR et al: Advances in the understanding of knee ligament injury, repair, and rehabilitation, *Med Sci Sports Exerc* 16:427-443, 1984.

169. Ruffoli R et al: Mechanoreceptors in the posterior cruciate and lateral collateral ligaments of the human knee, and the lateral collateral ligament of the canine knee, *J Sports Trauma Rel Res* 18:113-122, 1996.

170. Bodtker S et al: Blood flow of the anterior and posterior cruciate ligament in a canine model, *Scand J Med Sci Sports* 4:145-147, 1994.

171. Dunlap J et al: Quantification of the perfusion of the anterior cruciate ligament and the effects of stress and injury to suporting structures, *Am J Sports Med* 17:808-810, 1989.

172. Butler DL et al: On the interpretation of our anterior cruciate ligament data, *Clin Orthop* 196:26-34, 1985.

173. Yasuda K, Hayashi K: Changes in biomechanical properties of tendons and ligaments from joint disuse, *Osteoarthr Cartilage* 7:122-129, 1999.

174. Laros GS, Tipton CM, Cooper RR: Influence of physical activity on ligament insertions in the knees of dogs. *J Bone Joint Surg* 53A:275-286, 1971.

175. Noyes FR et al: Biomechanics of ligament failure. II. An analysis of immobilization, exercise, and reconditioning effects in primates, *J Bone Joint Surg* 56A:1406-1418, 1974.

176. Noyes FR: Functional properties of knee ligaments and alterations induced by immobilization: a correlative biomechanical and histological study in primates, *Clin Orthop* 210-242, 1977.

177. Bahniuk E: The effects of the tibial femoral angle and of disuse on the strength of canine anterior cruciate ligaments, *Bull Hosp Jt Dis Orthop Inst* 46:185-192, 1986.

178. Tipton CM et al: Influence of exercise on the strength of the medial collateral knee ligaments of dogs, *Am J Physiol* 218:894-901, 1970.

179. Keira M et al: Mechanical properties of the anterior cruciate ligament chronically relaxed by elevation of the tibial insertion, *J Orthop Res* 14:157-166, 1996.

180. Woo SL et al: The biomechanical and morphological changes in the medial collateral ligament of the rabbit after immobilization and remobilization, *J Bone Joint Surg* 69A:1200-1211, 1987.

181. Newton PO et al: Immobilization of the knee joint alters the mechanical and ultrastructural properties of the rabbit anterior cruciate ligament, *J Bone Joint Surg* 13A:191-200, 1995.

182. Vailas AC et al: Physical activity and hypophysectomy on the aerobic capacity of ligaments and tendons, *J Appl Physiol* 44:542-546, 1978.

183. Montgomery RD: Healing of muscle, ligaments, and tendons, *Semin Vet Med Surg Small Anim* 4:304-311, 1989.

184. Aoki M et al: Biomechanical and histologic characteristics of canine flexor tendon repair using early postoperative mobilization, *J Hand Surg Am* 22:107-114, 1997.

185. Woo SL et al: New experimental procedures to evaluate the biomechanical properties of healing canine medial collateral ligaments, *J Orthop Res* 5:425-432, 1987.

186. Woo S et al: Treatment of the medial collateral ligament injury. II. Structure and function of canine knees in response to differing treatment regimens, *Am J Sports Med* 15:22-29, 1987.

187. Piper TL, Whiteside LA: Early mobilization after knee ligament repair in dogs: an experimental study, *Clin Orthop* 150:277-282, 1980.

188. Inoue M et al: Treatment of the medial collateral ligament injury. I. The importance of anterior cruciate ligament on the varus-valgus knee laxity, *Am J Sports Med* 15:15-21, 1987.

189. O'Donoghue DH et al: Repair of knee ligaments in dogs. I. The lateral collateral ligament, *J Bone Joint Surg* 43A:1167-1178, 1961.

190. O'Donoghue DH et al: Repair and reconstruction of the anterior cruciate ligament in dogs, *J Bone Joint Surg* 53A:710-718, 1971.

191. Ogata K, Whiteside LA, Andersen DA: The intra-articular effect of various postoperative managements following knee ligament repair: an experimental study in dogs, *Clin Orthop* 150:271-276, 1980.

192. Barber-Westin SD, Noyes FR: The effect of rehabilitation and return to activity on anterior-posterior knee displacements after anterior cruciate ligament reconstruction, *Am J Sports Med* 21:264-270, 1993.

193. Gelberman RH, Woo SLY, Lothringer K: Effects of early intermittent passive immobilization on healing canine flexor tendons, *J Hand Surg* 7A:170-175, 1982.

194. Silva MJ et al: Effect of increased tendon excursion in vivo on the biomechanical properties of healing flexor tendons. In Anaheim, CA, 1999, *Proceedings of the 45th Annual Meeting*, Orthopaedic Research Society, p. 68.

195. Silva MJ et al: Effects of increased in vivo excursion on digital range of motion and tendon strength following flexor tendon repair, *J Orthop Res* 17:777-783, 1999.

196. Gelberman RH et al: The effect of gap formation at the repair site on the strength and excursion of intrasynovial flexor tendons: an experimental study on the early stages of tendon-healing in dogs, *J Bone Joint Surg* 81A:975-982, 1999.

197. Takai S et al: The effects of frequency and duration of controlled passive mobilization on tendon healing, *J Orthop Res* 9:705-713, 1991.

198. Gelberman RH et al: Healing of digital flexor tendons: importance of the interval from injury to repair, *J Bone Joint Surg* 73A:66-75, 1991.

199. Grewal R et al: Passive and active rehabilitation for partial lacerations of the canine flexor digitorum profundus tendon in zone II, *J Hand Surg* 24A:743-750, 1999.

200. Butler DL et al: Mechanical properties of primate vascularized vs. nonvascularized patellar tendon grafts; changes over time, *J Orthop Res* 7:68-79, 1989.

201. Kannus P et al: Effects of training, immobilization and remobilization on tendons, *Scan J Med Sci Sports* 7:67-71, 1997.

202. Butler DL et al: Biomechanics of ligaments and tendons, *Exerc Sport Sci Rev* 6:125-181, 1978.

203. Cherdchutham W et al: Effects of exercise on biomechanical properties of the superficial digital flexor tendon in foals, *Am J Vet Res* 62:1859-1864, 2001.

204. Tipton CM et al: The influence of physical activity on ligaments and tendons, *Med Sci Sports* 7:165-175, 1975.

205. Jarvinen TAH et al: Mechanical loading regulates tenascin-C expression in the osteotendinous junction, *J Cell Sci* 112:3157-3166, 1999.

206. Viidik A: Simultaneous mechanical and light microscopic studies of collagen fibers, *Z Anat Entwicklungsesch* 136:204-212, 1972.

207. Noyes FR et al: Effect of intra-articular corticosteroids on ligament properties: a biomechanical and histological study in rhesus knees, *Clin Orthop* 123:197-209, 1977.

208. Fredberg U: Local corticosteroid injection in sport: review of literature and guidelines for treatment, *Scand J Med Sci Sports* 7:131-139, 1997.

209. Seneviratne AM et al: The effect of corticosteroid induced osteoporosis on tendon insertion sites in a rabbit model. In Anaheim, CA, 1999, *Proceedings of the 45th Annual Meeting*, Orthopaedic Research Society, p. 68.

210. Albrechtsen SJ, Harvey JS: Dimethyl sulfoxide. Biomechanical effects on tendons, *Am J Sports Med* 10:177-179, 1982.

211. Williams RJ et al: The effect of ciprofloxacin on tendon, paratenon, and capsular fibroblast metabolism, *Am J Sports Med* 28:364-369, 2000.

212. Rodeo SA et al: Use of recombinant human bone morphogenetic protein-2 to enhance tendon healing in a bone tunnel. *Am J Sports Med* 27:476-488, 1999.

213. Grynpas MD et al: The effect of pamidronate in a new model of immobilization in the dog, *Bone* 17:225S-232S, 1995.

214. Waters DJ, Caywood DD, Turner RT: Effect of tamoxifen citrate on canine immobilization (disuse) osteoporosis, *Vet Surg* 20:392-396, 1991.

215. Sievanen H, Kannus P, Jarvinen TLN: Immobilization distorts allometry of rat femur: implications for disuse osteoporosis, *Calcif Tissue Int* 60:387-390, 1997.

216. Jee WS, Ma Y: Animal models of immobilization osteopenia. *Morphologie* 83:25-34, 1999.
217. Marotti G et al: Quantitative analysis of the bone destroying activity of osteocytes and osteoclasts in experimental disuse osteoporosis, *Ital J Orthop Traumatol* 5:225-240, 1979.
218. Uhthoff HK, Jaworski ZF: Periosteal stress-induced reactions resembling stress fractures: a radiologic and histologic study in dogs, *Clin Orthop* 199:284-291, 1985.
219. Uhthoff HK, Jaworski ZF: Bone loss in response to long-term immobilisation, *J Bone Joint Surg* 60B:420-429, 1978.
220. Waters DJ et al: Immobilization increases bone prostaglandin E: effect of acetylsalicylic acid on disuse osteoporosis studied in dogs, *Acta Orthop Scand* 62:238-243, 1991.
221. Uhthoff HK, Sekaly G, Jaworski ZF: Effect of long-term nontraumatic immobilization on metaphyseal spongiosa in young adult and old beagle dogs, *Clin Orthop* 192:278-284, 1985.
222. Li G, Patrick J: Blood flow in canine long bones using the radioactive labeled microsphere method, *Chinese J Sports Med* 6:209-212, 1987.
223. Schaffler MB et al: Alterations of bone tissue mechanical properties with immobilization, *Proc Orthop Res Soc* 40:31-36, 1994.[KL1]
224. Goethgen CB and others: Changes in tibial bone mass after primary cementless and revision cementless total hip arthroplasty in canine models, *J Orthop RES* 9:820-827, 1991.
225. Boyd SK et al: Changes in femoral bone mineral density in ACL deficient dogs using quantitative computed tomography. In *Proceedings of the Third North American Congress on Biomechanics*, 1998, Canadian Society for Biomechanics, American Society of Biomechanics.
226. Carter DR, Vasu R, Harris WH: The plated femur: relationships between the changes in bone stresses and bone loss, *Acta Orthop Scand* 52:241-248, 1981.
227. Leppala J et al: Effect of anterior cruciate ligament injury of the knee on bone mineral density of the spine and affected lower extremity: a prospective one-year follow-up study, *Calcif Tissue Int* 64:357-363, 1999.
228. Kannus P et al: A cruciate ligament injury produces considerable, permanent osteoporosis in the affected knee, *J Bone Miner Res* 7:1429-1434, 1992.
229. Kannus P et al: Reduced bone-mineral density in men with a previous femur fracture, *J Bone Miner Res* 9:1729-1736, 1994.
230. Kannus P et al: Osteoporosis in men with a history of tibial fracture, *J Bone Miner Res* 9:423-429, 1994.
231. Allison N, Brooks B: Bone atrophy. *Surg Gynecol Obstet* 33:250-260, 1921.
232. Turbes CC: Repair, reconstruction, regeneration and rehabilitation strategies to spinal cord injury, *Biomed Sci Instrum* 34:351-356, 1997.
233. Rodgers MM et al: Musculoskeletal responses of spinal cord injured individuals to functional neuromuscular stimulation-induced knee extension exercise training, *J Rehabil Res Dev* 28:19-26. 1991.
234. Stromberg L, Dalen N: Atrophy of cortical bone caused by rigid internal fixation plates. An experimental study in the dog, *Acta Orthop Scand* 49:448-456, 1978.
235. Woo SL et al: A comparison of cortical bone atrophy secondary to fixation with plates with large differences in bending stiffness, *J Bone Joint Surg* 58A:190-195, 1976.

236. Ferguson SJ, Wyss UP, Pichora DR: Finite element stress analysis of a hybrid fracture fixation plate, *Med Eng Phys* 18:241-250, 1996.
237. Liu JG, Xu XX: Stress shielding and fracture healing, *Zhonghua Yi Xue Za Zhi* 74:483-485, 1994.
238. Xu XX, Zhao YH, Liu JG: Blood supply and structural changes of canine intact tibia following plate fixation with different rigidities, *Chinese Med J* 104:1018-1021, 1991.
239. Sumner DR, Galante JO: Determinants of stress shielding: design versus materials versus interface, *Clin Orthop* 274:202-212, 1992.
240. Ijiri K et al: Remobilization partially restored the bone mass in a non-growing cancellous bone site following long term immobilization, *Bone* 17:213S-217S, 1995.
241. Kannus P et al: Effects of immobilization, three forms of remobilization, and subsequent deconditioning on bone mineral content and density in rat femora, *J Bone Miner Res* 11:1339-1346, 1996.
242. Kannus P et al: Effects of free mobilization and low-intensity to high-intensity treadmill running on the immobilization-induced bone loss in rats, *J Bone Miner Res* 9:1613-1619, 1994.
243. Kannus P et al: Expression of osteocalcin in the patella of experimentally immobilized and remobilized rats, *J Bone Miner Res* 11:79-87, 1996.
244. Smith EL, Gilligan C: Dose-response relationship between physical loading and mechanical competence of bone, *Bone* 18:45S-50S, 1996.
245. Kannus P, Sievanen H, Vuori I: Physical loading, exercise, and bone, *Bone* 18:1S-3S, 1996.
246. Westerlind KC et al: Effect of resistance exercise training on cortical and cancellous bone in mature male rats, *J Appl Physiol* 84:459-464, 1998.
247. Jarvinen TLN et al: Randomized controlled study of the effects of sudden impact loading on rat femur, *J Bone Miner Res* 13:1475-1482, 1998.
248. Millis DL et al: The effects of canine recombinant somatotropin on skeletal tissues in an unstable fracture gap model, *Vet Surg* 27:513, 1998.
249. Martin RK et al: Load-carrying effects on the adult beagle tibia, *Med Sci Sports Exerc* 13:343-349, 1981.
250. Puustjarvi K et al: Long-distance running alters bone anthropometry, elemental composition and mineral density of young dogs, *Scand J Med Sci Sports* 5:17-23, 1995.
251. Johnson KA, Skinner GA, Muir P: Site-specific adaptive remodeling of Greyhound metacarpal cortical bone subjected to asymmetrical cyclic loading, *Am J Vet Res* 62:787-793, 2001.
252. Fedle JM et al: Local skeletal effects of a lifetime of physical activity in the beagle: metacarpals and metatarsals. In *Transactions of the 37th Annual Meeting, Orthopaedic Research Society*, vol 16, p 428, 1991.
253. Liu CH, McCay CM: Studies of calcium metabolism in dogs, *J Gerontol* 8:264-271, 1953.
254. Meadows TH et al: Effect of weight-bearing on healing of cortical defects in the canine tibia, *J Bone Joint Surg* 72A:1074-1080, 1990.
255. Heikkinen E, Vihersaari T, Penttinen R: Effect of previous exercise on fracture healing: a biochemical study with mice, *Acta Orthop Scand* 45:481-489, 1974.
256. Caywood et al: Effects of 1 alpha,25-dihydroxy-cholecalciferol on disuse osteoporosis in the dog: a histomorphometric study, *Am J Vet Res* 40:89-91, 1979.
257. Nakamura T et al: Regulation of bone turnover and prevention of bone atrophy in ovariectomized beagle dogs by the administration of 24R,25(OH)2D3. *Calcif Tissue Int* 50:221-227, 1992.

Exercise Physiology

Robert Gillette

A good basic knowledge of exercise physiology is necessary when designing and implementing a rehabilitation or conditioning program. The definition of *training,* for the purposes of this chapter, refers to working with the dog in an obedience training program that addresses behavioral aspects, whereas *conditioning* refers to an exercise or workout program that addresses physiologic aspects. Exercise physiology is a discipline that examines how exercise affects the body and is very applicable in the field of physical rehabilitation.

The level of conditioning of a dog is constantly changing, and at any time the body performs at a specific metabolic level. The systems of the body are conditioned to maintain homeostasis at this level. If the demands placed on the body increase over time, the body adapts and conditions itself to maintain homeostasis at this new level. An understanding of the physiologic changes involved in this process helps in the development of programs that allow regulation of the conditioning or reconditioning of the body. These programs may be used to condition the entire body or to focus on individual body segments. In physical rehabilitation, programs may be developed to treat injuries, to stimulate healing of the injuries, and to enhance reconditioning of the injured segment. Because of the biomechanical forces acting on the body during the reparative phases of healing, certain segments may become stronger than other segments. Exercise programs should be implemented to remedy any conditioning imbalances of the body. The basic goals should be to allow the tissues to heal, then to recondition the tissues so that they can accept predetermined workloads, and finally to recondition the entire body to balance any conditioning deficits.

Muscle Physiology

Muscle is a tissue greatly affected by exercise or disuse associated with injury. Understanding muscle function and the molecular events of muscle contraction provides a basis for the concepts of physical rehabilitation and exercise physiology. There are three types of muscle in the body: skeletal, smooth, and cardiac. This chapter will focus on skeletal muscle. Skeletal muscles connect one bone to another. Each muscle consists of thousands of myocytes. A muscle fiber is long, fusiform, and surrounded by a plasma membrane called the sarcolemma. Inside these fibers are myofibrils, which consist of filaments composed of contractile proteins. These contractile proteins are arranged in units called sarcomeres.

Actin and myosin are two types of protein chains in the sarcomere. They interact as a result of enzymatic and chemical reactions to produce muscle contraction. Calcium and phosphate are chemical components involved with the production of muscle contractions. Phosphate is in the form of adenosine triphosphate (ATP). ATP is located at the end of the myosin leverage arm. The actin filament includes troponin, which is bound to strands of tropomyosin. A calcium ion attaches to the troponin molecule, which changes the shape of the tropomyosin. This action opens a receptor site on the actin protein chain. Energy is emitted when ATP releases a phosphate ion, producing adenosine diphosphate (ADP). The resultant energy allows the ADP to create a bond between the open actin receptor site and the myosin leverage arm. This bond changes the myosin structure, allowing leverage to produce a contraction between the two fibers. The ADP is released and the lever arm is freed

Thin Filament

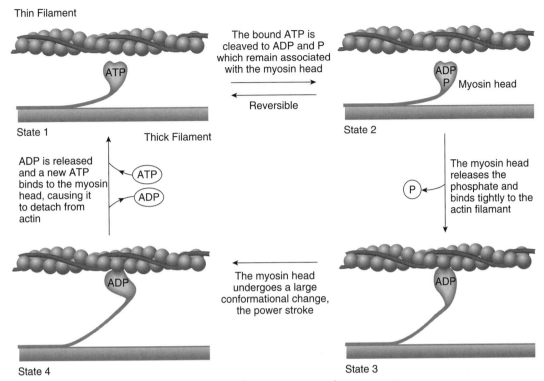

Figure 8-1   Actin and myosin interaction during contraction.

to reattach. Energy is then required to add a phosphate group to the ADP, recreating ATP, which is then used for further contractions (Figure 8-1).

Muscle Structure and Function

The accumulated contractions of the muscle fibers create contraction of an entire muscle. The innervation to a muscle controls the muscle contraction. A single motor nerve diverges to innervate many muscle fibers. The combination of a nerve and the muscle fiber it innervates is called a motor unit. Contraction of an entire muscle is a result of the cumulative contraction of many motor units. The muscle fibers are grouped together and organized with other fibers by a sheath of connective tissue that is named according to its level of organization. Endomysium covers each of the muscle fibers themselves, while perimysium separates discrete bundles of fibers. Epimysium is the connective tissue layer that surrounds the grouped bundles. Muscle fascia is the sheath that covers the epimysium and serves to protect each muscle from movement over hard structures or movement from adja-

cent muscles. The arrangement of these fibers plays a role in the function of each muscle. It is the combination of motor unit group and fiber arrangement that dictates the resultant type of muscular contraction.

In general, muscle contraction and work are transferred through the tendon and its attachment to a bone. The musculotendinous junction is a layered transition between muscle fibers and the collagen of the tendons. Tendons of origin and insertion may run throughout the length of the structure. Musculotendinous structures are closely tied to functional requirements. Structural shapes of muscle include fusiform and pennate forms. Pennate muscles may be divided into unipennate, bipennate, and multipennate forms. Pennate structures allow a muscle to lift great loads but through a small range of motion, such as in vertebrae. Fusiform structures have the ability to lift a small load at a great velocity through a large range of motion. These types of muscles include the biceps brachii and brachialis muscles in the antebrachium. These two forms of muscle shapes can work together if both strength and speed of movement are needed in a particular joint, such as the shoulder or hip joint.

Muscle Energy Systems

Muscles require energy to maintain basal metabolism, and additional energy during physical activity. The body uses three systems to provide this energy: (1) immediate energy sources, (2) glycolytic metabolism, and (3) oxidative metabolism. The type of activity the muscle is performing defines which of the systems will be used. The cellular environment must also be conducive to these processes. Factors affecting the cellular environment include pH, hydration status, temperature, and presence of the proper enzymes. Changes in any of these factors may alter the reactions needed for energy production. While energy production is occurring, waste products are simultaneously produced. Waste product removal is essential, because local accumulation of these substances alters the cellular environment.

The immediate energy source involves intracellular ATP, creatine phosphate (CP), and the ADP/myokinase reaction to provide energy for activity. Intracellular ATP is the first energy source used for contraction. A limited amount of ATP is stored at the myosin cross-bridges, near mitochondria, and beneath sarcolemma. ATP breakdown is a hydrolytic reaction and is highly regulated. The body does not allow large changes in ATP content. Creatine phosphate is a high-energy compound that is used to ensure that the ATP concentration does not become depleted. It is located near the actin-myosin filaments and in the mitochondrial membrane. The CP molecule donates a phosphate group to replenish the ATP used at the contraction site. The third immediate energy source comes from the myokinase reaction. Myokinase is the enzyme that allows two ADP molecules to combine to form ATP and adenosine monophosphate (AMP). This reaction provides little energy to the system, but AMP serves as one of the allosteric modulators to stimulate carbohydrate (glucose) breakdown in glycolytic metabolism. Energy from this system lasts anywhere from 5 to 10 seconds with high-intensity exercise and occasionally up to 20 seconds in some elite athletes.

The glycolytic pathway provides energy from 5 to 20 seconds up to 2 minutes as a result of the anaerobic breakdown of glucose. This is a more complex form of energy production, using multiple enzymes and reactions. In the first phase of glycolysis, a glucose molecule enters the cell where the enzyme hexokinase adds a phosphate group to the glucose molecule, which creates glucose 6-phosphate (G6P). G6P then enters a series of reactions to produce fructose 1,6-biphosphate. One of the reactions involves the enzyme phosphofructokinase, which adds another phosphate to the molecule. As a result, two ATP molecules are used in phase 1. In the first reaction of the second phase of the glycolytic pathway, fructose 1,6-biphosphate is converted into two three-carbon molecules. Glyceraldehyde 3-phosphate is then phosphorylated and oxidized, which releases two hydrogen molecules and two electrons. The two electrons and one hydrogen molecule combine with nicotinamide adenine dinucleotide (NAD$^-$) to form NADH, which can be used in oxidative metabolism. The four remaining reactions of phase 2 result in the production of two ATPs. Combined with two ATPs from the other three-carbon chain, this results in a total of four ATPs produced in phase 2. The end result of the glycolytic pathway is the production of pyruvate and two ATPs that may be used as energy (Figure 8-2).

If the pyruvate is not able to enter the oxidative energy system, it combines with NADH via the enzyme lactodehydrogenase (LDH) to produce lactic acid. When released into an environment with physiologic pH, lactic acid releases a proton and becomes lactate. Without a buffer, lactate production results in a decrease in cellular pH. Lactate production in itself is not necessarily detrimental to muscle metabolism. After bouts of intense exercise, lactate is oxidized back to pyruvate, which can be converted to glucose in the liver, or converted to pyruvate in muscle and other tissues for ATP production. Lactate concentrations coincide with the release of a proton and potential decreases in pH. It is this decrease in cell and blood pH that has detrimental effects on energy metabolism and enzyme activity.

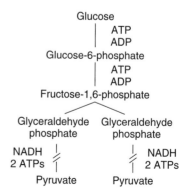

Figure 8-2 Glycolytic pathway with production of pyruvate and ATP.

Therefore, although associated with the release of protons, the lactate itself is not a problem, but the associated acidosis is.

The third energy source comes from oxidative metabolism, which predominate about 2 minutes after the beginning of exercise. It is the most complicated energy system and uses glycolysis, the citric acid cycle, and the electron transport chain. Each of these are complex multiple reaction cascades that result in the production of ATP and energy. Carbohydrates, lipids, and proteins are used as energy sources, and this is the system that is used to the greatest extent during long-term activity. Pyruvate is converted to acetyl-CoA by the enzyme pyruvate dehydrogenase, which also produces carbon dioxide and NADH. Free fatty acids are converted to acetyl-CoA by a process called β-oxidation. The resultant acetyl-CoA then enters the citric acid cycle. The products of this cycle are carbon dioxide, ATP, NADH, and FADH.

The use of oxygen occurs in the electron transport chain. The electrons acquired in NADH and FADH are added to hydrogen atoms and oxygen atoms to form water, along with energy to create ATP from ADP. The last electron receiver in the chain is oxygen. This process is termed oxidative phosphorylation. Three ATPs are produced for each NADH molecule, and two for each FADH molecule. If oxygen is not present to receive the electrons that flow down the chain, the chain stops, and the result is an accumulation of the components of the electron transport chain and the systems that produce them, halting energy production.

In a rehabilitation program, the conditioning program places energy demands on the muscles. The energy systems used depend on the forces required by the program and the duration of the workout. If the energy systems are insufficient to meet the demands required, the program will not benefit the patient and may actually harm the rehabilitative process. An understanding of muscle physiology will help in designing a conditioning program that is beneficial to the patient.

Musculoskeletal Conditioning

When the body performs at a level greater than its normal daily routine, there is a greater demand for energy. The systems must work together to provide energy to the areas of need, and at the same time maintain homeostasis. Therefore the fuel resources must be sufficient to meet this demand and be available to the body. In other words, energy must be stored in the body to perform physical activity, and the body's energy systems must be conditioned to efficiently produce, transport, and use this energy in the location where it is required. Homeostatic metabolism is associated with normal daily needs and allows the body to function properly throughout the day. If a short-term stress is placed on the system, the body is able to adapt, within reason, to meet this altered demand. If the stress is repeated on a daily basis, the daily routine is altered and the energy systems are conditioned to meet these new demands. Workout repetition results in adaptation to meet these demands, including pooling energy sources at the location of greatest need (e.g., intracellular ATP, CP, and glucose). The concentrations of enzymes required by the specific energy systems used the most may also increase. Workout repetition conditions the body to the stresses of the new demands and minimizes the chances of systemic or cellular injury.

The muscle response to different types of conditioning programs is determined by the muscle fiber type. The fiber types are divided into type I (slow-twitch) and type II (fast-twitch) muscle fibers. Type I muscle fibers are fatigue resistant, use aerobic metabolism, and have a low contractile force and less ATPase activity. Type II fibers are subdivided by their metabolic characteristics: type IIa (oxidative) and type II Dog (glycolytic) fibers. Type IIa muscle fibers use both the oxidative energy system (aerobic metabolism) and the glycolytic energy system (anaerobic metabolism). They may be trained to use one system preferentially according to the demands placed on them. Type IIb fibers primarily use the glycolytic system (anaerobic metabolism), although there is some disagreement over whether dogs have true type IIb muscle fibers as compared with other species.[1-3] These fibers are generally termed type II Dog. Some change in muscle fiber composition may occur with exercise and conditioning.[4]

How a dog responds to a conditioning program may be affected by its fiber type composition. The type I/type II ratio of the muscle fiber types in a particular muscle is genetically predetermined, although some change in muscle fiber composition may occur with specific conditioning.[5] Greyhounds bred for sprint activity tend to have a greater percentage of type II fibers than other breeds, whereas Foxhounds, which are bred for endurance, have a greater percentage of type I fibers.

In addition to genetic determination, the distribution of fiber types throughout the body and within individual muscles depends on the muscle's function. A higher percentage of type I fibers populate the deeper muscles, while a higher percentage of type II fibers are present in the more superficial muscles.[6] The deeper muscles are associated with postural activity, while the more superficial muscles are used in movement. Altering the muscle function can change the fiber type. Muscle fiber type changes have been produced by tenotomy, tendon transfers,[7] and altered training.[8] Knowing the breed of dog and the anatomical area of focus will help determine the type of conditioning program that will be most beneficial for the patient.

There are two general categories of conditioning programs: strength/power programs and endurance programs. In human exercise physiology, endurance events usually last longer than 2 to 4 minutes and are performed at intensities $\leq 90\%$ of maximal aerobic power (VO_{2max}). Strength/power events are of short duration (<2 minutes) and are performed at intensities that are maximal or supramaximal.[9] The metabolic changes that occur during a conditioning program depend on the principles of intensity, duration, frequency, and method of training. The program should incorporate these principles to result in proper system and organ adaptation. Central and peripheral physiological changes occur as a result of conditioning. Central changes include alterations to the cardiovascular, pulmonary, and endocrine systems. Peripheral changes occur in the musculoskeletal system. The conditioning program chosen should be specific to the type of activity the dog will be performing.

Short-duration, maximal-intensity workouts are recommended if the purpose of the program is to increase strength. This type of program affects peripheral conditioning more than central conditioning. If an increase in speed is the goal, the conditioning program should include sprint workouts at maximal intensity. Workouts that include exercises for the spinal muscles should be included, because it has been theorized that the spinal muscles are the first to fatigue during sprinting.[10] Uphill sprint running helps to strengthen and condition the spinal muscles. Running with resistance helps to build body strength. Running with a harness and pulling weights is an example of resistance running. In a strength program, the most important change to the muscles is an increase in cross-sectional area because of increased myofibrillar protein content. In addition, there is an increase in muscle resting glycogen and muscle buffering capacity.

If the purpose of the program is to increase endurance, long-duration workouts of submaximal intensity are recommended. Examples are distance running or swimming. An endurance conditioning program may also include some strength activities. Endurance conditioning improves aerobic capacity to provide energy and conditions the musculoskeletal system to use energy more efficiently. In humans, changes occurring in the cardiovascular system include increased stroke volume and cardiac output.[11] Pulmonary changes include an improved ventilation-to-perfusion ratio, tidal volume, and alveolar and arterial partial pressures of oxygen.[12] Peripheral changes that occur in skeletal muscle are improved capillary density, glycolytic and oxidative enzyme activity, and lactate transport and clearance.[13]

Tissue Injury

Injury of musculoskeletal tissues may occur when a sudden stress occurs that is too great for the body to overcome, or when chronic stresses are greater than the ability of the body to repair itself. This may occur in any of the musculoskeletal tissues, but the type and location of injury depend on the forces and the direction of the forces that cause the injury. For example, a sudden high-energy force exerted on a bone may cause a fracture, whereas chronic prolonged stresses may result in periostitis or stress fractures of the bone. These are examples of bone injuries, but similar stresses may also affect muscle, tendon, ligaments, or synovial tissue.

After injury occurs, the body adapts and the dog alters its movements according to limitations as a result of the injury. If pain is involved, gait is altered to minimize painful movement while allowing locomotion.[14,15] Injury also changes structure, which alters how forces are received by the body.[16,17] As the altered movement continues, the musculoskeletal system adapts to produce movement with minimal abnormal stress on the system.[18] However, the altered movement may create additional abnormal stresses that may lead to secondary and sometimes tertiary injuries at locations other than the initial insult.

The altered movement and forces resulting from a musculoskeletal insult should be addressed early before further injury occurs. The tissues involved should be determined by a proper diagnostic workup; then a treatment program that addresses the pain and altered structure is initiated. A physical rehabilitation regimen should be implemented soon after medical treatment is initiated for the initial injury to prevent biomechanical alterations that may result in secondary problems. Secondary injuries complicate the rehabilitative process and may prolong the recovery time.

Further injury may also occur during healing and rehabilitation. If the rehabilitation program places too much stress on the healing tissue, tissue healing may be impaired and the tissue may be reinjured. For this reason, return to normal function should be delayed until the original tissue insult has healed to a point that it can withstand normal activity. A properly managed rehabilitation program should minimize the time of restricted activity without creating further injury.

Disuse and Immobilization

Following injury and rest, the body adapts to deconditioning, with changes occurring as a result of disuse or immobilization. Disuse refers to the state where the segment is not used as a result of injury or dysfunction. Immobilization occurs when a limb is maintained in a fixed position by splints, casts, or external fixation. Both of these states result in disuse atrophy, which has effects on muscle, bone, ligaments, tendon, and cartilage.[19,20]

Disuse atrophy of muscle results in decreased circumference and muscle fiber size. Type I muscle fibers are more affected than type II fibers, with a decrease in overall muscle strength. Because of the decrease in strength and endurance, there is increased stress on the affected joints, abnormal movement, and an increased risk of injury. Bone responds with an increase in bone resorption and perhaps decreased bone deposition and is guided by the external forces exerted on the bone. Immobilization also decreases loads on ligaments. Ligament mass decreases after just a few weeks of immobilization, so that after 6 to 9 weeks of immobilization, the ligament complexes are only about 50% as strong as normal controls.[21,22] Tendons behave in a similar manner, with alterations in the balance of collagen synthesis and degradation. Articular

cartilage also responds by atrophy and thinning of the surface layer of cartilage. If the joint is immobilized in a weight-bearing position, changes similar to those that occur with osteoarthritis may develop.

Immobilization may nevertheless be indicated as part of the initial treatment of many musculoskeletal injuries to allow an adequate healing environment, in spite of the changes that may occur with disuse and immobilization. The detrimental effects of immobilization should be considered in designing the treatment protocol because the recovery pattern is related to the duration of immobilization.

Reconditioning

A reconditioning program should address aspects of tissue healing, musculoskeletal physiology, and joint anatomy. It must include not only the injured area, but also the entire body. Nutrition, psychological aspects, and the effects of tissue injury on the entire body must also be considered. The goals should be to maximize healing of injured tissue and minimize degradation of healthy tissue. The primary long-term goal of rehabilitation is to maintain the physical condition of the injured segment during healing and not cause further damage. The secondary goal is to return the tissues of the affected segment to normal strength and character after injury and therapy. The third goal is to recondition the entire body to increase strength, coordination, and endurance to balance any secondary biomechanical disturbances that developed during injury and recovery.

The goal of maintaining condition of the ligaments, tendons, and cartilage may be achieved to some extent by passive range of motion. These tissues maintain their strength or conditioning level by mechanical action or movement, and by the forces placed on them. Bone is more dependent on loading forces and less so on mechanical action and motion. Muscle requires active contractions to preserve tissue strength. In most instances, bone and muscle tissue are most affected during healing and rehabilitation.

After sufficient healing has occurred, the next step is to return strength to the involved tissues. The conditioning program should emphasize strengthening exercises. Before any reconditioning program is begun, the level of strength should be determined, and therapeutic goals should be set by the clinician and owner. The reconditioning program should then be designed to achieve these goals.

There are three types of strengthening exercises: isometric, isokinetic, and isotonic. Isometric exercises involve muscle contraction without movement. This type of exercise is difficult to achieve in dogs. Isokinetic exercises provide constant velocity throughout joint range of motion. Because of the equipment needed to perform this form of exercise, it has not been used in canine rehabilitation. Isotonic exercises involve forces of varying magnitude applied throughout the range of motion. This is the most common form of exercise in dogs.

Isotonic exercise involves the muscle contracting while it shortens (concentric) or the muscle contracting while it lengthens (eccentric) while it is loaded throughout a range of motion. Loading the muscle stimulates strength gains. The effort should be high-intensity submaximal loading. Strength gain in reconditioning is similar to that of a regular strength program, except that the initial conditioning status of the tissue is less than normal. Exercises should be focused on strengthening the limb that is most affected by the injury, taking care to avoid overloading the healing tissues to avoid further damage.

As rehabilitation progresses, the focus shifts from localized exercise to overall body conditioning. This includes strength workouts balanced with endurance workouts. The strength portion of the program may still be focused on the areas of weakness, while the endurance portion can act on the entire body.

Nutrition

An important component of any conditioning program is nutrition. Nutritional needs change throughout the treatment and time of rehabilitation. Initially, there is a decrease in energy use by the patient. This should be addressed to keep the patient from becoming overweight during rehabilitation. After reconditioning begins, nutritional components may be added to allow for the nutritional demands of increased physical activity. The basic feeding program should provide for the basic nutritional needs of the patient. The content of protein, carbohydrate, and fat in the feeding program is determined by the type of conditioning. For example, dogs that are performing strength workouts will use the immediate and glycolytic energy systems. Therefore

they require a lower percentage of fat in their diets.

Supplemental feeding should be timed to benefit conditioning. An important feeding strategy is a to provide a post-workout snack. This is the optimal time to replenish nutrients that become depleted during the workout. Immediately after the workout, the body is devoted to replenishing the deficits of the energy systems. Feeding a snack during this time promotes replenishment of the deficient nutrients. This snack should consist of simple carbohydrates, a meat protein source, calcium, and phosphorus.

Summary

A proper conditioning program provides a good healing environment for injured tissues. It should minimize the detrimental effects of injury to the healthy tissues and the entire body. As healing progresses, the program should recondition and strengthen the tissues that are affected by injury. It should also provide nutrients to allow proper healing and be designed to consider the psychological aspects of rehabilitation. An understanding of exercise physiology is necessary to design and implement rehabilitative programs that aid tissue healing and recovery of the patient.

REFERENCES

1. Braund KG, Hoff EJ, Richardson KEY: Histochemical identification of fiber types in the canine skeletal muscle, *Am J Vet Res* 39:561-565, 1978.
2. Snow DH R et al: No classical type IIb fibers in dog skeletal muscle, *Histochemistry* 75:53-56, 1982.
3. Rivero JLL et al: Enzyme-histochemical profiles of fiber types in mature canine appendicular muscles, *Anat Histol Embryol* 23:330-336, 1994.
4. Latorre R et al: Skeletal muscle fiber types in the dog, *J Anat* 182:329-337, 1993.
5. Rosenblatt JD et al: Fiber type, fiber size, and capillary geometric features of the semitendinosus muscle in three types of dogs, *Am J Vet Res* 49:1573-1576, 1988.
6. Newsholme SJ, Lexell J, Downham DY: Distribution of fiber types and fiber sizes in the tibialis cranialis muscle of beagle dogs, *J Anat* 160:1-8, 1988.
7. Castle ME, Reyman TA: The effect of tenotomy and tendon transfers on muscle fiber types in the dog, *Clin Orthop Rel Res* 186:302-310, 1984.
8. Puustjarvi K et al: Running training alters fiber type composition in spinal muscles, *Eur Spine J* 3:17-21, 1994.
9. Potteiger JA: Principles of applied exercise physiology and training. In *Proceedings of the Seventh Annual Central Veterinary Conference*, Central States Kansus City, MO. 1995.
10. Zebas CJ et al: Selected kinematic differences in the running gait of the greyhound athlete during the beginning and end of the race. In Tant CL, Patterson

PE, York SL, editors: *Biomechanics in sport IX*, Ames, Iowa, 1991, Iowa State University.

11. Hartley LH: Cardiac function and endurance. In Shepard RJ, Astrand PO, editors: *Endurance in sport*, Oxford, 1992, Blackwell Scientific.

12. Dempsey JA, Manohar M: The pulmonary system and endurance. In Shepard RJ, Astrand PO, editors: *Endurance in sport*, Cambridge, Mass, 1992, Blackwell Scientific Publishing.

13. Wells CL, Pate RR: Training for performance of prolonged exercise. In Lamb DR, Murray R, editors: *Perspectives in exercise science and sports medicine*, vol 1, Carmel, Ind, 1988, Benchmark Press.

14. Rumph PF et al: Vertical ground reaction force distribution during experimentally induced acute synovitis in dogs, *Am J Vet Res* 54:365-369, 1993.

15. Dueland R, Bartel DL, Antonson E: Force-plate technique for canine gait analysis of total hip and excision arthoplasty. *JAAHA* 13:547-552, 1977.

16. DeCamp CE et al: Kinematic evaluation of gait in dogs with cranial ligament rupture, *Am J Vet Res* 57:120-126, 1996.

17. Bennett RL et al: Kinematic gait analysis in dogs with hip dysplasia, *Am J Vet Res* 57:966-971, 1996.

18. Rumph PF et al: Redistribution of vertical ground reaction forces in dogs with experimentally induced chronic hindlimb lameness, *Vet Surg* 24:384-389, 1995.

19. Lieber RL et al: Differential responses of the dog quadriceps muscle to external skeletal fixation of the knee, *Muscle Nerve* March:193-201, 1988.

20. Shires PK et al: Effect of localized trauma and temporary splinting on immature skeletal muscle and mobility of the femorotibial joint in the dog, *Am J Vet Res* 43:454-460, 1982.

21. Woo SL-Y et al: The biomechanical and morphological changes in the medial collateral ligament of the rabbit after immobilization and remobilization, *J Bone Joint Surg* 69A:1200-1211, 1987.

22. Noyes FR: Functional properties of knee ligaments and alterations induced by immobilization: a correlative biomechanical and histological study in primates, *Clin Orthop* 123:210-242, 1977.

The Role of Chondroprotectants and Nutraceuticals in Rehabilitation

Brian S. Beale

Optimal recovery from musculoskeletal disorders requires attention to mechanical, environmental, and biologic factors. Characteristics associated with one factor often have an effect on another. For instance, proper attention to mechanical and environmental factors improves the biologic environment of injured joints. Mechanical factors that play a role in enhancing recovery may include an appropriate level of physical activity, the use of special exercises to promote joint range of motion, and use of aids to protect or alleviate pain of a joint or limb. Environmental factors that affect rehabilitation include patient compliance, pet-owner compliance, weather conditions, and the type of environment to which the pet is subjected. Biologic factors affect the local environment of the joint. Examples include the quality and quantity of synovial fluid, presence of degradative enzymes in the synovial fluid and articular cartilage, condition of the extraarticular matrix of articular cartilage, and the metabolic state of the chondrocytes. Nutraceuticals and chondroprotectants may play a beneficial role by providing favorable biologic factors, thus enhancing joint health and the ability to recover from injury.

Chondroprotectants and nutraceuticals have become attractive adjunctive or alternative treatments for cats and dogs suffering from osteoarthritis (OA). OA, also commonly referred to as degenerative joint disease (DJD), is characterized by varying amounts of joint pain and dysfunction depending on the severity and course of disease. Initially, clinical signs may be limited to occasional stiffness, difficulty rising, or reluctance to exercise. As the condition progresses, clinical signs such as lameness, loss of joint range of motion, and muscle atrophy become readily identifiable.

Clinical signs may be exacerbated by inappropriate exercise, long periods of rest or recumbency, and weather changes (particularly cold weather). Some pets show signs of a restricted, stiff gait rather than an obvious lameness. This is commonly seen in cats and dogs with mild DJD or those having multiple joints with degenerative changes. Pets may also have a history of previous joint trauma (intraarticular fracture, ligamentous injury, dislocation, and so forth), osteochondral disease (osteochondrosis, ununited anconeal process, fragmented coronoid process), or congenital deformity (patellar luxation, hip dysplasia). OA is now diagnosed in cats more frequently as a result of more critical observation and greater diagnostic effort. The osteoarthritic patient can be satisfactorily managed in most situations with a combination of optimal body condition, exercise modification, antiinflammatory therapy, and use of chondroprotectant agents. Chondroprotectants are available as oral nutraceuticals and oral and injectable pharmaceuticals. At present, recommendations cannot be made as to which chondroprotectant is best for a dog or cat afflicted with OA. Direct comparisons of these products have not been made. In addition, it is not known when the different mediators of OA play an important role. It is possible that mediators of pain and degradation (prostaglandins, free radicals, metalloproteinases, serine proteases, and so forth) may change during the course of disease. It would be ideal to know what the predominant mediators were in an individual suffering from OA to accurately select the best product to treat that individual patient. At present, the best recommendation is to use products having well-designed experimental and clinical research evaluating efficacy and safety, as well as products that are manufactured under the high-quality standards practiced by the pharmaceutical industry.

Definition of Chondroprotectants and Nutraceuticals

The term chondroprotectant has been applied to various compounds which are proposed to have a positive effect on the health and metabolism of chondrocytes and synoviocytes. This definition is quite broad and thus has been used to label a wide variety of products that differ considerably in their structure, function and degree of purity. Other terms have been used to describe these types of products, including slow-acting disease-modifying osteoarthritic agents (SADMOA), structure/disease modifying antiosteoarthritis drug (S/DMOAD), and symptomatic slow-acting drugs for OA (SYSADOA).[1-3] Because of the great variation in nomenclature and molecular structure of these compounds, care should be taken when attempting to compare one chondroprotectant agent to another. Where applicable, it is always preferable to use generic compound names rather than trade names or broad descriptive terms (e.g., chondroprotectant, SADMOA) when discussing the effects or comparing the merits of these agents. Nevertheless, the term chondroprotectant will be used in this chapter to help bridge the information presented here with that reported previously elsewhere. Chondroprotective agents are purported to have three primary effects:
1. To support or enhance the metabolism of chondrocytes and synoviocytes (anabolic)
2. To inhibit degradative enzymes in the synovial fluid and cartilage matrix (catabolic)
3. To inhibit formation of thrombi in the small blood vessels supplying the joint. (antithrombotic)

Many different types of compounds allegedly have chondroprotective effects. These include glycosaminoglycans (GAGs), amino sugars, structural proteins, enzymes, minerals, preparations of whole tissue, and semisynthetic compounds.[4,5] These compounds are available in oral and injectable forms. Most oral chondroprotectants are classified as dietary supplements. A subset of the oral chondroprotectant agents are designated as nutraceuticals. A veterinary nutraceutical has been defined by the North American Veterinary Nutraceutical Council as a nondrug substance that is produced in a purified or extracted form and administered orally to provide compounds required for normal body structure and function with the intent of improving health and well-being.[6] Injectable chondroprotectants are drugs, and these include GAG polysulfate ester, pentosan polysulfate, and hyaluronic acid.

Regulation of Chondroprotectants

In the United States, dietary supplements for humans are regulated under the Dietary Supplements Health and Education Act (DSHEA). This law was enacted to assist consumers with making purchasing decisions regarding supplements. Such products must be safe; however, no premarketing approval is necessary as is required for pharmaceuticals.

Unfortunately, DSHEA does not apply to veterinary dietary supplements. Strict interpretation of the Food, Drug, and Cosmetic Act classifies oral veterinary compounds as foods, food additives, or pharmaceuticals; therefore the same dietary supplements legally sold under DSHEA for human use are technically unapproved veterinary pharmaceuticals when sold for animal use. However, to date the Center for Veterinary Medicine has exercised discretion in the removal of veterinary dietary supplements from the market. Provided the product is safe, poses no risk to the human food supply, and does not claim to treat, cure, prevent, or mitigate a disease, veterinary dietary supplements have not been removed from the market. Chondroprotective agents administered by routes other than oral, such as topical or injectable, are considered drugs and fall under the regulation of the Food and Drug Administration.

Manufacturing and Quality Control of Chondroprotectants

The manufacturing process of chondroprotectant products can vary widely. Manufacturers should apply similar high-quality standards practiced by the pharmaceutical industry (Good Manufacturing Practice, GMP). The raw materials and finished product should be tested for purity and consistency by validated analytical methods to ensure the label accuracy of the product reaching the consumer. Problems with truth-in-labeling and quality control of oral chondroprotectant products have been documented.[7,8] Unfortunately the consumer cannot always be assured that the ingredients listed on the container are actually present in the product at the claimed concentration or purity. At present, the results of clinical and experimental research conducted on one product cannot be extrapolated to another similar product because of inconsistencies in manufacturing and quality control standards. Until regulation of these products improves, it is probably best to heed the recommendation found in the Arthritis Foundation's Guide to Alternative Therapies: "When a supplement has been studied with good results, find out which brand was used in the study, and buy that brand."

Chondroprotectants and Nutraceuticals: Mechanism of Action

The mechanism of action of many of these products is unknown or unproven. Some products, on the other hand, have demonstrated positive effects in experimental and clinical trials. Dietary supplements and nutraceuticals cannot be marketed with the intent to diagnose, treat, cure, or prevent disease. Instead, they must be marketed as nutrients necessary for supporting or improving normal structure and function of the joint. Chondroprotective agents presumably influence cartilage metabolism by providing substrate and upregulating chondrocytes to produce cartilage matrix. They also appear to inhibit degradative enzymes, including metalloproteinases, serine proteases, and free radicals. Finally, some of these products inhibit the formation of microthrombi in the periarticular vasculature, thus supporting normal blood supply to the joint tissues. The mechanism of action of specific products, if known, is discussed in the section addressing specific types of chondroprotectants.

Structure and Function of Normal Joints

Normal joints are composed of a joint capsule, synovial fluid, articular cartilage, and subchondral bone. Normal joint function requires normal structure and function of these tissues. The joint capsule is composed of an outer fibrous capsule and an inner synovial membrane. The integrity of the joint capsule is important for normal gliding function, production of hyaluronic acid, and defense mechanisms. Synovial fluid is an ultrafiltrate of plasma containing the GAG hyaluronic acid. Synovial fluid functions include lubrication, protection (through its viscoelastic properties and participation in defense mechanisms), and provision of nutrients and removal of metabolic waste products from the cartilage. Articular cartilage is composed of hyaline cartilage, which has specific viscoelastic properties that allow it to function at the low levels of friction that are needed to withstand the long-term forces experienced by the joint over a lifetime. Cartilage is a living tissue made up of chondrocytes embedded in an extracellular matrix composed of water, collagen, and proteoglycans. Proteoglycans are composed of small proteins, a hyaluronic acid backbone, and GAGs (keratin sulfate and chondroitin sulfate). GAGs are long chains of disaccharides. Glucosamine is a hexosamine sugar and is a precursor for the disaccharide units of GAGs. The GAGs play an important role in maintaining the proper concentration of water in the cartilage, which is essential for normal viscoelastic function. Chondrocytes are metabolically active cells, producing collagen and proteoglycans needed for the cartilage matrix. These cells have little mitotic ability. Thus it is imperative to support the health of chondrocytes. The subchondral bone plays an important role in dissipating concussive forces to the joint. This cushioning effect protects the overlying articular cartilage by decreasing the load on the cartilage. As OA progresses, the subchondral bone becomes denser, increasing the loads placed on the cartilage, resulting in damage. Disruption of any of these components can lead to suboptimal performance, pain, and progression of OA.

Pathophysiology of Osteoarthritis

OA may be broadly classified as primary (idiopathic) or secondary. Primary OA is often referred to as wear-and-tear joint disease, owing to its insidious onset, which is thought to be due to long-term use combined with aging. Primary OA is not associated with an identifiable predisposing cause; however, this may only be due to our inability to detect subtle abnormalities. Secondary OA, identified more commonly, results from an initiating cause such as joint instability, trauma, osteo-chondral defects, or joint incongruity.

OA is characterized by a low-grade inflammatory process resulting in progressive changes in the structure and function of the joint. Joint capsular thickening and inflammation lead to pain, decreased range of motion, and reduced function. Synovial fluid alterations cause pain, a change in joint biomechanics, and a reduction in the protective mechanisms of the joint. Loss of articular cartilage leads to pain and loss of function and establishes a mechanism for perpetuating low-grade inflammation and progressive OA. Increased density of the subchondral bone indirectly affects the joint by increasing the amount of force placed on the articular cartilage. The initial change occurring in OA involves changes in the structural components of articular cartilage, including the loss of proteoglycans from the extracellular matrix as a result of increased destruction and decreased production. This continued breakdown, along with the loss of collagen and chondrocytes as the disease progresses, leads to irreversible change.

Understanding the pathogenesis of OA is essential to develop a rational approach to manage this condition. Although OA is usually categorized as a noninflammatory joint disease, low-grade inflammation plays an important role in its pathogenesis. Inflammation of the synovial membrane leads to extravasation of inflammatory cells, primarily mononuclear cells, from synovial capillaries to synovial fluid. Leukocytes and synoviocytes release a variety of inflammatory mediators, including prostaglandins, leukotrienes, neutral metalloproteinases, serine proteases, oxygen-derived free radicals, lysosomal enzymes (proteases, glycosidases, and collagenases), oncoproteins, interleukins, tumor necrosis factor, and other cytokines. The neutral metalloproteinase stromelysin is thought to be the primary factor responsible for proteoglycan degradation in degenerative cartilage. Collagenase also plays a role in the destruction of cartilage.

Treatment of Osteoarthritis

Treatment of OA includes weight loss, exercise modification, physical rehabilitation, pharmacological therapy, and possibly surgery. In cases of secondary OA, the underlying cause must be identified and eliminated if possible to minimize the progression and long-term

effects of OA. Examples include removal of an osteochondral fragment or stabilization of a stifle after rupture of a cranial cruciate ligament. Weight loss decreases the clinical signs of OA because of decreased forces placed on abnormal joint surfaces. Weight reduction before surgery reduces postoperative stress placed on the surgical repair. Decreased body weight is an important factor in reducing the prevalence and severity of OA in dogs with hip dysplasia.[9] Enforced rest and restricted activity provide an opportunity for transient episodes of inflammation to resolve, in addition to decreasing stress placed on surgical repairs.

Pharmacological management of OA includes a wide variety of pharmaceuticals. Consideration should be given to drugs that inhibit the release or activity of prostaglandins, leukotrienes, neutral metalloproteases (stromelysin, collagenase), serine proteases, oncoproteins, interleukins, and tumor necrosis factor, such as nonsteroidal antiinflammatory drugs (NSAIDs). Other drugs, such as the chondroprotective agents, not only inhibit mediators of inflammation within joints, but may also stimulate metabolic activity of synoviocytes and chondrocytes. Examples of these drugs include GAG polysulfate ester, pentosan polysulfate, and hyaluronic acid. Nutraceuticals and other dietary supplements have also become an important tool in the management of OA in dogs and cats.

Nutraceuticals

Glucosamine

Glucosamine salt supplements are most commonly found as glucosamine hydrochloride or glucosamine sulfate. Although both forms are readily available, the hydrochloride form provides more glucosamine per unit weight than the sulfate form. Another form, *N*-acetylglucosamine, appears to have less activity than the hydrochloride and sulfate forms.[10] Glucosamine is commonly found in combination products containing other products, including chondroitin sulfate (CS) and manganese ascorbate. Glucosamine is an amino sugar that is a precursor to GAGs present in the extracellular matrix of articular cartilage. Normal chondrocytes have the ability to synthesize glucosamine. Osteoarthritic cartilage, however, appears to have a decreased ability to synthesize glucosamine.[4,11] Exogenous glucosamine stimulates the production of pro-teoglycans and collagen by chondrocytes in cell culture.[12,13] Glucosamine has good bioavailability when administered orally or parenterally, having good distribution to all body tissues and reaching highest concentrations in the liver, kidney, and articular cartilage.[14-16] Oral glucosamine has an intestinal absorption rate of 87%.[17] Glucosamine hydrochloride is absorbed in less than 2 hours, but does not accumulate over time.[14] Orally administered glucosamine sulfate has been associated with relief of clinical signs of OA and chondroprotection in clinical and experimental studies in humans.[18-21] Although glucosamine does not relieve clinical signs associated with OA as quickly as ibuprofen, two clinical trials in people found it to have equal long-term efficacy.[18] Oral glucosamine also improved clinical performance in humans with OA.[22] Use of this product as an individual agent in animals has been proposed, but adequately controlled clinical studies have not been performed to substantiate its efficacy.

Chondroitin Sulfate

CS is the predominant GAG found in the extracellular matrix of articular cartilage. Oral supplementation of exogenous CS has been advocated anecdotally for many years as a treatment for OA in humans and animals. This compound is often combined with other nutraceuticals, such as glucosamine and free radical scavengers. CS decreases interleukin-1 production, blocks complement activation, inhibits metalloproteinases and histamine-mediated inflammation, and stimulates GAG and collagen synthesis.[1,23] Oral absorption of CS has been reported using a variety of techniques. Some controversy exists regarding the fate of CS following oral administration. Although CS has the ability to be intestinally absorbed, uncertainty remains as to whether the majority of CS is absorbed intact or as a subunit of CS.[1,24,25] The fate of orally administered CS appears to be affected by the molecular weight of the molecule. A highly pure, low-molecular-weight form of CS has been found to have good absorption and bioavailability.[14] Low-molecular-weight CS is absorbed in approximately 2 hours and accumulates in the serum over time, having an estimated bioavailability of 200%.[14] Clinical studies have shown improvement in clinical signs associated with OA in human patients receiving CS supplementation.[2,24,25]

Glucosamine Hydrochloride/Chondroitin Sulfate/Manganese/Ascorbate

A combination of glucosamine hydrochloride, CS, manganese, and ascorbate is the most commonly used nutraceutical in osteoarthritic companion animals.[26] A patented combination of high-purity glucosamine, low-molecular weight CS, and manganese ascorbate (Cosequin, Nutramax Laboratories Inc., Edgewood, MD) has become an important part of the management strategy in dogs and cats affected with OA.

Cosequin is marketed as a GAG enhancer, capable of providing raw materials needed for the synthesis of endogenous synovial fluid and extracellular matrix of cartilage. Glucosamine has been described as a building block of articular cartilage matrix and is a preferential substrate and stimulant of proteoglycan biosynthesis, including hyaluronic acid and CS.[1] CS, mixed GAGs, and manganese ascorbate also promote GAG production. CS appears to inhibit degradative enzymes associated with OA including metalloproteases and collagenases. These degradative enzymes break down the cartilage and hyaluronan in synovial fluid. The combined actions of glucosamine and CS are synergistic.[27] Manganese is a cofactor in the synthesis of GAGs, and its supplementation may aid in cartilage matrix synthesis. Manganese is also necessary for the synthesis of synovial fluid. It is possible that manganese may have antioxidant properties as well. Overdose safety studies have been conducted with Cosequin in the dog, cat, and horse. No persistent abnormalities in hematology, serum chemistry, or hemostatic parameters were observed.[23,28,29] No serious side effects have been seen in cats or dogs.

Clinical and experimental studies support the use of these nutritional supplements, either combined or as individual components. Leeb et al[30] performed a metaanalysis of the clinical efficacy of CS in humans. A total of 16 published studies were examined, with seven trials of 372 patients selected for the metaanalysis. All selected studies were randomized, double-blinded designs in parallel groups. However, rescue medications (analgesics or NSAIDs) were permitted, which is typical of human clinical studies of OA. CS was shown to be significantly superior to placebo with respect to the Lequesne index (a validated, subjective assessment of pain associated with OA). Patients showed at least a 50% improvement in study variables in the CS group compared to placebo. A double-blind clinical study in horses showed Cosequin's efficacy for treatment of DJD associated with navicular disease.[31] Administration of Cosequin to dogs with experimentally induced OA via transection of the cranial cruciate ligament showed increased concentration of OA markers, possibly indicating cartilage matrix synthesis.[32] Glucosamine, CS, manganese, and ascorbate may act as signaling molecules for upregulation of the genes for aggrecan and collagen II, not just as substrates for cartilage production.[33] Cosequin has also been found to suppress the inflammatory effects of chemically induced acute synovitis and experimental immune-mediated arthritis.[34,35]

Other Mixed Glycosaminoglycan Products

Many other oral GAG or glucosamine products are available as either single- or multiple-ingredient products. Most of the GAG products contain CS or "mixed" GAGs. Different glucosamine salts are available. Much controversy exists regarding the necessary purity, concentration, and type of GAG or glucosamine product necessary to provide beneficial effects to cartilage.

The New Zealand green-lipped mussel (*Perna canaliculus*) is known to contain GAGs, omega-3 fatty acids, amino acids, vitamins, and minerals.[36] It is available as a sole dietary supplement or as an additive in canine diets. *P. canaliculus* is purported to have mild antiinflammatory and chondroprotective actions, but these effects remain to be unequivocally substantiated in humans and animals. Beneficial effects have been reported in one study of human beings suffering from rheumatoid arthritis or OA. A recent study in dogs found improvement in joint pain and swelling in arthritic dogs fed a complete diet containing 0.3% green-lipped mussel.[36] Joint crepitus, range of motion, or mobility scores were not improved. Although the study concludes that a diet supplemented with green-lipped mussel can alleviate signs of OA in dogs, several points may be questioned in the study. OA was not definitively diagnosed in the dogs. Joint swelling, which is not a consistent finding in osteoarthritic joints, was significantly improved. However, joint mobility, range of motion, and crepitus, all commonly associated with OA, were not improved.

Additionally, control dogs showed a marked worsening of joint pain and swelling over the 6-week period of the study, which is inconsistent with dogs selected for a chronic, slowly progressive condition, such as OA. This study also included a subjective scoring system. A total score for each dog was determined by adding the scores together for each joint. It is difficult to envision that certain scores, such as joint swelling of the hip and shoulder, could be accurately or consistently measured. Further study is warranted before this substance is unequivocally accepted as a chondroprotective agent or nutraceutical useful in osteoarthritic dogs.

Free Radical Scavengers

Another class of nutraceuticals that has been promoted to reduce inflammation is free radical scavengers, such as superoxide dismutase (SOD), bioflavonoids, glutathione, and dimethyl sulfoxide (DMSO). Oxygen-derived free radicals (superoxide, hydrogen peroxide, and hydroxyl radicals) are thought to play a role in the progression of OA through their ability to damage cells by oxidative injury. Oxidative injury leads to depolymerization of hyaluronic acid, destruction of collagen, and decreased production of proteoglycans.[37-39]

SOD and glutathione are endogenous antioxidants present in mammalian cells that inhibit production of oxygen-derived free radicals. SOD acts to stabilize white blood cell membranes and lysosomes and to reduce superoxide radical levels in tissues, with a resultant decrease in free radical generation.[38-40] The efficacy, bioavailability, and safety of many oral antioxidants are unknown. In addition, this product may have potential manufacturing or storage problems, resulting in less active ingredient being available to the pet than is labeled on the product. A recent study found discrepancies in certificate of analysis and labeled contents in six SOD products.[8] Since this study, several new products have become available that may have resolved this problem. One author recommends giving dogs 5 mg subcutaneously for 6 days, followed by alternate-day therapy for 8 days.[40] The manufacturer recommends giving 2.5 mg/kg subcutaneously five times a week for 2 weeks for treatment of spondylitis or disc disease.

DMSO, used as a topical agent to treat musculoskeletal problems, has the ability to penetrate most tissues, including skin.[40] Topical application of 20 ml/day of a medical-grade

DMSO (70% to 90% solution) every 6 to 8 hours for up to 14 days has been recommended to treat local inflammation.[40] Side effects with topical use are minimal but include a garlic odor to the breath and enhanced absorption of substances on the skin.

Bioflavonols are also purported to have strong antioxidant properties. Grape-seed meal is a rich source of bioflavonols. Bioflavonols are purported to scavenge free radicals, alleviate inflammation induced by oxidative damage, and inhibit degradative enzymes released by cells.[41-44] One double-blind, randomized study in dogs found improvement in clinical signs attributable to hip OA in dogs supplemented with a product containing bioflavonols, SOD and glutathione.[41] Other clinical studies also reported improved function and decreased pain in dogs and horses with OA.[42-44] These studies reported improvement after 2 to 3 weeks of product administration. Bioflavonols are available commercially, usually in combination with glucosamine and hydrolyzed collagen, or with an assortment of other antioxidants, including selenium, vitamin E, and SOD.

Methylsulfonylmethane

Methylsulfonylmethane (MSM) has been suggested as an agent for management of pain, inflammation, and as an antioxidant.[45] The rationale behind its use, according to the manufacturer and others, is the possibility of a dietary sulfur deficiency. MSM is a white, crystalline, water-soluble, odorless, and tasteless compound that is sold as a supplement. It is actually a metabolite of industrial-grade DMSO. MSM is found naturally in certain foods; however, it is destroyed during processing. DMSO is a by-product of the wood pulp processing industry and is also available as a medical-grade compound, which is only approved in the United States for the treatment of interstitial cystitis in people. Radiolabeled sulfur from MSM has been found in amino acids (methionine and cysteine) of proteins in guinea pigs following experimental oral administration. There are no controlled experimental or clinical studies available to support the use of MSM for the management of OA in dogs. Companies supplying MSM have based their claims of relief of pain and inflammation on results of studies conducted with DMSO. Little is known about safety of the product. MSM is available in powder form, tablets, and capsules for small animals and horses. Manufacturer recommen-

dations for dosage should be followed. Its use cannot be recommended at this time, however, because of the lack of efficacy and safety studies.

Omega-3 Fatty Acids

Omega-3 fatty acids have recently gained popularity for their potential use in pets with DJD. These products are available naturally in fish and plant sources and commercially as nutraceutical supplements. Omega-3 fatty acids are desaturated in the body to produce eicosapentaenoic acid, which is an analog of arachidonic acid. Prostaglandins, thromboxanes, and leukotrienes are produced from both of these compounds through the action of cyclooxygenase and lipoxygenase. The products resulting from arachidonic acid metabolism are proinflammatory, promote platelet aggregation, and are immunosuppressive, as compared to the metabolic by-products of eicosapentaenoic acid, which are less inflammatory, less aggregatory for platelets, and less immunosuppressive. The use of omega-3 fatty acids could theoretically benefit dogs and cats suffering from OA by decreasing inflammation and reducing the occurrence of microthrombi; however, objective data are lacking to attest to these effects. The ideal ratio of N6:N3 fatty acids for canine diets is controversial, but a current recommendation is between 10:1 and 5:1. A recent study reported lower PGE_2 and reduced clinical and radiographic signs of OA in experimental dogs undergoing cranial cruciate ligament transection while being fed a diet low in N6 fatty acids.[46]

Chondroprotectant Drugs

Polysulfated Glycosaminoglycan

Adequan (Luitpold Pharmaceuticals, Shirley, NY), a drug that is gaining popularity for use in dogs in the United States is a GAG polysulfate ester (GAGPS). It is purported to be both chondroprotective and chondrostimulatory. Chondroprotection is achieved by inhibiting various destructive enzymes and prostaglandins associated with synovitis and DJD. GAGPS has been found to inhibit neutral metalloproteinases (stromelysin, collagenase, elastase), serine proteases, hyaluronidase, and a variety of lysosomal enzymes.[39,47-50] The drug has also been found to inhibit PGE_2 synthesis, generation of oxygen-derived free radicals, and the complement cascade.[47,48] Protection of articular cartilage has also been seen on gross and histologic examination in numerous experimental studies.[49-51] GAGPS also stimulates anabolic activity in synoviocytes and chondrocytes.[52-56] Chondrostimulatory effects are characterized by enhanced proteoglycan, hyaluronate, and collagen production by articular chondrocytes and increased synoviocyte secretion of hyaluronate. GAGPS also has anticoagulant and fibrinolytic properties that facilitate clearing of thrombotic emboli deposited in the subchondral and synovial blood vessels.[39,56,57] While the majority of experimental and clinical studies support the premise that GAGPS possesses properties of chondroprotection and chondrostimulation, some studies have found GAGPS either to have no beneficial effect or to actually have a detrimental effect on cartilage metabolism.[39,56]

A clinical study of dogs with hip dysplasia found the greatest improvement in orthopedic scores occurred at a dose of 4.4 mg/kg given intramuscularly every 3 to 5 days for 8 injections.[58] Use in cats has also been reported at the same dose. Another study found twice-weekly intramuscular administration of 5.0 mg/kg GAGPS from 6 weeks to 8 months of age in growing pups that were susceptible to hip dysplasia resulted in less coxofemoral subluxation.[59] The longevity of relief provided by GAGPS is unknown. Most studies have evaluated its effect in the short term only. Anecdotal reports have indicated that improvement of clinical signs ranges from days to months. It is also not known whether another complete series of injections is needed after clinical signs return or whether a shorter regimen would suffice.

Side effects of GAGPS in dogs include short-term inhibition of the intrinsic coagulation cascade as well as inhibition of platelet aggregation when given at a dose of 5 mg/kg or 25 mg/kg intramuscularly.[60] Also, GAGPS has been found to inhibit neutrophils and complement, which may predispose dogs to infections, especially when GAGPS is injected intraarticularly under contaminated conditions.[61,62] GAGPS has caused sensitization reactions in people, but this has not been reported in dogs.

Pentosan Polysulfate

Pentosan polysulfate (Cartrophen-Vet, Biopharm Australia, Sydney, Australia) is a polysaccharide sulfate ester (mean molecular weight of 6,000 daltons) prepared semisynthetically from beech hemicellulose.[63] The drug is approved for use in dogs and horses in Australia and is used in much the same manner as Adequan for relieving clinical signs of OA. Pentosan polysulfate can be administered intraarticularly, intramuscularly, subcutaneously, or orally. The recommended dose for intraarticular use is 5 to 10 mg per joint weekly, as necessary. The intramuscular or subcutaneous dose in dogs is 3 mg/kg, once weekly for 4 weeks. This regimen may be repeated as necessary. A double-blind study evaluating the efficacy of this product for treatment of OA in dogs found this dose to be ideal.[63] Anecdotally, this dose has also been used in cats. Oral calcium pentosan polysulfate given at a dose of 10 mg/kg weekly for 4 weeks, then repeated every 3 months, was found to reduce the presence of cartilage breakdown products in osteoarthritic cartilage.[64]

Sodium Hyaluronate

Sodium hyaluronate has been touted to promote joint lubrication, increase endogenous production of hyaluronate, decrease prostaglandin production, scavenge free radicals, inhibit migration of inflammatory cells, decrease synovial membrane permeability, protect and promote healing of articular cartilage, and reduce joint stiffness and adhesion formation between tendon and tendon sheaths.[65,66] The molecule lines the synovial membrane and acts like a sieve, excluding bacteria and inflammatory cells from reaching the synovial compartment by steric hindrance.[65,66] The actions of exogenous and endogenous hyaluronan appear to be similar. At present, sodium hyaluronate is generally recommended for mild to moderate synovitis and capsulitis, rather than OA. The drug appears to have a chondroprotective effect, but it is unclear whether this is a direct effect or a result of its effect on the periarticular soft tissues. Sodium hyaluronate is administered intraarticularly or intravenously. Hyaluronate was used in experimental dogs at a dose of 7 mg per joint, intraarticularly, once weekly with success in slowing OA.[65,66]

Chondroprotectant Use During the Postoperative Period and Physical Rehabilitation

Rehabilitation programs are developed to improve function and decrease pain in dogs and cats having musculoskeletal compromise or following orthopedic surgery. Rehabilitation can involve many physical modalities designed to improve strength, flexibility, and coordination. Chondroprotectants may be used concurrently to accelerate and enhance recovery, possibly by several mechanisms:

1. Pain relief may increase patient willingness to perform rehabilitation exercises.
2. Reduction of degradative and inflammatory enzymes may help to protect cartilage.
3. Stimulation of synovial fluid, proteoglycan, and collagen production may promote cartilage matrix repair.

Agents that reduce the expression of inflammatory mediators or up-regulate normal chondrocyte expression may serve to provide a microenvironment favorable for optimal cartilage and connective tissue homeostasis. A recent study evaluated the effect of a nutraceutical on intraarticular graft organization in dogs undergoing unilateral cranial cruciate ligament transection. Cosequin appeared to have two primary effects in this study: a return of the joint capsule and intraarticular graft complex to a more physiological state, and a reduction in the severity of OA in operated joints.[67] Translation following transection of reconstructed cranial cruciate ligaments from the Cosequin group was similar to that of controls, which suggested preservation of a more normal, physiological joint capsule. Dogs not receiving Cosequin had less translation after resection of the reconstructed cranial cruciate ligament which suggests joint capsule thickening and fibrosis. OA was less in dogs receiving Cosequin, both subjectively as judged by morphologic observation, and objectively as measured with mean modified Mankin scores.

Limb immobilization may be performed postoperatively as adjunctive support, to restrict use, to reduce pain, to treat open wounds, or to control swelling. Whatever the indication, immobilization of joints can have adverse effects on joint health. Joint immobilization reduces synovial fluid production and leads to proteoglycan depletion due to decreased loading. Chondroprotectant treatment may help reduce deleterious effects on the joint during periods of immobilization. Immobilization should be limited to the shortest possible time to improve the chances of joint recovery.

REFERENCES

1. McNamara PS, Johnston SA, Todhunter RJ: Slow-acting, disease-modifying osteoarthritic agents, *Vet Clin North Am Small Anim Pract* 27:4:863-867, 951-952, 1997.
2. Verbruggen G, Goemaere S, Veys EM: Chondroitin sulfate: S/DMOAD (structure/disease modifying anti-osteoarthrosis drug) in the treatment of finger joint OA, *Osteoarthr Cartil* Suppl A:39-46, 1998.
3. Bucsi L, Poor G: Efficacy and tolerability of oral chondroitin sulfate as a symptomatic slow-acting drug for osteoarthritis (SYSADOA) in the treatment of knee osteoarthritis, *Osteoarthr Cartil* 6 (Suppl A):31-36, 1998.
4. Anderson MA: Oral chondroprotectant agents. I. *Compend Contin Educ Pract Vet* 21:601-609, 1999.
5. Boothe DM: Drug management of osteoarthritis, *Proc TNAVC* 12:586-591, 1998.
6. Boothe DM: Nutraceuticals in veterinary medicine. I. *Compend Contin Educ Pract Vet* 19:1248-1255, 1997.
7. Adebowale A et al: Analysis of glucosamine and chondroitin sulfate content in marketed products and the Caco-2 permeability of chondroitin sulfate raw materials, *JANA* 3: 1998, 37-44, 2000.
8. Beale BS: Evaluation of active enzyme in six oral superoxide dismutase products, *Proc Vet Orthop Soc*, p 65.
9. Smith G: Influence of diet and age on subjective hip score and hip OA: a life long study in Labrador retrievers. *Proc Vet Orthop Soc*, 2002, p 41.
10. Karzel K, Domenjoz R: Effect of hexosamine derivatives and uronic acid derivatives on glycosaminoglycan metabolism on fibroblast cultures, *Pharmacology* 5:337-345, 1971.
11. Jimenez SA, Dodge GR: The effects of glucosamine on human chondrocyte gene expression. *In Proc 9th Eular Symposium*, 1996, pp 8-10.
12. Hellio MP, Vigron E, Annefeld M: The effects of glucosamine on the human osteoarthritic chondrocyte: in vitro investigations, *Proc 9th Eular Symp*, 1996, pp 11-12.
13. Basleer C: Stimulation of proteoglycan production by glucosamine sulfate in chondrocytes isolated from human osteoarthritic articular cartilage in vitro, *Osteoarthr Cartil* 6:427-434, 1998.
14. Du J et al: Bioavailability and disposition of the dietary supplements, FCHG49 glucosamine and TRH122 chondroitin sulfate in dogs after single and multiple dosing, *AAPS Pharm Sci Suppl* 3:W417, October 24, 2001.
15. Davidson G: Glucosamine and chondroitin sulfate, *Comp Contin Educ Pract Vet* 22:454-458, 2000.
16. Setnikar I, Giacchetti C, Zanolo G: Pharmacokinetics of glucosamine in dog and in man, *Arzneim-Forsch/Drug Res* 36:703-705, 1986.
17. Setniker I, Giaccheti C, Zanolo G: Pharmacokinetics of glucosamine in the dog and in man. *Arzneimittelforschung* 36:729, 1991.
18. Vaz AL: Double-blind clinical evaluation of the relative efficacy of ibuprofen and glucosamine sulphate in the management of osteoarthrosis of the knee in outpatients, *Curr Med Res Opin* 8:145-149, 1982.
19. Hungerford D, Navarro R, Hammad T: Use of nutraceuticals in the management of osteoarthritis, *JANA* 3:23-27, 2000.
20. Leffler CT et al: Glucosamine, chondroitin and manganese ascorbate for degenerative joint disease of the knee or low back: a randomized, double-blind, placebo-controlled pilot study, *Military Med* 164:85-91, 1999.
21. Das AK, Hammad TA: Efficacy of a combination of FCHG49 glucosamine hydrochloride, TRH122 low

molecular weight sodium chondroitin sulfate and manganese ascorbate in the management of knee osteoarthritis, *Osteoarthr Cartil* 8:343-350, 2000.

22. D'Ambrosio E et al: Glucosamine sulfate: a controlled clinical investigation in arthrosis, *Pharmacotherapeutica* 2:504-508, 1981.

23. McNamara PS, Barr SC, Erb HN: Hematologic, hemostatic and biochemical effects in dogs receiving an oral chondroprotective agent for thirty days, *AJVR* 57:1390-1394, 1996.

24. Li Hirondel JL: Double-blind clinical study with oral administration of chondroitin sulfate versus placebo in tibiofemoral gonarthrosis, *Lit Rheumatol* 14:77-82, 1992.

25. Bourgeois P et al: Efficacy and tolerability of chondroitin sulfate 1200 mg/day vs 3 × 400 mg/day vs placebo, *Osteoarthr Cartil* 6(suppl A):25-30, 1998.

26. Hulse DS: Treatment methods for pain in the osteoarthritic patient, *Vet Clin North Am Small Anim Pract* 28:361, 1998.

27. Lippiello L et al: Chondroprotection and metabolic synergy of glucosamine and chondroitin sulfate, *Clin Orthop Rel Res* 381:229-240, 2000.

28. McNamara PS et al: Hematologic, hemostatic and biochemical effects in cats receiving an oral chondroprotective agent for thirty days, *Vet Ther* 1:108-117, 2000.

29. Kirker-Head RP: Safety of an oral chondroprotective agent in horses, *Vet Ther* 2:345-353, 2001.

30. Leeb, BF et al: A metaanalysis of chondroitin sulfate in the treatment of osteoarthritis, *J Rheumatol* 27:205-211, 2000.

31. Hansen RR et al: Oral treatment with a glucosamine-chondroitin sulfate compound for degenerative joint disease in horses: 25 cases, *Equine Pract* 19:16-22, 1997.

32. Johnson KA et al: Effects of an orally administered mixture of chondroitin sulfate, glucosamine hydrochloride and manganese ascorbate on synovial fluid chondroitin sulfate 3B3 and 7D4 epitope in a canine cranial cruciate transection model of osteoarthritis, *Osteoarthr Cartil* 9:14-21, 2001.

33. O'Grady CP, Marwin SE, Grande DA: Effects of glucosamine hydrochloride, chondroitin sulfate, and manganese-ascorbate on cartilage metabolism, *Proc AAOS 68th Annu Mtg*, 2001, p 157.

34. Beren J et al: The effect of pre-loading oral glucosamine/chondroitin sulfate/manganese ascorbate combination on experimental arthritis in rats, *Exp Biol Med* 226:144-152, 2001.

35. Canapp SO et al: Scintographic evaluation of glucosamine HCL and chondroitin sulfate as treatment for acute synovitis in dogs, *AJVR* 60:1552-1557, 1999.

36. Bui LM, Bierer TL: Influence of green lipped mussels *(Perna canaliculus)* in alleviating signs of arthritis in dogs, Vet Ther 2:101-111, 2001.

37. Simon SR: Oxidants, metalloproteases and serine proteases in inflammation. In Cheronis JC, Repine JE, editors: *Proteases, protease inhibitors and protease-derived peptides*, Basel, 1993, Birkhauser Verlag, 27-37.

38. Auer DE, NG JC, Seawright AA: Effect of palosein (superoxide dismutase) and catalase upon oxygen derived free radical induced degradation of equine synovial fluid, *Equine Vet J* 22:13-17, 1990.

39. Ghosh P, Smith M, Wells C: Second-line agents in osteoarthritis. In Dixon JS, Furst DE, editors: *Second-line agents in the treatment of rheumatic diseases*, New York, 1993, Marcel Dekker, pp 363-427.

40. Beale BS, Goring RL: Degenerative joint disease. In Bojrab MJ, editor: *Disease mechanisms in small animal*

surgery, Philadelphia, 1993, Lea and Febiger, pp 727-736.

41. Impellizeri JA, Lau RE, Azzara FA: A 14 week clinical evaluation of an oral antioxidant as a treatment for osteoarthritis secondary to canine hip dysplasia, *Vet Q* 20(suppl 1):S107-108, 1998.

42. Kuck JC, Mulnix JA: Clinical evaluation of an antioxidant joint nutrient and relief of the signs of pain associated with osteoarthritis in the dog. Proprietary data, Animal Health Options, Golden, CO, 2001.

43. Mulnix JA: ProMotion study, canine formula. Proprietary data, Animal Health Options, Golden, CO, 2001.

44. Kuck JC, Mulnix JA: Clinical evaluation of an antioxidant joint nutrient and relief of the signs of pain associated with osteoarthritis and gait irregularities in the horse. Proprietary data, Animal Health Options, Golden, CO, 2001.

45. Jones WE: MSM reviewed, *J Equine Vet Sci* 3:148,174-175, 1983.

46. Budsberg S et al: Effects of different N6:N3 fatty acid diets on canine stifle osteoarthritis, *Proc Vet Orthop Soc*, 2001, p 40.

47. Egg D: Effects of glycosaminoglycan polysulfate and two nonsteroidal anti-inflammatory drugs on prostaglandin E_2 synthesis in Chinese hamster ovary cell cultures, *Pharmacol Res Commun* 15:709-717, 1983.

48. Altman RD et al: Therapeutic treatment of canine osteoarthritis with glycosaminoglycan polysulfuric acid ester, *Arthr Rheum* 32:1300-1307, 1989.

49. Carreno MR, Muniz OE, Howell DS: The effect of glycosaminoglycan polysulfuric acid ester on articular cartilage in experimental osteoarthritis: effects on morphological variables of disease severity, *J Rheum* 13:490-497, 1986.

50. Hannen N et al: Systemic administration of glycosaminoglycan polysulphate provides partial protection of articular cartilage from damage produced by menisectomy in the canine. *Orthop Res* 5:47-59, 1987.

51. Altman RD et al: Prophylactic treatment of canine osteoarthritis with glycosaminoglycan polysulfuric acid ester, *Arthr Rheum* 32:759-766, 1989.

52. Verbruggen G, Veys EM: The effect of sulfated glycosaminoglycan on the proteoglycan metabolism of synovial lining cells, *Acta Rheumatol Belgica* 1:75-92, 1971.

53. von der Mark K: Collagen synthesis in cultures of chondrocytes as effected by arteparon. In *IX Eur Congr Rheumatol*, Basel, 1980, Euler, pp 39-50.

54. Nishikawa H, Mori I, Umemoto J: Influences of sulfated glycosaminoglycans on hyaluronic acid in rabbit knee synovia. *Arch Biochem Biophys* 240:146-148, 1985.

55. Smith MM, Ghosh P: The effect of polysulfated polysaccharides on hyaluronate (HA) synthesis by human synovial fibroblasts. *Agents Actions* 18:55-62, 1986.

56. Verbruggen G, Veys EM: Treatment of chronic degenerative joint disorders with a glycosaminoglycan polysulfate. *IX Europ Cong Rheumatol*, Basel, 1980, Euler, pp 51-69.

57. Dettmer N, Nowack H, Raake W: Platelet aggregation by heparin and arteparon, *Munch Med Wschr* 125:540-542, 1983.

58. de Haan JJ, Goring RL, Beale BS: Evaluation of polysulfated glycosaminoglycan for the treatment of hip dysplasia in dogs, *Vet Surg* 23:177-181, 1994.

59. Lust G et al: Effects of intramuscular administration of glycosaminoglycan polysulfates on signs of incipient hip dysplasia in growing pups, *Am J Vet Res* 53:1836-1843, 1992.

60. Beale BS, Clemmons RM, Goring RL: The effect of a semi-synthetic polysulfated glycosaminoglycan on coagulation and primary hemostasis in the dog, *Vet Surg* 19:57, 1990.

61. Rashmir-Raven AM et al: Inhibition of equine complement activity by polysulfated glycosaminoglycans, *Am J Vet Res* 53:87-90, 1992.

62. Tsuboi I et al: Effects of glycosaminoglycan polysulfate on human neutrophil function, *Jpn J Inflam* 8:131-135, 1988.

63. Read R, Cullis-Hill D: The systemic use of the chondroprotective agent pentosan polysulfate in the treatment of osteoarthritis: results of a double-blind clinical trial in dogs. *J Small Anim Pract* 37:108-114, 1996.

64. Innes JF, Barr AR, Sharif M: Efficacy of oral calcium pentosan polysulphate for the treatment of osteoarthritis of the canine stifle joint secondary to cranial cruciate ligament deficiency, *Vet Rec* 146:433-437, 2000.

65. Howard RD, McIlwraith CW: Sodium hyaluronate in the treatment of equine joint disease, *Compend Contin Educ Pract* 15:473-481, 1993.

66. Schiavinato A et al: Intraarticular sodium hyaluronate injections in the Pond-Nuki experimental model of osteoarthritis in dogs. II. Morphological findings. *Clin Orthop* 241:286-299, 1989.

67. Hulse DA et al: The effect of Cosequin in cranial cruciate deficient and reconstructed stifle joints in dogs, *Proc Vet Orthop Soc,* 1998, p 64.

PATIENT ASSESSMENT

■ C h a p t e r 1 0

Orthopedic and Neurologic Evaluation

Darryl L. Millis, Robert A. Taylor, and Michael Hoelzler

Detection and assessment of orthopedic and neurologic disorders may be challenging. Ideally, each person involved in the treatment and rehabilitation of the patient should be able to perform a physical examination for lameness detection and should have knowledge of the underlying condition and its assessment. The evaluator should develop a systematic approach to standardize the physical examination and to prevent omissions of important findings.

History

The patient's age, gender, and breed should be determined and recorded in the medical record. It is helpful to obtain information regarding the patient's general health. The owner should be questioned to determine if there are any signs of systemic disease, such as fever, anorexia, depression, vomiting, or diarrhea. The presence of any preexisting conditions that may produce or contribute to the lameness should be recorded.

Any known previous trauma should be recorded, along with the affected areas that were injured. The travel history of the affected animal or of other pets in the household should be assessed. Certain fungal diseases and some diseases transmitted by ticks, such as ehrlichiosis and Rocky Mountain spotted fever, are endemic in certain geographic areas, and travel to those regions may result in infection.

The owner or handler should be asked to state the chief complaint, or the reason why the dog is being evaluated. When questioning an owner or handler regarding the affected limb(s), it is important to be certain that the correct limb is identified. Sometimes, the owner may be confused and misidentify the affected leg(s). To eliminate any confusion, the owner should point to the limb that is the source of concern.

The progression of the condition should be addressed, including when it started, changes in severity over time, changes with weather, changes with exercise or rest, and any changes that occur over the course of a typical day. Information regarding any previous diagnoses should also be obtained. The results of any previous treatments should be assessed. In particular, any medications administered should be recorded, along with the dose, dosing interval, length of treatment time, and whether or not the treatment was effective. It is relatively common for inappropriate doses of medications, such as nonsteroidal antiinflammatory drugs, to be administered, and it may be inappropriate to conclude whether such treatment has been ineffective in the treatment of conditions such as osteoarthritis. If the history is lengthy or confusing, it may be helpful to construct a timeline.

The owner's impression of the degree of pain or lameness should be obtained, and whether there is multiple limb involvement. With regard to the lameness, the following short series of questions may be useful:

- Have other limbs been involved?
- Has the lameness increased/decreased in severity?
- Is the lameness worse in the morning or evening?
- Was the limb subjected to some traumatic event?
- How long has the lameness been present, and is it static, increasing, or decreasing in severity?
- Does the lameness change with weather or exercise?
- Have there been any previous related diagnoses or treatment?

During the gathering of historic information it is vital that the examiner also consider that certain neurologic or oncologic problems may mimic orthopedic diseases, and the converse is true as well. Dogs with bilateral cranial cruciate ligament ruptures may have gait and stance problems suggestive of neurologic disease. Oncologic conditions, such as osteosarcoma or multiple myeloma, may present with a lameness that mimics an orthopedic problem. Some neoplastic conditions may have paraneoplastic manifestations, such as hypertrophic osteopathy, in which a mass in another location may result in periosteal reaction of the bones of the distal limbs and lameness.

General Physical Examination

It is critical that a thorough general physical examination be performed by the attending veterinarian. Information concerning other body systems is vital to determine whether certain forms of therapy may be contraindicated, or if a systemic disease such as Lyme disease or systemic lupus erythematosus may be the underlying cause of a lameness. It is especially important if surgical intervention is possible or if long-term medication is anticipated to be certain that major body systems are healthy and able to tolerate the treatment. In particular, the cardiovascular, respiratory, gastrointestinal, hepatic, renal, and endocrine systems should be assessed to determine if underlying disease conditions are present that

may affect the selection and appropriate use of various medications or anesthetic agents. Thorough auscultation of the heart and lungs, abdominal palpation, lymph node palpation, evaluation of mucocutaneous junctions, and assessment of the skin are necessary. Ancillary tests may be needed for more thorough evaluation, including electrocardiogram, complete blood count, serum biochemistry profile, urinalysis, radiographs or sonograms of the thorax or abdomen, and other special tests.

Initial Observation

The dog should be carefully observed at rest and at several gaits before in-depth examination and palpation to avoid artificially accentuating lameness with manipulation of the affected area. If possible, observe the patient as it arises from a sitting or recumbent position. Often the lameness is more severe immediately after rising and then improves with ambulation; in some instances, the patient may not use the affected limb at all to help rise to a standing position.

With the patient standing, one should observe for weakness, limb trembling, asymmetry of regions of the limbs indicative of muscle atrophy, asymmetry of the head and neck, limb position, and conformation (Figure 10-1). It is common for standing animals to bear less weight on a limb afflicted with lameness. In this situation, the animal may not have the entire foot in contact with the floor. One method to assess the relative amount of weight placed on each limb is for the examiner to place a foot on the palm of each hand and allow the animal to bear weight on the observer's hands rather than on the floor. This is a semiquantitative method of assessing weight-bearing. Another method to assess weight-bearing is to use a sphygmomanometer cuff inflated to a certain pressure; the increase in pressure with the cuff placed under the foot is then recorded, and the difference between the two measurements is recorded. In many lamenesses there is also marked muscle atrophy of the affected leg. In some chronic lamenesses there may be abnormal foot pad wear and unequal weight-bearing that may be noticeable.

Gait

Gait evaluation is generally performed after observing the dog rising and at a stance. The

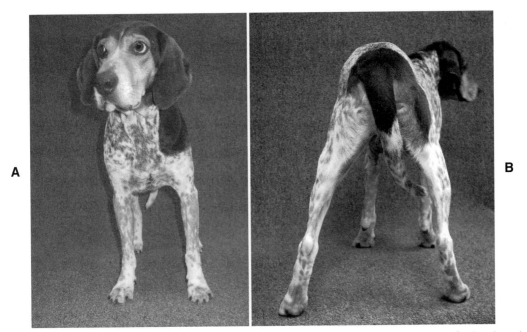

Figure 10-1   The animal should be observed from **(A)** the front and **(B)** the rear while standing for evidence of reduced weight-bearing on an affected limb, turning the toes out, and not bearing weight symmetrically in comparison to the contralateral limb. Note the reduced weight-bearing on the left rear limb indicated by less contact of the metatarsal pad with the ground and the more lateral position of the foot as compared with the other rear limb.

patient's gait is best observed in a large, enclosed exercise area from a distance of at least 30 to 40 feet. In addition, it is beneficial to have an area in which observations may be made with the dog off leash. Gaiting begins with the handler moving the patient past the examiner first at a walk, then at a trot. The patient should be evaluated while moving directly away from, and then toward the examiner (Figure 10-2). The patient should then be evaluated from the side at a distance (Figure 10-3). Evaluation at a lope or gallop may be performed if the patient is able, but this gait is less useful for evaluation of most lameness because of the speed of limb motion and the fact that these gaits are asymmetrical. It may be helpful to capture the gait with a video camera and then evaluate the gait in slow motion. The degree of lameness may be subjectively evaluated using a lameness scoring system to allow comparison of the lameness over a period of time (Box 10-1).

Observation of the patient while it is walking is beneficial for those patients with severe lameness that may be unwilling to trot. Because the walk is a slow four-beat gait, each limb may be separately evaluated. This is particularly beneficial to help differentiate lameness in diagonal forelimbs and hindlimbs in some difficult lamenesses that are detected at a trot. In many cases, the head will nod up and down if a lameness is present. In general the head will nod up when the affected leg is placed on the ground if a forelimb lameness is present, and the head will nod down when the affected limb is placed on the ground if a hindlimb lameness is present. The reason for this is to reduce weight-bearing and force on the lame limb by using the head and neck as a lever arm to shift weight from the painful limb to the opposite end of the body.

The patient should also be evaluated at a trot, which is a symmetric two-beat diagonal gait. While forelimb and hindlimb lameness may be differentiated at a walk because the pattern of footfalls is separated, differentiation of forelimb and hindlimb lameness is more challenging at a trot. The reason for this is that diagonal forelimbs and hindlimbs strike the ground at the same time. As an example, consider a head that nods up when the left forelimb strikes the ground. This may indicate a left forelimb lameness. However, it may also be indicative of a left hindlimb lameness, because as the left hindlimb strikes the ground, the head will nod down; as the right hindlimb and left forelimb strike the ground immediately after, the head will nod back up.

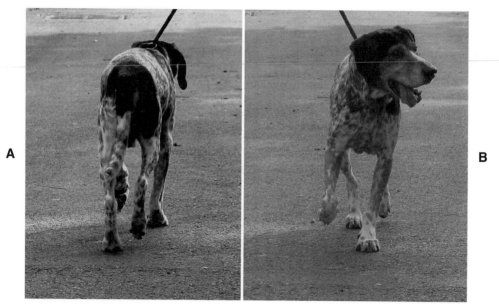

Figure 10-2   The animal should be observed going **(A)** away from and **(B)** toward the evaluator at both a walk and a trot.

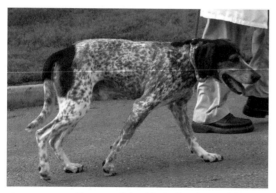

Figure 10-3   The animal should also be observed from the side.

■ ■ ■ **BOX 10-1** Lameness Score That May Be Applied to Dogs at a Walk and at a Trot

0: Normal
1: Slight, intermittent lameness
2: Obvious weight-bearing lameness
3: Severe weight-bearing lameness
4: Intermittent non–weight-bearing lameness
5: Continuous non–weight-bearing lameness

Careful observation of other features of gait may help distinguish between forelimb and hindlimb lameness at a trot, in conjunction with other features of the physical examination. Careful observation at a walk may also help to distinguish the lame limb because of the separate pattern of footfalls. It may also be helpful to place each major joint through a full range of motion, and then reassess the lameness. Stresses placed on joints as they are flexed and extended may accentuate a subtle lameness.

In addition, other factors such as stride length, limb carriage, joint motion, and side bending of the spinal column are useful in evaluating lameness. The affected limb may have a shortened stride length and reduced flexion and extension of the affected joints. Most dogs will walk with the normal limb centered under the body during the weight-bearing phase of gait on that limb, while a lame limb may be carried further laterally during weight-bearing. The affected limb may also circumduct during gait. Animals with hip or stifle conditions may have increased lateral flexion of the spinal column toward the affected side in an attempt to advance the limb by using the back, especially if the stride is shortened on that side. In all cases, symmetry of movement should be evaluated. Abnormal proprioception, dragging of the nails, knuckling over on the dorsum of the paw, and hypermetria indicate neurologic disease.

When possible, the patient should be walked and trotted in a large circle. In many cases, lameness of the inside limb will be accentuated. Stairs and steps may also be helpful in observing lameness and subtle neurologic problems. Dogs may skip up steps

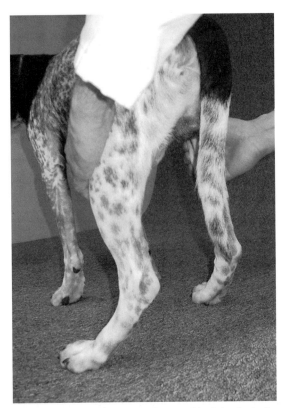

Figure 10-4   Simultaneous palpation of both hindlimbs for evidence of muscle atrophy and asymmetry.

with the affected limb rather than pushing off the limb to ascend a flight of stairs, or may knuckle over on the dorsum of the paw of a limb afflicted with a neurologic condition.

General Palpation for Symmetry and Atrophy

Following observation of the patient for lameness during ambulation, a brief examination is performed while the dog is still standing to assess symmetry and to assess relative muscle mass and the presence of muscle atrophy. Simultaneous palpation of both forelimbs and then both rear limbs will allow the examiner to detect subtle differences between limbs that are normally symmetrical (Figure 10-4). Fractures and neoplasia of the musculoskeletal system are usually obvious. Individual regions are evaluated for swelling, abnormal shape, heat, and sensitivity and pain.

Beginning with the forelimb, the dorsal border of the scapula is palpated to be certain that one side is not higher than the other. The spine of the scapula is assessed for fractures and prominence of the spine of the scapula,

which might indicate muscle atrophy if it is readily palpable and differs from the other side. The acromion and greater tubercle of the humerus are palpated next. The distance between the two landmarks and the amount of soft tissue between the two points should be equal on both sides. The shaft of the humerus is palpated next to locate any areas of swelling or muscle atrophy.

The elbow is a difficult joint to assess because many structures are present in a relatively small area, including the medial and lateral epicondyles of the humerus and the flexor and extensor muscles that arise from them, the head of the radius, the region of the medial coronoid process of the ulna, the joint capsule, and other soft-tissue structures in the area. The task is made easier by standing behind the dog and placing the forefingers of each hand on the lateral epicondyles. The middle fingers are then placed on the head of the radius. The thumbs are placed in the region of the medial coronoid process of the ulna. The lateral and cranial joint compartments are assessed for joint effusion, swelling, and increased or decreased soft-tissue mass. The caudolateral joint compartment is assessed next between the lateral epicondyle and the olecranon process for joint effusion or swelling, which might indicate osteoarthritis or an ununited anconeal process. This swelling is usually palpable caudal and parallel to the lateral epicondyle, and compression forces the effusion medially. The thumbs are used to palpate the medial joint compartment and the region of the medial coronoid process. Following assessment of swelling and joint effusion, the area is firmly pressed to assess for pain and discomfort, which may indicate a fragmented medial coronoid process. By palpating the elbows simultaneously with the dog standing, subtle abnormalities may be detected by assessing the area for asymmetry. It may also be helpful in certain cases to pronate and supinate the distal extremity when evaluating each individual elbow. These maneuvers help to concentrate the forces in the medial or lateral joint compartment, accentuating any subtle discomfort.

The shafts of the radius and ulna are palpated from proximal to distal to assess the bones for any pain or swelling. The carpi and digits are usually best assessed with the dog in lateral recumbency, although the standing angle of the carpus should be observed to be certain that carpal hyperextension is not present.

The hindlimbs are evaluated next. The dorsal aspect of the wings of the iliums are located to be certain that one is not located further cranially or dorsally than the other, which might indicate a sacroiliac luxation. The gluteal muscles are assessed for atrophy throughout the ilium. The area between the greater trochanter and the tuber ischium is located and compared to the other side. Asymmetry may indicate the presence of muscle atrophy on the side that has less soft tissue between the two points, or a hip luxation if the distance between the two points differs. The thigh musculature is evaluated for atrophy. The stifles are simultaneously palpated in a manner similar to that of the elbows to assess for joint effusion, the presence of firm tissue on the medial aspect of the distal femur (often referred to as a medial buttress) that might indicate a chronic rupture of the cranial cruciate ligament, and the position of the patellas.

The tibias are assessed for any asymmetric swelling or pain, and the angle of the tarsus is observed to evaluate the integrity of the common calcaneal tendons. The tarsus and digits are best evaluated with the patient in lateral recumbency.

Orthopedic Examination

It is helpful to use a systematic approach to reduce the risk of missing a condition and to create an evaluation that can be consistently repeated. In many cases the contralateral limb may be used as a reference for comparison of limb circumference, range of motion, and sensitivity to palpation. Comparison to the contralateral limb may be especially helpful when a subtle condition exists and there is uncertainty regarding an abnormality. Concentrating on anatomy during the examination, and referring to an anatomy book as necessary, helps in confusing or unusual situations.

Rear Limbs

Evaluation of the rear limbs first may be safer for the examiner while the patient is becoming accustomed to the examiner. The phalanges and metatarsals of the distal limb are evaluated first. The toes are spread apart to evaluate the nail beds, webbing between the toes, and the pads for any infection, trauma, or cracks. The phalanges, interphalangeal joints, metatarsal bone, and metatarsophalangeal joints are individually palpated and assessed for pain,

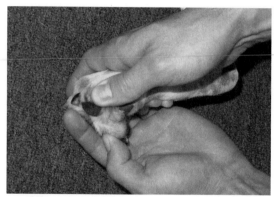

Figure 10-5   The interdigital areas, pads, phalanges, and metatarsal bones should be palpated and the joints placed through a range of motion.

crepitus, swelling, fractures, luxations, or collateral ligament instability (Figure 10-5). The range of motion of the joints is also assessed. The area over the plantar sesamoid bones is palpated for pain and proliferative changes that might be associated with an old fracture or arthritis. Joint stability is further assessed by flexing and extending individual joints and placing varus and valgus stresses on the joints. It is helpful to be familiar with the origin and insertion of the interphalangeal ligaments to properly evaluate instability (see Box 10-2).

The tarsus is a complex series of joints. It is first assessed for joint effusion and instability. Palpation of the dorsal aspect of the tarsocrural joint is especially rewarding in cases of joint effusion. The joint is placed through a full range of motion to assess the joint for limitations, crepitus, and pain. The examiner's finger is used to palpate the tarsal bones, with particular attention to the central, third, and fourth tarsal bones. The tarsus has short and long components of the medial and lateral collateral ligaments that are taut in different degrees of flexion and extension. To assess the long components of the collateral ligaments, valgus and varus stresses are applied while the tarsus is placed in full extension (Figure 10-6). Normally, there should be little varus or valgus movement with the hock extended. The short portions of the collateral ligaments are assessed by placing varus and valgus stresses on the tarsus with the tarsocrural joint flexed to 90 degrees. Assessment of these structures while the hock is flexed is more difficult because there is some normal motion in this position. After stabilizing the metatarsus with one hand and the tuber calcis with the other, dorsal and plantar stresses are placed

BOX10-2 Common Conditions of the Hindlimbs

Common Conditions of the Digits, Pads, and Feet
- Paronychia
- Lacerations of the interdigital skin or foot pads
- Luxations of the interphalangeal joints
- Luxations of the tarsometatarsal joint
- Fractures of the metatarsal bones
- Fractures of the phalanges
- Fractures of the sesamoid bones

Common Conditions of the Tarsus
- Osteochondritis dissecans of the talus
- Fracture of the calcaneus
- Fracture of the central tarsal bone
- Fracture of the third or fourth tarsal bones
- Luxations of the tarsus with damage to the short or long tarsocrural ligaments
- Osteoarthritis
- Disruption of the common calcaneal tendon
- Rupture of the plantar ligaments

Common Conditions of the Tibia and Fibula
- Fractures of the tibia and fibula
- Panosteitis
- Traumatic periostitis
- Osteosarcoma

Common Conditions of the Stifle
- Cranial cruciate ligament disruption
- Osteochondritis dissecans of the femoral condyles
- Injuries to the medial/lateral collateral ligaments
- Medial/lateral patellar luxation
- Medial/lateral meniscal damage
- Fractures
- Congenital absence of the patella
- Caudal cruciate ligament disruption
- Osteoarthritis

Common Conditions of the Femur
- Fracture of the femur
- Panosteitis
- Osteosarcoma

Common Conditions of the Coxofemoral Joint
- Hip dysplasia
- Fracture of the acetabulum
- Fracture of the femoral head or neck
- Fracture/separation of the proximal capital femoral physis
- Legg-Calvé-Perthes disease
- Traumatic luxation of the coxofemoral joint
- Osteoarthritis

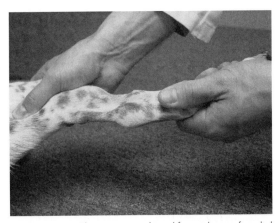

Figure 10-6   The tarsus is evaluated for evidence of medial or lateral collateral ligament damage by applying varus and valgus stresses to the joint.

be little ability to flex the tarsus. Excessive flexion may indicate that there has been a fracture of the calcaneus or damage to the common calcaneal tendon. It is also helpful to palpate the insertion of the tendon on the calcaneus to rule out partial avulsion injuries, which may be manifested as a firm swollen area. It is valuable to compare the suspected limb to the contralateral limb to assess subtle findings.

Palpation of the tibia is relatively easy because the medial aspect has little muscle covering. The metaphyseal and diaphyseal regions are palpated for periosteal or bone pain, which might indicate panosteitis, hypertrophic osteodystrophy, fractures, neoplasia, or traumatic periostitis (Figure 10-7). It is helpful to palpate the head of the fibula and the medial and lateral malleoli.

The stifle joint is a joint that is frequently afflicted with orthopedic conditions. Sedation may be necessary in some larger patients that are tense. The joint is initially assessed for swelling. The tibial tubercle is located first, and the path of the patellar ligament is traced proximally. The joint is palpated medial and lateral to the patellar ligament. Normally, the ligament feels like a pencil and the medial and lateral edges can be distinctly felt, but with joint effusion, the patellar ligament is less distinct and fluid may be palpable in cases of moderate to severe joint effusion. The femoral condyles and the region of the trochlear ridges are palpated next. In some cases, osteophytes or joint capsule thickening may be palpable. Thickening of the medial aspect of the distal femur is often present in dogs with chronic rupture of the cranial cruciate ligament. This is easily felt by placing the examiner's hand and

on the hock to determine if subluxation is present or if there has been damage to the supporting plantar structures. With the stifle maintained in an extended position, the hock is flexed to evaluate the calcaneus and common calcaneal tendon. Normally, there should

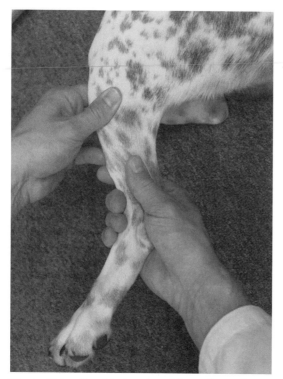

Figure 10-7   The tibia is palpated for evidence of pain, swelling, or inflammation.

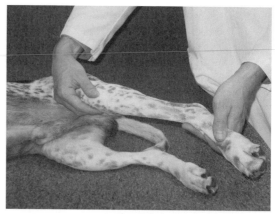

Figure 10-8   To evaluate the stifle for medial patella luxation, the stifle is extended, the tibia is internally rotated, and an attempt is made to push the patella medially out of the trochlear groove.

fingers across the stifle so that the fingers rest over the medial surface of the joint. The other stifle may be simultaneously palpated to compare the two limbs. Swelling of the craniolateral joint in a young dog might indicate the presence of an avulsion of the long digital extensor tendon, although this condition is rare. The stifle is flexed and extended to evaluate for crepitus, grating, clicking, or snapping, which might indicate osteoarthritis, a damaged meniscus, or joint instability. The examiner's hand may be placed on the patella to assess crepitus. Often dogs with chronic osteoarthritis secondary to cranial cruciate ligament rupture have marked pain with full stifle extension.

The patella is assessed for medial or lateral luxation. To test for medial patella luxation, the stifle is extended, the distal limb is internally rotated, and pressure is applied to the lateral aspect of the patella to try to displace it medially (Figure 10-8). While maintaining pressure, the limb is slowly flexed and extended to be certain that luxation does not occur with the limb in a position other than full extension. Medial patella luxation is common in toy and miniature breeds and in larger breeds such as Labrador retrievers. In small dogs, the patella may be difficult to locate if

patella ectopia exists. In these cases, the tibial tubercle is located and the path of the patellar ligament is traced proximally until the patella is located. To test for lateral patella luxation, the stifle is placed in extension or slight flexion while the distal limb is externally rotated. Pressure is applied to the medial aspect of the patella, trying to force it laterally. Although medial patella luxation is most common in all breeds, if a lateral patella luxation is present, it is most likely a large dog or a Basset hound.

Instability of the medial collateral ligament is assessed with the stifle in extension. While holding the distal femur with one hand and the proximal tibia with the other, a valgus stress is placed on the tibia. In normal dogs, little motion occurs with this maneuver. Lateral collateral ligament integrity is assessed by holding the limb as if checking for medial collateral instability, but a varus stress is placed on the tibia.

Injury to the cranial cruciate ligament is common, and this structure should be carefully evaluated. Large dogs may be tense and require sedation for a thorough examination. The most common method of assessing rupture of the cranial cruciate ligament rupture is the cranial drawer test (Figure 10-9). To perform this test, place one index finger on the tibial tubercle and stretch the soft tissues caudally with the thumb until the head of the fibula is reached. Place the other index finger on the patella and stretch the soft tissues with the thumb until the lateral fabella is palpated. Now place the stifle in mild flexion and quickly and gently try to move the tibia cranially and caudally (slide the drawer open and closed). The examiner should avoid inter-

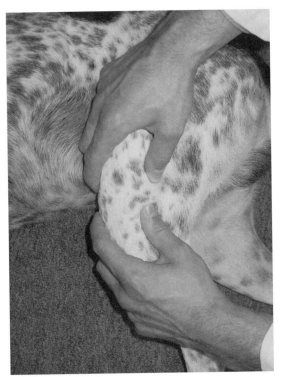

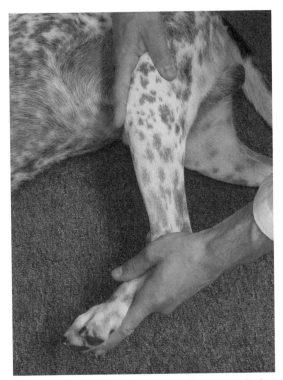

Figure 10-9   Cranial drawer motion is assessed by placing one forefinger on the patella, one thumb on the lateral fabella, the other forefinger on the tibial tuberosity, and the other thumb on the head of the fibula. An attempt is then made to slide the tibia cranially in relation to the femur, while holding the femur in a steady position.

Figure 10-10   The tibial compression test is a method to indirectly create cranial drawer motion. To perform this maneuver, the stifle is placed in a slightly extended walking position and firmly maintained in this position. The examiner places a forefinger on the tibial tuberosity and the thumb and remaining fingers on the medial and lateral condyles of the femur. The other hand is used to flex the hock. The forefinger on the tibial tuberosity detects any cranial shift of the tibia in relation to the femur as a result of an insufficient cranial cruciate ligament.

nally rotating the limb while performing the drawer maneuver. Because the cranial cruciate ligament also limits excessive internal rotation and hyperextension, in addition to cranial drawer, excessive internal rotation or hyperextension may be helpful in diagnosing injury to the ligament. In some cases, partial drawer may be detected. This may result from a partial cranial cruciate rupture, a torn meniscus that has become wedged between the tibia and femur, or a chronic cranial cruciate ligament rupture with periarticular fibrosis providing partial stability of the stifle. In some cases of partial cranial cruciate ligament rupture, there may be drawer motion in flexion but not extension.

An indirect method of evaluating the integrity of the cranial cruciate ligament is the tibial compression test (Figure 10-10). The stifle is flexed to an approximately 90-degree angle. One hand is placed on the stifle with the forefinger resting on the tibial tuberosity. The tarsus is slowly flexed with the other hand. This causes tension in the gastrocnemius muscle and common calcaneal tendon

that compresses the femur and tibia. In the absence of the cranial cruciate ligament, cranial movement of the tibial tuberosity in relation to the distal femur is detected.

Injury to the caudal cruciate ligament is rare and is usually due to trauma. Other structures are also commonly injured, such as the cranial cruciate ligament, the medial collateral ligament, or the medial meniscus. To assess the caudal cruciate ligament, the limb is held as for testing cranial drawer, but the tibia is displaced caudally rather than cranially. Diagnosis of tears of the caudal cruciate ligament can be difficult and requires excellent knowledge of the spatial anatomy of the stifle joint.

The femur is evaluated next. The quadriceps, biceps femoris, semimembranosus, and semitendinosus muscles are palpated for atrophy, swelling, and pain. Although muscle tears are rare in breeds other than sight hounds, the tensor fascia lata and gracilis muscles should be examined. The shaft of the femur is

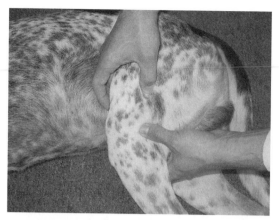

Figure 10-11   The femur is palpated for any pain, inflammation, or swelling, while minimizing excessive compression of the muscles.

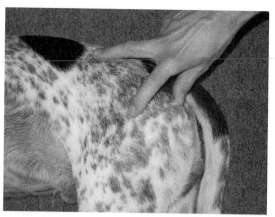

Figure 10-12   The relationships of the dorsal border of the wing of the ilium, the greater trochanter of the femur, and the ischiatic tuberosity are established. A triangle should be formed when these structures are outlined. In this photo, the thumb is on the tuber ischium, the forefinger is on the greater trochanter, and the middle finger is on the dorsal border of the wing of the ilium. If the greater trochanter is in a line with the dorsal wing of the ilium and the ischiatic tuberosity, a craniodorsal luxation of the coxofemoral joint may be present.

palpated between muscle bellies, being careful not to confuse bone pain with pain from pinching muscles (Figure 10-11). Bone pain and swelling in the distal femur may indicate osteosarcoma in a large breed, whereas pain in the diaphysis of the bone in a young dog may indicate panosteitis.

The coxofemoral or hip joint is another joint that is commonly afflicted with orthopedic conditions. The hip joint should be assessed for luxation in dogs with acute lameness of a rear limb as a result of trauma. To do this, fingers are placed on the tuber sacrale, greater trochanter, and tuber ischium (Figure 10-12). The greater trochanter should be below a line drawn from the tuber ischium to the tuber sacrale; if not, then a hip luxation should be suspected. Next, a thumb is placed in a notch between the greater trochanter and the tuber ischium, and the femur is externally rotated. With a normal hip, the thumb will be displaced out of the notch as the femur is rotated. With a hip luxation, the thumb is not displaced because the greater trochanter is typically displaced cranially and dorsally and does not rotate caudally to displace the thumb from the notch. Another method of evaluating the possibility of a hip luxation is to measure the length of the affected leg. The affected leg will be shorter with the hip extended and will be longer with the hip flexed as compared with the normal contralateral leg. It should be noted that fractures of the femoral neck and capital femoral physeal fractures may give similar physical examination findings.

Next the hip should be placed through a range of motion, including flexion, extension, and rotation of the hip joint to determine if pain, crepitus, or decreased range of motion

exist. In most cases the toes are able to reach the ipsilateral olecranon with full hip flexion. Patients with osteoarthritis of the hip have pain with hip extension. Subluxation of the hip commonly occurs in young dogs with hip dysplasia. The Ortolani sign may be performed to determine whether subluxation of the coxofemoral joint is present (Figure 10-13). To perform this test, the dog is placed in lateral or dorsal recumbency. The palm of one hand is placed over the region of the sacrum to support the dog and the fingers of that hand are placed on the greater trochanter and rim of the acetabulum. The femur is grasped with the other hand, and the femur is adducted and pushed dorsally. The examiner may feel the femur displace from the acetabulum. The femur is then slowly abducted while palpating for a change in the relation of the greater trochanter and acetabulum. If the hip was subluxated, a distinct "clunk" will be felt as the hip spontaneously reduces itself as the femur is abducted. An Ortolani maneuver may be performed in a standing dog by placing the dog's pelvis and sacrum against the examiner's chest and using one hand to create a dorsal force while adducting the hip.

Forelimbs

Evaluation of the digits, pads, interdigital skin, metacarpal bones, phalangeal joints, and metacarpophalangeal joints is similar to that

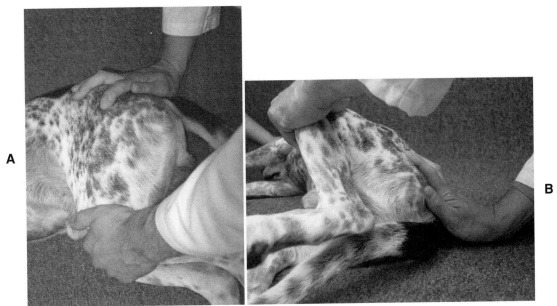

Figure 10-13   A, To perform the Ortolani test, the patient is placed in lateral recumbency, the palm of one hand is placed over the area of the acetabulum, the forefinger of that hand is placed on the greater trochanter, and the femur is adducted while the femur is pushed dorsally with the other hand. **B,** The femur is then abducted, and if subluxation of the hip has occurred, the reduction will be felt with the forefinger on the greater trochanter as it is reduced.

conducted in the rear limbs (Figure 10-14 and Box 10-3). Careful digital palpation on the dorsal surface of these bones may reveal point pain or tenderness often associated with stress periostitis.

The carpus is evaluated next. The antebrachial carpal, middle carpal, and carpometacarpal joints are assessed for effusion. The areas of each carpal bone are individually palpated for pain, swelling, and discomfort that may indicate chip fractures or other injuries. The carpus is placed through a complete range of motion to assess for restricted motion, pain, or crepitus. Normally, the carpus should flex so that the pads on the bottom of the foot contact the caudal aspect of the antebrachium. The carpus should extend approximately 10 to 20 degrees beyond vertical. The collateral ligaments of the carpus are evaluated by placing varus and valgus stresses with the carpus in full extension. The carpus should be placed in a normal walking position and pressure placed on the foot to evaluate for carpal hyperextension syndrome, which is associated with damage to the palmar fibrocartilage and intercarpal ligaments (Figure 10-15). In early hyperextension injuries, there may be pain and reduced flexion of the carpus. The accessory carpal bone should be evaluated for fractures or changes associated with chronic osteoarthritis.

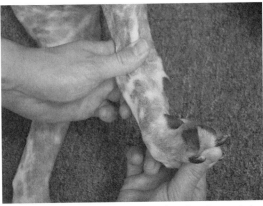

Figure 10-14   The phalanges are flexed and extended to determine if any pain or decreased range of motion is present. Here, the digits are flexed as a group.

The radius and ulna are assessed for angular limb deformities, and their entire lengths are palpated for pain and swelling. The examiner should palpate the medial and lateral styloid processes. Swelling and pain in the metaphyseal region may indicate hypertrophic osteodystrophy in a young, large-breed dog. Lameness and pain on palpation of the diaphyseal region of the radius or ulna in a young large-breed dog may indicate panosteitis (Figure 10-16).

BOX10-3   Common Conditions of the Forelimbs

Common Conditions of the Digits, Pads, and Feet
- Paronychia
- Lacerations of the interdigital skin or foot pads
- Luxations of the interphalangeal joints
- Luxations of the carpometacarpal joint
- Fractures of the metacarpal bones
- Fractures of the phalanges
- Fractures of the sesamoid bones
- Stress periostitis
- Periosteal bone formation associated with hypertrophic osteopathy

Common Conditions of the Carpus
- Fractures of the accessory, radial, ulnar, or numbered carpal bones
- Carpal hyperextension injury
- Collateral ligament injuries
- Stress tendinitis of the ulnar lateralis
- Osteoarthritis

Common Conditions of the Radius, Ulna, and Elbow
- Fragmented coronoid process of the ulna
- Ununited anconeal process
- Incongruity of the elbow joint
- Fracture of the lateral/medial condyle of the humerus
- Luxation of the elbow joint, usually lateral
- Panosteitis
- Hypertrophic osteodystrophy
- Osteoarthritis
- Luxation of the antebrachicarpal joint
- Fracture of the radius and ulna

Common Conditions of the Humerus
- Fracture of the humerus
- Panosteitis
- Osteosarcoma

Common Problems of the Scapulohumeral Joint
- Avulsion fracture of the supraglenoid tubercle
- Luxation of the scapulohumeral joint
- Fracture of the scapulohumeral joint
- Biceps tenosynovitis
- Mineralization of the supraspinatus tendon
- Contracture of the infraspinatus muscle
- Osteochondritis dissecans of the caudal head of the humerus
- Osteoarthritis

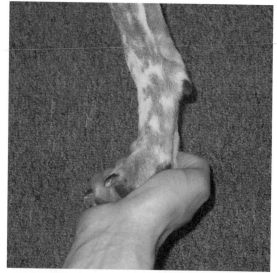

Figure 10-15   The carpus is placed through a range of motion. With the limb placed in a walking position, dorsal pressure is placed on the bottom of the foot to test for carpal hyperextension syndrome.

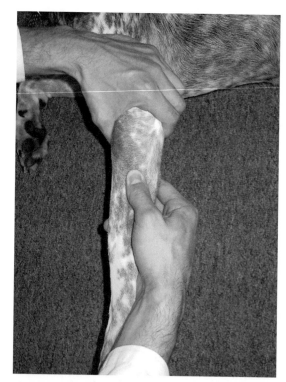

Figure 10-16   The radius and ulna are palpated. If pain is elicited in the midshaft of the radius in a skeletally immature large-breed dog, panosteitis is suspected.

The elbow is a difficult joint to assess because three bones are articulating together, and many soft-tissue structures originate in the region of the elbow. It is helpful to simultaneously palpate both elbows to detect subtle differences between them, such as mild joint effusion (Figure 10-17). The range of motion in flexion and extension is determined, and the joint is evaluated for crepitus. The medial and lateral humeral epicondyles and heads of the radius and ulna are palpated. The collateral ligaments of the elbow joint are evaluated with the elbow and carpus flexed to 90

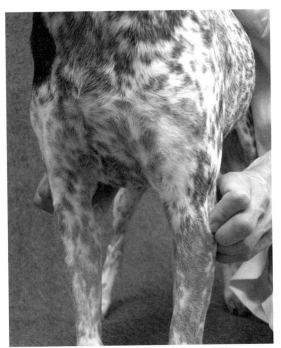

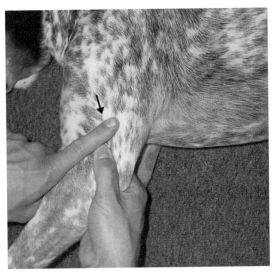

Figure 10-18 Caution should be exercised when palpating the distal humerus to be certain that compression of the radial nerve by the examiner is not causing pain and discomfort. The general area of the radial nerve is indicated by the finger and arrow.

Figure 10-17 Simultaneous palpation of both elbows allows for the detection of subtle abnormalities, such as mild joint effusion. The placements of hands and fingers are essentially mirror images of each other on the right and left elbows. Effusion of the caudolateral compartment in a 6-month-old large-breed dog may indicate the presence of an ununited anconeal process, whereas effusion of the craniomedial joint compartment may indicate a fragmented medial coronoid process or osteochondritis dissecans of the medial condyle of the humerus.

degrees. The distal extremity is grasped, and medial, and then lateral, stress is applied to evaluate the collateral ligaments. With this maneuver, it is possible to internally rotate the distal extremity and increase pressure on the medial portion of the joint. In many dogs with coronoid problems, pain may be elicited. Swelling in the caudolateral aspect of the elbow may indicate joint effusion associated with an ununited anconeal process; swelling on the medial aspect of the elbow joint may indicate osteochondritis dissecans of the medial humeral condyle or a fragmented medial coronoid process of the ulna. With digital pressure, the effusion may be displaced, but the effusion reappears after the digital pressure is released.

The humerus is palpated for swelling and pain that may result from panosteitis or neoplasia. Caution should be exercised in interpreting pain when palpating the region of the radial nerve (Figure 10-18). Direct pressure on the nerve may elicit a painful response unre-

lated to any pathology of the humerus. Anatomically, an imaginary line drawn along the dorsal border of the antebrachium and continued to the humerus with the elbow held in mild flexion will approximate the location of the radial nerve as it crosses over the humerus.

The scapulohumeral or shoulder joint should be flexed and extended. In addition, varus and valgus stresses should be applied to the shoulder to check the collateral support. In some dogs with chronic scapulohumeral instability, it is possible to elicit a drawer motion of the humerus in relation to the scapula. The relationship of the acromial process to the greater tubercle of the humerus should be palpated. An abnormality of this relationship may indicate a shoulder luxation, either medial or lateral. In the absence of trauma, pain on extension of the shoulder joint of a young dog is almost pathognomonic for osteochondritis dissecans of the caudal aspect of the humeral head (Figure 10-19). Similarly, pain may be elicited in a dog with osteochondritis dissecans if the shoulder joint is simultaneously flexed and internally rotated. Pain may be elicited with simultaneous flexion of the shoulder joint and extension of the elbow if biceps tenosynovitis is present (Figure 10-20). This maneuver places increased stress on the biceps tendon as it traverses the bicipital groove in the proximal humerus. Direct palpation of the biceps tendon in this region, located cranial and medial to the greater tubercle, may also elicit pain.

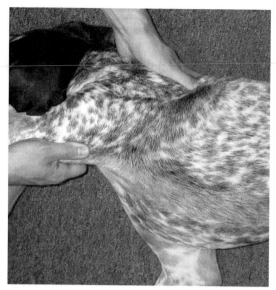

Figure 10-19   Pain caused by extension of the shoulder joint in a skeletally immature large-breed dog is consistent with osteochondritis dissecans of the caudal head of the humerus.

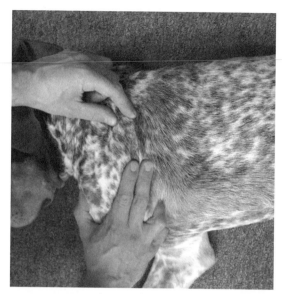

Figure 10-21   Palpation of the scapula is performed to evaluate for fractures or, rarely, luxation of the scapula.

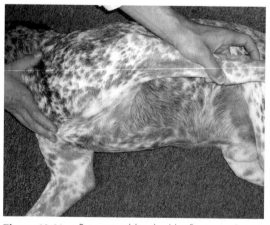

Figure 10-20   Pain caused by shoulder flexion and simultaneous extension of the elbow is likely due to biceps tenosynovitis. Direct palpation of the region of the biceps tendon just medial to the greater tubercle of the proximal humerus may also be painful.

The scapula should be palpated for fractures or pain, especially the spine of the scapula (Figure 10-21). The body of the scapula should be moved in a dorsal direction to determine if a scapular luxation exists, although this is a rare condition.

Other Tips

The best systematic approach to the orthopedic examination is to examine the normal limbs first and the affected limb last. In many cases subtle problems in other limbs may be masked or not detected if attention is initially placed on the most obvious problem. Also, many animals become tense throughout the body if they experience discomfort as a result of palpating a painful area on the affected limb, and a thorough, accurate examination may no longer be possible. Tranquilization and sedation should be avoided until after the initial examination has been completed so that discomfort during palpation is not masked. Similarly, it is best to avoid antiinflammatory drugs for 24 to 48 hours before examination. Diagnostic joint blocks should also be considered. These can be helpful in prioritizing problems if more than one joint is involved, such as in osteoarthritis of the tarsocrural joint and chronic rupture of a cranial cruciate ligament. Tranquilization may facilitate examination of large, athletic dogs in which muscle tone or an anxious patient results in difficulty in assessing certain aspects of the examination, such as an Ortolani sign or cranial drawer motion.

Arthrocentesis

In some cases, arthrocentesis of one or more joints may be performed by a veterinarian. The joint should be identified and will typically have some effusion or an increased quantity of synovial fluid. The area should be clipped and prepared using aseptic technique.

■ ▓ ▓ **Table 10-1**   Synovial Fluid Changes in Canine Arthritis

Condition	Nucleated cells/mm³	Differential mononuclear cells	Differential neutrophils
Normal	250-3000	94-100	0-6
DJD	1000-5000	88-100	0-12
Erosive (rheumatoid-like)	8000-38,000	20-80	20-80
Nonerosive	4400-371,000	5-85	15-95
Septic	40,000-267,000	1-10	90-99

From Piermattei DL, Flo GL: *Brinker, Piermattei, and Flo's handbook of small animal orthopedics and fracture repair*, ed 3, Philadelphia 1997, WB Saunders.

A 20- or 22-gauge needle and 3-cc syringe are used. The affected joint should be flexed and extended several times before arthrocentesis. This helps to dislodge any bacteria from the synovium if an infection is suspected. The needle is inserted without the syringe attached, and the veterinarian waits for synovial fluid to drop into a small EDTA tube. This avoids direct aspiration of the joint and iatrogenic hemorrhage. If no synovial fluid drips from the needle, then the syringe is attached and gentle aspiration is attempted. The fluid should be cultured if sepsis is suspected. Two samples are obtained, one for immediate culture, and the other for culture in blood culture media for 24 hours. This will allow the recovery of relatively low numbers of bacteria to be detected. Synovial fluid analysis is most useful to differentiate inflammatory and noninflammatory joint disease. Table 10-1 indicates the most common general joint conditions and the characteristics of synovial fluid analysis.

Neurologic Examination

During evaluation of small animals for lameness or other musculoskeletal abnormalities, the neurologic system must always be examined because some "lamenesses" are actually neurologic conditions. A complete neurological examination should be performed to help determine the contribution of the nervous system to the condition being evaluated, and to help identify other problems that may be occurring concurrently. In addition, a neurologic evaluation should be performed in trauma patients, and owners should be made aware of conditions before undertaking any treatment of musculoskeletal conditions. A neurologic examination should be performed in a systematic, sequential manner. By always performing a neurologic evaluation in

a consistent fashion, the examiner can ensure that all aspects of the nervous system are evaluated and that nothing is omitted. The neurologic examination should always be performed in a calm, quiet place with minimal distractions. It is important that the patient not be sedated or tranquilized before the examination to help minimize erroneous interpretations of pain sensation or reflexes.

General Neurologic Examination

The neurologic examination begins when an animal is initially presented to the hospital. The general appearance of the patient may initially be evaluated at the time the history is taken, even before a physical examination is performed. Behavior, posture, and voluntary movements should be noted as the animal is allowed to freely move around the examination room. An animal's behavior may be normal, aggressive, excited, apathetic, or depressed. A change in mentation should be noted because this may indicate abnormal brain function or other problems. Posture and voluntary movement may also indicate abnormal brain function, but may also indicate a spinal cord lesion or other neurologic conditions. For an animal to have normal posture, normal peripheral sensory inputs must be processed in the higher centers of the brain including the cerebrum, the cerebellum, and the brain stem. Conditions such as head tilts, tremors, or falling to one side may indicate a problem in any one of these locations.

Nonambulatory animals may be paretic or paralyzed. Either condition causes obvious and markedly abnormal posture in patients. Paretic animals cannot walk without assistance, and although patients can still voluntarily move their legs, limb motion is weak. A lesion causing paresis is considered less severe than one causing paralysis where voluntary movement is no longer possible. Although paresis may be caused by many conditions, it is often a sign of a less severe lesion than would be seen in a paralyzed animal. If a paretic lesion worsens, the condition often progresses to complete paralysis. When examining quadrupeds with spinal lesions, the examiner should keep in mind that paresis and paralysis do not always affect all four limbs equally. When an animal is unable to use or move its limbs, it is said to be paralyzed. When an animal is unable to walk because of paresis in all four limbs, the term tetraparesis is used. Hemiparesis and paraparesis are terms used to describe paresis on one side of the body or of the hindlimbs, respectively, while other limbs have normal function. These presentations are typically seen when a lesion affects nerves to a particular limb without affecting the innervation of other limbs. A typical example would include a thoracolumbar spinal fracture leading to paraparesis or paralysis of both hindlimbs while forelimb function remains unaffected.

After the history is recorded and the general appearance of the animal is evaluated, the patient's gait should be evaluated. A harness should be used for any patient in which head or neck lesions are suspected. In preparation for this aspect of the evaluation, a handler is instructed to gait the animal at a walk and a trot. Although an ataxic or circling animal may not need to be trotted, other conditions such as hypometria or hypermetria may not be evident until the speed of the gait is increased. Gait evaluation should always be performed on a surface with adequate traction and should involve evaluation while the patient ambulates toward and away from the examiner. Several passes at a walk and trot should be performed to detect any minor deficits that may be present. Special attention should focus on each limb and not just the limb or limbs in question to help ensure that all four limbs are properly examined.

After behavior, posture, voluntary movements, and gait have been assessed, the physical examination is initiated. Palpation allows the examiner to inspect muscles, bones, and other soft tissues for subtle abnormalities. Palpation is performed in a systematic way beginning at the head, moving down the neck, and proceeding to the trunk and extremities. Again, by following the same procedure for each patient, the examiner minimizes omissions and is able to perform a consistent evaluation. One side of the body is compared to the other to evaluate symmetry. Careful attention should be paid to muscle size, tone, and strength. Deviation of joints or limbs, abnormal body carriage, or worn toenails could indicate a neurologic problem. Since intervertebral disc herniation and other forms of spinal cord trauma may be painful, the presence of pain during physical examination not only may help identify possible differential diagnoses for a condition, but also may help to localize the lesion.

Spinal Reflexes

Spinal reflexes are used to test the sensory and motor components of a reflex arc. In general, reflexes may be (1) decreased or absent (hyporeflexia), indicating either partial or complete loss of sensory or motor nerve function to a particular region of the body (lower motor neuron disease, LMN); (2) normal, indicating that no neurologic abnormalities exist within the reflex arc; or (3) increased or exaggerated (hyperreflexia), indicating that the inhibitory neurons from the brain and spinal cord cranial to the lower motor neurons have been affected (upper motor neuron disease, UMN). In general, spinal reflexes are graded using the following scheme: absent (0); decreased (+1); normal (+2); exaggerated (+3); or very exaggerated or clonus (+4).

MYOTATIC REFLEXES

Myotatic reflexes are stretch reflexes that cause muscle contraction after the muscle is stretched. These are local reflex arcs that are used for body posture and movement and do not rely on cerebral input for function. The reflex arc consists of a sensory neuron that responds to the stretch of a muscle, and a motor neuron that in turn causes muscle contraction. In general, if only one limb is affected, a peripheral nerve injury is suspected, whereas a spinal cord lesion usually produces bilateral deficits. The most reliable myotatic reflex is the patellar reflex. This reflex is performed with a relaxed patient in lateral recumbency and the pelvic limb held in a slightly flexed position. With the knee supported, the patellar ligament is briskly tapped with a pleximeter (Figure 10-22). As long as the leg is not already in full extension, suddenly stretching the patellar ligament evokes a reflex arc that causes sudden extension of the stifle. Typically, if this reflex is diminished or absent, a LMN lesion is localized to spinal cord segments L4 to L6 or to peripheral sensory or motor nerves. If hyperreflexia is present, an UMN lesion involving the spinal cord cranial to L4 is suspected. Although other myotatic reflexes such as the gastrocnemius, sciatic, triceps, and biceps reflexes have been described, these reflexes are generally less consistent than the patellar reflex. If these reflexes are present, the reflex arc is intact. However, the inability to obtain a reflex does not necessarily indicate that there is no intact pathway.

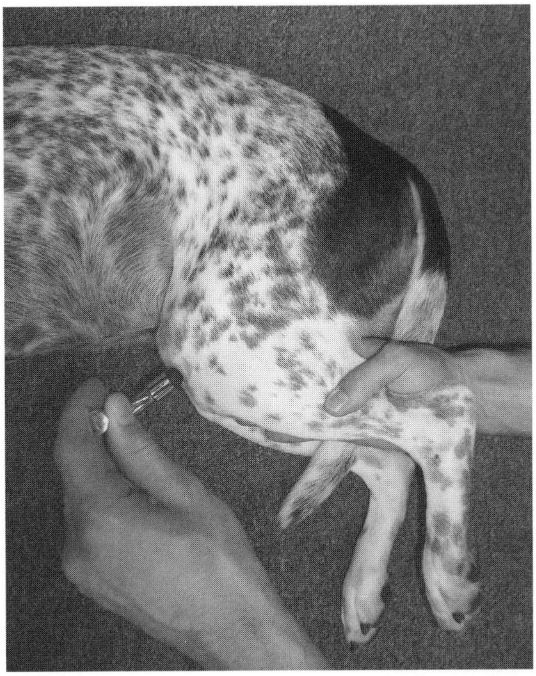

FLEXOR REFLEXES

Flexor reflexes are used to evaluate nerve function in both the thoracic and pelvic limbs. These reflexes are useful in the normal animal to help prevent injury from noxious stimuli and to allow withdrawal of the limb away from a noxious stimulus. Briefly, the animal is positioned in lateral recumbency and the limb is positioned in a neutral position. The animal should be relaxed and comfortable. A noxious stimulus is applied to the foot, stimulating sensory neurons (Figure 10-23). Only the amount of stimulus required to elicit a response should be used. Initially, the skin on a toe is pinched. If no response is elicited with a mild stimulus, a hemostat placed across the nailbed of a toe is used before concluding that there is a negative response. The motor pathways of flexor reflexes are more complex than those of myotatic reflexes because motor neurons for all flexor muscles in the affected limb are activated and the entire limb is flexed. An example would include a flexor reflex of the pelvic limb of a dog, which causes flexion of the hock, stifle, and hip.

Figure 10-22   A patellar reflex is elicited with the patient relaxed and in lateral recumbency by tapping the patellar ligament with a pleximeter.

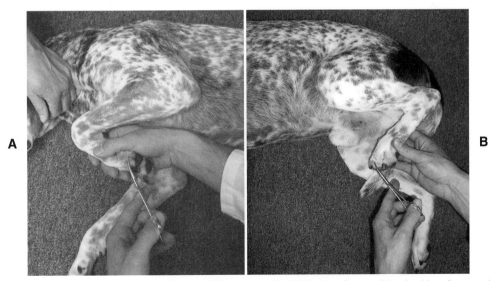

A   B

Figure 10-23   Eliciting a flexor reflex of a forelimb **(A)** and a hindlimb **(B)**. Note flexion of the shoulder, elbow, and carpus in the forelimb, and the hip, stifle, and hock in the rear limb.

AUTONOMOUS ZONES

Because specific peripheral sensory nerves innervate various portions of the limbs, the peripheral nerves and their spinal cord segments may be evaluated to determine the level of injury. In the thoracic limb, the dorsal surface of the foot is innervated by the radial nerve (C7-T1), the medial surface of the antebrachium is innervated by the median nerve (C8-T1), and the caudolateral surface of the foot is innervated by the ulnar nerve (C8-T2). In the pelvic limb, the most medial toe is innervated by the saphenous nerve, a branch of the femoral nerve (L4-L6), whereas the rest of the foot is innervated by the sciatic nerve (L6-S1). Variable responses to noxious stimuli in different regions of the limb help to localize the lesion to a particular region.

CROSSED-EXTENSOR REFLEX

The crossed-extensor reflex is a normal reflex in a standing animal. The reflex causes extension of one limb when the contralateral limb is flexed. In a recumbent animal, this reflex is normally inhibited by descending inhibitory pathways. To elicit the reflex, the animal is placed in lateral recumbency, and the flexor reflex is evoked. Extension of the contralateral limb while the patient is in lateral recumbency signals a lesion in the inhibitory pathways or UMN pathology.

PERINEAL REFLEX

The perineal reflex is elicited by tactile stimulation of the perineal region. The normal response of this reflex consists of contraction of the anal sphincter (anal winking) and ventral flexion of the tail. The sensory and motor components of this reflex are innervated by the pudendal nerve; thus an absent or decreased response indicates a lesion of the pudendal nerve or sacral spinal cord segments S1-S3. Lesions in the sacral spinal cord or pudendal nerves also often result in decreased urethral sphincter tone and an LMN bladder.

CUTANEOUS TRUNCI REFLEX

The cutaneous trunci reflex (sometimes called the panniculus reflex) is a relatively complex reflex elicited by applying a noxious stimulus to the skin, which stimulates the superficial spinal nerves innervating a particular region or autonomous zone (dermatome) of the dermis and elicits a motor response, which is seen as a skin twitch. Typically, fingers or hemostats are used to pinch the skin and dermis just lateral to the dorsal midline, beginning in the cranial thoracic region and moving caudally to the sacrum. When the cutaneous trunci reflex is elicited, a reflex arc is initiated, with the afferent nerves of that particular region of the skin stimulated and a signal transmitted to the spinal cord. The signal is transmitted cranially to the C8-T1 spinal cord segments, where the nerves synapse with the efferent nerves of the lateral thoracic nerve. The impulse causes contraction of the cutaneous trunci muscles to elicit a skin twitch. Spinal nerve roots to autonomous zones travel from cranial to caudal; therefore this reflex usually tests spinal cord segments or nerves approximately two vertebral bodies cranial to the noxious stimulus. Thus a deficit in the cutaneous trunci response at a specific location indicates a spinal cord lesion approximately two vertebral bodies cranial to the site of the skin pinch. The cutaneous trunci reflex is most reliable in the middle of the back. Testing over the cervical, caudal lumbar, and sacral regions is far less reliable.

Sensation

The presence or absence of sensation in each appendage must be assessed. Unless peripheral nerve injury is suspected, pain sensation is usually absent only when voluntary motion is also absent. This typically occurs in the presence of severe spinal cord injury. In general, if an animal can move its limbs, sensation is usually present. In paralyzed animals the presence or absence of pain sensation is very important because absence of deep pain sensation may indicate severe and often irreversible spinal cord damage.

Deep pain sensation is assessed concurrently with the flexor reflexes. Animals with severe damage to the spinal cord cranial to the nerve cell bodies and peripheral nerves of the tested flexor reflex may still have an intact flexor reflex, but may not transmit the signal to the brain for the interpretation of pain. Intact pain perception is indicated by a cerebral response to the pain, such as vocalization, turning the head toward the stimulated limb, or an attempt to move away from the stimulus. The absence of deep pain perception usually indicates severe spinal cord damage, but it does not indicate whether the lesion is UMN or LMN. The presence of a hyporeflexic or hyperreflexic flexor reflex indicates whether the lesion is UMN or LMN. It must be emphasized that a patient may still retain a positive flexor reflex, but have loss of deep pain sensation. This situation occurs relatively commonly in dogs with serious intervertebral disc extrusion in the thoracolumbar region.

Postural Reactions

Postural reactions are used by animals to maintain an upright position and normal body posture. Under normal circumstances, an animal knows the position of each limb in space and will appropriately shift its weight to avoid falling. Postural reactions involve spinal reflexes, as well as input from higher centers, such as the brain and spinal cord, to maintain proper body position. Several postural reactions should be tested during a complete neurologic examination. Although these tests involve different limbs, all test the integration of brain, spinal cord, and peripheral nerves. Abnormal postural reactions indicate a neurological abnormality, but provide the examiner with limited information regarding the specific location of the lesion. Other portions of the neurologic examination will help to localize the lesion. Common postural reaction tests are described below.

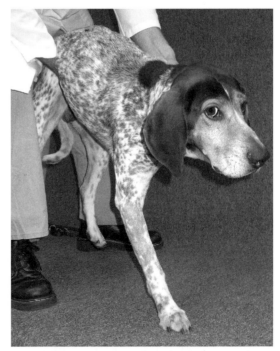

Figure 10-24 Hopping performed to assess postural reactions in a forelimb.

HOPPING

Hopping may be performed on thoracic and pelvic limbs. The animal is supported, and weight is placed on one limb with the other limbs supported so they bear no weight (Figure 10-24). The animal is then moved laterally in a smooth and quick fashion. The animal should hop on the limb to prevent falling and collapse. Caution should be used in animals with muscle weakness because these animals might have a normal postural reaction to hopping, but may not have the muscle strength to support their weight. In these situations, the animal may be supported to allow hopping, even if it is weak.

WHEELBARROWING

Wheelbarrowing is performed by lifting the caudal abdomen and pelvic limbs of an animal and allowing weight-bearing on the forelimbs (Figure 10-25). In this position, an animal with normal neurologic function should be able to

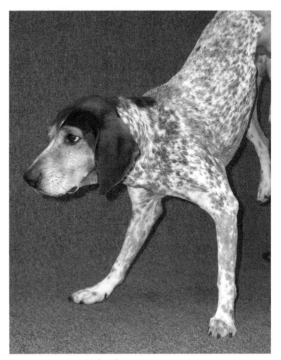

Figure 10-25 Wheelbarrowing to assess proprioceptive function of the forelimbs.

move forward as the animal is pushed forward. Muscle weakness may affect wheelbarrowing and postural reactions, requiring some support.

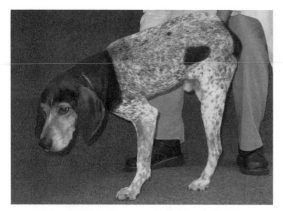

Figure 10-26   Hemiwalking.

HEMIWALKING

The hemiwalking test is performed by lifting ipsilateral forelimbs and hindlimbs of the patient, forcing weight-bearing on the other two contralateral limbs (Figure 10-26). The animal is moved laterally and should be able to walk on two legs without falling. Weak animals may require some support.

KNUCKLING (CONSCIOUS PROPRIOCEPTION)

Conscious proprioception is used to test an animal's awareness of limb position in space without visual input. It is unnatural for an animal to walk or stand on the dorsum of the paw. To test conscious proprioception, a knuckling test is performed on each of the four limbs. With the animal supported, the paw is picked up and turned over so that the dorsum of the paw contacts the ground (Figure 10-27). Generally, normal animals immediately pick up the paw and place it into a normal position. Normally, a patient will not stand on the dorsum of the paw to support weight. If the paw is not properly replaced, a neurologic deficit is usually present. In general, animals with mild neurologic lesions may have proprioceptive deficits, but may not show other obvious abnormal signs; in some cases, motor activity may remain relatively normal until the lesion progresses.

TACTILE PLACING

Tactile placing tests are performed by covering an animal's eyes, lifting it off of the ground, and bringing the forelimbs toward a table or stable surface. After sensing the surface, the normal response to a tactile placing test is to immediately place both forelimbs

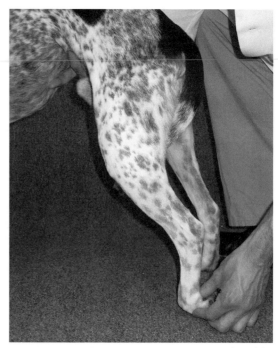

Figure 10-27   Conscious proprioception is evaluated by knuckling over the dorsum of the paw. A normal patient will quickly right the paw to a proper position.

onto the surface in a weight-bearing position. A normal tactile placing response relies on normal sensory and motor pathways of the thoracic limbs. Also, normal cerebrocortical function is required to receive and process the information.

Visual placing tests are performed in the same manner as a tactile placing test except that the patient's eyes are not covered. During this test, it is normal for a suspended animal to reach for a surface even before touching it. Although this test still relies on a normal cerebral cortex and intact motor function to the thoracic limbs, sensory input is via the visual pathways rather than the tactile sensation of the paw.

Cranial Nerve Examination

A brief cranial nerve examination should be performed during a neurologic evaluation. Animals possess 12 cranial nerves (Table 10-2). These nerves are mainly involved with functions of the head, and abnormal function may indicate a brain lesion. As with other neurologic tests, cranial nerve examination should be performed in a systematic manner and usually does not add more than a few minutes to the examination. Cranial nerve examination will be briefly discussed with the nerves being

■ ■ ■ **Table 10-2** Cranial Nerves and Their Functions

CN I: Olfactory nerve	Sensory pathway for the sense of smell
CN II: Optic nerve	Sensory pathway for vision and pupillary light reflexes
CN III: Oculomotor nerve	Motor pathway to all extrinsic ocular muscles except the lateral rectus, retractor bulbi, and dorsal oblique muscles
	Motor pathway for pupillary constriction
CN IV: Trochlear nerve	Motor pathway to the dorsal oblique muscle of the eye
CN V: Trigeminal nerve	Motor pathway to masticatory muscles
	Sensory pathway to the mouth and face
CN VI: Abducent nerve	Motor pathway for the lateral rectus and dorsal oblique muscles of the eye
CN VII: Facial nerve	Motor pathway to the muscles of facial expression
	Sensory pathway for taste to the rostral two thirds of the tongue and the palate
CN VIII: Vestibulocochlear nerve	Vestibular portion—Proprioceptive role for equilibrium and posture
	Cochlear portion—Sensory role in hearing
CN IX: Glossopharyngeal nerve	Sensory and motor innervation for swallowing and the gag reflex
	Sensory pathway for taste to the caudal third of the tongue
CN X: Vagus nerve	Sensory and motor innervation for swallowing, the gag reflex, laryngeal function, and vocalization
CN XI: Spinal accessory nerve	Motor pathway to the muscles of the neck
CN XII: Hypoglossal nerve	Motor innervation to the muscles of the tongue

evaluated indicated in parentheses after each portion of the test.

The patient's head is inspected for muscle atrophy and abnormal jaw tone (cranial nerves VII [facial nerve] and V [trigeminal nerve], respectively). While the eyes are covered, the skin around the ears, eyes, and nose is stimulated to elicit a twitch or other facial movement (cranial nerves V and VII). The lateral and medial canthus of each eye is stimulated to elicit a blink response. A menace response is elicited by quick hand movements toward each open eye. In adult animals, anticipation of ocular injury should cause momentary closure of the affected eye (cranial nerves II [optic nerve] and VII). A pupillary light response is tested by shining a bright light into each eye while monitoring for pupillary constriction (cranial nerves II and III [oculomotor nerve]). Direct and consensual pupillary light responses should be tested. To elicit a physiologic nystagmus response, the patient's head is moved from side to side. The fast phase of the nystagmus should be in the direction of the movement (cranial nerves III, IV [trochlear nerve], VI [abducens nerve], and VII). The mouth is then opened and the gag reflex is tested (cranial nerves IX [glossopharyngeal nerve], X [vagus nerve], XII [hypoglossal nerve]). Palpation of the neck muscles for the presence of atrophy helps to evaluate cranial nerve XI (accessory nerve). Rubbing of the nose typically causes a licking response (cranial nerve XII). The sense of smell may be tested by monitoring for a response to a food odor such as a favorite treat positioned near the nose (cranial nerve I [olfactory nerve]).

Interpreting the Neurologic Examination

After the neurologic examination is complete, the results of each individual test should be reviewed to help determine the presence or absence of a neurologic abnormality and to help the examiner to localize the lesion. In general, animals with progressive neurologic disease will initially have decreased proprioception, followed by loss of motor function, and in severe cases, a patient may progress to loss of deep pain. If patients recover, deep pain sensation generally returns first, followed by return of some motor function, and with near-complete recovery, proprioceptive function returns last.

Interpretation of the neurologic examination is important to localize the lesion so that additional diagnostic tests can be performed to evaluate a particular area. The hallmarks of LMN signs are hyporeflexia, weakness and reduced resting tone of muscles, and a decreased ability to generate tone with limb movement. The indications of UMN signs are hyperreflexia, maintenance of strength and increased resting tone of muscles, and spasticity of the limbs.

Lesions of spinal cord segments or nerves of C1-C5 will result in UMN signs to all four

C1-C5	C6-T2	T3-L3	L4-S3
UMN Forelimbs UMN Rear Limbs	LMN Forelimbs UMN Rear Limbs	Normal Forelimbs UMN Rear Limbs	Normal Forelimbs LMN Rear Limbs

			- If lesion is L4-L5, LMN
			  signs to femoral nerve
			  distribution
			- If lesion L6-S2, Normal
			  femoral nerve function, LMN
			  to sciatic nerve

Figure 10-28   Appearance of upper motor or lower motor neuron signs associated with lesions of various spinal cord segments or their nerve roots.

limbs (Figure 10-28). In some cases, the clinical signs may be more obvious in the hindlimbs because the spinal tracts to these limbs are located more peripherally in the ventral spinal cord, where compression by a space-occupying mass, such as a protruding disc, may occur. Lesions of spinal cord segments or nerves of C6-T2 will cause LMN signs to the forelimbs and UMN signs to the hindlimbs. The forelimbs will be normal if the lesion is caudal to T2. Lesions between T3 and L3 will result in UMN signs to the hindlimbs. Lesions located from L4 to S3 will result in LMN signs to the hindlimbs.

Ancillary Tests

Thorough orthopedic and neurologic examinations help to isolate the area of interest to a smaller region. This will ultimately save time and expense and will likely result in a more accurate diagnosis. Ancillary tests to aid in a definitive diagnosis include radiographs, magnetic resonance imaging, computerized tomography, and nuclear medicine studies.

Radiographs are the most commonly used test. It is important to always take at least two views at 90-degree angles. Most commonly, lateral and cranial-caudal views are obtained of the region of interest. Comparison films of the opposite limb may be useful to evaluate subtle lesions. Occasionally, stress views of the tarsus or carpus may be helpful. Specialty clinics and university teaching hospitals may have the capability to perform advanced diagnostic tests such as MRI or CT. These studies may give enhanced resolution and information, particularly of soft tissue structures, and of the three-dimensional nature of conditions. Nuclear studies may indicate regions of inflammation and metabolic activity in soft tissues or bone, but are available in only a few locations.

Chapter 11

Gait Analysis

Robert Gillette

Gait analysis is a common term used for the study of locomotion. Gait analysis may be used to identify alterations in gait and assist in diagnosing disorders of locomotion (Figure 11-1). Locomotion has been compared to a symphony orchestra in that "all parts must blend into a harmonious pattern—from the gentle sway of the head and tail for balance to the coordinated efforts of each limb and body muscle to accomplish its special function. Conversely, also like an orchestra, if all movements are not attuned to the whole, a major fault should be evident."[1] Gait analysis plays a very important role in helping to understand how the body is functioning.

Kinesiology is the study of motion. There are two fields within the science of kinesiology. Kinetics describes the forces involved in motion. Kinematics describes the motion of body parts. The descriptions are characterized in linear or angular measurements.

Normal Gait

Gait describes a series of limb and body movements used for locomotion. A gait is made up of a series of repeated strides. A stride is defined as the cycle of body movements that begins with the contact of one foot and ends when that foot again contacts the ground. There are various gaits that are defined by how the body moves during each stride.[2,3] Within a stride, each individual limb goes through a step cycle. A step cycle is the most basic unit of gait and includes a stance phase and a swing phase.

The stance phase is the period when the foot is in contact with the ground (Figure 11-2). The first part of the stance phase is when the braking forces occur as a result of surface contact. This is followed by the second part of the stance phase when there is a period of propulsion. The swing phase is the period when the foot is in the air (Figure 11-3). It is divided into three parts. The leg first swings caudally as a result of the propulsive action, the muscles then swing it cranially for locomotion, and then bring it caudally and down as it returns to the ground. The muscle activity and resultant skeletal movement apply forces to the limbs to create each of these phases. Abnormalities in these phases may help the clinician to diagnose lameness.

Symmetrical gaits include the walk, trot, and pace. The walk is a slow four-beat gait. The sequence of footfalls is left hind (LH), left fore (LF), right hind (RH), and right fore (RF). The trot is a two-beat diagonal gait, where the movements of one stride have the diagonal forelimbs and hindlimbs in support while the other two diagonal limbs are in the swing phase (Figure 11-4). In other words, the left forelimb and right hindlimb move in unison, as do the right forelimb and left hindlimb. The pace is a two-beat lateral gait in which the ipsilateral forelimb and hindlimbs enter the swing and stance phases together. There is more side-to-side rolling of the body, and there is less total joint motion as compared to the trot.

The intermediate-speed gait for most dogs is the trot; however, a small percentage of dogs will preferentially pace. Dogs that pace may appear to have a stiff, stilted gait to the untrained eye, but this is a normal characteristic of the pace. Occasionally, dogs with arthritis will adopt the pace as the preferred intermediate-speed gait to decrease the joint range of motion needed to advance the body.

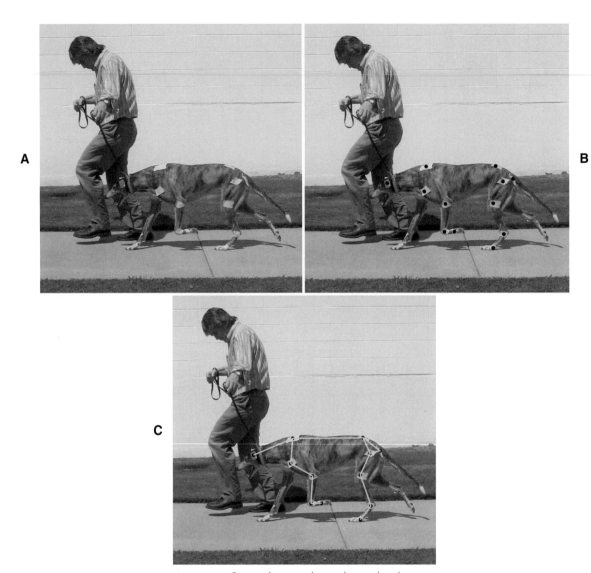

Figure 11-1 Gait analysis may be used to analyze locomotion.

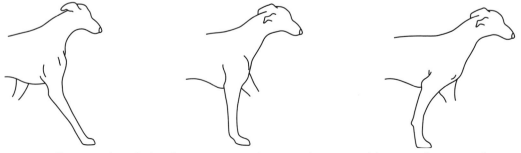

Figure 11-2 The stance phase. Braking forces occur at initial impact and continue until the center of gravity transfers over the fulcrum. Propulsive forces predominate for the remainder of the stance phase until the foot leaves the surface.

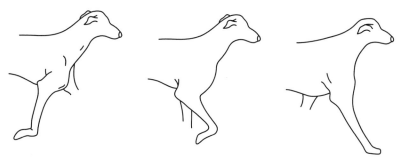

Figure 11-3   The swing phase. Initially the leg swings caudally, after the foot leaves the ground. It then swings cranially, until it begins the last caudal swing, which ends when the foot touches the surface.

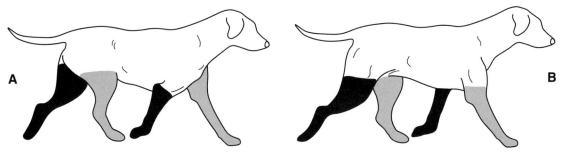

Figure 11-4   The trot. The limbs in gray are in the stance phase, while the black limbs are in the swing phase.

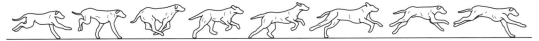

Figure 11-5   The gallop, with the dog in the right lead.

Many dogs also display a gait called the amble, which is an irregular four-beat gait in which the limbs on either side move almost as a pair, similar to a pace. This is often a transitional gait that dogs use in going from a walk to a faster gait, but should not be confused with a pacing gait.

Asymmetrical gaits include the canter and gallop. The canter is slower than the gallop and is a three-beat gait, characterized by a "lead" forelimb, with two limbs moving separately and two as a diagonal pair. The pattern of footfalls with a dog cantering in a left lead is right hind, left hind, and right fore together, followed by the left forelimb reaching furthest forward. The opposite series of footfalls would occur when a dog is cantering on the right lead. There is only one flight phase in the canter when all four limbs are off the ground, and it occurs just after the forelimbs leave the ground. The canter, sometimes called a lope, is an endurance gait and is sometimes used by

sled dogs. Some of the larger dogs that have a wider body structure, such as the Rottweiler or Saint Bernard, use the canter as their preferred running gait.

The gallop is the gait typically used by dogs that are running at high speeds and is characterized by powerful propulsion from the hindlimbs and a four-beat rhythm.[4] It has two support phases and two flight phases in each stride (Figure 11-5). Similar to the canter, the gallop can have either a right lead or a left lead. There are four possible footfall sequences that occur in galloping dogs. In a diagonal gallop on the left lead, the left hind leg comes into contact first, followed by the right hind foot in the hindlimb support phase. The dog then leaves the ground in a flight phase. The next foot to make contact is the right forelimb followed by the left forelimb in the forelimb support phase. The dog then propels forward, leaving the ground a second time in a flight phase, after which the sequence is repeated. A right-lead dog goes though a similar but opposite sequence. Most dogs have a rotary footfall sequence during the gallop. The sequence of footfalls in a dog galloping on the left lead with rotary footfall is left hind, right hind, right front, and left front. The opposite footfall sequence occurs for dogs galloping on the right lead. This gait is also sometimes described as a double suspension–rotary gallop.

Structural Definitions

Movement is balanced throughout the body in dogs with normal locomotion. In the neuro-musculoskeletal system, the two sides of the body are symmetrical. An understanding of body symmetry is the key to analyzing gait

abnormalities and lameness (Figure 11-6). Whether by palpating the dog during a physical examination or by observing the dog's movement, the right side of the body should be symmetrical to the left side.

The canine musculoskeletal system consists of axial and appendicular segments (Figure 11-7). The axial segment consists of many joints and is divided into anatomical segments consisting of the head, cervical, thoracic, abdominal, and tail segments. The appendicular segments are the forelimbs and the hindlimbs. These are subdivided into smaller segments, including the shoulder, elbow, carpus, hip, stifle, tarsus, and phalanges of the hindlimbs and forelimbs. Locomotion is a result of the individual movements of each of these segments. How each of the segments and joints is used is determined by the relationship of the dog's

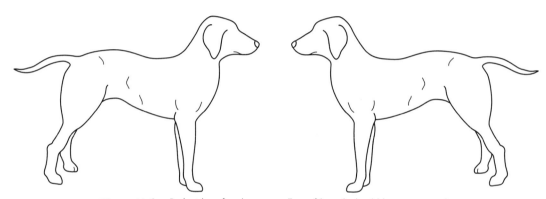

Figure 11-6 Both sides of a dog, regardless of breed, should be symmetrical.

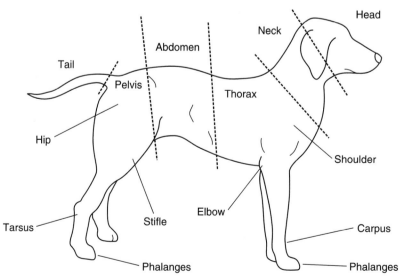

Figure 11-7 The axial skeleton includes the head, neck, thorax, abdominal, and tail segments. The appendicular skeleton is divided into shoulder, elbow, carpus, and phalanges segments in the forelimb; and hip, stifle, tarsus, and phalanges segments in the hind leg.

center of gravity to the ground and the type of movement being performed.

Center of Gravity

In the dog, 60% of the weight is carried by the forelimbs and 40% is carried by the hindlimbs while standing.[4] The center of gravity (COG) is located at the mid-chest level behind the scapula (Figure 11-8). The location of the COG, along with normal gait, results in the forelimbs undergoing more braking than propulsive forces and the hindlimbs undergoing more propulsive than braking forces when ambulating on a level surface.

Traveling uphill shifts the balance of forces toward the hindlimbs, and moving downhill shifts the forces toward the forelimbs (Figure 11-9). An uneven or varying surface will produce a variety of force alterations, which depend on the body's position. For this reason, gait analysis should be performed on a level surface that provides proper traction.

A number of factors influence the forces transmitted to the limbs during impact, including the gait, the velocity and acceleration of the dog, the dog's body weight, and the dog's conformation or musculoskeletal structure. The forelimbs of a galloping dog receive high impact forces as the limbs contact the ground. This is because as they contact the ground, the entire weight of the body, as well as the added braking and propulsion forces, must be absorbed by the limbs. In dogs that use the canter, the impact forces are distributed differently, being more evenly distributed between the forelimbs and hindlimbs. These forces are greater on the lead forelimb than the other forelimb because the lead limb is the sole limb in contact with the ground during its stance phase, whereas the other forelimb shares part of the load with the contralateral hindlimb during its stance phase.

Another factor that affects how the body moves and receives forces is conformation. Faulty conformation predisposes structures to injury. Gait analysis reveals certain

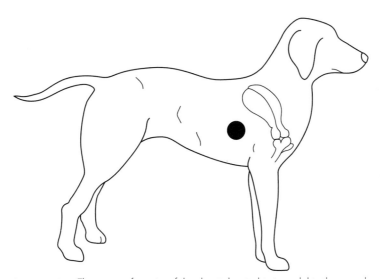

Figure 11-8   The center of gravity of the dog is located just caudal to the scapula.

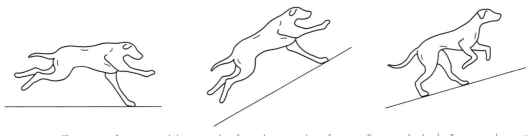

Figure 11-9   The center of gravity and the ground surface determine how forces will act on the body. For example, vertical forces on the forelimbs decrease as a dog goes up an incline and are transferred to the hind legs.

characteristics of a dog's conformation that are displayed during motion. Sound movement contributes to the health and normal lifespan of dogs.[5] Locomotion may vary in different breeds,[3] but during symmetrical gait, such as the trot, the movements of one side should still mirror the movements of the other side. A conformational abnormality usually creates an abnormal gait. An abnormal gait should initially be assessed for a conformational cause. A lameness due to a conformational abnormality may be related, not to pain, but to a structural fault. If incorrect movement is not a result of compensation due to conformational abnormalities, there may be other factors influencing the movement, including musculoskeletal and neurologic conditions. Treatment of a lameness as a result of conformation problems may require a different therapeutic course than treatment of a lameness related to a pathologic cause. Dogs with conformational abnormalities that may result in musculoskeletal problems should be eliminated from breeding programs.

Gait Analysis

The study of animal movement has been an intense subject of research.[6] Both qualitative and quantitative gait analysis have been used to analyze dogs and horses.[7,8] Subjective gait analysis has traditionally been performed by skilled clinicians. With recent advances in computer and video technology, there has been an increased interest in canine kinesiology research. Kinetic studies[9-13] have focused on the mechanical stresses involved in movement. Kinematic studies[3,14,15] have described motion analysis of dogs. Currently the cost of these diagnostic tools may be prohibitive to most veterinary clinics. In the future, some of these techniques may become available as a result of the rapid technological advancements in this field.

Kinetic Analysis

A force plate may be used to analyze gait. Force plates measure ground reaction forces (GRFs) of the limb during the stance phase of the gait. The forces are measured in three orthogonal components (Figure 11-10), including the vertical (z) plane, braking-propulsion (y) plane, and medial-lateral (x) plane. The force plate is usually embedded in a pathway for the test subjects to pass over. As the paw

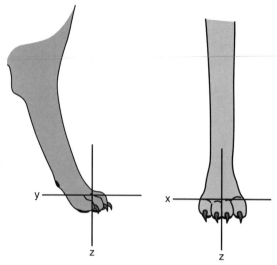

Figure 11-10   Ground reaction forces act on the foot in three orthogonal planes (x, y, and z).

comes into contact with the plate, the GRFs are measured. The force plate is connected to a computer that acquires the data for analysis. A software program then converts the information obtained from the force plate to the three planes of GRFs. For analysis, the data from one limb can then be compared to data collected over time or to other limb data from the subject.

Measurements obtained may include peak forces and impulses. The contact time of the foot depends on the velocity of the subject. As the velocity increases, the contact time of the foot decreases. For example, the foot contact time at the walk is longer than the contact time at the trot. The data from a walking gait demonstrate a biphasic z force, which is similar to that of humans. This is also seen in the y force, where the first peak indicates the braking phase, and the second peak, which is directed opposite the first peak, indicates propulsion. The x force plays a minimal role in gait analysis and is usually not evaluated. The biphasic z force is not seen at the trot, probably because of decreased contact time. Vertical forces demonstrate a single loading peak (Figure 11-11, A). The y force still has braking and propulsive components (Figure 11-11, B). The contact time of the walk is longer than that of the trot, but the z force of the trot is approximately twice the z force of the walk. These differences are because of changes in velocity and the differences in the stance phases between the two gaits.

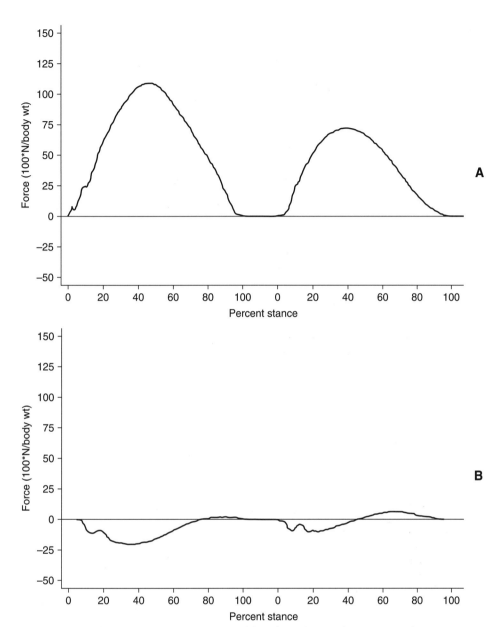

Figure 11-11   **A,** Force plate data showing measurement of the *z* force during surface contact at the trot. **B,** Measurement of *y* force taken during the trot.

A technique has been reported for measuring ground contact pressure on individual foot pads of dogs.[13] The force plate measures the GRFs transferred to the entire foot. To assess how the foot receives the GRFs, each individual digit may be assessed. This is accomplished by attaching a force-sensing resistor to each individual weight-bearing pad. An unexpected finding in one study was that the greatest forces were measured on digital pads 3 and 5, and pads 2 and 4 had less measured forces. It has been traditionally believed that digits 3 and 4 were the pads receiving the greatest force. This measurement technique may be useful to evaluate bandaging methods, prosthetic devices, and surgical procedures.

Kinematic Analysis

Kinematic analysis is one of the oldest methods to evaluate movement of the musculoskeletal system. In 1888, Muybridge used stroboscopic photography to show the stride of racing Greyhounds and hound dogs running at various speeds.[16] Subjective gait analysis may be used as an aid in the diagnosis of lameness. Quantitative kinematic analysis of canine movement has been performed using electrogoniometry, film, or videotape.[3,14,15] Current analytical methods use computer-assisted videography.

Subjective gait analysis is the most common diagnostic tool to assess lameness. To describe the components that make up a stride, the movements of each individual segment must be assessed, including the distance, speed, and consistency of movement of each of the segments. In a normal symmetrical gait the movements of one side mirror the movements of the other side. The trot, which is a symmetrical gait, provides the best visual presentation of movement for the clinician to diagnose lameness. If a gait abnormality is present, the movements of one side will be different from those of the other side.

Observations should be made before any physical palpation. The animal is initially observed at rest, looking for conformational abnormalities or abnormal stance. For example, the dog may hold one limb up or put most of its body weight on a particular limb(s). After these observations are noted, the animal is evaluated while moving. The patient is trotted in a straight line moving toward and away from the clinician. Next, it should be assessed moving in a straight line from the right side and then the left side. Then it should be observed moving in a circle, both clockwise and counterclockwise.

Movements of the entire body should be assessed for major gait deficits. Then, the step cycle of each leg should be evaluated to determine if a phase of the cycle is deficient. If the lameness appears at foot contact only, or if the stance phase is shortened, the lameness may be associated with impact or support. If the gait deficit is associated with the swing phase or a combination of the swing and stance phase, the lameness may be associated with structures responsible for advancing the limb forward.

Most clinical abnormalities may be detected with subjective gait analysis. A dog with a lesion causing severe constant pain may carry the limb and not lie on that limb when recumbent. A dull aching pain may produce a weight-bearing lameness during gait. A lesion that produces mild pain during certain phases of locomotion causes the dog to alter its gait to alleviate the pain. Quadrupeds have the ability to minimize pain by altering movement in such a way that the abnormality may be nearly imperceptible.[17] However, this altered gait may lead to compensatory orthopedic problems. For example, joint range of motion is usually symmetrical between the left and right sides at a trot (Figure 11-12). Minor pain, such as synovitis of the right carpal joint, may create an imbalance in the system and affect not only the carpus, but also the right shoulder and both tarsi (Figure 11-13).

Abnormal gait alters the pattern of forces acting on the musculoskeletal structure to produce movement. In addition to appendicular changes, the axial skeleton may be affected. Because the axial skeleton is the frame though which alterations in gait are transferred, secondary or tertiary biomechanically induced injury may occur to the back or other limbs. Psychologically, chronic pain may lead to behavioral problems.

Computer-assisted videographic (CAV) gait analysis may also be used to assess the effects of lameness on the musculoskeletal system.[8,15,18] Recent advances in video and computer technology have improved the potential applications of gait analysis.[8,15,18] Three-dimensional CAV–motion analysis systems give the most accurate and comprehensive information. Data obtained may provide information regarding the structure of the musculoskeletal system, lameness, and evaluation of surgical and medical treatments.

Three-dimensional CAV systems are expensive and are limited to a few academic institutions at this time. Two-dimensional CAV gait analysis systems are less expensive but are limited in their ability to provide accurate data because rotation and circumduction cannot be accounted for in two-dimensional systems. However, they may be an economical alternative for routine clinical applications.

With CAV gait analysis, reflective markers are attached to the subject at specific anatomic locations (Figure 11-14). For example, markers may be placed on the ear, lateral aspect of the distal fifth digit of the front foot, the carpus, the elbow, the acromion/greater tubercle of the humerus, the dorsal border of the scapular spine, the lateral aspect of the distal fifth digit

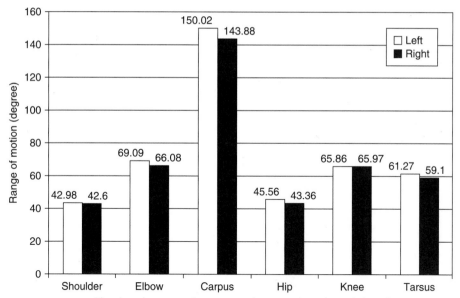

Figure 11-12 The chart shows actual joint range-of-motion values of sound dogs during a trot.

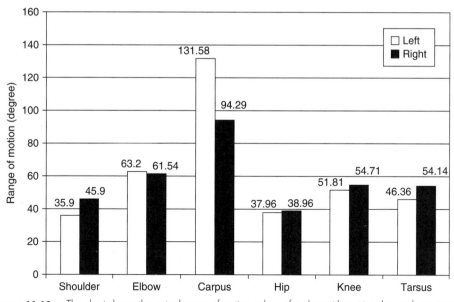

Figure 11-13 The chart shows the actual range-of-motion values of a dog with restricted carpal movement.

of the hind foot, the tarsus, the stifle, the greater trochanter of the femur, and the iliac crest. The subject is then trotted with its right side to the camera and then with its left side to the camera. The movement is filmed by a video camera system. Computer software is then used to convert the motion of the reflective markers into digital images. Software is then used to quantify limb and joint movement, as well as stride characteristics.

The information may be used for diagnostic or research purposes. A parameter on one side

of the body may be compared to the same parameter on the opposite side. When assessing gait and joint movement at the trot, differences between the two sides may be useful to help diagnose lameness.

Future kinematic studies should address breed characteristics and how conformation and structure affect function. Analysis of normal dogs helps to provide normal ranges of limb and joint motion. These factors may be useful when analyzing gait clinically. Furthermore, gait characteristics of dogs with

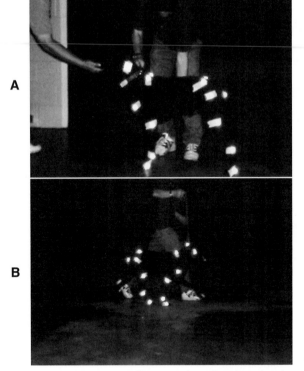

Figure 11-14   A, Reflective markers placed on the dog before filming. **B,** Markers seen during locomotion.

musculoskeletal pathology may allow study of certain interventions and allow evaluation of their efficacy.

Summary

Gait analysis is a useful analytical tool for clinicians, technicians, handlers, and owners. It is an indicator of the status of the neuromusculoskeletal system and its function. The evaluator should have a thorough understanding of the individual components of the gait cycle and the underlying anatomy. New technologies have advanced our abilities to evaluate gait. Veterinarians, physical therapists, owners, and patients may all benefit from the recent advances in gait analysis. Improved capabilities for data collection, storage, and analysis, in combination with the advancements in personal computer technology, have provided an opportunity for the development of powerful analytical techniques.

REFERENCES

1. Roy WE: Examination of the canine locomotor system, *Vet Clin North Am* 1:53-70, 1971.
2. Grogan JW: The gaits of horses, *J Am Vet Assoc* 118:112-117, 1951.
3. Hildebrand M: Symmetrical gaits of dogs in relation to body build, *J Morphol* 124:353-360, 1968.
4. Zebas CJ et al: Kinematic descriptors of the running gait in the greyhound athlete. In Marshall RN, Wood GA, Elliott BC, et al, editors: *XIIIth International Conference on Biomechanics),* Perth, Australia, 1991, University of Western Australia.
5. Elliot RP: *The new dogsteps,* New York, 1983, Howell Book House.
6. Leach DH, Dagg AI: Evolution of equine locomotion research, *Equine Vet J* 15:87-92, 1983.
7. Leach DH, Dagg AI: A review of research on equine locomotion and biomechanics, *Equine Vet J* 15:93-102, 1983.
8. DeCamp CE: Kinetic and kinematic gait analysis and the assessment of lameness in the dog, *Vet Clin North Am* 27:825-840, 1997.
9. Deuland R, Bartel DL, Antonsen E: Force-plate technique for canine gait analysis of total hip and excision arthroplasty, *J Am Anim Hosp Assoc* 13:547-552, 1977.
10. Cavagna GA: Force platforms as ergometers, *J Appl Physiol* 39:174-179, 1985.
11. Budsberg SC, Verstraete MC, Soutas-Little RW: Force plate analysis of the walking gait in healthy dogs, *Am J Vet Res* 48:915-918, 1987.
12. McLaughlin R, Roush JK: Effects of increasing velocity on braking and propulsion times during force plate gait analysis in Greyhounds, *Am J Vet Res* 56:159-161, 1995.
13. Rumph PF, Marghitu DB, Gillette RL, et al: A technique for measuring ground contact pressure on individual paw pads of dogs. In *Proc Annu Mtg Am Assoc Vet Anatomists* Blacksburg, Va, 1998. (abstract)
14. Adrian MJ, Roy WE, Karpovich PV: Normal gait of the dog: an electrogoniometric study, *Am J Vet Res* 27:90-95, 1966.
15. DeCamp CE et al: Kinematic gait analysis of the trot in healthy Greyhounds, *Am J Vet Res* 54:627-634, 1993.
16. Muybridge E: In Brown, LS, editor: *Animals in motion,* New York, 1957, Dover Publications.
17. Nunamaker DM, Blauner PD: Normal and abnormal gait. In Newton CD, Nunamaker DM, editors: *Textbook of small animal orthopaedics,* Philadelphia, 1985, Lippincott.
18. Gillette RL, Zebas CJ: A comparison of limb symmetry in the trot of the Labrador Retriever, *J Am Anim Hosp Assoc* 35:515-520, 1999.

Assessing and Measuring Outcomes

■ Darryl L. Millis

Assessing the outcome of treatments, including physical rehabilitation, is essential to determine how an animal is progressing and to determine the effectiveness of treatment protocols. Review of outcome data and evaluation of protocols are necessary so that changes can be initiated to improve outcomes. Assessments should consist of objective data whenever possible because owners and veterinarians often believe a patient is doing better than the data suggest. In addition, documentation of progress is important to provide incentive for owners to continue rehabilitation return to function, and to justify continued treatment.

Several measurements are important for assessing outcomes, including the ability to perform functional activities of daily living, gait analysis, joint function, muscle mass and strength, body composition, return to function, impressions of owners and veterinarians.

Activities of Daily Living

Despite the best treatments, rehabilitation facilities, and personnel, some conditions are so serious that complete recovery cannot be expected. In these situations, the owner must be informed of a reasonable expected outcome. The rehabilitation goals should be realistic and should concentrate on performing basic life functions, such as eating and drinking with no or minimal assistance, changing body positions without assistance, rising from a sitting position, and walking outside to urinate and defecate with no or minimal assistance. In some cases, even these goals may not be met. Progress may be slow, but it should be recorded, and rehabilitation plans should concentrate on activities to help achieve these rehabilitation goals.

Gait Analysis

Weight-Bearing at a Stance

Evaluation of a dog's stance gives information regarding willingness to place complete weight on an affected limb. Many dogs may have no visible or only very mild lameness at a walk or trot, but will not bear equal weight on the limbs when standing. Weight-bearing at a stance may be assessed by observing the placement of a foot in relation to the contralateral front or rear foot. In severe cases, the dog may hold the foot completely or partially off the ground. More commonly, the dog places a moderate amount of weight on the foot, but not complete weight. The toes may point out, and when the limb is gently pushed forward, it may be moved more easily than the contralateral limb when it is gently pushed. Alternatively, the evaluator may place both hands under the fore or rear feet with the palm facing the pads, and the relative amount of weight-bearing may be assessed. Weight-bearing at a stance may be incorporated into global lameness scores.

An inexpensive method of acquiring more quantitative information regarding weight-bearing at a stance is to have a dog stand with each limb on a common household scale. It is important to be certain that the dog is standing squarely in a standard position. Dogs should also undergo a period of acclimation to the scales so that data collection is valid. Scales should periodically be calibrated to standard weights to be certain that accurate weights are recorded.

Evaluation at a Walk
0 Walks normally
1 Slight lameness
2 Obvious weight-bearing lameness
3 Severe weight-bearing lameness
4 Intermittent non–weight-bearing lameness
5 Continuous non–weight-bearing lameness

Lameness Evaluation at a Trot
0 Trots normally
1 Slight lameness
2 Obvious weight-bearing lameness
3 Severe weight-bearing lameness
4 Intermittent non–weight-bearing lameness
5 Continuous non–weight-bearing lameness

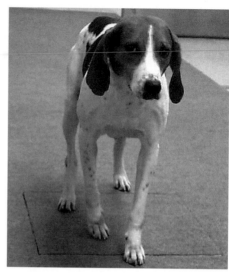

Figure 12-1   Measurement of ground reaction forces using a force plate.

Lameness Scores

Lameness scores are a vital clinical outcome assessment tool. The walk and trot are the gaits most commonly evaluated because the speed of the limbs during movement is easier to assess without specialized equipment, and these gaits are symmetrical, making identification of a lame limb easier. The reader is referred to the chapter on orthopedic and neurologic evaluation for information regarding identification of lameness. It is important to separate the walk from the trot when scoring lameness: Dogs are generally less lame at a walk because less force is placed on the limb at this less strenuous gait. Trotting may accentuate a lameness that is mild to moderate at a walk because of the greater forces placed on the limb with increased velocity. Having separate lameness scores for the walk and trot allows finer discrimination of gait analysis and may be more sensitive for detecting subtle improvements during rehabilitation (Box 12-1).

Kinetic (Forceplate) Analysis of Gait

Kinetic evaluation of gait involves the measurement of ground reaction forces with a force plate or platform (Figure 12-1). It is an objective, repeatable measure of weight-bearing on limbs when proper technique is used for data collection. Lameness can be compared over a period of time without relying on memory of previous assessments because data may be stored on a computer. Although measurement of ground reaction forces is a reliable and well-accepted method of determining the degree of weight-bearing on the limbs, it is an artificial situation, and some dogs may display different clinical signs in a home environment. Force platform systems are available at many veterinary colleges and some private practices. It is important that appropriate software for quadruped animals be used.

Force plates use either strain gauges or piezoelectric crystals. The force plate is either mounted on a platform or embedded in the floor so that it is even with the surface. A runway of adequate length is essential. Most systems have timer lights that are triggered as the handler and dog approach and cross the force plate to allow the calculation of mean velocity and acceleration. Control of velocity and acceleration within appropriate parameters is essential for repeatable data collection, because these greatly affect the force placed on each limb. The force plate is connected to a computer that calculates ground reaction forces.

The most useful forces measured are the peak vertical force (Z_{Peak}) and vertical impulse ($Z_{Impulse}$) (Figure 12-2). Other forces that may be useful are the peak braking ($Y_{A\ Peak}$) and propulsion ($Y_{B\ Peak}$) forces and braking ($Y_{A\ Impulse}$) and propulsion ($Y_{B\ Impulse}$) impulses (Figure 12-3). Medial-lateral forces (X_{Peak}) and impulse ($X_{Impulse}$) are likely too small and variable to be clinically useful. Forces may be measured during stance, walking, or trotting.

It is essential that appropriate technique be used during data collection. In addition to consistent velocity and acceleration targets, an

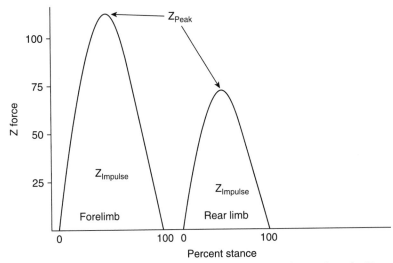

Figure 12-2 Graphic depiction of peak vertical force (Z_{Peak}) and vertical impulse ($Z_{Impulse}$).

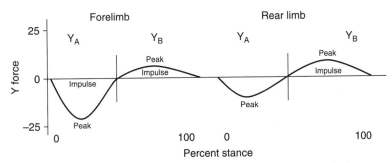

Figure 12-3 Graphic depiction of peak braking ($Y_{A\ Peak}$) and propulsion ($Y_{B\ Peak}$) forces and braking ($Y_{A\ Impulse}$) and propulsion ($Y_{B\ Impulse}$) impulses.

experienced handler is necessary to minimize intertrial variability, although there is little or no difference in measured forces between experienced handlers. The handler should be between the dog's head and shoulder, and the dog should be gaited without undue tension or pulling on the leash. The dog should not alter the gait, throw its head, turn the head, lunge, or make other sudden movements as it approaches and crosses the force plate. The head carriage should be in a neutral position to avoid shifting weight to the front or rear limbs.

In general, dogs bear 30% of their body weight on each front limb and 20% on each rear limb while in a standing position with the limbs placed squarely under the body. Walking at a velocity of 0.7 to 1.0 m/sec results in forces equivalent to 60% of body weight on each forelimb and 40% on each rear limb in a medium to large dog. Increasing the velocity to a trot of 1.7 to 2.0 m/sec results in weight-bearing of 100% to 120% of body weight on each forelimb and 65% to 70% of body weight on each hindlimb in a similar-size dog. Reduced weight-bearing on an individual limb may result in mild weight shifts to the other limbs.

Kinematic (Motion) Analysis of Gait

Kinematic or motion analysis of gait is a powerful tool that can be used to measure flexion and extension angles of joints during gait, stride length, and other parameters of stride. It is usually combined with kinetic gait analysis. There is limited availability of three-dimensional kinematic gait analysis because the necessary equipment is sophisticated and expensive. Two-dimensional systems are less expensive, but the data have limited usefulness because joints rotate and limbs circumduct during gait.

Attention to detail is critical for kinematic gait analysis. Most systems use a number of reflective devices that are attached to the dogs at very specific anatomical points to allow repeatable data collection at different times. Motion of the markers in relation to the joints is determined with a series of cameras interfaced with a computer. Software for quadruped animals allows reconstruction of a walking "stick figure" on the computer screen. The software is then used to calculate a number of measurements, including flexion and extension angles of joints during gait, angular velocity of joints, and stride length and frequency.

Noninvasive, computer-assisted, three-dimensional kinematic gait analysis was used in one study to describe lameness associated with cranial cruciate ligament rupture in dogs.[1] Dynamic flexion and extension angles and angular velocities were calculated for the hip, stifle, and hock joints. Distance and temporal variables were also determined. Mean flexion extension curves were developed for all joints, and the changes in movement that occurred over time after cruciate rupture were compared. Each joint had a characteristic pattern of flexion and extension movement that changed with cruciate rupture. The stifle joint angle was more flexed throughout stance and early swing phase of stride and failed to extend in late stance. Angular velocity of the stifle joint was damped throughout stance phase, with extension velocity almost negligible. The hip and hock joint angles, in contrast to the stifle joint angle, were extended more during stance phase. Stride length and frequency also varied significantly after cruciate rupture. A change in the pattern of joint movement appeared to occur in which the hip and hock joints compensated for the dysfunction of the stifle joint.

Knowledge of kinematic parameters may allow more effective rehabilitation of patients following surgery or those with chronic conditions. In particular, changes that are noted during the course of treatment may allow for stepping up the level of activity, or more importantly, may signal changes that occur in other joints as a result of fatigue or overuse. Knowledge of these data may help prevent injuries to other joints or limbs.

Pedometers

Most outcome assessment measurements are performed in a clinic where equipment and personnel are located. However, in many cases, the animal temporarily becomes more active as a result of traveling, exposure to other animals, and being in a strange environment. In these situations, the dog often appears to be better than has been reported in the home environment. A pedometer may give some indication of a dog's activity level in its home environment. Most pedometers have a pendulum that swings back and forth with the normal gait cycle and indicates the number of steps taken. Pedometers may be up to 85% to 90% accurate with regard to counting the number of steps taken by a dog.

Proper placement of the pedometer is crucial. We have found that placing the pedometer just proximal to the elbow most accurately indicates the number of steps taken (Figure 12-4). Pedometers are not accurate in all dogs, however. It is recommended that the dog be walked 100 steps; the number of steps indicated by the pedometer is compared to see if the pedometer is reasonably accurate to record a dog's activity level. An additional test to

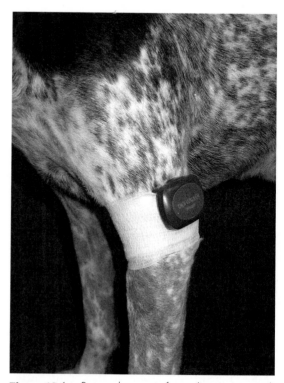

Figure 12-4 Proper placement of a pedometer is crucial. Placing the pedometer just proximal to the elbow is one method that has been used to count the number of steps taken.

determine accuracy is to place the pedometer and then allow the dog to have free activity while 100 steps are counted. The pedometer may double-count when the dog is trotting, running, or going up and down stairs, so it is used only as a semiquantitative indicator of home activity. Environmental conditions are another major factor in the activity of dogs. Dogs that spend some time outdoors may not be as active if it is raining or cold, or if the weather is otherwise inclement. Therefore comparative assessments should be made on days when the weather is as similar as possible.

Joint Function

Joint motion may be evaluated using both objective and subjective assessments. The primary motion of a joint is the movement of bones as a whole, such as occurs with stifle flexion, and is termed physiologic or osteokinematic motion. The quantity of joint flexion and extension motion is measured using a goniometer (Figure 12-5). Unlike human range-of-motion measurements, the actual geometric angles are measured in dogs because the many different body types and conformation in individual dogs make estimation of the neutral or "0-degree" position difficult. Measuring the actual angle eliminates the need to estimate the "normal" standing angle. Therefore there are no negative angles.

The maximum angles of extension and flexion are those angles of greatest joint excursion. Normal angles of maximum flexion and extension have been reported for the Labrador retriever (Appendix 1).[2] Excellent intertester and intratester reliability was reported in that study. In addition, measurements made in dogs had very good correlation with measurements made from radiographs.

Measuring maximum angles may involve some discomfort. An animal experiencing discomfort is unlikely to use the limb at those angles while ambulating. Therefore measuring the comfortable range of motion may be more clinically applicable. To measure the comfortable range of motion, the joint is slowly flexed until the first indication of discomfort, such as tensing the muscles, pulling the limb away, or turning the head slightly, is noted. The joint is then slowly extended until the first indication of discomfort is noted. These angles are recorded. The mean of three independent measurements is used to be certain that the measured angles are reproducible. Physical rehabilitation may influence the return of joint motion following surgery, such as cranial cruciate ligament stabilization surgery.

The quality of joint motion is more subjective and involves the assessment of joint biomechanics, crepitus, and pain during motion. The more subtle motions occurring at the surface of the joints are termed accessory or arthrokinematic motions. Examples of these motions are glide (slide), roll, spin, distraction or traction, and compression or approximation. Glides are shear or sliding motions of opposing articular surfaces. A normal amount of glide occurs in normal functioning joints. Glides at joint surfaces often are imposed interventions using joint mobilization techniques to regain normal motion in a joint with pathology. Joint surface geometry, soft tissue resistance, and external forces all affect glide. Rolls involve one bone rolling on another, such as the femoral condyles rolling on the tibial plateau. Gliding motion in combination with rolling is needed for normal joint motion. Spins are joint surface motions that result in continual contact of a single area of articular

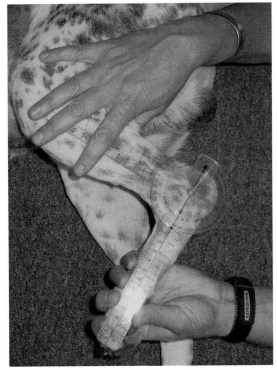

Figure 12-5 Joint angles of flexion and extension are measured using a goniometer.

cartilage on adjacent articular cartilage within a joint. Distraction or traction accessory motions are tensile (pulling apart) movements between bones. Compressive or approximation accessory motions are compressive (pushing together) movements between bones. The quality of the end feel during joint motion may indicate abnormalities such as restriction by fibrous tissue, excess joint capsule, bone, or cartilage. Crepitus is often associated with surface irregularities in articular cartilage or periarticular changes, such as occur in osteoarthritis. The sensations of crepitus palpated during joint motion have been described as being similar to crinkling a piece of cellophane. Other sensations such as cracking, snapping, or popping may indicate abnormalities, such as a torn meniscus.

Joint Laxity

Assessment of joint laxity in dogs is generally limited to qualitative evaluation, although some quantitative evaluations have been performed. In general, joint laxity may occur as a result of developmental conditions (such as hip dysplasia), trauma, or pathologic degeneration of ligaments, such as the cranial cruciate ligament.

Damage to collateral supporting structures is most easily assessed by placing varus and valgus stresses on the affected joint. The most joints most commonly affected with collateral ligament damage include the hock, stifle, carpus, elbow, and shoulder. The digits are occasionally involved. Assessment is most accurate when the joint is placed in full extension to prevent inadvertent internal or external rotation of the joint that may be mistaken for varus or valgus movement. Breed and age differences exist regarding normal varus and valgus motion, especially in young animals, so comparison with the contralateral normal limb is helpful.

Hip joint laxity is most commonly assessed in young, growing dogs as an indication of early hip dysplasia. Subjective assessment is commonly performed using the Ortolani maneuver to create subluxation of the hip joint. A more quantitative method of assessing hip joint laxity is the use of PennHip, in which controlled pressure is applied to the hip joint to create subluxation. A radiograph is made with the coxofemoral joint in this position, and measurements are made to quantify the degree of laxity, known as the hip distraction index. The hip distraction index has correla-

tion with the development of hip dysplasia in some breeds of dogs.

Stifle joint laxity is clinically assessed by palpating for cranial drawer motion. There should be no drawer motion in normal dogs. Methods to quantify drawer motion, which are not commonly used in dogs, include measurement of direct cranial drawer, quantitative cranial tibial thrust, and use of instrumented devices.[3] Direct cranial drawer is determined by simply marking the position of the tibial tuberosity with the stifle in reduction on a piece of graph paper, and then remarking the position of the tibial tuberosity with full cranial drawer. Caution must be used to prevent motion of the femur and to keep the marking device perpendicular to the graph paper. Quantitative cranial tibial thrust is measured in a similar fashion, except that the stifle is kept extended while the hock is flexed. This results in cranial displacement of the tibial tuberosity if the cranial cruciate ligament is ruptured. Marks are made on graph paper with the tibia in a reduced position, and with the tibia in full cranial tibial thrust. Care is taken to keep the caudal aspect of the femur in contact with a solid surface, so that the only motion that occurs is the cranial displacement of the tibia.

Instrumented devices for knee-drawer tests have been used in humans to measure shifts of the tibial tuberosity relative to the patella.[4-6] The total anterior and posterior displacement produced by anterior and posterior loads of 20 lb is measured from a reference position. Studies have evaluated the effects of variables on the accuracy and reproducibility of anterior-posterior drawer measurements. Reproducibility is principally affected by deviations in subject positioning. In addition to drawer motion, inadvertent knee flexion and tibial rotation may occur and result in incorrect measurements, despite attempts to prevent these. The effects of different observers, time sequences, different days, and muscle relaxation have been studied and contribute to error rates of 5% to 15%. Stress radiography, a relatively sensitive method of measuring drawer motion, has been used to compare instrumented systems in humans with tears of the anterior cruciate ligament (ACL). In one study, stress radiography was superior to instrumented arthrometer testing for determining cruciate ligament status.[7] Similar studies have not been performed in dogs, but instrumented knee-drawer devices are difficult to use in dogs and require practice to obtain reproducible results. Pediatric devices may be easier to use because the smaller size may allow a better fit of the instrument to the dog's limb.

Muscle

Assessment of muscle is important in physical rehabilitation. Muscle mass, muscle strength, and muscle injury may be assessed to help evaluate the patient's progress. Regaining muscle mass and strength following injury is important to help improve function and prevent further injury to joints and other soft tissues. The degree of muscle atrophy is also a reasonable indication of limb use. Therefore careful attention to muscle assessment provides a great deal of information regarding the progress of the rehabilitation patient.

Muscle Mass

Muscle mass measurements are a useful outcome measure in veterinary rehabilitation. Muscle mass indicates limb use and is associated with muscle strength. Muscle mass may be estimated with limb circumference measurements, ultrasound, computerized tomography (CT), magnetic resonance imaging (MRI), and dual-energy X-ray absorptiometry (DEXA).

Measurement of limb circumference is an indirect method of assessing changes in muscle mass and is inexpensive, quick, and easily performed on clinical patients. Acceptable results depend on using standard, repeatable methods of measuring limb circumference. A measuring tape with a spring tension device is useful in measuring limb circumference to improve consistent placement of tension on the tape when making measurements (Figure 12-6).

One study evaluated the effect of limb position, clipping hair, sedation, and different evaluators on thigh circumference measurements at two different locations before and after stifle stabilization surgery.[8] Thigh length was determined by measuring from the tip of the greater trochanter to the distal aspect of the lateral fabella. Circumference was determined at points equal to 50% and 70% of thigh length. Measurements were technically easier when made at the 70% location because the skin of the flank did not impede measurements (Figure 12-7). Clipping had little effect on thigh circumference measurements, but

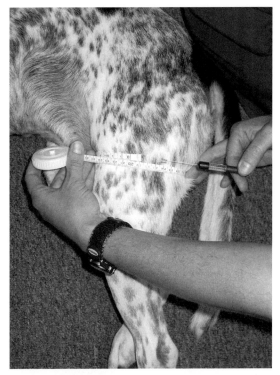

Figure 12-6   A measuring tape with a spring tension device is used to measure limb circumference. Use of this instrument allows the consistent placement of tension on the tape when making measurements.

dogs with short hair coats were used (Figure 12-8). Measurements may be affected to a greater extent in dogs with long hair.

Limb position is also important. Full flexion of the stifle results in greater thigh circumference measurements as compared with measurements made with the limb placed at a functional standing angle or with the stifle fully extended (Figure 12-9). Extension of the joint causes the muscle bellies to elongate, whereas flexion results in shortening and bunching of muscle bellies, creating greater thigh circumference. Measurements made in awake dogs with the stifle extended are not significantly different from those made following heavy sedation, as long as the dogs are not very tense, probably because the muscles are in an elongated position when the stifle is extended (Figure 12-10). Thigh circumference measurements are sensitive enough to detect muscle atrophy 2 weeks after stifle surgery (Figure 12-11). Similar measurements may be obtained by independent evaluators as long as standard technique is used and the evaluators practice before obtaining actual measurements.

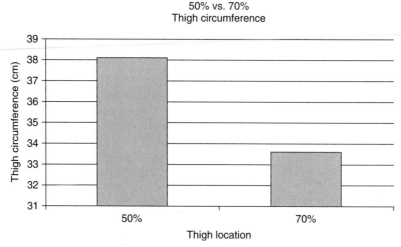

Figure 12-7   Thigh circumference measurements at the 50% and 70% thigh length. Although the 50% leg has greater thigh circumference because of greater muscle mass in that location, the measurements are technically more difficult at that location in some dogs because of the presence of the skin of the flank.

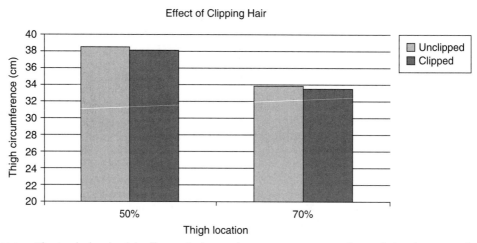

Figure 12-8   Clipping the hair has little effect on thigh circumference measurements in dogs with short hair coats. The effect of clipping would likely be greater in dogs with long hair.

The association of limb circumference with actual muscle mass is important if it is to be useful in the evaluation of rehabilitation patients. Human male cadavers were subjected to comprehensive anthropometry and weighing of all skeletal muscle.[9] Limb circumference had good correlation with total skeletal muscle mass for the forearm ($r = 0.96$), mid-thigh ($r = 0.94$), calf ($r = 0.84$), and midarm ($r = 0.82$).

Thigh circumference also has significant correlation with actual muscle mass in dogs (Figure 12-12). Even greater correlation may be obtained when thigh length is also considered and the volume of a cylinder is calculated. Although this method is simplistic because the thigh is not a true cylinder, the volume of a cylinder is easy to calculate and this estimate of muscle mass may be more clinically useful. Similar principles likely exist for circumference measurements of other limbs. Currently, we prefer performing thigh circumference measurements with the hair short or clipped, the limb held in an extended position, at 70% of the length of the thigh, and with the animal relaxed, but not necessarily sedated.

Limb circumference measures are commonly used in people to assess muscle atrophy, but relatively little is known regarding circumference measurement changes following knee injury and subsequent surgery. One

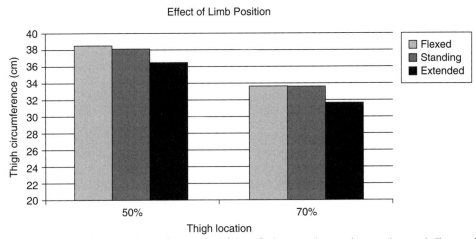

Figure 12-9 Thigh circumference is less with extension of the stifle because the muscles are elongated. Flexion of the limb results in greater thigh circumference, but the measurements are more difficult because of shortening of the hamstring muscles and difficulty in applying the tape measure.

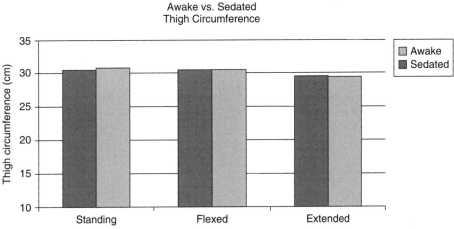

Figure 12-10 Measurements made in awake dogs with the stifle extended are not significantly different from those made following heavy sedation if the patient is not very tense, probably because the muscles are in an elongated position when the stifle is extended.

study compared thigh and calf circumference measurements of affected and unaffected extremities before and after knee surgery for patients with acute and chronic knee injuries.[10] There were significant differences between affected and unaffected extremities at both the presurgery and postsurgery time periods of the acute and chronic groups. The bulk of the circumference measurement differences existed before surgery for both groups. In another study, the intrarater and interrater reliability of lower extremity circumference measurements in humans recovering from ACL reconstructive surgery demonstrated high correlation (0.82 to 1.0 and 0.72 to 0.97, respectively) for both the involved and uninvolved sides in several locations.[11]

Measurement of thigh circumference may also be biased by the expectations of observers.[12] Use of a tape measure with a spring tension device may help to minimize bias of the evaluator because the end tension of the tape can be standardized. A relatively small change in limb circumference may indicate much greater loss of muscle mass. A study of people with chronic unilateral patellofemoral pain indicated that although symptomatic limbs had significant reductions in limb circumference, very small reductions in thigh circumference (1%) were associated with significant reductions in muscle size (13%).[13]

The thickness of the skin and subcutaneous tissues may be another factor affecting thigh

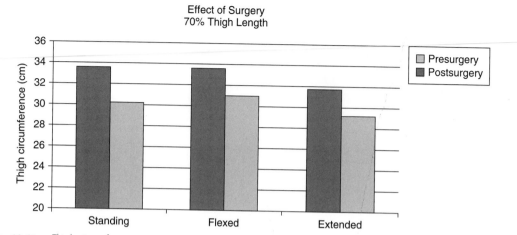

Figure 12-11   Thigh circumference measurements are sensitive enough to detect muscle atrophy 2 weeks after stifle surgery, indicating that this technique may be useful as a simple, cost-effective method of assessing limb mass.

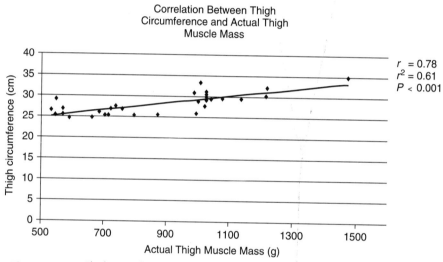

Figure 12-12   Thigh circumference has significant correlation with actual thigh muscle mass in dogs.

circumference measurements.[14] One investigation developed an equation using circumference and skinfold measurements for estimating anatomical cross-sectional area (CSA) of the quadriceps, hamstrings, and total thigh muscles.[15] Derived equations using midthigh circumference and anterior thigh skinfold assessment may be of value for estimating muscle CSA values when more sophisticated procedures are not available. Other studies have made similar assumptions that a cross section of the thigh could be represented as a circle with concentric layers of skin, fat, muscle, and bone.[16] However, approximations of thigh muscle CSA may underestimate the fat-plus-skin compartment when calipers are used.

Although thigh circumference has been used as an effective method of measuring muscle size to evaluate the effect of an injury or effectiveness of an intervention, some studies in humans have shown this technique to be unreliable under certain conditions. Therefore other methods of measuring muscle size may be useful. Such modalities include ultrasound scans, dual energy X-ray absorptiometry, computerized tomography, or magnetic resonance imaging of muscles.

One study investigating the validity and reliability of measuring quadriceps CSA with ultrasound scanning at the level of the midthigh found it to be a reliable method.[17] In a similar study, thigh circumference and segment volumes of the thigh were more strongly correlated to anterior versus posterior thigh musculature (when corrected for skinfold thickness) when B-mode ultrasound scanning was used.[14]

The question of whether various evaluation techniques are sensitive enough to detect changes in muscle mass was addressed in a training study on men.[18] Men were exposed to conditions designed to elicit differential hypertrophic adaptations following 21 sessions of squat training. A control group did no formal physical training. Tests used to evaluate muscle size included thigh circumference and quadriceps femoris and hamstring thicknesses via B-mode ultrasound. Thigh circumference and quadriceps femoris thickness were greater in groups that trained to a greater degree than in controls. Changes in the groups subsequent to training were similar for hamstring thickness.

MRI and CT are promising reference methods for quantifying whole body and regional skeletal muscle mass. In people, arm and leg skeletal muscle CSA estimates obtained by standard MRI and CT methods had good correlation with corresponding cadaver values.[19] MRI used to estimate muscle CSA also had good correlation with actual cross-sections of anatomic specimens in other studies.[16,20] These findings strongly support the use of MRI and CT as a method to determine appendicular skeletal muscle in vivo.

Neurogenic muscle atrophy induced by crushing the sciatic nerve was examined using CT in dogs.[21] The CT number and CSA in denervated muscles decreased 1 to 2 weeks after denervation and were significantly less after 3 weeks. Examination with CT may be useful to evaluate neurogenic muscular atrophy.

Some work has compared various methods of muscle mass estimation in people. For example, the CSA and volume of the quadriceps femoris muscle using MRI was compared with B-mode ultrasound.[22] The CSA was estimated at the junction of the proximal one third and distal two thirds of the thigh, and several sections of the thigh were obtained in order to estimate muscle volume by both modalities. There was no significant difference in the CSA estimates or volume estimates when ultrasound and MRI were compared.

DEXA is another noninvasive method of measuring lean tissue mass, but the estimations are limited to the whole body or an entire limb because it is difficult to determine lean tissue mass of relatively small regions.

Although CT and MRI have been used to measure limb circumference and have the advantage that the area of large muscles may be measured, the equipment is expensive and interpretation must be performed by a person trained in these diagnostic modalities. DEXA is somewhat less expensive, and less training is required for interpretation of data, although patient positioning is critical to obtain accurate results.

The accuracy of DEXA for measuring total body fat-free mass and leg muscle mass at four leg regions was assessed in people.[23] Computed tomography of the legs was also performed. Fat-free mass and muscle mass by DEXA was positively associated with CT at all four leg regions (r^2 = 0.86 to 0.96), but the correlation of muscle mass by DEXA was higher than by CT in three regions. A comparison of DEXA with MRI to evaluate estimates of muscle and adipose tissue in human lower limb sections indicated high agreement between DEXA and MRI for muscle, but less so for adipose tissue.[24]

Muscle Strength

Little investigation has been performed in dogs regarding muscle strength estimates, likely because of the difficulty in making such measurements in animals. One study of Beagle dogs measured muscle strength as indicated by measuring maximum isometric extension torque of the hindlimb.[25] This required general anesthesia, a surgical approach to the thigh of the dog, placement of a stimulating electrode near the femoral nerve, and instrumentation of the limb to measure muscle torque while the muscle was electrically stimulated. Such invasive procedures are not clinically applicable. However, maximum isometric extension torque had strong correlation with muscle fiber diameter obtained from biopsies of the vastus lateralis muscle. Obtaining muscle biopsies is an invasive procedure, although less so than the technique for determining muscle torque, and less instrumentation is required.

Other studies of muscle strength of humans may provide information that may be applicable to dogs. One study determined the relationship between selected anthropometric dimensions and strength in resistance-trained athletes.[26] Athletes were measured following the completion of a 10-week resistance training program for one-repetition maximum lifts. The highest relationships existed between estimates of regional muscle mass (arm circumference, arm muscle CSA, and thigh circumference) and lifting performance. The fewer joints and muscle groups involved in a lift, the greater the predictive accuracy from structural dimensions.

Although muscle mass is clearly associated with muscle strength, the type and strength of this relationship is less clear. The use of limb circumference measurements as an indication of muscle strength in humans is somewhat controversial. A predictive model was developed to evaluate the relationship of peak knee flexion and extension torque production to thigh circumference.[27] Stepwise regression analyses indicated that peak knee torque production can be predicted with statistically significant accuracy ($r^2 = 0.78$ to 0.87). A similar study assessed the correlation of maximal isometric force production of leg extensor muscles of elite human weight lifters with thigh circumference.[28] Maximal isometric force had significant correlation with thigh circumference, but surprisingly not with the mean muscle fiber area of the vastus lateralis muscle. The CSAs of fat, muscle, and bone tissues of limbs as well as maximal voluntary isokinetic strength were measured in men and women in another study.[29] Anatomical CSAs were determined by ultrasound of the upper arm and thigh. The isokinetic strength of the elbow and knee extensor and flexor muscles were measured using an isokinetic dynamometer. There was significant correlation between CSA and strength in all muscle groups except for the elbow extensors of the men and the elbow flexors of the women.

Another study correlated thigh circumference, muscle CSA by MRI, and isokinetic strength in patients 48 months after surgery for ACL injury.[30] There was a significant 1.8% decrease in thigh circumference, an 8.6% decrease in quadriceps CSA area by MRI, and a 10% decrease in average quadriceps torque in the involved extremities as compared with the uninvolved extremities. A positive correlation was found between MRI CSA and quadriceps and hamstring peak torque in involved and uninvolved extremities. A positive correlation between thigh circumference, quadriceps, and hamstring peak torque was found in uninvolved extremities but not in operated extremities. Another study assessed whether measurements of thigh circumference of patients undergoing unilateral meniscectomies and rehabilitation exercises would be an indicator of muscle power.[31] In this study,

muscle power was not predicted from thigh circumference measurements. Another study also found that the changes in muscle strength are not directly correlated to limb circumference. In this study, isometric quadriceps strength and thigh circumference were determined in humans before and after a unilateral strength-training protocol of the quadriceps muscles for 5 weeks.[32] There were no significant changes in the untrained thighs. The trained quadriceps increased their isometric strength by 15% while they changed their CSA by only 6%. Quadriceps hypertrophy was underestimated by measurements of thigh circumference. Nevertheless, CSA measurements may indicate improvement in strength produced by training.

Although limb circumference may be associated with muscle power and strength in some situations, other factors may affect muscle strength besides muscle size. A single measurement of circumference in both thighs of subjects with unilateral injury may not be adequate to assess muscle function, but serial measurements over time may be of value as an index of muscle power. One study assessed the relationship between thigh circumference and muscle strength and power in noninjured and injured subjects.[33] The correlation between the torque produced at the knee by the knee extensors and flexors and a single thigh circumference measurement was not significant. In contrast, repeated measurements over a 6- to 8-month period showed a significant relationship between change in thigh circumference and change in quadriceps power.

Muscle Injury

Evaluation of muscle injury during rehabilitation may provide important information, especially as it pertains to prevention of overuse injuries. Magnetic resonance spectroscopy (MRS) and MRI are powerful tools to study tissue biochemistry and to provide precise anatomical visualization of soft tissue structures.[34] These techniques may be used to study exercise-induced muscle injury. MRS measurements show an increase in the ratio of inorganic phosphate to phosphocreatine (Pi/PCr) after eccentric exercise. This increase could be due to either increases in extracellular Pi or small increases in resting muscle metabolism. Increased Pi/PCr is also seen during training programs and may indicate persistent muscle injury. Increased resting Pi/PCr with injury is not associated with altered metabolism during exercise. Elevations in resting Pi/PCr have been used to show increased susceptibility of dystrophic muscle to exercise-induced injury. Progressive clinical deterioration in dystrophic dogs is marked by impaired muscle metabolism, and the presence of low oxidative muscle fibers not seen in normal dogs. Unfortunately, MRS is not commonly available for use in animals.

MRI shows changes following eccentric exercise that last up to 80 days after injury and can reflect muscle edema as well as longer lasting changes in the characteristics of cell water. MRI shows the precise localization of the injured area. Thus MRS can provide information on the metabolic response to injury, while MRI provides information regarding the site and extent of the injury. These tools are promising as aids in understanding exercise-induced muscle injury.

Body Composition

Assessment of body condition is important in rehabilitation patients because obesity has been associated with the exacerbation of some conditions, such as osteoarthritis. In addition, many companion animals are obese or overweight, and this may affect performance. Conversely, poor muscle mass may indicate inadequate nutrition, pathologic conditions, injuries, or poor conditioning. Morphometric techniques, such as body condition scoring systems, commonly used in clinical practice, are simple, inexpensive, and generally reasonably accurate. Body conformation is assessed from the side and the dorsal aspect and the animal is also palpated over certain regions. These profiles are then compared to a standard and a body condition score is assigned (Figure 12-13). Other morphometric measures, including tape measurements of body areas,

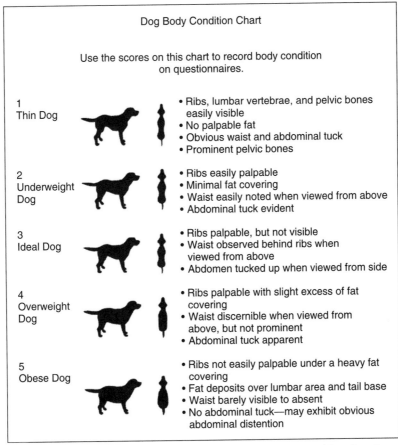

Dog Body Condition Chart

Use the scores on this chart to record body condition
on questionnaires.

1
Thin Dog
- Ribs, lumbar vertebrae, and pelvic bones easily visible
- No palpable fat
- Obvious waist and abdominal tuck
- Prominent pelvic bones

2
Underweight Dog
- Ribs easily palpable
- Minimal fat covering
- Waist easily noted when viewed from above
- Abdominal tuck evident

3
Ideal Dog
- Ribs palpable, but not visible
- Waist observed behind ribs when viewed from above
- Abdomen tucked up when viewed from side

4
Overweight Dog
- Ribs palpable with slight excess of fat covering
- Waist discernible when viewed from above, but not prominent
- Abdominal tuck apparent

5
Obese Dog
- Ribs not easily palpable under a heavy fat covering
- Fat deposits over lumbar area and tail base
- Waist barely visible to absent
- No abdominal tuck—may exhibit obvious abdominal distention

Figure 12-13   Body condition scores may be assigned to patients. The patient is assessed from the side and the dorsal aspect and the conformation is compared to a standard. (Body condition score courtesy Iams Co., Dayton, OH).

such as the cranial thoracic region and abdomen, are somewhat useful for assessing body composition, but because of the variation in body type in dogs, they may not be better than body condition scores.[35]

Although body condition scores are clinically useful, they are not as precise as other methods of noninvasive body composition assessments, such as DEXA analysis.[35] These units (Figure 12-14) measure lean body mass, fat, and bone mineral and are accurate within 2% of actual measurements. In addition, many software programs allow the generation of body composition of various portions of the body, such as the left and right forelimbs and rear limbs. Although generally considered the gold standard for the noninvasive assessment of body composition, animals must be heavily sedated or anesthetized to obtain information. DEXA units are relatively expensive and are limited to institutions at this time.

Skin caliper measurements, while having relatively good correlation to body composition in humans, are generally not very useful in dogs, perhaps because of differences in subcutaneous tissues and fat distribution.[35] Other methods of assessing body composition, such as diagnostic ultrasound, electrical impedance, and isotope dilution using the deuterium oxide method, have not been adequately investigated, require specialized equipment, or are limited to research institutions.

Pain Assessment

Assessment of pain and discomfort is important in the physical rehabilitation of animals.

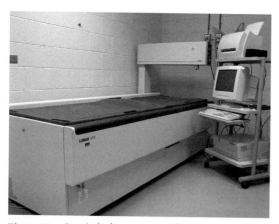

Figure 12-14   A dual-energy x-ray absorptiometer may be used to measure lean body mass, fat mass, and bone mineral content.

Excessive discomfort may prevent or slow progress during treatment, but objective measurement of pain is difficult in animals because they do not verbalize the level of pain that they may be experiencing. Therefore pain assessment scores are generally used to evaluate behaviors that are believed to be associated with pain and discomfort (Box 12-2). In addition, ordinal or visual analog scales are sometimes used in which owners are asked how painful they believe their pet is. Some physiologic parameters, such as heart rate, respiratory rate, and blood pressure, have been used to evaluate pain in the acute postoperative period, but these are generally not as useful for assessing pain in chronic conditions.

Painful behavior in dogs may be indicated by whining, crying, or other forms of vocalizing when the animal moves or the affected body part is manipulated. Holding an affected limb in a tightly flexed or guarded position is frequently noticed after surgery. Animals may be particularly resentful of palpation and manipulation of the area. Painful behavior may also be exemplified by lying quietly in the back of a run or in the corner of a room with little desire to rise and move about. This may be a protective mechanism to avoid further injury and pain from moving about. The degree of pain in these patients is frequently underestimated because of their quiet nature.

Impressions of Owners and Veterinarians

Dogs and cats have different personalities and may respond very differently to various therapies. It is important for individuals who best know patients to evaluate their progress. For example, owners are often very aware of subtle changes in their pet's behavior. Although it is somewhat difficult to quantify these changes, these subjective findings often provide the therapist with important information

---

■ ■ ■ **BOX 12-2** Pain Assessment Score

0 No signs of pain during palpation of affected joint
1 Signs of mild pain during palpation of joint
2 Signs of moderate pain during palpation
3 Signs of severe pain during palpation
4 Dog will not allow examiner to palpate joint

regarding patient progress. If possible, the changes should be as objective as possible, such as recording the amount of time a pet spends playing rather than resting, measuring the distance that an animal is able to walk before needing to rest, or evaluating the length of time a neurologic patient is able to stand unassisted.

Owners should keep a log of daily activities to further define the progress of the patient at home. This may also provide incentive for owners to continue a home rehabilitation program if they can see the progress that is made from week to week and month to month. Poor compliance is a common reason for failure of a patient to progress. Regularly checking the log gives the veterinarian and owner an opportunity to evaluate the patient's progress, as well as make alterations to the rehabilitation program that account for an owner's ability to provide continued home care. In addition, videotaping the patient's activity on a regular schedule will allow comparisons to be made over relatively long periods of time.

Return to Function

Return to function is perhaps the best indication of a successful outcome following treatment of an acute or chronic condition. The desired level of function depends on the intended use of the patient, which varies from a highly trained working dog or racing Greyhound to a house pet. Some outcomes are relatively easy to quantify, such as winning a race in the same class that the animal raced in before an injury or being able to perform a particular task in the case of a working dog. Others are more nebulous, such as a return to acceptable house-pet function. Regardless of the desired outcome, reasonable expectations must be set based on the severity of the condition being treated, and this must be conveyed to the owner to avoid future disappointment when a higher level of function is expected than may be achieved.

For example, it is unreasonable to expect an elderly arthritic dog to return to competitive coursing, but it may be reasonable to expect the dog to be able to play ball for short periods of time. In addition, expectations may need to be altered if the response to treatment is better or worse than expected. In severely affected neurologic patients, reasonable expectations should center around functional activities of daily living, such as being able to climb stairs to get in and out of the house, able to go outside to eliminate with minimal or no assistance, and able to take short walks with the owner.

Functional scoring systems for specific injuries may be useful, such as a functional stifle score. Such scoring systems have been used for outcome assessment in people recovering from ACL surgery because an ACL may result in functional disability. The optimal method to measure the degree of functional disability is unknown in dogs. A useful system in dogs likely should incorporate limb use, lameness, stance, pain, muscle atrophy, range of motion, joint effusion, drawer motion, and functional activities to evaluate limb function following cranial cruciate ligament surgery (Box 12-3). A subjective and functional rating system in people related six activity levels to pain, swelling, giving-way and overall activity.[36] In this study, activity level, symptoms, clinical laxity, meniscal damage, lower limb alignment, tibiofemoral crepitus, patellofemoral factors, rehabilitation, and patient compliance were identified as risk factors for future joint arthrosis.

Other functional tests that have been used in humans may be applied to dogs, with modification. For example, one study of people assessed the sensitivity of four different types of one-legged hop tests to determine alterations in lower limb function in ACL-deficient knees.[37] Comparisons were made between limb symmetry as measured by the hop tests and muscle strength, symptoms, and self-assessed function. Statistical trends were noted between abnormal limb symmetry on the hop tests and low-velocity quadriceps isokinetic test results. The time and distance that a dog will walk on the rear limbs with the forelimbs elevated (dancing) may provide similar information.

Summary

Assessment of patients is important to document the benefits of a rehabilitation program and to help improve protocols. Assessment techniques may be relatively simple and inexpensive, or more elaborate with expensive equipment. New assessment techniques must be developed to allow adequate comparison of a patient's progress over time, and to make specific changes in protocols to achieve the best possible outcome.

■ ■ ■ **BOX 12-3**   Functional Stifle Score

Limb Use

Trot

10 No lameness and weight-bearing on all strides
6 Lame but weight-bearing on >95% of strides
4 Lame but weight-bearing on >50% and <95% of strides
2 Lame but weight-bearing on <50% and >5% of strides
0 Continuous non–weight-bearing lameness or weight-bearing on <5% of strides

Walk

10 No lameness and weight-bearing on all strides
6 Lame but weight-bearing on >95% of strides
4 Lame but weight-bearing on >50% and <95% of strides
2 Lame but weight-bearing on <50% and >5% of strides
0 Continuous non–weight-bearing lameness or weight-bearing on <5% of strides

Lameness

Trot

10 Trots normally
8 Slight lameness
6 Obvious weight-bearing lameness
4 Severe weight-bearing lameness
2 Intermittent non–weight bearing lameness
0 Continuous non–weight bearing lameness

Walk

10 Walks normally
8 Slight lameness
6 Obvious weight-bearing lameness
4 Severe weight-bearing lameness
2 Intermittent non–weight bearing lameness
0 Continuous non–weight bearing lameness

Stance

10 Stands with equal weight on both rear limbs
6 Favors affected limb while standing
2 Toe touches while standing
0 Does not bear weight on affected limb while standing

Activities

Stairs

5 No difficulty
3 Slight difficulty
1 Skips steps or bunny hops
0 Unable

Sit

5 Sits and rises squarely with no difficulty
4 Sits and rises with slight difficulty
2 Sits and rises with difficulty
0 Unable to sit or rise on own

Weight-Bearing on Rear Limbs (Dancing)

5 Able to move freely forward and backward
3 Resists moving forward and backward
0 Unable to bear weight on rear limbs to move forward and backward

Pain

5 None
3 Mild
2 Moderate
0 Severe

Stifle Swelling

5 None
3 Mild
2 Moderate
0 Severe

Thigh Muscle Atrophy

10 None
6 1-2 cm
4 2-4 cm
0 More than 4 cm

Range of Motion

Extension

5 155-170 degrees
3 135-154 degrees
1 110-134 degrees
0 Less than 110 degrees

Flexion

5 30-45 degrees
3 44-50 degrees
1 51-60 degrees
0 More than 60 degrees

Drawer Motion

5 Less than 2 mm
3 2-4 mm
1 5-7 mm
0 More than 7 mm
     Total

REFERENCES

1. DeCamp CE et al: Kinematic evaluation of gait in dogs with cranial cruciate ligament rupture, *Am J Vet Res* 57:120-126, 1996.
2. Jaegger G, Marcellin-Little D, Levine D: Reliability of goniometry in Labrador retrievers, *Am J Vet Res* 63:979-986, 2002.
3. Peacock J, Millis DL, Weigel JP: A comparative analysis of two methods of cranial drawer quantitation in the canine stifle. In *Proc 26th Annu Conf Vet Orthoped Soc*, Sun Valley, Idaho, 1999, p 30.
4. Edixhoven P et al: Accuracy and reproducibility of instrumented knee-drawer tests, *J Orthop Res* 5:378-387, 1987.
5. Doupe MB et al: A new formula for population-based estimation of whole body muscle mass in males, *Can J Appl Physiol* 22:598-608, 1997.
6. Daniel DM et al: Instrumented measurement of anterior laxity of the knee, *J Bone Joint Surg Am* 67:720-726, 1985.

7. Hewett TE, Noyes FR, Lee MD: Diagnosis of complete and partial posterior cruciate ligament ruptures: stress radiography compared with KT-1000 arthrometer and posterior drawer testing, *Am J Sports Med* 25:648-655, 1997.

8. Millis DL, Scroggs L, Levine D: Variables affecting thigh circumference measurements in dogs. In *Proc 1st Int Symp Rehab Physical Ther Vet Med*, 1999, p 157.

9. Martin AD et al: Anthropometric estimation of muscle mass in men, *Med Sci Sports Exerc* 22:729-733, 1990.

10. Ross M, Worrell TW: Thigh and calf girth following knee injury and surgery, *J Orthop Sports Phys Ther* 27: 9-15, 1998.

11. Soderberg GL, Ballantyne BT, Kestel LL: Reliability of lower extremity girth measurements after anterior cruciate ligament reconstruction, *Physiother Res Int* 1:7-16, 1996.

12. Maylia E et al: Can thigh girth be measured accurately: a preliminary investigation, *J Sport Rehab* 8: 43-49, 1999.

13. Doxey GE: Assessing quadriceps femoris muscle bulk with girth measurements in subjects with patellofemoral pain, *J Orthop Sports Phys Ther* 9: 177-183, 1987.

14. Doxey GE: The association of anthropometric measurements of thigh size and B-mode ultrasound scanning of muscle thickness, *J Orthop Sports Phys Ther* 8:462-468, 1987.

15. Housh DJ et al: Anthropometric estimation of thigh muscle cross-sectional area, *Med Sci Sports Exerc* 27:784-791, 1995.

16. Knapik JJ, Staab JS, Harman EA: Validity of an anthropometric estimate of thigh muscle cross-sectional area, *Med Sci Sports Exerc* 28:1523-1530, 1996.

17. Howe TE, Oldham JA: The reliability of measuring quadriceps cross-sectional area with compound B ultrasound scanning, *Physiother Res Int* 1:112-126, 1996.

18. Weiss LW, Coney HD, Clark FC: Gross measures of exercise-induced muscular hypertrophy, *J Orthop Sports Phys Ther* 30:143-148, 2000.

19. Mitsiopoulos N et al: Cadaver validation of skeletal muscle measurement by magnetic resonance imaging and computerized tomography, *J Appl Physiol* 85: 115-122, 1998.

20. Beneke R, Neuerburg J, Bohndorf K: Muscle cross-section measurement by magnetic resonance imaging, *Eur J Appl Physiol* 63:424-429, 1991.

21. Orima H, Fujita M: Computed tomographic findings of experimentally induced neurogenic muscular atrophy in dogs, *J Vet Med Sci* 59:729-731, 1997.

22. Walton JM, Roberts N, Whitehouse GH: Measurement of the quadriceps femoris muscle using magnetic resonance and ultrasound imaging, *Br J Sports Med* 31: 59-64, 1997.

23. Visser M et al: Validity of fan-beam dual-energy X-ray absorptiometry for measuring fat-free mass and leg muscle mass: Health, Aging, and Body Composition Study—Dual-Energy X-ray Absorptiometry and Body Composition Working Group, *J Appl Physiol* 87: 1513-1520, 1999.

24. Fuller NJ et al: Assessment of limb muscle and adipose tissue by dual-energy x-ray absorptiometry using magnetic resonance imaging for comparison, *Int J Obes Relat Metab Disord* 23:1295-1302, 1999.

25. Lieber RL et al: Growth hormone secretagogue increases muscle strength during remobilization after canine hindlimb immobilization, *J Orthop Res* 15: 519-527, 1997.

26. Mayhew JL, Piper FC, Ware JS: Anthropometric correlates with strength performance among resistance trained athletes, *J Sports Med Phys Fitness* 33:159-165, 1993.

27. Gross MT et al: Relationship between multiple predictor variables and normal knee torque production, *Phys Ther* 69:54-62, 1989.

28. Hakkinen K, Komi PV, Kauhanen H: Electromyographic and force production characteristics of leg extensor muscles of elite weight lifters during isometric, concentric, and various stretch-shortening cycle exercises, *Int J Sports Med* 7:144-151, 1986.

29. Kanehisa H, Ikegawa S, Fukunaga T: Comparison of muscle cross-sectional area and strength between untrained women and men, *Eur J Appl Physiol* 68: 148-154, 1994.

30. Arangio GA et al: Thigh muscle size and strength after anterior cruciate ligament reconstruction and rehabilitation, *J Orthop Sports Phys Ther* 26:238-243, 1997.

31. Maylia E et al: Can muscle power be estimated from thigh bulk measurements: a preliminary study, *J Sport Rehab* 8:50-59, 1999.

32. Young A et al: The effect of high-resistance training on the strength and cross-sectional area of the human quadriceps, *Eur J Clin Invest* 13:411-417, 1983.

33. Cooper H et al: Use and misuse of the tape-measure as a means of assessing muscle strength and power, *Rheumatol Rehabil* 20:211-218, 1981.

34. McCully K et al: The use of nuclear magnetic resonance to evaluate muscle injury, *Med Sci Sports Exerc* 24:537-542, 1992.

35. Burkholder WJ: Precision and practicality of methods assessing body composition of dogs and cats, *Compend Contin Educ Pract Vet* 23:1-10, 2001.

36. Noyes FR, McGinniss GH, Mooar LA: Functional disability in the anterior cruciate insufficient knee syndrome: review of knee rating systems and projected risk factors in determining treatment, *Sports Med* 1:278-302, 1984.

37. Noyes FR, Barber SD, Mangine RE: Abnormal lower limb symmetry determined by function hop tests after anterior cruciate ligament rupture, *Am J Sports Med* 19:513-518, 1991.

THERAPEUTIC MODALITIES

■ **C h a p t e r   1 3**

Range-of-Motion and Stretching Exercises

Darryl L. Millis, Angela Lewelling, and Siri Hamilton

Range of motion (ROM) and stretching exercises are very important to achieve improved motion of joints after surgery or in patients afflicted with chronic conditions. They are also important to help increase flexibility, prevent adhesions between soft tissues and bones, remodel periarticular fibrosis, and improve muscle and other soft tissue extensibility to help prevent further injury to joints, muscles, tendons, and ligaments.

As with many types of rehabilitation activities, it may be beneficial to administer analgesic medication 30 to 60 minutes before beginning any rehabilitation exercises to allow peak absorption of the medication and take advantage of its maximal analgesic effect.

Range of Motion

The full motion that a joint may be moved through is termed the ROM. The structure of the joint and the volume, integrity, and flexibility of the soft tissues that pass over the joint affect joint motion.[1] ROM is commonly measured with a goniometer, and each joint has characteristic angles, such as flexion and extension of the stifle and flexion, extension, abduction, adduction, and internal and external rotation of the hip (Appendix 1).

Muscles also have a ROM, which is termed the functional excursion of muscles.[1] This is the distance that a muscle is able to shorten after it has maximally elongated. The functional excursion may be affected by the joint it crosses, particularly if joint motion is restricted. Some muscles, such as the biceps brachii and the rectus femoris muscles, cross two joints. In general, muscles that cross multiple joints may lose functional excursion easier than those that cross only one joint.

ROM exercises are useful to diminish the effects of disuse and immobilization.[2] To maintain ROM, the joints and muscles must be periodically moved through their available ranges. Movement may be passive, active assisted, or active. In each situation, a load is produced on the soft tissues that helps to maintain the articular cartilage, muscles, ligaments, and tendons in a healthy state. It is generally appropriate to initiate passive ROM as soon after injury or surgery as possible provided there are no contraindications. Progression through active assisted and active ROM follows, and when appropriate, some resistance to motion may be introduced for strengthening.

Passive Range of Motion

Passive ROM is motion of a joint that is performed without muscle contraction within the available ROM, using an external force to move the joint. Additional pressure at the end of the available ROM is stretching. Both passive ROM and stretching can be performed in conjunction with each other to help maintain and improve joint ROM. In animals, passive ROM is performed by the therapist.

The benefits of continuous passive ROM immediately after joint surgery were initially described by Salter and include decreased pain and improved rate of recovery.[3] However, it is critical that the therapist maintain a ROM that is comfortable to the patient and not injure tissues by exceeding the limits of the tissues.

Tissues limiting passive ROM may be normal or pathologic and include joint capsule, periarticular soft tissues, muscles, ligaments, tendons, and skin. For example, open wounds over joints that are allowed to heal secondarily by contraction and epithelialization may result in limitations to passive ROM. Surgical incisions may result in adhesions and fibrosis between skin, subcutaneous tissues, fascia, muscles, and bone, limiting the ability of tissues to glide over one another. Musculotendinous tissue may also be relatively shortened as a result of spasm or contracture. Any restriction of motions may result in resistance to movement and pain.

Passive ROM is used whenever a patient is unable to move joints on its own, or if active motion across a joint may be deleterious to the patient, such as with a tenuous articular fracture repair. Passive ROM is sometimes used to help relax an anxious patient. The most common indication for passive ROM exercises is immediately after surgery, before active weight-bearing, to help prevent joint contracture and soft tissue adaptive shortening, maintain mobility between soft tissue layers, reduce pain, enhance blood and lymphatic flow, and improve synovial fluid production and diffusion.[2]

Another indication for passive ROM is the prevention of joint contracture during healing and recovery in paralyzed patients. Ideally, exercises should be performed two to six times per day to help maintain normal joint mobility. However, if the patient does not regain functional neuromuscular control, it is likely that joints will undergo some degree of contracture despite aggressive efforts. Passive ROM will not prevent muscle atrophy, increase strength, improve endurance, or be as effective in improving vascular and lymphatic flow as active ROM techniques.

Proper technique for performing passive ROM is important. The patient should be relaxed and comfortable. If active muscle contraction is not desired, it is especially important to be gentle and not create pain or discomfort. The bones proximal and distal to the joint should be supported to avoid excessive stress on the joint. The therapist should gently grasp the limb and avoid painful areas, such as incisions and wounds. The motion should be smooth, slow, and steady with motion occurring with movement of the distal limb with the proximal limb held steady. The patient should be continually monitored for any discomfort, and the technique altered if necessary to enhance comfort.

Active Assisted Range of Motion

Active assisted ROM occurs when the therapist guides joint motion and some degree of the patient's muscle activity assists joint motion. In animal patients, the amount of muscle activity provided by the patient is difficult to control. In reality, because it is difficult to avoid muscle activation in patients that are not paralyzed, most ROM exercises in small animal patients involve a degree of active assisted ROM. In anxious patients or in those with upper motor neuron conditions, muscle contraction of antagonist muscle groups may oppose joint ROM exercises.

Active assisted ROM exercises are most useful for those patients that are weak or recovering from lower motor neuron conditions. In addition to assisted ROM with the patient in lateral recumbency, exercises may be performed with the patient supported by a sling, with the therapist assisting limb movement and joint ROM during ambulation. This may be performed while the patient is slowly walked on the ground or a ground treadmill. Another form of active assisted ROM exercise is performed while swimming. Patients with limited ability to ambulate on the ground may benefit from controlled swimming, during which the therapist assists movement of the animal's limbs and joints while in the water with the patient. The buoyancy of the water helps to support the weight of the limbs while the therapist concentrates on assisting the limb through a normal cycle of movement.

Active assisted ROM helps to combat the negative effects of immobilization on limbs, similar to those achieved with passive ROM. Some degree of active muscle contraction allows muscle strengthening and strengthening of bone at muscle origin and insertion sites. In addition, some neuromuscular reeducation, and proprioceptive and gait training may be achieved.

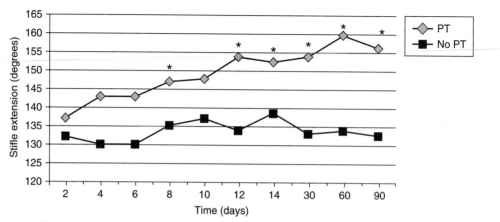

Figure 13-1 Effect of physical rehabilitation on stifle extension. Note the return of normal stifle extension by 2 weeks after surgery, in those dogs receiving rehabilitation and the loss of complete stifle extension in some dogs not receiving postsurgical rehabilitation. *$P < 0.05$.

Active Range of Motion

Active ROM is the motion of a joint that may be achieved by active muscle contraction. In addition to increasing strength, coordination between muscle groups is necessary because the guidance of assisting the patient through ROM is no longer provided. The active ROM may be performed during a regular gait cycle, in which the excursion of joint motion is relatively limited, or under special conditions designed to expand motion and more completely use the full available ROM. Examples of these activities include swimming; walking in water, tall grass, snow, or sand; climbing stairs; crawling through a tunnel; and negotiating cavaletti rails.

As the patient improves flexion and extension of a joint, it is helpful to continue to perform passive ROM and stretching to achieve as complete ROM as possible, and then perform active ROM through this increased motion to emphasize more complete use of the limb. Greater strength is required for patients to perform active ROM, and some of the special conditions require more muscle strength than normal ambulation during walking or trotting. Therefore, for those exercises, a transition between active assisted and active ROM may be necessary. Active ROM exercises may be a prelude to other strengthening activities. Owners may also be involved with active ROM exercises in helping with a home care program for their pet.

Precautions and Contraindications to Range of Motion

All forms of ROM exercises are contraindicated when motion may result in further injury or instability. Such examples include unstable fractures near joints and unstable ligament or tendon injuries. Communication between the surgeon and therapist is critical to be certain that appropriate ROM exercises are performed and that the limits of the range are not exceeded, which might result in damage to the tissues. In most cases, early passive ROM is felt to be beneficial if the therapist stays within a ROM that is reasonable for the patient and condition being treated. In addition, the therapist should perform the exercises at a reasonable speed that is not painful for the patient.

Range-of-Motion Studies

In some canine conditions, active ROM is a prerequisite to a successful outcome. For example, it is critical that puppies with distal femoral physeal fractures have early active ROM exercises to avoid fracture disease and tiedown of the quadriceps muscle group.[4] Similarly, dogs with condylar fractures of the distal humerus must begin active ROM to prevent permanent joint stiffness.

In one study of dogs following surgery for cranial cruciate ligament rupture, patients not receiving early passive and active ROM exercises had reduced stifle extension (Figure 13-1).[5] This loss of motion appeared to be permanent in some dogs if extension was not achieved within 2 weeks. In contrast, those dogs receiving appropriate rehabilitation had return of near-normal stifle extension. There also appears to be an association of stifle extension with weight-bearing, with improved weight-bearing in dogs with near-normal stifle extension (Figure 13-2). However, the cause and effect of this relationship are unknown.

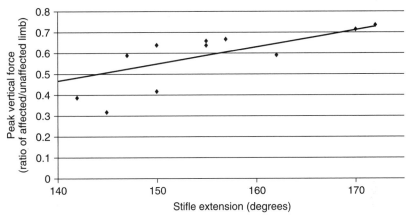

Figure 13-2 Relationship of comfortable angle of stifle extension to peak vertical force in dogs 10 weeks after cranial cruciate ligament transection and stifle stabilization. Dogs with normal stifle extension have greater weight-bearing on the limb at a trot than those with limitation to stifle extension. Although a cause-and-effect relationship cannot be definitively identified from these data, there is a significant relationship. $r = 0.78$; $P < 0.001$.

The functional and structural consequences of remobilization of the shoulder joint after 12 weeks of immobilization were studied in 10 beagle dogs.[6] It was found that after 12 weeks of immobilization, the passive ROM was markedly impaired, intraarticular pressure increased during movement, and the filling volume of the joint cavity was reduced. Histologically, the capsule showed hyperplasia of the synovial lining and vascular proliferation in the wall, but there was no increase of collagen in the capsular wall. Both the functional and structural changes were unaltered after 4 weeks of remobilization, but after 8 weeks they began to reverse, and they returned to normal after 12 weeks, indicating that functional and structural changes after immobilization of an uninjured shoulder joint are potentially reversible.

Another study of dogs evaluated the effects of joint mobilization treatment on carpal joints of dogs.[7] The right carpal joints of 12 dogs were immobilized for 6 weeks resulting in joint hypomobility. The treated group received mobilization therapy daily during the 4 weeks after immobilization. In control and treated groups, passive ROM, peak angles of extension and flexion of the carpal joint, and the amount of time required in the gait cycle to reach these peak points were evaluated cinematographically during gait before immobilization and once weekly for 4 weeks after immobilization. The treated group had improved passive ROM and motion during gait.

Continuous passive ROM has been assessed in several studies to evaluate its use in the management of cartilage defects. Salter et al demonstrated that young rabbits with a full-thickness defect in the articular cartilage managed with continuous passive motion had healing of 52% of the defects with hyaline-type cartilage.[8] Similar results were obtained in adult rabbits, in which 44% of the defects were repaired with hyaline cartilage. Passive motion may also help to reduce cartilage destruction following infection of a joint.[9,10] The optimal daily dose of passive ROM and the total duration of treatment are unknown. However, one study of rabbits found that at least 8 hours of passive motion per day was necessary to achieve the level of healing obtained by Salter.[11] The effect of active motion on cartilage healing is unknown in animals because of the difficulty in achieving consistent limb use after cartilage injury.

Continuous passive motion has also been recommended to prevent contracture of periarticular tissues and to restore joint function. Immobilization results in shortening of fibrous tissues and loss of motion, depending on the position of immobilization. There is a loss of collagen mass after immobilization, and there is collagen cross-linking of periarticular connective tissues, which may lead to increased stiffness. Passive motion may reduce these changes and prevent joint stiffness. In one study, 16 hours or more of continuous motion prevented increased joint stiffness following articular cartilage damage.[12] Longer durations of passive motion may be necessary to help maintain normal quantities and turnover of collagen and glycosaminoglycans, as well as to help maintain the normal alignment of collagen fibers and prevent shortening and cross-linking.

The duration of daily passive motion treatment has varying effects. For example, relatively short daily passive motion may reduce stiffness immediately after treatment, but there may be greater long-term stiffness.[12] In fact, shorter durations of passive motion may be detrimental.[12,13] One study indicated more stiffness with 10 to 30 minutes of passive motion per day than if the joints were immobilized,[12] while another indicated increased stiffness with less than 8 hours of daily passive motion.[13] Although somewhat surprising, these results suggest that there may be increased trauma associated with breakdown of soft adhesions that form when motion is not occurring, and that very frequent motion is necessary to keep the tissues mobile.

Both continuous motion and as little as 4 hours of daily passive motion help to preserve muscle mass in rabbits.[12,14] In fact, 5% to 15% greater limb muscle mass may occur in rabbits with passive motion as compared with those that are immobilized.

The effects of passive motion on bone loss are less clear. It is well-documented that immobilization results in loss of bone mineral; however, 16 or 24 hours of passive motion resulted in the loss of greater bone mineral than immobilization.[12] It was suggested by these authors that the increased joint stiffness that resulted from less than 16 hours of motion may have increased the bending stresses and load on the bones, while greater duration of passive motion maintained normal joint stiffness and prevented the additional loading on the bones.

In people, the use of active and passive knee motion in the immediate postoperative period and a treatment plan for early postoperative limitations in knee motion has proven highly effective in restoring motion after anterior cruciate ligament reconstruction.[15] In this study of 207 knees, 91% regained full ROM. The remaining patients did not regain motion as rapidly and were placed in an early postoperative phased treatment program of serial extension casts, early gentle manipulation under anesthesia, or arthroscopic treatment of intraarticular adhesions and scar tissue. Most of these patients regained full ROM. Those patients who failed to follow the rehabilitation program had permanent and significant limitation of motion. The incidence of postoperative motion problems was related to the extent of the surgical procedure. Patients who had more extensive surgery, such as a concurrent meniscus repair or a medial collateral ligament repair, had a higher incidence of restricted motion.

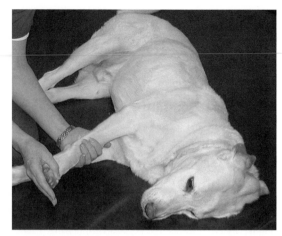

Figure 13-3 Before performing ROM or stretching exercises, the patient should be placed in lateral recumbency with the affected limb up.

Clinical Application of Range of Motion

Passive Range of Motion

The treatment should be administered in a quiet and comfortable area, away from distractions, such as loud noises, other pets, and other people who are not helping with the treatment. This will allow the patient to be calm, relaxed, and more receptive to the treatment.

It is recommended that patients have a muzzle applied for the initial treatments, or if they are painful, resistant to treatment, or overly anxious. The patient should be placed in lateral recumbency with the affected limb up (Figure 13-3). Help may be required to restrain the animal and to help keep it quiet and relaxed. In all forms of ROM activities, therapists should be comfortable and use proper body mechanics to avoid injury to themselves.

After the animal has relaxed, gently place both hands on the injured limb and begin a very gentle massage to help further relax the patient. Massage for 2 to 3 minutes, and then gently move one hand to the portion of the limb above the joint. Place the other hand on a portion of the limb below the affected joint. Be certain that the entire limb is supported to avoid any undue stress to the involved joint.

After the hands are in the correct position and the limb is supported, begin by slowly and gently flexing the treated joint (Figures 13-4 to 13-7). The other joints of the limb should be allowed to remain in a neutral posi-

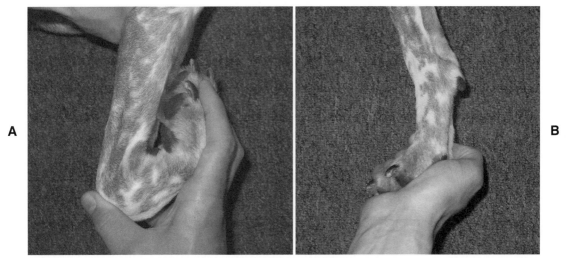

Figure 13-4   A, Carpal flexion. While supporting the radius and ulna in one hand and the foot in the other, the carpus is gently flexed. **B,** Carpal extension. While supporting the radius and ulna in one hand and the foot in the other, the carpus is gently extended.

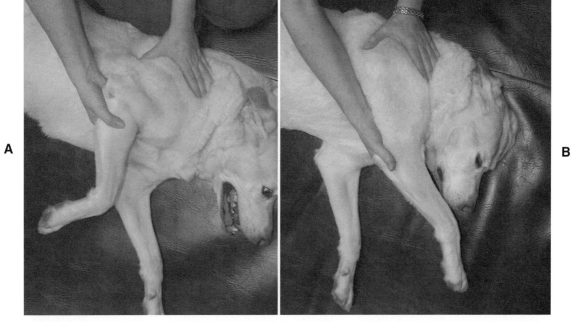

Figure 13-5   A, Shoulder flexion. While supporting the distal scapula in one hand and the humerus in the other, the shoulder is gently flexed. **B,** Shoulder extension. While supporting the distal scapula in one hand and the humerus in the other, the shoulder is gently extended.

tion (a position as if the animal were standing). Try not to move the other joints while working on the affected joint because some joints may be restricted by the position of the joints above or below the target joint. In these situations, the other joints should be placed in a position that will allow as complete a

ROM as possible to the target joint. For example, maximal hock flexion cannot be obtained while the stifle is maintained in an extended position. In this case, placing the stifle in a flexed position allows more complete flexion of the hock. Slowly continue to flex the joint until the patient shows initial signs of

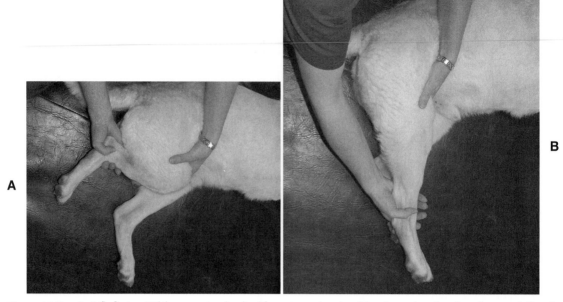

Figure 13-6   A, Stifle flexion. While supporting the distal femur in one hand and the tibia in the other, the stifle is gently flexed. **B,** Stifle extension. While supporting the distal femur in one hand and the tibia in the other, the stifle is gently extended.

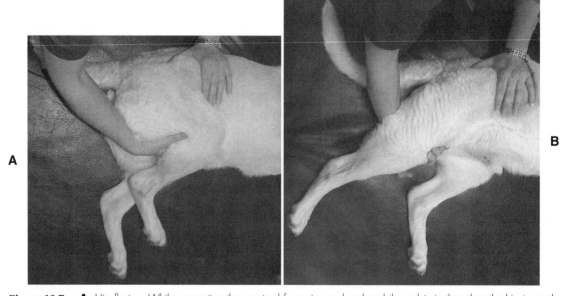

Figure 13-7   A, Hip flexion. While supporting the proximal femur in one hand and the pelvis in the other, the hip is gently flexed. **B,** Hip extension. While supporting the proximal femur in one hand and the pelvis in the other, the hip is gently extended.

discomfort, such as tensing the limb, moving, vocalizing, turning the head toward the therapist, or trying to pull away, but do not cause undue discomfort.

With the hands maintained in the same positions, slowly extend the joint. Again, try to keep the other joints in a neutral position and minimize any movement of the other joints.

Slowly continue to extend the joint until the patient shows initial signs of discomfort.

Alternatively, a number of joints may be simultaneously placed through a ROM, a technique sometimes referred to as ROM though functional patterns. This form of ROM exercises may be appropriate as an animal nears active use of a limb. Flexing and extending all

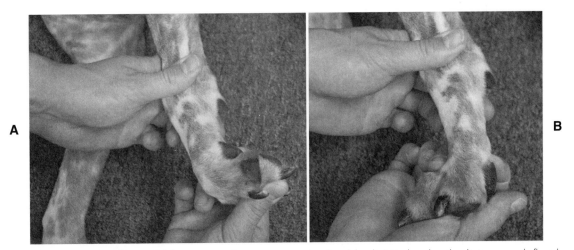

Figure 13-8   A, Digit flexion. While supporting the carpus in one hand and the digits in the other, the digits are gently flexed. **B,** Digit extension. While supporting the carpus in one hand and the digits in the other, the digits are gently extended.

of the joints of a limb in a pattern that mimics a normal gait pattern may also be beneficial for neuromuscular reeducation.

The number of ROM repetitions and the frequency of the treatments depend on the condition treated. In general, for most routine postoperative conditions, 15 to 20 repetitions performed two to four times per day are likely adequate. As the ROM returns to normal, the frequency may be reduced. For more challenging conditions, such as articular fractures, physeal fractures in young dogs, joints with contracture, or joints that have been immobilized for a period of time, an increase in the number and frequency of repetitions may be necessary.

It is also important to maintain normal ROM in the other joints of the affected limb. After completing ROM of the affected joint, keep the limb in a neutral position and slowly move the hands distally to the digits (or if already working on the digits, move proximally). Be certain to keep the injured joint supported. Performing ROM of the digits requires additional consideration because it is difficult to passively flex and extend a single joint at a time because of the proximity of the other joints of each digit. In addition, it is more efficient to perform ROM in all joints simultaneously (Figure 13-8). Place the fingers or palm on the pads of the patient's foot and slowly extend the toes until the point of initial discomfort. Then place the fingers or palm on the dorsal surface of the digits and slowly flex the digits until the point of initial discomfort. After ROM is performed on the digits, ROM exercises are performed on the other joints.

The ROM session may be ended with a gentle massage to the injured limb. Gently and slowly massage for approximately 5 minutes. This helps to maintain a relaxed state. An ice pack may be applied to the injured joint after the ROM and massage.

Active Assisted Range of Motion

Active assisted ROM is the next step in the progression of joint motion during rehabilitation. In most situations, veterinary patients will have some muscle tension during ROM activities, and there is an equally likely chance that an agonist or antagonist muscle group, or likely a combination of both, will contract with joint movement. Patients with neurologic conditions may benefit from assisted movement of limbs while in lateral recumbency, or while standing and generating a gait pattern.

Active assisted ROM may be performed while the patient is ambulating on a ground treadmill or during swimming activity, during which the therapist helps move the limb at the appropriate phase of the gait cycle. Similarly, placing the animal in an ambulatory sling and slowly pushing the sling while assisting the animal to advance the limb are appropriate active assisted ROM activities.

Active Range of Motion

When the animal is able to ambulate and move the affected limb, active ROM exercises may be initiated. Joint ROM is limited during normal walking and trotting, so the joints do not go through a complete normal ROM. If joint restriction is present, patients may benefit by performing activities which encourage a more complete ROM. Swimming or walking in water result in greater flexion of joints. Decreased joint extension may occur with swimming, but walking in water maintains relatively normal active joint extension while increasing joint flexion, resulting in greater overall joint ROM. Other activities that may be performed include walking in snow, sand, or tall grass, and crawling through a play tunnel. Climbing stairs may increase joint excursion, while also increasing strength. Walking over cavaletti rails is an excellent method of achieving normal limb extension for walking, while increasing joint flexion as the patient negotiates the rails. In addition, the rails may be raised or lowered to encourage increased or decreased joint flexion, based on the needs of the individual patient.

Stretching

Stretching techniques are often performed in conjunction with ROM exercises to improve flexibility of the joints and extensibility of periarticular tissues, muscles, and tendons.[2] Conditions that result in adaptive shortening of tissues, including immobilization, reduced mobility, injury and fibrosis of periarticular tissues, or neurologic conditions, may respond favorably to stretching.[1] Muscle weakness may occur with adaptive shortening of tissues because peak muscle tension cannot occur, and joint ROM may be decreased as a result of periarticular fibrosis.

Flexibility refers to the ability of tissues, particularly muscle, to relax and respond to an elongation force. Overstretching refers to the elongation of tissues beyond normal limits to allow greater joint ROM than normal. Overstretching may be detrimental if there is inadequate soft tissue support to maintain joint stability and prevent injury. Tightness implies mild shortening of a musculotendinous unit, with no specific pathologic etiology. Two-joint muscles, such as the rectus femoris and gastrocnemius muscles, are especially susceptible to tightness. The unit may be lengthened with stretching exercises.

Contracture occurs when muscles or other soft tissues that span a joint shorten and limit ROM. Contractures may be defined by the types of soft tissues involved.[1] Myostatic contractures have a musculotendinous junction that has adapted to a shortened position.

There is no pathology, but the joint has significant loss of motion. Scar tissue adhesions between normal tissues, such as muscles and fascia, tie down the tissues and prevent normal gliding motion between the tissues, resulting in reduced ROM. Most scar tissue adhesions may be prevented with appropriate stretching, exercise, and massage in the early tissue healing phase following injury. If the adhesion continues to mature without tissue modification, a fibrotic adhesion may form. These types of adhesions dramatically reduce joint ROM, and the resultant contracture is very difficult to treat and restore normal function to the joint. When there is an excessive amount of fibrous tissue, cartilage, and bone, there may be permanent loss of soft tissue extensibility. Damage to the central nervous system with upper motor neuron signs may result in hypertonic muscles, and a pseudomyostatic contracture. In this situation, the muscle seems to be in a chronic state of contraction, resulting in reduced ROM. Appropriate ROM and stretching may help to improve this form of contracture.

The various tissues that are involved, such as muscle, ligaments, tendons, joint capsule, and skin, respond to stretching differently. Interestingly, in a study of rat denervated gastrocnemius muscle-tendon units, the muscle tissue accounted for 95% of the total increase in length of the unit with loading, while the tendon contributed only 5% to the length.[16] Therefore the therapist must consider which tissues are most likely limiting mobility and choose the appropriate techniques to help achieve more normal function. If stretching occurs within the normal physiologic limits of the tissue, elastic deformation occurs in which the tissues return to their normal resting length after the stretch is completed. If the tissue is stretched beyond its limits, permanent deformation of the tissue(s) remains after the stretch is completed, resulting in an increased resting length; this is called plastic deformation.

Stretching is a general term that is used to indicate maneuvers to elongate pathologically shortened tissues, and to increase flexibility and joint motion in normal and abnormal tissues. Stretching differs from ROM exercises in that stretching takes tissues beyond the normal ROM. Passive ROM only takes structures through the available range. Passive stretching techniques are most commonly used in veterinary medicine because of the inability to verbally communicate instructions to the patient to selectively relax and contract various muscle groups. It may be possible, in some situations, to apply neuromuscular electrical stimulation to various muscle groups to mimic active muscle contraction of an individual muscle for certain active stretching techniques. But this requires exquisite coordination of efforts, and usually two or three people must be involved in the treatment session.

Several stretching techniques have been described, including static stretching, prolonged mechanical passive stretching, ballistic stretching, and proprioceptive neuromuscular facilitation stretching. The acute effect of stretching is an immediate elongation of the elastic component of the musculotendinous unit. A chronic stretch may be applied with the limb immobilized with the target tissues in an elongated position. Chronic stretching over a period of time may result in sarcomeres being added to lengthen muscle tissue.[17] The number of sarcomeres in series increases, resulting in an increased resting muscle length. This form of stretching is used to lengthen shortened tissue and to decrease muscle stiffness.[2] Immobilization of a muscle in a shortened position results in a decrease in sarcomeres and increased connective tissue.

The muscle spindle monitors the velocity and degree of muscle stretch. When a muscle is stretched very quickly, the muscle spindle contracts, which stimulates the primary afferent fibers and results in increased muscle tension. This is termed the monosynaptic stretch response. Caution should therefore be used to avoid stretching too rapidly, which may cause stimulation of the muscle spindle and an increase in muscle contraction instead of relaxation.[1] The Golgi tendon organ senses muscle tension during a muscle contraction and provides a protective function to the muscle by inhibiting contraction of the muscle. When excessive muscle tension develops during muscle contraction, the Golgi tendon organ responds, and the muscle relaxes.

Noncontractile soft tissues, such as tendons and ligaments, are composed primarily of collagen. Initial stretch applied to these tissues results in straightening of the collagen fibers with relatively little force. As the tissue is stretched to the end of a ROM, the tissue remains elastic, and release of the stretch results in return of the collagen to its normal resting position. If the stress on the tissues continues, the bonds between the collagen fibrils and fibers may be damaged, resulting in plastic deformation. Caution must be used during stretching to avoid tissue damage in most instances. Low-magnitude forces placed on the tissues over a period of time allow collagen fibers to rearrange, perhaps resulting in a safer mode of tissue elongation. In people, 15 to 20 minutes of low-intensity sustained stretch, repeated for 5 days, has increased the length of the hamstring muscles.[18] Cyclic submaximal loading may also increase resting tissue length through tissue remodeling. Hamstring length was increased in people following a series of 10-second stretches and 8-second rest periods for 15 minutes per day, for 5 days.[18]

Clinical experience suggests that in uncomplicated cases of muscle tightness, 5 to 10 degrees of ROM may be gained per week, and 3 to 5 degrees may be gained in cases with joint capsule tightness. Other factors may alter these expected responses, including the animal's weight-bearing status, other medical conditions such as Cushing's disease, the extent of trauma to the tissues, and the type of surgical procedure performed.

There is no consensus regarding which stretching technique is most effective, and some controversy exists regarding the efficacy of some stretching techniques for certain conditions. However, if benefits are achieved, the effects of a consistent stretching program may be maintained over a period of time, even if stretching is temporarily discontinued. A stretching program performed three to five times per week may result in measurable increases in flexibility in patients with stiffness. After flexibility improves, the frequency of stretching may be reduced. In fact, stretching too frequently may be harmful in some situations. The natural cycle of stress and adaptive remodeling may be interrupted if adequate time is not allowed for healing between intense stretching sessions. Additional caution is required in aged animals because collagen becomes less elastic, and less stretch is tolerated before plastic deformation.

Static Stretching

Static stretching involves placing the joint(s) in a position so that the muscles and connective tissues are stretched while held in a static position with the tissues at their greatest length. Stretches should be held for 15 to 30 seconds. There is probably little advantage to stretching for longer periods.[19] One advantage of this form of stretching is that less force is applied, reducing the possibility of iatrogenic damage to the tissues. There is also less stimulation of the Ia and II spindle afferent fibers, which increase the muscle's resistance to stretch.[2] It is important to be certain that the stretch is gentle, comfortable, and tolerated by the patient. A low-intensity stretch applied for a longer duration may be more comfortable for some patients. A slow static stretch is less likely to induce tension in the muscle being stretched.[1] The gains in ROM are relatively transient with static stretching, and the increases are generally attributed to elastic changes in actin-myosin overlap.[1]

When performing this form of stretching, it is important to have the patient as relaxed as possible to allow the maximal stretching of the muscle and tissues with as little resistance as possible. It is important to properly support the limb and perform the stretch with the joints in the proper alignment with the limb to reduce any abnormal stresses on the joints. After the stretching period, the tissues are allowed to return to a neutral position, and then the stretch is reapplied for up to 20 times in a session.

Prolonged Mechanical Stretching

This form of stretching is similar to static stretching in that a low-intensity stretch is applied. It differs, however, in that the stretch is prolonged. The stretch, applied for a minimum of 20 minutes and up to several hours, is effective in increasing ROM in many patients.[20] In people, a low-intensity prolonged stretch applied 1 hour per day was more effective than static stretching over a 4-week period in patients with chronic knee flexion contractures.[21]

In animals, an effective manner of achieving prolonged mechanical stretching is the use of splints or other coaptation devices to provide prolonged stretch to tissues. For example, dogs with a fracture of the radius and ulna treated with a cast often have contracture of the carpus following fracture healing (Figure 13-9). Pain and reduced limb use are frequent sequelae. A dorsal fiberglass splint, which has been contoured to the normal contralateral side, may be placed on the affected limb over several rolls of cotton cast padding that have been placed over the limb. Gauze bandaging material may then be used to help pull the foot up to the contoured splint with mild tension, applying controlled prolonged gentle stretch to the palmar carpal tissues. The wrap may be changed several times per day, and static stretching and ROM exercises performed. When the wrap is replaced, additional stretch may be applied by increasing the tension on

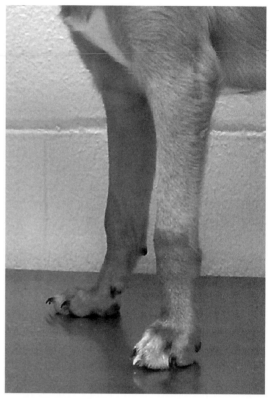

Figure 13-9 A dog with contracture of the left carpus and digits after immobilization of the forelimb as a result of a fracture. Note the upright stance of the foot in comparison to the normal contralateral side.

the gauze bandaging material. At no time should the patient feel undue discomfort.

Other devices to provide prolonged mechanical stretch in veterinary medicine include the use of a dynamic flexion apparatus to apply flexion stretch to the stifle in patients with fracture disease and quadriceps contracture.[22,23] In some instances, it may be necessary to surgically release adhesions and scar tissue. A dynamic flexion apparatus may then be applied to help prevent recurrence of the contracture. The apparatus consists of transcutaneous pins placed in the pelvis or proximal femur, and in the tibia, with elastic bands placed between the pins to provide prolonged stretch with the stifle in flexion. In addition, the patient may also actively extend the stifle against the resistance of the elastic band, but when the quadriceps muscle relaxes, the elastic band applies stretch to the stifle in flexion.

It is believed that when muscles are maintained in a lengthened position for several weeks, sarcomeres are added.[17,24] This increase in length persists if the new length is actively used. Other connective tissues may lengthen as a result of plastic deformation of the tissue.

Ballistic Stretching

This form of stretching differs from static stretching in that a series of quick movements are used to stretch the muscles and connective tissues.[2] This is a high-intensity, short duration of bouncing stretch.[1] The stretch that occurs often results in of contraction of the muscles antagonistic to the tissues being stretched. Although effective stretching may occur with this form of stretching, there is a risk of tissue injury, and this form may not be appropriate for patients early in the postoperative period. In fact, the muscle tension that occurs with ballistic stretching is approximately twice that obtained with low-intensity prolonged stretching.[25]

Proprioceptive Neuromuscular Facilitation Stretching

This form of stretching is more complex and takes advantage of neuromuscular stretch activation. The stretches use a contract-relax sequence, an agonist muscle contraction, or a contract-relax-agonist muscle contraction sequence.[2] Unfortunately, these stretches require the patient to actively and consciously contract a muscle group. Because we cannot verbally communicate to an animal when the muscle should contract, the therapist must use the other forms of stretching. There is a possibility that neuromuscular electrical stimulation may be used to provide active muscle contraction of a particular agonist muscle group, but clinical experience in this technique is lacking.

Precautions and Contraindications to Stretching

Joints should not be forced into an uncomfortable position beyond the ROM. Patients should not be painful during or after stretching. Caution should be exercised if a limb has been immobilized for a length of time. The goal should be to stretch and realign connective tissue, not rip and tear tissues. Stretching should not be performed if a ligament or tendon has been injured until the fibrous tissue can withstand some stress. Similarly, caution should be exercised during stretching in regions of relatively new fractures after repair has been performed.

Stretching Studies

Although there is a relative paucity of data and scientific knowledge regarding stretching to improve flexibility, it is a widespread practice in both human and animal rehabilitation. Studies of stretch behavior of normal human muscle have yielded interesting results. One study evaluated the passive properties of the hamstring muscle group during stretch, while measuring passive hamstring resistance and electromyographic activity.[26] Resistance to stretch was defined as passive torque of the hamstring muscle group during passive knee extension. The knee was passively extended to a predetermined final position where it remained stationary for 90 seconds (static stretch). Alternatively, the knee was extended to the point of discomfort (stretch tolerance). Passive energy and stiffness were calculated. Torque decline in the static phase was considered to result from viscoelastic stress relaxation of the tissues. A single static stretch resulted in a 30% viscoelastic stress relaxation. With repeated stretches, muscle stiffness temporarily decreased, but returned to baseline values within 1 hour. Stretching over a 3-week period increased joint ROM because of a change in stretch tolerance rather than in the passive properties of the muscle. Strength training resulted in increased muscle stiffness, which was unaffected by daily stretching. Inflexible and older subjects have increased muscle stiffness, but a lower stretch tolerance compared to subjects with normal flexibility and younger subjects.

Another study evaluated the effects of one 10-minute stretch on muscle stiffness in subjects with short hamstrings.[27] The subjects were unable to touch the floor when bending forward. One group performed static stretching exercises for 10 minutes interspersed with relaxing, while an untreated group served as controls. One 10-minute stretch resulted in a significant increase in passive muscle moment, ROM, and elongation of the hamstrings. There was no significant change in passive muscle stiffness, however, with respect to the prestretch stiffness curve. The authors also concluded that one session of static stretching does not influence muscle stiffness, and the increased ROM and extensibility of the hamstrings resulted from an increase in stretch tolerance.

Acute changes in the flexibility of hamstring muscles were evaluated in elderly people.[28] A single 32-second stretch was performed by men and women with a mean age of 65 years. Although the changes were moderate, the increase in flexibility was significantly greater in the stretch group as compared to the controls (4 degrees vs. 1 degrees).

While most muscle stretching studies have focused on defining the biomechanical properties of isolated elements of the muscle-tendon unit or on comparing different stretching techniques, one group of investigators evaluated stretching properties in an entire muscle-tendon unit.[29] Rabbit long digital extensor and cranial tibialis muscle-tendon units were evaluated using commonly used stretching techniques. The effect of varying stretch rates was also evaluated. Similar to other studies, the muscle-tendon units responded viscoelastically to tensile loads. Both cyclic and static stretching resulted in sustained muscle-tendon unit elongations, suggesting that greater flexibility can result if these techniques are used clinically. With repetitive stretching, there was little additional alteration of the muscle-tendon after four stretches, implying that a minimum number of stretches leads to most of the elongation in repetitive stretching. Also, greater peak tensions and greater energy absorptions occurred at faster stretch rates, suggesting that the risk of injury in a stretching regimen may be related to the stretch rate. Indeed, one group of investigators found that during slow (or static) muscle stretching, factors inhibiting motor neurons contributed to the lengthening of the muscle.[30]

Passive stretching may also help to prevent muscle atrophy by allowing constant change in the length of the muscle fibers. Intermittent muscle stretching helped to prevent atrophy and loss of sarcomeres in muscles of mice that were immobilized in a shortened position.[31] In this model, a static stretch for as little as 30 minutes per day helped to preserve sarcomeres. In addition, there was less development of intramuscular connective tissue with some stretching. In a study of rat tail tendons, a low force stretch over a prolonged period resulted in effective elongation of the tendon.[32] Also, the proportion of prolonged tendon lengthening was greater with low-force, long-duration stretching.[20] Heating tissue before stretching has been advocated to help improve the effectiveness of stretching. Elevating the tissue temperature before stretching the rat tail tendons resulted in significantly less tissue damage, and lower loads applied with heating for a prolonged period resulted in significantly greater elongation. One researcher concluded that approximately three times as much force is needed to elongate tendons at temperatures of 20° to 30° C than at 43° C.[33]

Therapeutic ultrasound is frequently mentioned as an adjunctive treatment to improve the effectiveness of stretching through its ability to warm tissues. However, the specific effects of heating on tissues and the manner in which stretch is affected is unclear. In a study of ultrasound treatment of the common calcaneal tendon of dogs, it was found that pulsed-mode ultrasound was not effective in increasing tendon temperature, but continuous-mode ultrasound was.[34] The amount of heating with 3-MHz continuous-mode ultrasound was related to the power, with 1.5 W/cm^2 increasing tendon temperature more than did 1.0 W/cm^2. Interestingly, the greatest temperature increase occurred within 3 minutes, with little increase thereafter. Tendon cooling occurred very rapidly, with return to baseline temperature within 1 minute after stopping ultrasound. A 4-kg stretch applied to the tendon immediately after ultrasound treatment (10 minutes of 3-MHz continuous ultrasound heating at 1.5 W/cm^2) resulted in a 5-degree increase in hock flexion, while two bouts of stretching of the contralateral nontreated calcaneal tendon within 5 minutes did not result in increased hock flexion. The increased hock flexion was lost within 5 minutes after the ultrasound was discontinued, however (Figure 13-10). Clearly, methods of maintaining the increased stretch are needed to improve tissue extensibility.

One study performed in people also evaluated the effects of (1) static stretch and ultrasound, (2) static stretch alone, or (3) no treatment, on triceps surae muscle extensibility.[35] Static stretch and ultrasound consisted of 7 minutes of continuous ultrasound at 1.5 W/cm^2 to the muscle with stretch applied during the seventh minute. Static stretch alone consisted of a 51-lb load applied for 1 minute. Static stretch and ultrasound treatment increased flexion an average of 1.2 degrees, or 20% more than static stretch alone, while static stretch alone increased flexion an average of 1.3 degrees, or 27%, more than no treatment. Both increases were statistically significant.

A similar study in people confirmed the short-term benefit of heating with ultrasound before stretching.[36] One group received ultrasound (1.5 W/cm^2) to the musculotendinous junction of the triceps surae and then stretching, while another group received stretching alone. Ultrasound and stretch increased mean ROM more than did stretch alone, but there were no long-term residual effects.

Another study evaluated whether heating with continuous-mode ultrasound would augment the effect of stretching of the medial collateral ligament of the knee in normal humans.[37] Treatment consisted of 3-MHz, 1.25 W/cm^2 continuous ultrasound or sham treat-

Tarsal Angle

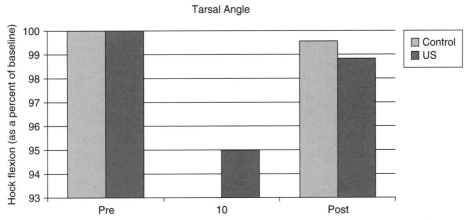

Figure 13-10   A mild stretch applied to the common calcaneal tendon immediately after ultrasound treatment (10 minutes of 3-MHz continuous ultrasound heating at 1.5 W/cm²) resulted in a 5-degree increase in hock flexion, but this increased flexion was lost within 5 minutes after the ultrasound was discontinued. Repeated stretching of control tendons without ultrasound resulted in no increase in hock flexion.

ment over the medial collateral ligament. A valgus stretch of the knee (10 ft-lb for 2.5 min) was performed after ultrasound treatment. Stretching alone resulted in a 1-degree valgus displacement of the knee, whereas stretching with ultrasound resulted in a displacement of 1.24 degrees. However, these differences were not statistically significant.

Clinical Application of Stretching

In preparation for stretching, it is beneficial to perform some low-intensity active exercise if possible. In addition, application of superficial heat or therapeutic ultrasound before stretching may improve tissue extensibility. There may be less damage to tissues, and less force may be required to attain increased tissue length with stretching if the tissues are warmed. The combination of muscles, tendons, skin, and joint capsule should be considered and their relative contributions to restricted motion assessed. For example, the target tissue for lengthening a muscle that is contracted is the muscle belly, not the tendon. The patient should be in a comfortable position, which is generally in lateral recumbency, and should be on a padded surface. It is important that the patient be as relaxed as possible, and in some cases, mild sedation or tranquilization may be beneficial.

Static Stretching

The affected limb and joint should be slowly placed through one end of a ROM (usually

beginning in flexion) until a restriction to motion is felt. One hand should stabilize the bone proximal to the joint, and the other should stabilize the bone distal to the joint. The distal bone should be moved relative to the proximal bone. Very gentle traction may be applied to the joint while slowly stretching to the point of initial restriction. The patient may indicate that it feels mild discomfort, such as by turning the head or mildly tensing the muscles in the affected limb. Under no circumstances should more severe pain be inflicted, which might be indicated by vocalizing, trying to move away, or attempting to bite. The stretch should be prolonged, ideally for at least 15 seconds. During the stretch, a conscious effort should be made to try to increase the joint excursion without increasing the level of discomfort. There should be no bouncing motions during the stretch. Following the stretch at one end of the motion range, the pressure is slowly released and the opposite end of the ROM should be stretched.

In some situations, muscles that cross two joints, such as the rectus femoris and biceps brachii muscles, may be restricted. In these situations, it is beneficial to put an individual joint through a stretching session, and then place the other joint through a stretching session. As ROM and flexibility improve, both joints may be simultaneously placed through stretching exercise. For example, the hip and stifle joints may be stretched in extension. This is more challenging, and there will usually be less joint excursion with simultaneous extension of both joints than if each joint is individually stretched in extension. However, these motions more completely reflect the use of these joints and muscles during normal gait, and it is valuable to perform these maneuvers.

The therapist should be patient and not try to achieve full ROM in one or two sessions. The ideal daily frequency of stretching is unknown for dogs. In general, two to four sessions per day may initially be required, with the frequency decreased as normal ROM and tissue extensibility improve. The process must be applied consistently and regularly to obtain good results, and it may take 2 to 3 weeks to see noticeable improvement.

Prolonged Mechanical Stretching

The most problematic joints that are affected with immobilization of a limb in a cast or splint are the digits, which may develop flexural contracture. This may occur in either the front or the rear limbs as a result of fractures of the radius and ulna or tibia and fibula, or with surgical fusion (arthrodesis) of the carpus or tarsus. After 4 weeks in a coaptation device, the digits are often contracted in a flexed position and are painful when attempts are made to place them in a functional walking position.

Normal static stretching of the affected joints should be performed. It is usually only practical to stretch all of the digits at the same time. Between stretching sessions, a dorsal fiberglass splint, molded to the normal contralateral side, is placed on the affected limb to help maintain prolonged mechanical stretching. The splint may be manufactured using fiberglass casting material folded back and forth on itself, using the normal limb as a template. Several rolls of cotton cast padding are placed over the affected limb. The dorsal splint is applied, and gauze bandaging material is rolled on to the limb under mild tension to pull the foot up to the splint, applying controlled prolonged gentle stretch to the restricting tissues. The wrap is changed several times per day, and static stretching and ROM exercises performed. When the wrap is replaced, additional stretch may be applied by increasing the tension on the gauze bandaging material. In general 7 to 14 days is adequate to regain normal ROM of the digits. Similar principles may be applied to more proximal joints, such as the elbow and stifle. In some situations, it may be difficult to use a fiberglass splint, and placement of transcutaneous pins in the bones proximal and distal to the affected joint may be necessary to provide good fixation. Elastic bands may be placed to achieve flexion or extension as needed.

Ballistic Stretching

To perform ballistic stretching, the patient should be comfortable and the affected limb stabilized. The joints are positioned until a gentle stretch of the target tissues occurs, and then the therapist applies gentle "bouncing" of the tissues. The therapist should be careful to use only gentle movements to avoid damage to the tissues and pain. Because of the risk of tissue injury, this technique should not be performed in traumatized tissues, after surgery, or on tissues that are inflamed or edematous. Ballistic stretching may be beneficial to normal dogs that undergo ballistic-type activities, such as agility dogs that jump and turn sharply, or dogs that play Frisbee.

Summary

ROM and stretching exercises are basic parts of a complete physical rehabilitation program. The goals of ROM and stretching should be to lengthen muscles, improve joint ROM, increase tissue mobility, and improve functional use of the affected joint(s) and limb.

The therapist must be patient and be satisfied with small gains and slow improvement. To properly monitor patients, frequent measurement of ROM should be obtained using goniometry, and the results should be recorded to chart the patient's progress. Impatience and overzealous treatment may ultimately slow improvement and may actually reduce joint motion and worsen contracture of soft tissues. This is because tissue damage and pain may delay the active use of a limb through the available ROM, resulting in increased fibrosis of tissues and decreased flexibility.

REFERENCES

1. Kisner C, Colby LA: Range of motion. In Kisner C, Colby LA, editors: *Therapeutic exercise: foundations and techniques*, ed 4, Philadelphia, 2002, FA Davis.
2. Brody LT: Mobility impairment. In Hall CM, Brody LT, editors: *Therapeutic exercise: moving toward function*, ed 1, Williams & Wilkins, 1999, Philadelphia.
3. Salter RB et al: Clinical application of basic research on continuous passive motion for disorders and injuries of synovial joints: a preliminary report of a feasibility study, *J Orthop Res* 1:325-342, 1984.
4. Bardet JF: Quadriceps contracture and fracture disease, *Vet Clin North Am Small Anim Pract* 17:957-973, 1987.
5. Millis DL et al: A preliminary study of early physical therapy following surgery for cranial cruciate ligament surgery in dogs, *Vet Surg* 26:434, 1997.

6. Schollmeier G et al: Structural and functional changes in the canine shoulder after cessation of immobilization, *Clin Orthop* 323:310-315, 1996.
7. Olson VL: Evaluation of joint mobilization treatment. A method, *Phys Ther* 67:351-356, 1987.
8. Salter RB et al: The biologic effect of continuous passive motion on the healing of full-thickness defects in articular cartilage. An experimental investigation in the rabbit, *J Bone Joint Surg* 62A:1232-1251, 1980.
9. Salter RB, Bell RS, Keeley FW: The protective effect of continuous passive motion in living articular cartilage in acute septic arthritis: an experimental investigation in the rabbit, *Clin Orthop* 159:223-247, 1981.
10. Mooney V, Stills M: Continuous passive motion with joint fractures and infections, *Orthop Clin North Am* 18:1-9, 1987.
11. Shimizu T et al: Experimental study on the repair of full thickness articular cartilage defects: effects of varying periods of continuous passive motion, cage activity, and immobilization, *J Orthop Res* 5:187-197, 1987.
12. Gebhard JS, Kabo JM, Meals RA: Passive motion: the dose effects on joint stiffness, muscle mass, bone density, and regional swelling, *J Bone Joint Surg* 75A: 1636-1647, 1993.
13. Grauer D et al: The effects of intermittent passive exercise on joint stiffness following periarticular fracture in rabbits, *Clin Orthop* 220:259-265, 1987.
14. Dhert WJ et al: Effects of immobilization and continuous passive motion on postoperative muscle atrophy in mature rabbits, *Can J Surg* 31:185-188, 1988.
15. Noyes, FR, Mangine, RE, Barber SD: The early treatment of motion complications after reconstruction of the anterior cruciate ligament, *Clin Orthop* 217: 217-228, 1992.
16. Stolov WC, Weilepp TG, Riddell WM: Passive length-tension relationship and hydroxyproline content of chronically denervated skeletal muscle, *Arch Phys Med Rehabil* 51:517-525, 1970.
17. Tabary JC et al: Physiological and structural changes in the cat's soleus muscle due to immobilization at different lengths by plaster casts, *J Physiol* 224:231-244, 1972.
18. Starring D et al: Comparison of cyclic and sustained passive stretching using a mechanical device to increase resting length of hamstring muscles, *Phys Ther* 68:314-320, 1988.
19. Madding SW et al: Effect of duration of passive stretch on hip abduction range of motion, *J Orthop Sports Phys Ther* 8:409-416, 1987.
20. Sapega AA et al: Biophysical factors in range of motion exercises, *Physician Sports Med* 9:57-63, 1981.
21. Light KE et al: Low-load prolonged stretch vs high-load brief stretch in treating knee contractures, *Phys Ther* 64:330-333, 1984.
22. Wilkens BE, McDonald DE, Hulse DA: Utilization of a dynamic stifle flexion apparatus in preventing recurrence of quadriceps contracture, a clinical report, *Vet Comp Orthop Traumatol* 4:219-223, 1993.
23. Liptak JM, Simpson DJ: Successful management of quadriceps contracture in a cat using a dynamic flexion apparatus, *Vet Comp Orthop Traumatol* 13:44-48, 2000.
24. Williams PE, Goldspink G: Changes in sarcomere length and physiological properties in immobilized muscle, *J Anat* 127:459-468, 1978.
25. Walker SM: Delay of twitch relaxation induced by stress and stress relaxation, *J Appl Physiol* 16:801, 1961.
26. Magnusson SP: Passive properties of human skeletal muscle during stretch maneuvers: a review, *Scand J Med Sci Sports* 8:65-77, 1998.
27. Halbertsma JP, van-Bolhuis AI, Goeken LN: Sport stretching: effect on passive muscle stiffness of short hamstrings, *Arch Phys Med Rehabil* 77:688-692, 1996.
28. Feland JB, Myrer JW, Merrill RM: Acute changes in hamstring flexibility: PNF versus static stretch in senior athletes, *Phys Ther Sport* 2:186-193, 2001.
29. Taylor DC et al: Viscoelastic properties of muscle-tendon units: the biomechanical effects of stretching, *Am J Sports Med* 18:300-309, 1990.
30. Guissard N, Duchateau J, Hainaut K: Le stretching musculaire: aspects neurophysiologiques et biomecaniques (Muscle stretching exercises: neurophysiological and biomechanical aspects). *Ann Kinesither* 15:469-474, 1988.
31. Williams PE: Use of intermittent stretch in the prevention of serial sarcomere loss in immobilised muscle, *Ann Rheum Dis* 49:316-317, 1990.
32. Warren CG, Lehmann JF, Koblanski JN: Heat and stretch procedures: an evaluation using rat tail tendon, *Arch Phys Med Rehabil* 57:122-126, 1976.
33. Gersten JW: Effect of ultrasound on tendon extensibility, *Am J Phys Med* 34:368, 1955.
34. Loonam JE et al: The effect of therapeutic ultrasound on tendon heating and extensibility. In *Proc Vet Orthoped Soc*, Steamboat Springs, Colo, March 2003, p 69.
35. Wessling KC, DeVane DA, Hylton CR: Effects of static stretch versus static stretch and ultrasound combined on triceps surae muscle extensibility in healthy women, *Phys Ther* 67:674-679, 1987.
36. Draper DO et al: Immediate and residual changes in dorsiflexion range of motion using an ultrasound heat and stretch routine, *J Athletic Train* 33:141-144, 1998.
37. Reed BV et al: Effects of ultrasound and stretch on knee ligament extensibility, *J Orthop Sports Phys Ther* 30:341-347, 2000.

■ C h a p t e r   1 4

Therapeutic Exercises

Siri Hamilton, Darryl L. Millis, Robert A. Taylor, and David Levine

Therapeutic exercise is perhaps one of the most valuable modalities used in canine physical rehabilitation. Some of the common goals of therapeutic exercise are to improve active pain-free range of motion, muscle mass and muscle strength, balance, performance with daily function, and aerobic capacity; to help prevent further injury; and to reduce weight and lameness. Common activities include standing exercises, controlled leash activities, stair climbing, treadmill activity, "wheelbarrowing" (for forelimb activity), and "dancing" (for rear limb activity). Other activities include jogging, sit-to-stand exercises, pulling or carrying weights, walking and trotting across cavaletti rails, playing ball, taping a bottle or syringe cap to the bottom of an unaffected foot to encourage weight-bearing, slinging the contralateral good limb, and using balance balls or rolls. Therapeutic exercise is an important method to assist an animal's return to the best function possible. In addition, the equipment needed is relatively inexpensive, and similar principles apply to a variety of individuals and conditions. Therapeutic exercise programs designed for the home environment also provide an opportunity for owners to become actively involved in their pets' rehabilitation.

When designing a therapeutic exercise program, several factors must be considered. A problem list is developed based on an initial evaluation of the rehabilitation patient, and a treatment plan is formulated to address the identified problem(s). Realistic outcome goals are then established. Therapeutic exercise is a significant component of the treatment plan. Appropriate exercises are those that can be performed safely and effectively and accomplish the therapeutic goals. When prescribing

therapeutic exercise, the therapist should understand the diagnosis, identify the structure or structures involved, and recognize the stage of tissue recovery with the resultant functional limitations. The exercise plan should target the affected muscles and other structures. The type of injury or repair must be considered when formulating a treatment plan. For example, the postoperative treatment of hip dysplasia differs depending on whether a femoral head and neck excision or a total hip replacement was performed. With this knowledge and understanding, appropriate decisions can be made regarding therapeutic exercise choices.

Treatment considerations and choice of exercises vary with each stage of tissue repair and endurance. As the animal improves clinically and tissue healing progresses, the exercise plan should be altered to match the animal's progress and appropriately challenge the involved tissues. The intensity of an exercise may be increased or reduced by changing the *duration* of time that an animal performs an exercise, the *frequency* with which an exercise is performed, and the rate of *speed* at which a particular exercise is performed. Any of these may be altered to fine-tune an exercise prescription to achieve the expected outcome goals. For example, a realistic initial goal for a morbidly obese, deconditioned patient with degenerative joint disease may be to increase the amount of time the dog is able to comfortably tolerate walking, thus improving endurance and promoting weight reduction. Increasing the speed at which the dog walks may not be a realistic initial goal for this animal. A contrasting example may be an athletic animal recovering from injury that must be challenged to improve speed and frequency to meet the goal to return to performance activity. It is important for the therapist to have an understanding of exercise intensity and what is appropriate for each patient during rehabilitation treatment. Routine reevaluation of the patient is recommended to assess the adaptations that are occurring with the rehabilitation treatment plan and to determine the appropriate rate of progression.

Therapeutic exercise routines should be monitored at regular intervals by a trained individual who is familiar with the patient and the exercise techniques. Inappropriate exercise or improper technique may result in inappropriate stresses, further injury, or exacerbation of an existing condition. Certain exercises may not be safe for the strength, flexibility, or endurance level of the animal performing the exercise, or an exercise may not be the correct one to accomplish the intended goal.

Assisted Standing Exercises

Patients with severe injuries or debilitating conditions may not be able to stand and support their own body weight. A period of standing, either completely or partially assisted, may strengthen the patient, aid in proprioceptive training, improve circulation and respiration, provide an opportunity to eliminate, and enhance the patient's psychological well-being. The purposes of assisted standing exercises are to encourage neuromuscular function, reeducate muscles, develop strength and stamina of supporting muscles, and enhance proprioception.

Animals with multiple orthopedic injuries, neurologic conditions, or severe debilitation are excellent candidates for assisted standing exercises (Figure 14-1). Assisted standing exercises are among the first therapeutic exercises prescribed for severely afflicted animals that are not able to completely bear weight and may begin in patients that are receiving adequate pain control following injuries which are stable. Animals in pain resist standing and may further injure themselves or the therapist while struggling.

It is appropriate to begin assisted standing exercises in patients with adequate muscle tone and some ability of the limb(s) to resist motion (adequate upper motor neuron function). Patients with lower motor neuron signs have little or no muscle tone and flaccidity of

the limbs. Although patients with lower motor neuron conditions will likely benefit from standing exercises, it is unlikely that they will be able to fully support their weight and some additional assistance will be required.

Body Slings

Nonambulatory patients may benefit from placement in a body sling or harness to provide support for standing (Figure 14-2). An advantage of a sling is that the patient is able to maintain a body position with the limbs placed under the body in a standing position, which may provide an opportunity for limb strengthening and early proprioceptive training. Frequent episodes of supported standing also help to relieve pressure on bony prominences and may reduce the chances of decubital ulcer formation. Excessive congestion of the lungs that may result from spending long periods in lateral recumbency may be prevented with early implementation of standing in a sling. The body sling must be adjusted properly so that respiration is not compromised and the limbs are not compressed in the openings of the sling. Proper padding is also important for comfort. The skin should be inspected after each session in the sling to identify areas of potential skin irritation or breakdown. Rubber bungee cords may be used to secure the sling to the supporting frame. This may aid in the facilitation of

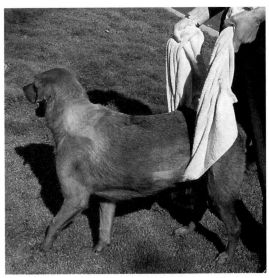

Figure 14-1 Support while standing is beneficial for patients with limited ability to stand and bear body weight.

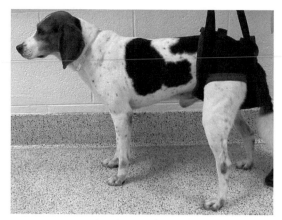

Figure 14-2 A sling that may be used to provide support for maximal assisted standing of a patient.

weight-bearing and movement during the sling sessions. The elasticity of the cord permits some gentle up-and-down movement that encourages the animal to safely bear partial weight on its limbs. It also may allow some attempts to move forward, backward, and side to side. A gentle bouncing motion may be manually introduced by the therapist to initiate rhythmic stabilization of muscle groups throughout the trunk and limbs.

Maximal Assisted Standing

Maximal assisted standing is appropriate for patients that are unable to support their body weight as a result of paralysis, paresis, pain, trauma, postoperative precautions, or general debilitation. Maximal assistance may be defined as support of 75% to 100% of the patient's body weight by the handler to maintain a standing posture. Maximal assisted lifts and standing are initially required for patients that are unable to independently rise from a recumbent position or support their own body weight.

Depending on animal size and weight, the handler can manually lift or use an assistive device such as a sling or towel to assist the animal from a recumbent to a supported standing position. To perform standing exercises, a sling or towel is placed under the cranial thorax, caudal abdomen, or both for conditions affecting the forelimbs, rear limbs, or both, respectively. After the animal is in a supported standing position, the handler or a second person manually places the animal's limbs in a normal stance position, with the feet posi-

tioned squarely on the ground. Even distribution of the animal's weight on the ground may provide position sense, which is proprioceptive input facilitating the animal's awareness of its joints at rest.

The animal should be encouraged to support its body weight as it is able, and the therapist gives only the necessary assistance to maintain the standing position (Figure 14-3, A). While supporting the animal, the handler slowly releases tension on the assistive device, allowing the animal to continue weight-bearing as much as it is able. Because the animal is encouraged to accept and support a portion of its weight, strength, balance, coordination, and proprioception are challenged. If the dog begins to collapse, the sling is gently pulled up to assist the patient back into the standing position and the exercise is repeated (Figure 14-3, B).

During a treatment session, the animal may need periods of rest and should be allowed to lie down during these times. Although the duration of each session should match the animal's tolerance, an initial starting goal is 10 to 15 repetitions two to three times daily, gradually increasing to 5 minutes per session. Individual patients progress at different rates. The therapist can keep track of and document the amount of time the animal is able to stand and how much assistance was needed.

Active Assisted Standing

As the animal becomes stronger and regains neuromuscular function, maximal assistance from the handler is not required. The progression from maximal assisted standing to active assisted standing occurs when the animal is able to actively support some of its weight, requiring only partial assistance from the handler (less than 75% of body weight). The animal should be encouraged to support as much of its weight as possible. The handler provides only the additional assistance required to maintain a standing position. The amount of assistance required is documented by recording the actual weight the handler is required to support for the animal to maintain a standing position, as well as the length of time the animal can maintain a standing position. The animal may require periodic rests during a treatment session. As the animal's strength and endurance improve, the duration of each session may be increased, the number of rest

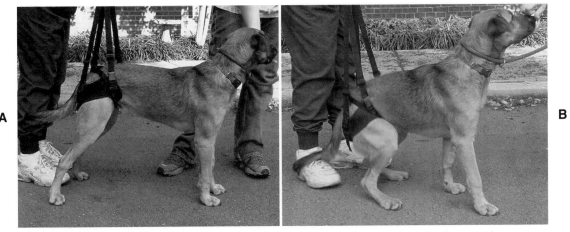

A

B

Figure 14-3   A, Use of a sling to help provide support for standing. **B,** As the patient begins to fatigue and attempts to sit, the therapist lifts the dog back into a standing position.

periods decreased, and the amount of assistance decreased.

Active Assisted Standing With Carts and Slings

Mobility carts and slings may be used as assistive devices for active assisted activities. Carts allow the animal to have some degree of independence and reduce the lifting and support needed from a caregiver. Two-wheeled carts may be used for patients with active forelimb function and four-wheeled carts for patients with all limbs affected. Slings may be used if animals are not ambulatory or only minimally ambulatory (Figure 14-4). The devices should be adjusted to the patient's height so the feet may be placed (either manually by the therapist or independently by the animal) in a normal weight-bearing position on the ground. The patient should not dangle above the ground in the cart because this may compromise circulation and place undue pressure on soft tissues that are in contact with the supporting structures of the cart.

Active Assisted Standing Using Exercise Rolls

A properly fitted inflatable exercise roll (Physio-roll) may also be used to actively assist the animal with stance, weight-bearing, and weight-shifting (Figure 14-5). Using the roll as an assistive device also relieves stress

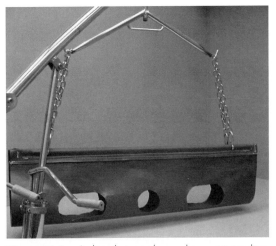

Figure 14-4   A sling that may be used to assist standing. Standing helps the patient develop stamina and endurance with minimal assistance required from a therapist.

on the handlers. Unless the animal is small, this technique may require two people to properly assist the patient.

The animal is placed in a standing position over an appropriately sized exercise roll (the roll provides greater lateral support and stability than a round exercise ball). The size should allow the animal to touch the ground with all four feet. If the roll is too tall, it may be deflated to meet the animal's height. Rolls that are slightly deflated are softer, more stable, and easier to work with than those that are fully inflated and very firm. The softer roll conforms to the animal's body better and is more comfortable. After the animal is secure

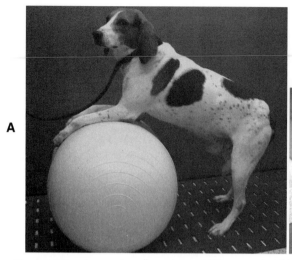

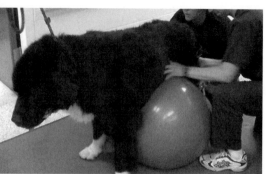

Figure 14-5   An exercise roll may be used **(A)** to provide additional challenges or increase weight-bearing on the front or rear limbs or **(B)** to assist standing.

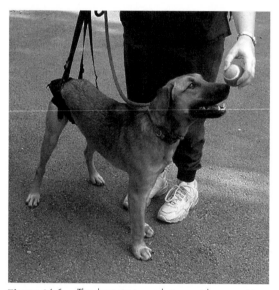

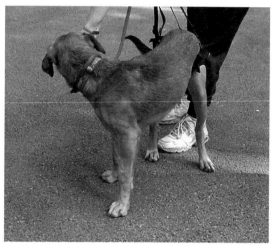

Figure 14-7   The therapist encourages weight shifting to help develop improved proprioception by moving a treat side to side.

Figure 14-6   The therapist is ready to provide support to a patient in the event of a loss of balance.

on the roll, one person stabilizes the front of the animal and another stabilizes the rear. While the animal is supported in a standing position with paws on the ground, the handler can generate a very gentle up-and-down bouncing motion through the patient and the inflated roll. This provides proprioceptive input and may stimulate contraction of the supporting limb muscles.

Weight-bearing in the thoracic or pelvic limbs may be promoted as the therapists shift

the roll forward and backward. As the animal becomes stronger, these same techniques may be performed at faster speeds to provide greater challenges to neuromuscular function and balance.

Standby Assisted Standing

The next progression in standing activities is *standby assisted standing*. At this point of the recovery, the animal has the strength and motor control necessary to support itself against gravity in a standing position. However, it may still experience ataxia or weakness and have an occasional loss of balance, requiring standby assistance. The therapist should be at the animal's side, ready to guard against a fall due to a loss of balance (Figure 14-6). The therapist does not assist the dog unless support is needed to prevent a fall. As strength improves, the patient will be more willing to advance the limbs if motor function is present.

Proprioceptive Training

When an animal is able to stand independently (without assistance) and safely, activities to improve balance may begin. *Dynamic balance* is the animal's ability to maintain balance while the body is moving, such as while walking. The following exercises may be performed to challenge the animal's dynamic balance. These exercises should be conducted on a nonslip surface to provide adequate traction and reduce the risk of falling.

Weight-Shifting

While the animal is standing, a treat or ball may be used to encourage weight-shifting. The interested dog will follow the treat up and down and side to side (Figure 14-7). Start with small movements and progress to larger, more challenging movements. The movement of the head causes the dog's center of gravity (COG)

to shift. As the COG shifts, the dog must shift its weight to maintain its balance. To maintain the unassisted standing position, the animal is required to use strength, coordination, and balance.

If the dog is motivated by ball play, a more challenging form of this exercise is close-distance ball tossing from above and the sides. During early attempts at these exercises it may be necessary to have someone available for standby assistance as the dog may be over-challenged, lose its balance, and fall.

The handler may also attempt to disturb the animal's balance by gently pushing the animal at the hips or shoulder or lifting the unaffected limb. The goal is to disturb its balance just enough so the animal can recover, being careful not to push with a force that may cause the animal to fall. Generally, pushing the animal to the more affected side challenges the animal sufficiently to allow the activity to have the desired effect. Some dogs become conditioned to this activity, however, and shift their weight toward the therapist to prevent being pushed toward the affected side. In this case, a *rebound weight shift* may be effective. For this maneuver, the therapist gently pushes the animal toward the affected side (Figure 14-8, *A*). When the animal shifts its weight to resist the movement, the therapist suddenly releases pressure, and simultaneously pushes gently toward the unaffected side (Figure 14-8, *B*). This results in a sudden

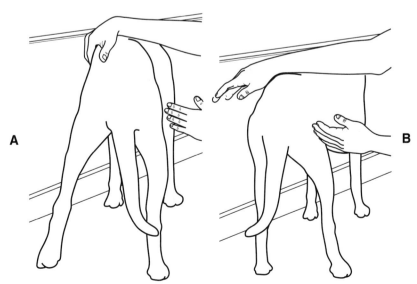

Figure 14-8 **A,** Rebound weight shift to encourage an animal to bear weight on the affected limb. The dog's weight is initially shifted toward the normal (right) limb. **B,** Pressure is suddenly released, resulting in a shift in weight toward the affected (left) limb to maintain balance.

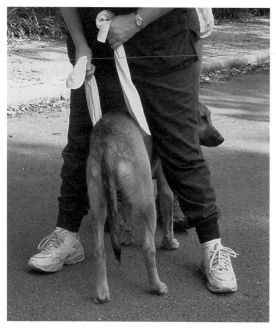

Figure 14-9 Shifting weight from side to side by moving a towel back and forth under the abdomen.

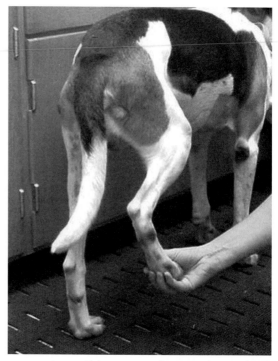

Figure 14-10 Shifting an animal's center of gravity by lifting a limb off the ground and forcing the patient to redistribute its weight.

unbalancing; the animal initially shifts its weight toward the unaffected side, but to keep from falling, it immediately shifts its weight back toward the affected side.

Additional challenges may be added by slowly moving a supporting towel back and forth ("shoe buff" maneuver), in a motion similar to buffing a shoe, to force the dog to shift its weight back and forth (Figure 14-9).

Weight shifts may also be performed during walking. As the animal is walked in a straight line, the handler gently bumps or pushes the animal to one side to challenge the dog to maintain its balance. Caution should be used to tailor the force of the push to the animal's stage of recovery to avoid falls and injury.

Manual Unloading of One Limb During Stance

Lifting and holding a single limb off the ground while the dog is standing causes a shift in the animal's COG (Figure 14-10). The animal shifts its body weight and COG to maintain the standing position. During a session, the handler may lift each leg separately to see where the animal is the weakest and focus on that area in successive sessions. If the animal is unable or unwilling to perform this exercise, it will not shift its weight prop-

erly, but instead will bear the weight on the handler's hand or collapse to the ground. A technique to avoid bearing all of the weight on the handler is to slowly abduct the raised limb, which allows transfer of weight from the handler to the desired limb to avoid falling.

Balance Board

A platform on rockers may be used to rock the dog forward and backward, side to side, diagonally, and 360 degrees. This is similar to a human Biomechanical Ankle Platform System (BAPS) board. In fact, a BAPS board may be used to help the animal practice proprioceptive positioning on just the forelimbs or the hindlimbs by placing the desired limbs on the board while the other limbs remain on the ground (Figure 14-11). If the goal is to have the animal exercise using all four limbs, then a specially made platform must be used that accommodates quadrupeds. It is important to have one person help support the dog while another person slowly and gently rocks the platform to allow the animal an opportunity to shift its weight and exercise its proprioceptive mechanism (Figure 14-12).

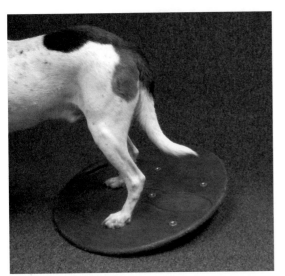

Figure 14-11   Use of a human Biomechanical Ankle Platform System (BAPS) board under a patient's hindlimbs to assist with proprioceptive training.

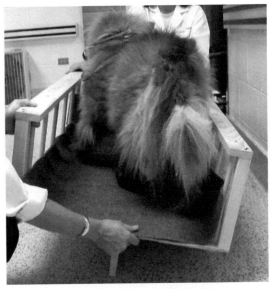

Figure 14-12   Using a balance platform to help quadruped animals develop improved proprioception.

Exercise Balls and Rolls

Therapeutic exercise balls and rolls designed for human use may be employed to improve an animal patient's balance, coordination, and strength. Balls and rolls may also be used for general stretching. The forelimbs are placed on the ball and supported by the handler, requiring the dog to maintain static balance of the caudal trunk and rear limbs. Dynamic balance may also be challenged as the ball or roll is slowly moved forward, backward, and side to side, challenging the rear legs to maintain balance while movement occurs. To address the cranial trunk, head, neck, and forelimbs, the rear limbs are placed over the ball as the forelimbs are asked to balance the body weight during both stance (static) and gentle movements (dynamic).

Dynamic Ambulation Activities

Assisted Ambulation/Gait Training

If a dog is unable to walk independently, an assistive device may be used to support the animal as needed. Gait training should begin with the use of a sling, towel, harness, or canine cart. The handler should assess the animal's needs before choosing the appropriate device. Encourage the dog to move slowly, allowing time for the dog to advance the limbs as independently as possible. Allow adequate time for the feet to come in contact with the ground with each step during the stance phase of gait. It may be necessary for the handler to manually assist the dog in the sequencing and placement of the limbs as the animal relearns the walking gait. If the animal moves too quickly, it will often avoid bearing weight on a painful limb, adopting an abnormal gait, such as a three-legged lameness, hopping, or dragging of a limb. The emphasis is on weight-bearing with each and every step, encouraging a slow gait. It is important for each person handling the dog to be consistent and not allow the dog to move too quickly.

Walking Slings

Commercially available canine slings should be durable, flexible, and washable and should conform to the body. They are available for the forelimbs and hindlimbs and for trunk support. Rear slings should have a recessed area so bowel and bladder function is not obstructed (Figure 14-13). Adjustable-length handles for the therapist to grip make a sling a more ergonomic choice of assistive device than a bath towel because the sling allows the handler to stand erect without bending forward while carrying the weight of the dog. This is an important concern especially if the handler will be assisting a large dog several times a day for any length of time. It is important for persons handling the animal to practice proper body mechanics while assisting the

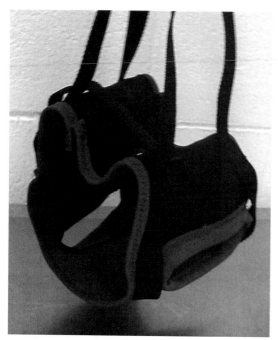

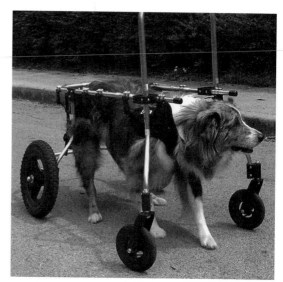

Figure 14-14   A 4-wheeled cart may be used for assisted ambulation in patients with tetraparesis.

Figure 14-13   Example of a commercially available sling that may be used for assisted ambulation and gait training.

canine patient to avoid injuring themselves. The sling may be used for both orthopedic and neurological patients in need of assisted ambulation.

Towels

A long towel may be used to support an animal that requires assistance with standing or ambulation. Towels are readily available, inexpensive, and washable. When assisting the dog's hindlimbs, the handler should place the towel around the abdomen just in front of the hindlimbs in the inguinal region. Nylon straps may be sewn on to the ends of the towel to provide added length so the handler can maintain proper body mechanics.

A disadvantage of towels on larger dogs with urinary incontinence is that it puts pressure on the urinary bladder and may cause it to be expressed. This is less likely to happen with a properly fitted commercial sling. Also, towels may not be as comfortable for the handler.

Canine Carts

Several manufacturers offer supportive carts for dogs and cats. These carts are designed to assist with independent ambulation of ani-

mals that are unable to support adequate weight for ambulation. Common indications for cart use are paralysis, paresis, severe arthritis, trauma in multiple limbs, and generalized weakness affecting one or more limbs. Commercially available custom carts are available in four-wheel and two-wheel models for animals of all sizes and a variety of conditions (Figure 14-14).

Mobility carts are appropriate for temporary use as the animal regains its ability to ambulate independently, as well as for permanent use for animals that will not regain full function. After a period of acclimation for both the animal and owner, a properly fitted cart may result in a positive change in the quality of life for both. When the animal is mobile in a cart, that mobility fosters independence that may have a profound positive effect on the animal's attitude.

It is important that the cart be properly sized and fitted to ensure comfort and adequate function. Most manufacturers provide specific instructions regarding proper measurements to provide a custom fit. The therapist can assist with the measuring and fitting process. In addition, the cart should have adequate padding for comfort and to prevent chafing or breakdown of skin, but it should not interfere with use of functional limbs.

The home environment may need to be altered to allow the animal to freely ambulate in the cart without encountering dangerous conditions. The animal's exercise area should be free of obstructions that could hinder the animal's ability to safely ambulate in the cart. Particular caution should be taken to prevent falls down stairs.

Independent Ambulation

Leash Walking

Slow leash walks are perhaps the most important exercise in the early rehabilitative period, and they are commonly performed incorrectly. Walking the animal slowly encourages the use of all limbs in a sequenced gait pattern. Walks must be slow enough to allow weight-bearing; if the dog is walked too fast, the tendency is to simply hold the intended limb up in a flexed position and not bear any weight on it. Slow leash walking is indicated when the animal is reluctant to use a limb as a result of pain, weakness, or proprioceptive deficits. Slow leash walks encourage placement of each limb on the ground, increasing stance time and weight-bearing.

If there are no contraindications to weight-bearing, slow leash walks may begin very soon after most orthopedic procedures. Behavior modification is important. The dog should be praised when touching the limb to the ground, and not praised when the leg is held up. As the animal regains use of the affected limb and is consistently able to place the limb at a slow leash walk, the pace of the walk may be increased. Faster walks further challenge balance, coordination, proprioception, and cardiorespiratory endurance, as well as functional muscle strengthening and endurance. When appropriate, the therapist may alter the exercise treatment plan to include fast walking, slow jogging, and running on a long lead.

Inclines and Declines

Walking or jogging the dog up inclines aids in strengthening of the quadriceps, semitendinosus, semimembranosus, and gluteal muscles with relatively low-impact activity (Figure 14-15). Muscle strength in the hips and stifles is required for the dog to propel itself up an incline. Walking should be done slowly and on leash; otherwise the dog may only toe-touch with the limb or hop in a non–weight-bearing fashion. In addition, if the head is held up slightly, the weight will be shifted caudally, requiring the animal to drive up the hill with the rear limbs and use the muscles to a greater extent.

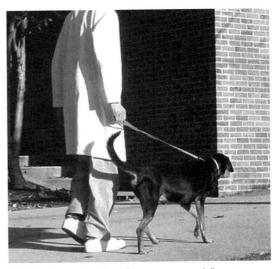

Figure 14-15   Leash walking up ramps or hills encourages muscle strengthening and cardiovascular endurance.

Weight-bearing while climbing promotes extension at the knee and hip. When the limb is in the stance phase of gait and the body is traveling forward, the knee and hip must extend to propel the animal forward. If extension is painful, the dog's stance time on the limb is shortened and an altered gait results. Inclines and declines should be introduced slowly, beginning with gradual inclines. As the dog's range of motion and strength improve, the dog may be challenged by walking up longer, steeper slopes and by increasing the duration and speed of the climbing exercise.

Walking down inclines is typically more difficult because it requires the dog to reach under the body with the hindlimbs, requiring flexion of the hock, stifle, and hip. Start with gently sloping, short declines and progress to steeper ones as the dog is able.

Standing or Walking on Foam Rubber, Mattresses, Air Mattresses

Altering the texture of the ground surface over which the animal walks provides a challenge to the animal's functional walking proprioceptive ability. Standing or walking on foam-rubber Egg-Crate mattresses, normal bed mattresses, air mattresses, and trampolines allows the animal to negotiate various surfaces that have some resiliency (Figure 14-16). Having different surfaces on either side of the animal while walking or changing the type of surface the animal must negotiate with all limbs during a walk provides additional challenges that may be integrated into the rehabilitation program.

Stair Climbing

As the dog consistently begins to use the affected limb or limbs at a walk with decreasing lameness and is able to walk inclines and

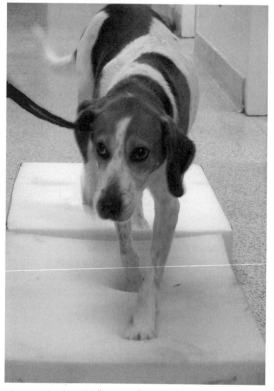

Figure 14-16 Walking on foam rubber mats provides a challenge to an animal recovering proprioceptive function.

declines with minimal difficulty, stairs may be added to the treatment plan. Climbing stairs is useful to improve power in the rear limb extensors, range of motion, coordination, and balance (Figure 14-17). Quadriceps and gluteal muscle groups are strengthened as the animal pushes off, extending both hips and knees while propelling the body weight up the steps. Stair climbing may begin if the repair is stable and the dog is consistently using the limb at a walk with progressively decreasing lameness. The dog must begin slowly climbing stairs to encourage proper use of the rear limbs, as opposed to simply carrying the limb, hopping with both hindlimbs, or skipping up stairs. Encourage the dog to go slowly and deliberately, climbing the stairs in a reciprocal stepping gait. Stairs should be introduced slowly because this is a challenging exercise for both the musculoskeletal and cardiovascular systems and the animal may fatigue quickly. Initially, some dogs may require assistance from the handler. Begin with five to seven steps, and gradually increase to two to four flights of stairs once or twice daily.

Treadmill Walking

Walking on a treadmill is very useful in rehabilitation. Most dogs trained to a leash readily take to treadmill walking in one or two sessions. A variety of treadmills are available for use, including commercial canine treadmills (Figure 14-18). A number of models available for human use may be modified for canine use by adding an overhead bar with a support system to which a canine harness can attach. A harness is useful to help support the dog in case it stumbles or falls. Side rails or fences

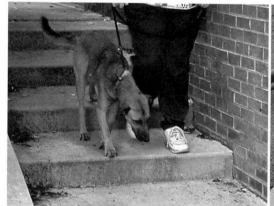

A

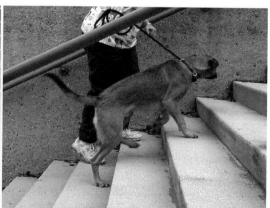

B

Figure 14-17 Stair climbing should begin on stairs with a gradual rise **(A)** and progress to steeper stairs **(B)**. Care should be taken to be certain that the dog pushes symmetrically off of both rear limbs.

placed on both sides of the treadmill are useful if a dog tends to step off to the side. Other useful features include variable speed control, a timer, and the ability to change the incline of the surface.

Treadmills are useful for patterning gait and encouraging initial weight-bearing following surgery. When the dog stands with the foot carried near the ground, it will generally begin to weight-bear when it is walked on a treadmill. It is important that the treadmill not face toward a wall; rather, it should face toward a hallway or the middle of a room to encourage unimpeded walking. Having one person standing in front of the dog with words of encouragement or treats and one person straddling the dog behind is helpful in the early training stages to keep the dog walking straight.

Walking on a treadmill for the first time is a new and sometimes awkward experience. Animals are not used to the ground moving under them, so when they walk on a moving belt, proprioception, coordination, and balance are challenged. The ground moving underneath the dog often encourages a dog that is non–weight-bearing on a limb as a result of an orthopedic condition to begin using the limb. In many instances, the animal will continue to use the limb even after the treadmill session is over. For patients with neurological conditions, the therapist may stand beside a dog and manually advance a foot during the normal gait sequence to encourage gait reeducation.

Treadmills may be useful during the initiation of rehabilitation programs for conditions in which extension of the hip or stifle is painful, such as hip dysplasia or postoperative recovery from cranial cruciate ligament surgery. Normally, patients are reluctant to perform activities such as climbing stairs, because extension of these joints is painful. Treadmill walking is less painful in some patients because the belt provides assistance with hip and stifle extension by helping to pull the rear limb back. There is less need for active contraction of the gluteal and quadriceps muscles for joint extension when walking on a treadmill than when walking on land.

The treadmill may be angled up or down to reduce or increase the forces placed on the forelimbs or hindlimbs. A syringe cap placed on the bottom of the contralateral, unaffected foot pad often encourages weight-bearing in patients that are reluctant to place weight on a limb. A sling may be used to support a paraparetic animal. To add resistance to limbs during treadmill activity to aid with muscle strengthening, an elastic band may be used to provide resistance to specific muscle groups (Figure 14-19). The band is secured to the involved extremity and the handler provides stability on the opposite end. For example, the band may be tied around the forearm with the line of pull from the rear, providing resistance and strengthen-

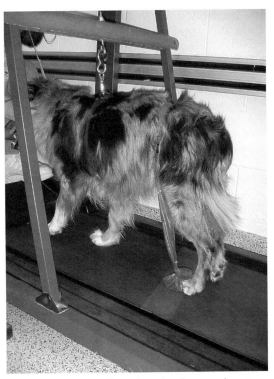

Figure 14-19   Use of an elastic band to provide resistive activity during treadmill walking.

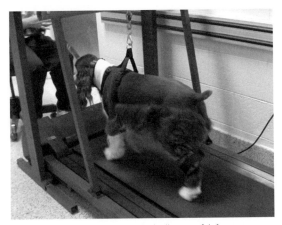

Figure 14-18   A canine treadmill is useful for patterning gait and encouraging early limb use following surgery.

ing of the elbow flexors and shoulder extensors during the swing phase of gait.

Assisted active advancement of a limb during the swing phase of gait can also be performed by using an elastic band. An animal with conscious proprioceptive deficits or muscle weakness that is unable to lift its foot off the ground during the swing phase of gait can be assisted using an elastic band. After one end of the elastic band is attached to the foot, the other end is secured to the body with the direction of pull designed to assist active advancement of the limb during gait. The handler may also manually place the foot as the animal walks on the treadmill.

Dancing and Wheelbarrowing

Dancing is a technique to increase weight-bearing and force on the rear limbs, while also challenging proprioception, coordination, and balance. When the dog's front legs are lifted off the ground, this shifts the weight to the hindlimbs and also promotes stifle, hock, and hip extension. The higher the dog is elevated off the ground, the more extension is required in the rear limb joints. It is important for the therapist or veterinarian to evaluate available range of motion in the rear limb joints before attempting this exercise to identify any potential limitations that may prevent the animal from safely performing the exercise.

When a dog is using its affected limb consistently at a walk with minimal lameness, dancing may begin. Muzzle dogs before exercise. The forelimbs are lifted off the ground, allowing the patient to bear weight only on the hindlimbs (Figure 14-20). Dogs with normal proprioception will naturally move the rear limbs as the handler moves and the animal "dances" backward and forward. Some dogs may resist dancing forward if the handler stands in front of the dog; dogs may plant their hindlimbs and stretch out as the handler moves until the forelimbs reach the ground. In this situation, the handler should stand behind the dog, placing their arms under the axillary region to support the dog, and walk forward. How far the dog is elevated off the ground depends on the amount of stress the animal is able to comfortably handle on the hindlimbs. Dogs may be elevated as high as possible and also dance up and down inclines or hills to place additional stress on the hindlimbs.

Wheelbarrowing is an exercise similar to dancing, except that the forelimbs are tar-geted. This exercise encourages increased use of the forelimbs and challenges proprioception, coordination, and balance. The dog's orthopedic condition must be adequately stable to handle the stresses of this exercise.

The handler should place a muzzle on the dog. To perform the wheelbarrow exercise, the handler places the hands under the caudal abdomen and lifts the rear limbs of the dog off the ground, and the dog is moved forward (Figure 14-21). Dogs with normal proprioception will move the forelimbs so they do not fall. Some dogs may require sling support if they are weak. Dogs may be wheelbarrowed up and down inclines for greater muscle strengthening. Theoretically, the higher the animal is lifted, the greater the forces placed on the forelimbs. However, the increase in weight-bearing may not be as great as anticipated because the stride length is much shorter when the animal is wheelbarrowed from a height (Figure 14-22). The shortened stride results in less force placed on the limbs while wheelbarrowing as compared with walking or trotting at a faster speed.

Jogging

Jogging may be initiated in cases with stable surgical repairs when the dog is walking on the limb with minimal lameness and pain.

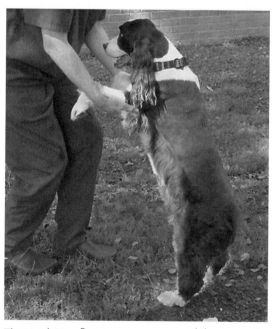

Figure 14-20 Dancing encourages weight-bearing on the rear limbs.

Begin slowly, jogging 0.5 to 3 minutes one to three times daily, and work up to 20 minutes two to three times daily. Be certain that lameness is not worse after jogging.

Sit-to-Stand Exercises

Sit-to-stand exercises help strengthen hip and stifle extensor muscles and improve active range of motion. The act of sitting, then standing up, requires muscle strength of the quadriceps, hamstring, and gastrocnemius muscle groups. Some training will be necessary, and low-calorie treats may be offered as a training aid to provide motivation to perform the

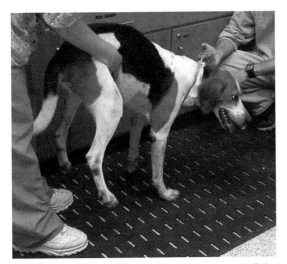

Figure 14-21   Wheelbarrowing encourages use of the forelimbs.

movement. It is important to perform these exercises correctly. Attention should be paid to sitting and standing straight, with no leaning to one side, and the joints of both rear limbs should be symmetrically flexed so that the dog sits squarely on its haunches (Figure 14-23). While on the leash, after a sufficient warm-up period of walking, the handler asks the dog to sit squarely for a few seconds and then asks the dog to stand, take a few steps forward, and then again sit. The sit-to-stands may be repeated a number of times before the dog is allowed to rest. It may be easier in some cases to back the dog into a corner, with the affected limb next to a wall so that the dog cannot slide the limb out while rising or sitting. Start with 5 to10 repetitions once or twice daily, and work up to 15 repetitions three to four times daily.

This exercise may be particularly beneficial for dogs with osteoarthritis of the hips. These patients generally feel pain when the hip joints are extended. In addition, there may be atrophy of the gluteal muscles. The sit-to-stand exercise allows active contraction of the gluteal muscles, but the hip joint is not generally extended to the point that results in pain. This allows strengthening without creating undue pain. Of course, each patient must be assessed to be certain that sit-to-stands are not too stressful or painful for that individual.

Down-to-Stand Exercises

A variant of the sit-to-stand exercise is the down-to-stand. With this exercise, the dog is

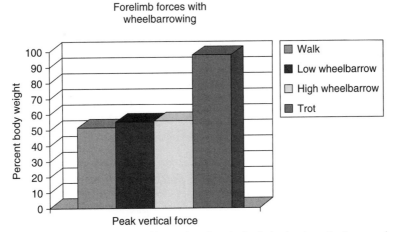

Figure 14-22   Bar graphs indicating the amount of force placed on the forelimb of a dog wheelbarrowed across a force platform. Note that there is little increase in vertical force placed on the forelimb while wheelbarrowing, likely because of the shortened stride during wheelbarrowing as compared to walking or trotting.

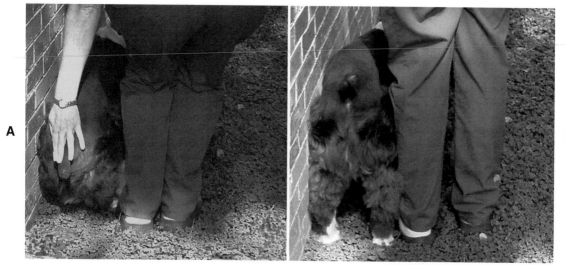

Figure 14-23   Sit-to-stand exercises. **A,** Note the symmetrical position of the dog in the sitting position. Placing the affected limb toward a wall will help the dog to sit in a square, symmetrical position. **B,** As the dog rises, it should push off equally with both rear limbs.

allowed to rise from a ventrally recumbent position to a standing position. It is important to have the dog rise symmetrically and push off equally with all four limbs. This exercise may require some additional time and training to perform correctly.

Cavaletti Rails

Cavaletti rails are poles that are spaced apart on the ground at a low height. Cavaletti rails may be used to encourage greater active range of motion and lengthened strides in all limbs. They may also be used to challenge proprioception, balance, and coordination in animals returning to function following neurological impairment. An alternative to cavaletti rails is to use a ladder and allow the rungs of the ladder to act as the low rails. Although ladders are readily available in most households, they have limited flexibility to change the distance between the rungs and the height that the animal steps over the rungs. This exercise can be beneficial for either orthopedic or neurological patients in need of improved voluntary motor control and accuracy in placement of the limbs. One or more poles may be used and should be spaced at appropriate distances apart, determined by the dog's natural stride length (Figure 14-24). After the animal becomes accustomed to the task, the handler can further challenge the dog by making simple modifications such as adding more poles, increasing the height of all the poles to encourage greater active flexion and extension of joints, and alter-

ing the heights of alternating poles to encourage dogs to negotiate different situations. Begin with walking and progress to trotting.

Walking in Tall Grass, Sand, or Snow

Walking a dog through a field of tall grass enhances muscle strengthening and endurance because of the resistance provided by the grass, as well as coordination to navigate varying terrain. In addition, dogs have a tendency to flex their joints to a greater extent as they negotiate the grass. Some caution should be used in dogs with allergies, which may be aggravated in such conditions, and in dogs with conjunctivitis, which might also be exacerbated.

Walking in deep sand or snow provides resistance to limb movement during walking and jogging and strengthens the flexor muscles, which must contract more to advance the limbs. Exercising in sand and snow minimizes concussive forces placed on arthritic joints, while allowing strengthening of supporting periarticular muscles. Standing in sand may also be beneficial to dogs in rehabilitation following neurologic conditions.

Pole Weaving

Weaving between vertical poles helps to promote side bending of the dog's trunk and also challenges proprioceptive functioning and strengthening of limb abductor and adductor muscles. The distance between poles should be

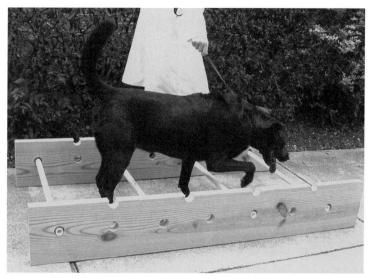

Figure 14-24   Cavaletti rails help increase active flexion and extension of joints as the dog negotiates the rails. Stride length may also be altered by placing the rails closer together or farther apart.

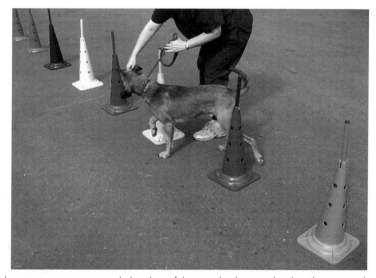

Figure 14-25   Pole weaving encourages side bending of the spinal column and aids with paraspinal muscle strengthening.

adjusted so that sufficient side bending results; in general, the distance between poles should be slightly less than the body length of the dog. In addition, the handler must lead the animal so that the head, neck, and body actually flex as the poles are negotiated (Figure 14-25).

Tunnels

Agility training tunnels or children's play tunnels may be used to promote flexion in the forelimbs and hindlimbs. The size of the tunnel opening should be appropriate for the size of the dog, that is, just shorter than the dog's standing height. The dog is encouraged to crouch low and "crawl" through the tunnel, which requires greater limb flexion and strength than that needed for normal walking. Greater challenges may be instituted by using tunnels that are less tall as dogs strengthen their muscles.

Pulling or Carrying Weight

A variety of harnesses are available for dogs to attach to carts or sleds for pulling weight. The

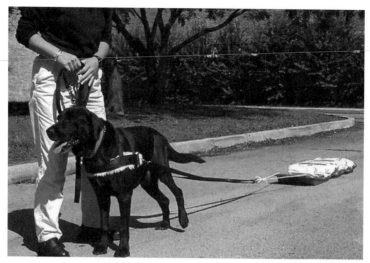

Figure 14-26   Pulling a sled with added weight helps with muscle strengthening.

harness should be well padded and comfortable. Pulling a cart with a large wheel diameter is easier than pulling a sled that slides along the ground (Figure 14-26). The positions of the head and neck are important in determining whether a dog pulls the weight forward with the forelimbs or the hindlimbs. If the dog carries its head and neck low to the ground, it is likely pulling with the forelimbs. A dog with the head and neck held high will shift some of the weight caudally and tend to use the hindlimbs to drive the body forward. A variety of sleds and carts are commercially available. In all cases, the harness should be adjustable and properly fit the animal and cart or sled to avoid abnormal pressure where the harness contacts the animal; a poorly fitted rig may result in pressure sores and alter the manner in which the dog pulls the weight.

Dogs may also wear leg weights. Leg weights may be fashioned from lead strips, or commercially available leg weights for people may be used (Figure 14-27). In general, ½-lb leg weights may be used on dogs that weigh 10 to 20 lb, 1-lb weights on dogs weighing 20 to 40 lb, 1½-lb weights for 40- to 60-lb dogs, and 2-lb weights for dogs weighing more than 60 lb. Caution should be used when first applying the weights because some dogs may shake the limb or have exaggerated limb motion because of the altered sensation. It is possible that injury may occur, so it is important to gradually introduce the weight to allow a period of accommodation.

Some leg weights designed for people may not fit properly. Many of these are filled with sand, and when the weight is applied to the

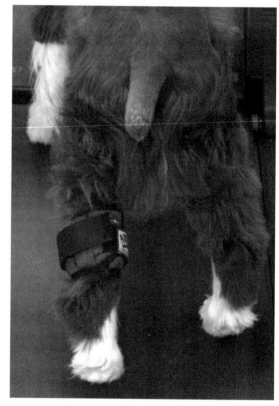

Figure 14-27   Leg weights may be fastened to the distal limbs to help with muscle strengthening. They may also be useful to encourage limb use.

thinner dog limb, the fastening straps may not provide a snug fit, allowing it to slip off. Removal of some of the sand may solve this problem. Another factor to consider is location of the limb weight. Biomechanically, greater

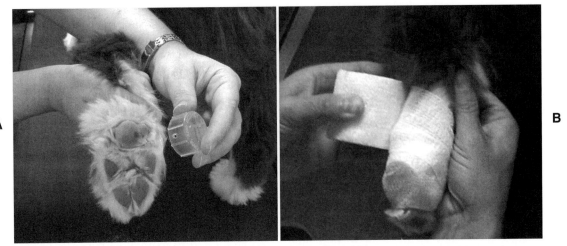

Figure 14-28   A, Placement of a syringe cap on the bottom of an unaffected foot to act as a minor irritant and encourage weight-bearing on an affected limb. **B,** Taping the syringe cap to the bottom of the foot.

force is required to move a limb if the weight is located more distally on the limb. Likewise, a distally placed limb weight may place additional torque on the joints, which may be undesirable if the animal is recovering from joint surgery. In this situation, placing the weight more proximally reduces the forces on the limb and joints. Dogs may also perform chronic "weight lifting" by wearing a canine backpack filled with weights. Weights may be loaded unequally or equally on both sides. When a dog wears a weighted backpack during down-to-stand or sit-to-stand exercises, greater muscle force is required to rise to a standing position.

Controlled Ball Playing

Ball playing is a fun and effective form of therapeutic exercise that dogs and their owners enjoy. It also has the potential to cause damage to surgical repairs. Controlled activity is the key. The degree of activity depends on the surgical procedure performed, the condition of the tissues, and the stage of tissue healing. Ball playing should begin on a relatively short leash to avoid explosive activity in the early postoperative period. As the patient progresses, the dog graduates to ball playing in an enclosed area, such as a run. As the animal nears full return to function, off-leash activity may be performed in a large fenced field free of irregular surfaces. The main benefits of ball playing are to increase power, speed, and muscle strength. In most conditions, jumping should be avoided to reduce the risk of injury.

Methods to Encourage Weight-Bearing

A syringe cap or coin may be placed on the bottom of the uninjured foot and held in place with adhesive tape to encourage weight-bearing on the affected limb (Figure 14-28). In many instances, weight-bearing continues on the affected limb even after the item is removed from the good foot. Some dogs will build up a tolerance to the item; therefore continuous application is not recommended. In some particularly difficult cases, a sling may be placed on the nonaffected limb to force the animal to bear weight on the affected limb. In our experience, this technique is less effective because many animals simply lie down and will not attempt to walk. Hemiwalking is sometimes useful to encourage weight-bearing on a particular limb. This exercise is performed by elevating the ipsilateral fore and rear limbs off the ground and shifting the weight to the contralateral limbs. The animal must move the contralateral fore and rear limbs laterally to avoid losing balance and falling. Although this is generally more successful than placing a sling on a limb, some animals may still resist and simply lie down.

Other Techniques to Encourage Limb Use

Some dogs and most cats provide special challenges for rehabilitation after injury. Additional activities may encourage limb use. Many cats will readily chase the spot of light from a flashlight around a room. Care should be taken to have good footing, such as carpeting, and to move the light at a speed appropriate for the animal's stage of recovery. In addition, stretching may be employed by moving the light along a vertical surface, such as a wall. Some dogs and cats will also chase a laser pointer light.

Many cats and dogs have been well conditioned to the sound of a can opener or other audible cues such as a door opening to go for a walk. The animal may be placed in another room and the sound made. In many instances, the animal disregards a lame leg and ambulates to the sound.

Most cats and some dogs will play with a toy such as a string or other object that they are used to "stalking" or chasing. Engaging the owner to identify some favorite playthings is important, because some animals will not react to toys in a strange environment such as a clinic. It is equally important to instruct the owner regarding the length of playtime, how to use the toy to maximize the rehabilitation process, and limits of play to reduce the chance of fatigue and injury.

Yet another technique that is sometimes useful to encourage limb use in difficult cases is to have a treat and encourage the animal to follow the treat while the owner holds it in front of the animal and moves about. This technique is also useful to encourage side bending in animals that are stiff in the neck and other portions of the spine. With the animal in a standing position, the treat can be moved from right to left and up and down to encourage mobility of the spine and surrounding muscles. This technique is contraindicated in animals with an unstable spinal canal or those with unstable intervertebral disks.

Progression of Exercises

Many variables must be considered in the design of a therapeutic exercise program, including the type and severity of the condition, the stability of any surgical repairs, the number of involved limbs and joints, the size of the animal, the preexisting physical condition of the patient, the available facilities, the skill and experience of the therapist, and whether the exercises will be administered by a professional, the owner, or a combination of the owner and a professional. Unfortunately, it is impossible to have a single protocol for each specific condition. Some basic guidelines may be applied, however.

The goal of any therapeutic exercise program should be to restore the animal to as full and active use as possible. The goal may need to be periodically adjusted if the patient progresses to a greater or lesser degree than expected. The initial goal should be to have the patient bear its full weight while standing. The next step should be assisted active ambulation. Proprioceptive training should occur concurrently with active ambulation, with the goal to have unassisted active ambulation while maintaining balance. As the animal nears return to house-pet function, strategies should be developed to encourage increased weight-bearing and muscle mass.

It is very important to perform the exercises correctly and to maintain a consistent level of activity daily or every other day. In most cases, several short sessions per day will be more effective than a single long session early in the recovery period. Overdoing activity on the weekends with relatively little activity during the rest of the week will likely be detrimental to the animal's recovery; regular, daily activity will avoid the "weekend warrior" syndrome.

If pain or lameness increases during or several hours after stepping up an activity, the level of activity should be reduced by 50% for 3 to 7 days. If the lameness and pain resolve, the activity may be slowly increased back to the pre–step-up activity level over 3 to 5 days, with careful observation to be certain that the activity is not increased too aggressively or rapidly. The rate of subsequent step-up activity should be half of what it originally was to avoid a recurrent episode of exacerbated lameness and pain.

It is also important to vary the routine for the animal's and the owners' sake to avoid boredom, and to allow incorporation of function-specific activities in the animal's home or work environment. During chronic management of the patient, weight control is extremely important. It is also important to continue to oversee the protocol and document improvement. Progress will occur at a slower rate during the chronic phase of recovery, but continued rehabilitation is just as important to achieve as full a return to activity as possible.

Several medications may be appropriate for use in the chronic rehabilitation period, including nonsteroidal antiinflammatory agents and chondroprotective agents. Caution should be used, however, to be certain that any analgesic medications do not mask pain and discomfort associated with the level of activity. They should facilitate rehabilitation and recovery rather than allow rehabilitation to progress faster than normal conditions and tissue healing should allow. When stepping up the level of an activity, antiinflammatory or pain medication should be withheld on the day of step-up and for the day after, to be certain that there is no additional tissue damage. If pain or lameness increases, the level of activity should be reduced 50% for 1 week; then the activity is stepped up again at a slower rate.

Summary

Beginning a rehabilitation program need not be elaborate or costly. Consideration should be given to the patient's needs, the owner's needs, and the therapist's needs. Also, although protocol development greatly depends on the available facilities and equipment, the willingness of the owners to help with rehabilitation, and the education level of the staff, some rehabilitation is better than none at all.

Therapeutic exercises are undoubtedly the most important aspects of rehabilitation. They may (and should) be incorporated with other modalities to enhance recovery, but it is the exercises that help improve muscle strength, joint mobility, limb use, proprioceptive training, and endurance to maximize function. Although a variety of techniques have been described, the ingenuity of the rehabilitation team, including the owner, will allow the development of other exercises that are specific to a patient's recovery. The keys to a successful therapeutic exercise program are to have site- and condition-specific exercises whenever possible, to use a variety of exercises and techniques to keep the therapy team and patient from becoming bored, and to allow the animal to appropriately progress so that tissues are adequately challenged for strengthening, but not so rapidly as to result in complications and tissue damage.

■ C h a p t e r   1 5

Aquatic Therapy

David Levine, Lauren Rittenberry, Darryl L. Millis

Principles of Aquatic Therapy

It is necessary to understand the basic principles and properties of water including relative density, buoyancy, viscosity, resistance, hydrostatic pressure, and surface tension to appreciate the benefits of aquatic therapy. These are important components to consider when planning an aquatic rehabilitation program.

Relative Density

The relative density of an object is the ratio of the weight of the object to the weight of an equal volume of water.[1] Relative density depends on the composition of an object. Densities of various substances are defined by a pure number value called specific gravity. The specific gravity of pure water is 1.0.[2] The specific gravities of fat, lean muscle, and bone are 0.8, 1.0, and 1.5 to 2.0, respectively.[3] The relative density and specific gravity of an object determine how well an object will float. If the ratio of an object's specific gravity to that of water is greater than 1, the object will tend to sink, and if the ratio is less than 1, the object will tend to float.[4] The specific gravity of an object also determines how much of the object's volume will float under water.[4] For example, the specific gravity of ice is approximately 0.92; therefore 92% of ice will be submerged to displace enough water so that the upward force of buoyancy will equal the downward force of gravity, and 8% will float above the surface of water.[2,5]

A lean person's specific gravity may be as high as 1.10, whereas an obese person's specific gravity may be as low as 0.93.[4] An object whose specific gravity is equal to that of pure water (1.0) will float just below the surface of the water. If a person's specific gravity is greater than 1.0, that person will tend to sink. The greater the specific gravity, the faster the sinking velocity.[2] Thus a lean animal that is not moving will have a tendency to sink faster than an obese animal.

Buoyancy

A body immersed in water is subjected to two forces, gravity and buoyancy. Buoyancy is defined as the upward thrust of water acting on a body that creates an apparent decrease in the weight of a body while immersed.[2] Buoyancy stems from Archimedes' principle: When a body is fully or partially submerged in a fluid at rest, it experiences an upward thrust equal to the weight of the fluid displaced.[1,2,4,6] The amount of water displaced depends on the density of the body immersed relative to the density of water.[2] An immersed limb or body with a relative density less than that of water will be assisted to the surface by buoyant forces.[7] An object with a relative density less than 1 floats because the weight of the object is less than the weight of the water displaced.[5,8] Buoyancy acts directly through the center of buoyancy.[3] The center of buoyancy is the centroid of the displaced volume of water and is dependent on the distribution of the displaced volume of fluid relative to the body.[9] Problems arise when the center of gravity and the center of buoyancy are not in the same vertical line. This can occur with the use of improperly placed floating devices, which can disrupt the vertical line causing an animal to tilt or flip over in order to reach a state of equilibrium.[3] The location of the center of buoyancy varies depending on the percent of body fat and distribution of adipose tissue.[10]

Fill to Level of Lateral Malleolus

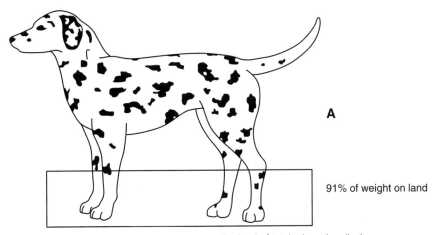

A

91% of weight on land

Figure 15-1   **A,** Dog in water to the level of (a) the lateral malleolus.

The more caudal the distribution of adipose tissue (which tends to occur more often in human females than in males), the closer the center of buoyancy is located to the center of mass.

Buoyancy aids in the rehabilitation of weak muscles and painful joints. It allows the patient to exercise in an upright position and may decrease pain by minimizing the amount of weight-bearing on joints. For example, the percentage of weight borne by human females when immersed in water is approximately 5.9% to 8.7% at the seventh cervical vertebral level, 25% to 31% at the level of the xiphoid, and 40% to 51% at the level of the anterior superior iliac spine.[11] Males bear 6.8% to 10%, 30% to 37%, and 50% to 56% of their body weight in the upright position at these same levels.[11] Other studies of humans have also found similar percentages of weight-bearing at these same levels.[12] In a similar study performed on dogs, the amount of body weight borne when immersed in water (as a percentage of body weight on dry ground) was approximately 91% when the water was at the level of the ateral malleolus of the tibia, 85% at the level of the lateral condyle of the femur, and 38% at the level of the greater trochanter of the femur (Figure 15-1).[13] This information may be particularly useful when treating patients with arthritis because joints may be unloaded as a result of the buoyant properties of water.

Hydrostatic Pressure

Pascal's law states that fluid pressure is exerted equally on all surfaces of an immersed body at rest at a given depth. This fluid pressure is directly proportional to both the depth and the density of the fluid.[4] Therefore the deeper a body is immersed in water the greater the pressure exerted. The atmospheric pressure at the surface of water is 1.00 kPa (15.7 psi) and fluid pressure increases by 0.029 kPa (0.43 psi) per foot of depth.[3] It can be estimated that the pressure exerted on a part of the body immersed 3 feet below the surface will experience a fluid pressure of 1.09 kPa (17 psi). Because hydrostatic pressure provides constant pressure to a body or limb immersed in water, it may provide an improved environment for working with swollen joints or edematous tissues.[7] Hydrostatic pressure opposes the tendency of blood and edema to pool in the lower portions of the body and can therefore aid in reducing swelling.[3] The benefits of edema reduction due to hydrostatic pressure are used by pregnant women who exercise in water to help minimize swelling in their lower extremities during exercise. The reduction in edema is probably due to several factors, including a general increase in circulation with exercise, and the prevention of further pooling of fluids in the lower extremities by the pressure exerted on them by water.

Fill to Level of Femoral Condyles

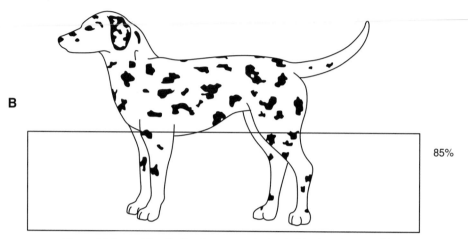

85%

Figure 15-1 cont'd   **B,** Dog in water to the level of the lateral epicondyle.

Fill to Level of Greater Trochanter

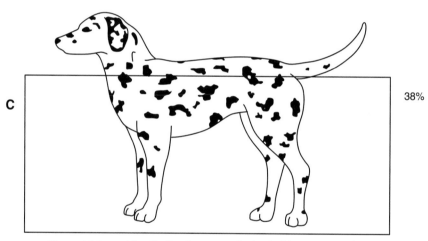

38%

Figure 15-1 cont'd   **C,** Dog in water to the level of the greater trochanter.

Hydrostatic pressure may also decrease pain during exercise. It is theorized that hydrostatic pressure provides phasic stimuli to the skin afferents (sensory receptors) that cause a decrease in nociceptor hypersensitivity. This acts to decrease a person's or animal's pain perception, which may allow the patient to perform a variety of movements with less pain.[7,14]

Viscosity and Resistance

Viscosity is a measure of the frictional resistance caused by cohesive or attractive forces between the molecules of a liquid.[15] The viscosity, or resistance to fluid flow, is significantly greater in water than in air,[7] making it harder to move through water than to move through air. Water can therefore provide resistance that may strengthen canine muscles and improve cardiovascular fitness. Viscosity is important in aquatic therapy for several other reasons. Viscosity may increase sensory awareness and assist in stabilizing unstable joints.[7] It can also help prevent falling by increasing the time span for patients to react,[7] which may reduce patient anxiety. For example, a dog with paraparesis may be more willing to walk in water than on land because of water's combined properties of buoyancy and viscosity, which help to support the dog.

Any body movement occurring in water must overcome water viscosity.[16] The resistance created by the viscosity of the liquid is proportional to the velocity of movement through a liquid. With increased velocity of movement in water, there is a uniform increase in resistance.

Various movements in water may increase or help reduce resistance. Streamline flow is the steady, continuous movement of fluid. There is little friction between layers of fluid in streamline flow because the layers separate to move around the object and smoothly rejoin behind it.[5] Turbulent flow consists of irregular movements of the layers of fluid.[1,5] The irregular movement in turbulent flow causes increased friction between the molecules of the fluid and between the object and the fluid.[5] Eddies are a form of turbulent flow where the layers of fluid following a moving object in water move in circular directions.[5] Eddies resist an object's movement in water by pulling the object backward. Because of all these factors, resistance in aquatic exercise may be increased by increasing the velocity of movement of the patient, increasing the surface area of the object or body part moving in water, or by increasing the length of the lever arm of the object moving in water.[16]

Surface Tension

The tendency for water molecules to adhere to each other is known as cohesion.[2] Water molecules have a greater tendency to adhere together on the surface. Resistance to movement is slightly greater on the surface of water because there is more cohesion on the surface of water.[2] Surface tension is the force of attraction between surface molecules of a fluid.[3] Surface tension is not a factor if the moving body part is completely submerged in water. It becomes a significant factor when a limb breaks the surface of the water. Therapeutically, if a patient is extremely weak, movements may be performed more easily in the water just beneath the surface rather than at or on the surface.

Therapeutic Benefits of Aquatic Exercise

There are many benefits of aquatic therapy. Exercising in water is effective for improving strength, muscular endurance, cardiorespiratory endurance, range of motion (ROM), agility, and psychological well-being, while minimizing pain.[17-19] The purpose of this section is to provide the reader with information regarding human studies of the benefits of aquatic therapy. Table 15-1 provides a summary of these studies. It is likely that similar principles apply to animals.

Gravity is the primary resistant force to exercise on land, whereas viscosity, friction, and turbulence are the primary resistant forces to exercise in water; these properties have a direct effect on heart rate and oxygen uptake.[20] Arm exercises on land produced an increase in heart rate from a resting rate of 77 beats per minute to 92 beats per minute in men (ages 21 to 27) and from 74 to 96 beats per minute in women (ages 20 to 29). Exactly the same arm exercises in water produced an increase in heart rate from 60 to 99 beats per minute in men and from 60 to 98 beats per minute in women. Compared to the subjects exercising on land, the subjects exercising in water exercised at slightly higher heart rates and had a greater overall increase in heart rate because of the initial lower resting heart rate. Subjects in this study had lower resting heart rates in water than on land because of two factors: the reflex response of the cardiovascular system to the cold receptors of the skin, and the effect of hydrostatic water pressure exerted on the submerged body.[20] The water temperature ranged from 26° to 26.5° C (78.8° to 79.7° F) during aquatic exercise. As discussed later, water temperature directly affects heart rate. Leg exercises further increased heart rate during water exercises: 76 (resting) to 124 (exercise) beats per minute for men on land versus 60 (resting) to 139 (exercise) beats per minute in water, and 73 (resting) to 126 (exercise) beats per minute for women on land versus 60 (resting) to 126 (exercise) beats per minute in water. The increased weight of legs as compared to arms may increase the necessary energy expenditure for exercises performed on land because of the increased mass and pull of gravity. This study demonstrated that heart rate and oxygen uptake were greater when performing exercises in water compared to performing the same exercises on land.[20]

The metabolic requirements are also greater for exercises performed in water than for exercises performed on land. In a study by Johnson et al,[20] men and women performed the same arm and leg exercises in water and on land.

■ ▨ ▨ **Table 15-1**   Summary of Human Studies on the Benefits of Aquatic Therapy

Study	Study subjects	Study parameters	Outcome
Cardiovascular Studies in Aquatic Therapy			
Avellini et al, 1983	Three groups of five men	Subjects trained on cycle ergometer 5 days/wk for 1 hr at 75% $V_{O_{2max}}$; group 1 exercised on land and groups 2 and 3 exercised in water at temperatures of 32° C and 20° C, respectively	Water groups exercised at a lower heart rate than land group
Bravo et al, 1997	77 postmenopausal women	Exercised in waist-deep water for 60 min 3 days/wk × 12 months	Improved functional fitness and psychological well-being
Choukroun & Varene, 1990	11 healthy volunteers (four women, seven men)	Subjects were immersed to neck in 25° C, 34° C, and 40° C water; cardiovascular demands measured at rest	Cardiac output increased significantly at 40° C versus lower temperatures
Evans et al, 1978	Six men	Walked and jogged at similar metabolic intensities on a treadmill in waist-deep water	Only one third to one half of the normal walking and jogging speed was required to work at the same level of energy expenditure in water as compared with on land (on a treadmill)
Hall et al, 1998	Eight women (mean 30.25 yo)	Submaximal exercise on land and on a treadmill in chest-deep water at water temperatures of 28° C and 36° C	Heart rate higher at 36° C compared to 28° C; walking in chest-deep water yields higher energy costs than walking at similar speeds on land
Johnson et al, 1977	Four men (mean 24 yo) and four women (mean 24.5 yo)	Same exercises performed by the same subjects on land and in water: shoulder ABD/ADD and hip flexion/extension with limbs extended	Decreased resting heart rate in water and increased V_{O_2} demands when exercising in water
Melton-Rogers et al, 1996	Eight adults with adult-onset rheumatoid arthritis (30-40 yo)	Graded maximal exercise test on a stationary bike on land and running in water wearing a flotation device	Higher maximum perceived exertion and respiratory rate were seen in water running; water provides a means for exercise for individuals with rheumatoid arthritis
Perk et al, 1996	20 stable COPD patients	Cardiorespiratory parameters were measured on land and in temperature-controlled water (32° C) at rest and during a 15-min submaximal upper-body exercise program	At rest in water there was a decrease in systolic and diastolic BP
Whitley and Schoene, 1987	12 healthy female college students	Heart rate was measured immediately after walking in waist-deep water and then on treadmill at same speed, duration, and distance	Heart rates were higher at each speed when walking in water vs walking on land

Continued

■ ■ ■ **Table 15-1**   Summary of Human Studies on the Benefits of Aquatic Therapy—cont'd

Study	Study subjects	Study parameters	Outcome
Range of Motion and Strength Studies in Aquatic Therapy			
Suomi and Lindauer, 1997	17 women with arthritis	Exercise subjects participated in three 45-min aquatic training sessions/wk for 6 wk; control subjects were asked to refrain from participating in any organized physical activity	Greater increase in strength and ROM occurred in the aquatic therapy subjects
Tovin et al, 1994	14 men and six women (16-44 yo) with ACL reconstructions	10 subjects participated in traditional rehabilitation protocol (stationary cycling, gait training, steps, hip flex/ext, ABD/ADD in standing, and knee flexion in sitting) while other 10 subjects performed same exercises in a pool; performed over first 8 postoperative wk	Rehabilitation program for patients with intraarticular ACL reconstruction performed in a pool was more effective in reducing joint effusion and facilitating recovery of lower extremity function as indicated by Lysholm scores; rehab in water is equally effective as on land for restoring knee ROM and quadriceps strength

ABD, Abduction; *ACL*, anterior cruciate ligament; *ADD*, adduction; BP, blood pressure; ROM, range of motion.

Oxygen uptake during exercise in water was 34% greater in men and 27% greater in women as compared with the same exercises on land.[20] The differences between men and women are probably due to different body compositions (male body composition tends to be more muscular, which requires more oxygen) and heights (men tend to be taller and have longer extremities, thereby having a longer lever arm, which requires more exertion to move). Another study found that subjects could walk or jog at slower speeds in water than on land while expending the same amount of energy as measured by oxygen consumption. In this study, subjects walked at 2.6 to 3.5 km/hr (1.6 to 2.2 mph) in water while subjects on land walked or jogged at speeds of 5.5 to 13.4 km/hr (3.4 to 8.3 mph). Both expended the same amount of energy, despite the greater velocity of people walking on land.[21] A study by Whitley and Schoene[19] supports these data with the observation that various types of exercise performed in water (aquatic calisthenics, shoulder and leg exercises, bicycle ergometry exercises, walking and jogging) require a significantly greater amount of energy expenditure compared to the same exercises performed on land. Subjects in a study by Hall et al[22] also expended more energy walking in water than on land at speeds greater than 4 km/hr (2.5 mph).

When aerobic exercise is used in the rehabilitation process, it may aid in improving cardiovascular fitness and weight reduction. Melton-Rogers et al[23] compared exercise during land bicycle ergometry with running in water with a flotation device in individuals with rheumatoid arthritis. Higher ratings of perceived exertion (RPE) by the subjects and respiratory exchange ratios were seen during water running.[23] These studies demonstrate that walking in water at specific speeds may be sufficient to meet heart rate requirements for developing and maintaining cardiorespiratory fitness.

Aquatic exercises are also beneficial for muscle strengthening. Bravo et al[17] performed a study on postmenopausal women who exercised in a pool with waist-deep water for 60 minutes, three times a week for 12 months. The average strength gain as a component of functional fitness was approximately 18%. Because of buoyancy, water walking can provide an excellent alternative method of achieving and maintaining muscle strength and ROM in individuals with lower limb joint problems such as osteoarthritis (OA). Although exercise in water may not be as effective in achieving maximum muscle performance as land exercises, rehabilitation in water may minimize the amount of joint effusion and lead to greater functional improvement.[24] Closed-chain exercises such as walking in water are more closely associated to movements in everyday activities than open-chain exercises because they recruit muscles in a more functional manner.[25] Performing closed-chain exercises in an environment where weight-bearing forces are decreased may minimize or eliminate damage and inflammation to the soft tissues, while maximizing functional training. The aqueous environment may also aid in reducing knee pain and joint effusion,[24] which may facilitate the recovery of lower-extremity function after cranial cruciate ligament (CCL) stabilization in dogs.

Water's buoyancy can ease the performance of exercise activities while also providing proprioceptive feedback to aid in the rehabilitation process. The effect of buoyancy allows for gentler active exercises by decreasing the loads placed on the injured tissues compared to exercises performed on land.[18] Aquatic exercises may be used as a transition to land-based exercises in postsurgery or postinjury rehabilitation. Water exercises are generally less painful than land exercises because of the support that buoyancy provides. Therefore water exercises may result in less discomfort and provide a better sense of security when initiating active movements.[18] This helps maintain ROM and functional movement before the strength gains needed to perform the same movements on land are achieved.

There are many physiologic effects resulting from exercise in heated water. Among them are increased circulation to muscles, increased joint flexibility, and decreased joint pain.[26] Templeton et al performed a study to determine whether subjects with rheumatic diseases experienced changes in joint flexibility and functional ability following an aquatic therapy program.[26] Subjects exercised in water for 8 weeks. Exercises consisted of therapeutic games emphasizing both isotonic and isometric exercises of the trunk, neck, and upper and lower extremities. Water temperature was maintained at 32.9° C (91.3° F) and the air temperature was maintained at 31.7° C (89° F). Active ROM and a Functional Status Index test that recorded the degree of assistance, pain, and difficulty experienced in the performance of 18 tasks were measured before and after the 8-week aquatic therapy session. The results of the study indicated that pain decreased with therapy, and active ROM and functional ability increased. The decreased pain and improvement in performing daily activities had a significant impact on the over-all increased functional ability of the subjects.[26] These findings support aquatic therapy as an effective rehabilitation technique for increasing functional ability and joint flexibility in people with severe joint disease. Osteoarthritic and rheumatoid arthritic patients participated in a study of the effects of aquatic exercise on ROM and strength.[27] Control subjects were asked to refrain from participating in any new physical activity throughout the duration of the study while the exercise group participated in an aquatic exercise program. After 6 weeks, hip strength and ROM were measured. Hip strength in the aquatic exercise group increased 10.9%, while ROM increased 11.8% as compared to the control group.[27]

Water temperature may also have a significant effect on the cardiovascular response to exercise. Subjects in cool water exercise at lower heart rates than those exercising on land at the same workload for several reasons.[28] If the water temperature is low, peripheral vasoconstriction occurs, blood moves centrally, venous return is enhanced, and stroke volume increases. Therefore to maintain the same cardiac output, heart rate decreases. In one study, subjects training in cool water (20° C [68° F]) had enhanced stroke volume and decreased heart rate, thereby increasing exercise efficiency.[28] It is also our experience that dogs exercise at lower heart rates walking on underwater versus land treadmills at the same velocity and length of time (unpublished data, Millis DL, 2000).

Blood pressure is also affected by water temperature. In a study of subjects at rest while submerged in 32° C (89.6° F) water, systolic blood pressure decreased 14 ± 14 mm Hg and diastolic pressure decreased 6 ± 10 mm Hg because of peripheral arterial dilation.[29] On the other hand, exercising in water at temperatures that exceed body temperature may increase cardiovascular demands above those of exercise alone.[12] In one study, cardiac output was measured at rest while people were immersed in water temperatures of 25°, 34°, and 40° C (77°, 93.2°, and 104° F).[30] Cardiac output of those immersed in 40° C water increased significantly. The authors of this study recommend that elite athletes train in water temperatures between 26° C and 28° C (78.8° F and 82.4° F) to prevent any heat-related complications.[30] This temperature range is also recommended by the authors for pools in which healthy dogs are training. Lower temperatures are also apparently tolerated quite well by dogs, especially those with thicker hair coats.

All of the benefits of aquatic therapy in humans (improved strength, muscle endurance, cardiorespiratory endurance, increased ROM, decreased stress on healing tissues, and minimized pain) may also apply to dogs. The type of aquatic therapy used by therapists, veterinarians, and owners depends on the specific rehabilitation needs for each individual. An understanding of the benefits of aquatic therapy will aid in the prescription of specific protocols.

Aquatic Therapy Equipment

This section provides the reader with information concerning the types of aquatic therapy and equipment currently available for dogs. The anticipated use, size of the dogs receiving therapy, and funds available help determine the type of equipment best suited for rehabilitation. Some of the available forms of aquatic therapy include whirlpools, pools of various sizes, and underwater treadmills (Figure 15-2).

Several options must be considered when installing a pool. Some of the features include whether jets or propellers used to circulate the water and add resistance to exercises will be useful, the location of the jets, the possibility of adding an underwater treadmill into the pool, hooks on the inner walls to which safety straps may be attached, manual versus computer-controlled water treatment and heating systems, above-ground versus in-ground pools,

and stairs, lifts, or ladders to enter the pool. In addition, the physical aspects of the enclosure and surrounding area must be considered. For example, the humidity and condensation associated with a heated indoor pool must be considered. The floor surface around the pool must also be carefully designed to avoid slipping and falling by both patients and handlers.

Other forms of aquatic therapy include hot tubs or whirlpools used in hospitals (Figure 15-3). Cost-effective forms of aquatic therapy for smaller dogs include bathtubs, large basins, and plastic pools. Taking a dog to a lake or river is also a cost-effective means of providing aquatic therapy, but caution must be exercised when swimming dogs with recent incisions in these environments. Strong water currents and natural hazards must also be avoided.

Equipment used in aquatic therapy for dogs can be relatively simple and inexpensive. One useful piece of equipment is a pet life preserver (Figure 15-4). These are designed to support the dog and allow free breathing. They may

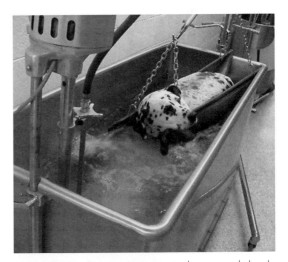

Figure 15-3 Dog receiving aquatic therapy in whirlpool.

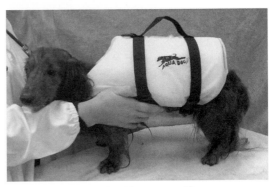

Figure 15-4 Dog wearing life vest.

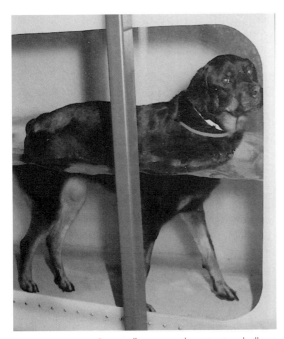

Figure 15-2 Dog walking on underwater treadmill.

include quick-release buckles with adjustable straps and handles for an attendant to assist the dog while swimming. Various sizes are available. Other devices used in aquatic therapy are balls and sticks for fetch games, a lift for entering or exiting the water (Figure 15-5), and harnesses to direct and maintain contact with the dogs if the attendant is not in the pool.

Persons working in the water with dogs may also benefit from specialized equipment such as wetsuits or other protective clothing to guard against prolonged exposure to pool chemicals or cold water (Figure 15-6). Those working from outside the pool with dogs in water should also expect to get wet and should take precautions.

The equipment required to clean and maintain tanks and pools includes disinfectant solutions, protective gloves, buckets, a water hose, brushes with handles to enable scrubbing of crevices, and clean, dry towels.[2] According to Hecox et al, there is no conclusive evidence regarding clear advantages of any one specific type of disinfectant over another.[2] Studies and reported observations suggest sodium hypochlorite (5.25%), sold as household laundry bleach, is an inexpensive and effective disinfectant. However, bleach may corrode the surface of stainless steel over time.[31] Although manual scrubbing with standard germicidal detergents may reduce bacterial contamination, complete removal of bacteria from the drains, edges, and bottom of the tank may not be possible.[2]

Dogs that defecate or urinate in the water or are incontinent pose additional problems in maintaining the cleanliness of tanks or pools. If an animal eliminates or is in incontinent in the water, the best way to minimize cross-contamination is to drain the pool after each use and sanitize it. It is also recommended that this precaution be taken with dogs that have open wounds. If draining the pool is not possible because of its size, the pool should be shocked with chemical disinfectant, and dogs that have open wounds should not use the pool for a period of time recommended by the manufacturer to ensure that the water has been sanitized. Although soiling the water poses potential problems, screening dogs before aquatic therapy may help to reduce or avoid this problem.

Aquatic Therapy for Dogs

Conditions Benefiting From Aquatic Therapy

There are many conditions for which aquatic therapy may be beneficial, including rehabilitation of postoperative fractures, CCL stabilization, neurologic conditions, tendinitis, conditioning, and other disorders in which a dog is reluctant to use the limb or there is a lack of strength, ROM, proprioceptive ability, or weight-bearing status.[32] The potential benefits such as strengthening, cardiovascular endurance, and improved function have been documented in humans, and aquatic therapy is now becoming more common in veterinary medicine. Outcome assessments of aquatic therapy programs are important for documenting progress and to determine the effectiveness of programs.

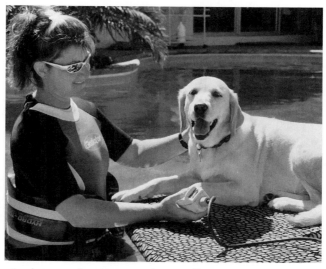

Figure 15-5   Dog being transferred into a pool using a lift. (Courtesy Trish Penick, San Diego, Calif.)

Contraindications and Precautions to Aquatic Therapy

Some dogs fear water or are reluctant to swim, and this must be considered before attempting treatment. If a dog panics, the dog and handler could be placed in a potentially dangerous situation. The dog may injure itself with excessive thrashing. The handler may be injured trying to restrain a panicked dog, or may also risk attack by the animal. Questioning the owner regarding a dog's history of swimming is critical, in addition to prudent safety and handling techniques. If possible, dogs that will be receiving aquatic therapy following nonemergency surgical procedures should be introduced to aquatic therapy before surgery. This allows for evaluation of the dog's disposition toward swimming and will also allow the dog to be introduced to the therapy received postoperatively. Preoperative evaluation is not possible for some traumatic injuries, such as fractures. When receiving aquatic therapy, dogs should never be left unattended in the water.[33]

Some veterinarians believe it is better to wait until incisions or open wounds are healed before placing the animal in water to minimize the risk of infection; others may begin aquatic therapy after the incision is sealed, but before the incision is completely healed. A safe recommendation is to wait until after suture removal if there are no wound complications, including discharge from the incision, gapping of the wound edges, or any evidence of infection. However, there may be conditions that warrant earlier use of aquatic therapy. Regardless of when therapy is started, the wound should be sealed before initiation. The cleanliness of the water may influence this decision, as well as the animal's overall health and medical history.

The cardiovascular fitness of the dog must be considered because many dogs are initially unable to swim more than a few minutes before fatiguing. Swimming the dog several times daily for only 2 to 5 minutes may still result in significant gains in strength, ROM, function, and overall cardiovascular fitness.[33,34]

Specific Exercises

Reluctance to use a limb following injury is a common problem. Dogs that are reluctant to use a limb on land may use it in water to swim or walk on the bottom. Dogs that may benefit from extra buoyancy because of weakness may be assisted by placing a life jacket or other flotation device around the dog's trunk, or by the use of an overhead harness.[33] Owners may provide additional motivation to encourage dogs to swim. Having the animal fetch a ball or other object may have the same motivational effect. If possible, swimming with the dog is another excellent way of encouraging therapy, in addition to ensuring that someone is present if the animal has any trouble. Caution must be used when swimming injured dogs in lakes and rivers.

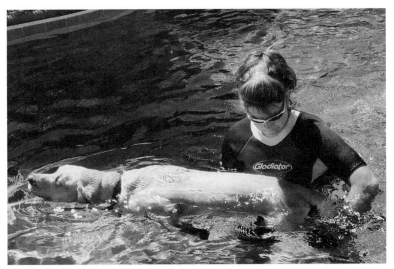

Figure 15-6   Dog swimming in a pool. (Courtesy Trish Penick, San Diego, Calif.)

Dogs must be prevented from diving or lunging off of docks or the shore when entering the water to prevent injury. Wading into the water with the dog until the dog is buoyant is recommended. Maintaining contact with the dog at all times is important. In addition, water sanitation and natural hazards must be considered.

Walking in the water, either on the bottom of the pool or on an underwater treadmill, is an excellent way to allow a dog with painful joints to exercise more comfortably because of the buoyancy provided by the water. This type of exercise may be used as a progression to swimming if the animal is either too weak or in too much pain to initially swim.

In addition to the buoyancy effects of swimming or walking in water, joint kinematics are also altered during aquatic therapy. Knowledge of aquatic kinematics is useful in designing specific exercise programs. For example, in one study comparing swimming with ground treadmill walking, dogs that swam had significantly greater stifle flexion and total stifle ROM compared with ground treadmill walking.[35] However, stifle extension was lower in swimming dogs than in dogs undergoing ground treadmill activity. In addition, dogs had less stifle flexion, extension, and total ROM following stifle surgery as compared with normal dogs.

Rehabilitation of dogs in an underwater treadmill may provide additional benefits regarding joint kinetics. The relative degree of buoyancy and resistance to walking in water can be adjusted by changing the water level. In addition, adjusting the water level to the level of various joints may further influence joint kinematics because those particular joints must gain the necessary momentum and force to break through the water surface and overcome surface tension of the water. One study compared dogs walking on a ground treadmill to dogs walking in an underwater treadmill at the same velocity (Table 15.2).[36] In addition, the water level was adjusted to the greater trochanter (level 1), stifle (level 2), hock (level 3), or the bottom of the foot (level 4). Joint motion was determined in both front and hindlimbs, with each limb in a fully flexed non–weight-bearing position, with each limb in the final propulsion stage of weight-bearing. and with each limb in the initial braking stage of weight-bearing. Unlike swimming, there was no significant reduction in joint extension with underwater treadmill walking during the initial braking phase of stance with water levels at and distal to the stifle. Therefore dogs had full active extension of all joints during a limb cycle, unlike joint motion during swimming. However, hip, stifle, and hock extension during the late phase

■ ■ ■ **Table 15-2** Conditions for Achieving Maximum and Minimum Joint Flexion and Extension During Walking on Either a Ground or an Underwater Treadmill

Joint	Maximum joint motion		Minimum joint motion	
	Extension	**Flexion**	**Extension**	**Flexion**
Forelimb				
Shoulder	142 degrees—ground	93 degrees—water (level 1)	132 degrees—water (level 1)	125 degrees—ground
Elbow	159 degrees—water (level 3)	70 degrees—water (level 3)	124 degrees—ground	98 degrees—water (level 4)
Carpus	193 degrees—water (level 4)	97 degrees—ground	185 degrees—water (level 1)	119 degrees—water (level 4)
Hindlimb				
Hip	141 degrees—ground	93 degrees—water (level 2)	120 degrees—water (level 1)	115 degrees—ground
Stifle	141 degrees—ground	64 degrees—water (level 2)	113 degrees—water (level 1)	109 degrees—ground
Hock	156 degrees—water (level 3)	81 degrees—water (level 2)	135 degrees—water (level 1)	115 degrees—ground

Values indicate the mean maximum and minimum joint flexion or extension angles of 8 dogs that occur under the indicated conditions during walking.
Ground, Walking on a ground treadmill; *water,* walking on an aquatic treadmill; *level 1,* water level at the greater trochanter; *level 2,* water level at the stifle joint; *level 3,* water level at the hock joint; *level 4,* water level at the bottom of the foot.

of propulsion was decreased when water was filled to the level of the greater trochanter. Joint flexion was increased with underwater treadmill walking. In general, joint flexion was greatest with water levels at or higher than the joint of interest. Therefore the advantages of additional joint flexion achieved with swimming are also present with underwater treadmill walking, but full extension of joints also occurs with treadmill walking, which is not the case with swimming.

A flotation device, such as a children's water wing, applied to a limb may also be used to alter joint kinematics. For example, if additional motion of all joints of a particular limb is desired, the device may be placed on the distal limb. If additional joint extension and increased stance time are desired, the device may be placed on the collateral limb. The altered sensation and unbalanced buoyancy of opposite limbs contribute to altered joint kinematics and may used to achieve certain goals during rehabilitation.

The following case demonstrates the usefulness of aquatic therapy in restoring physical condition to a dog that had lost a great deal of function.

Case Report

Blackie, a 2-year-old hound dog, was presented with a nonunion fracture of the left femur. The fracture was a short oblique fracture of the midshaft of the femur. The original repair consisted of an intramedullary pin and cerclage wire. The fixation devices were prematurely removed 2 months after surgery. Blackie refractured the same bone 4 weeks later. At this time, an external skeletal fixator was placed. Complications associated with pin loosening and continued instability of the fracture site resulted in placement of an intramedullary pin. At this point, the stifle was stiff. A recheck examination 2 weeks after surgery indicated that the dog was not using the leg. The dog was barely weight-bearing while standing and was non–weight-bearing at a walk. Twelve weeks after the last surgery, all fixation devices were removed. Following pin removal, instability of the fracture site was palpated.

Seven months after the original fracture, Blackie was examined at a surgery referral clinic. At that time, the dog would occasionally toe-touch the limb during walking, but would hold the affected limb up most of the time. In addition, the leg was painful, and the stifle had only 5 to 10 degrees ROM. The quadriceps muscles were adhered to the fracture callus and the femur. Adhesions and excessive callus were removed to increase the stifle ROM. A bone plate was applied to stabilize the fracture and align the bone. Following surgery, maximum flexion of the knee was 85 degrees and maximum extension was 160 degrees.

The day after surgery, a nonsteroidal antiinflammatory drug was administered twice daily. ROM and stretching exercises were performed on the hip, stifle, and hock for 20 repetitions, holding each stretch for 10 seconds. These were performed four to five times daily. Following ROM exercises, an ice pack was applied to the area for 10 minutes. Two days after surgery, stifle extension was 155 degrees and flexion was 70 degrees. Three days after surgery, Blackie was discharged from the hospital with instructions to limit activity to leash walks only and to perform ROM exercises four to five times daily. The therapy sessions were to be preceded by hot packs, and cold packs were to be applied after therapy. Following suture removal, swimming was recommended. The owner was warned that Blackie might never regain full function of the limb, because of the stiff stifle.

For 2 months the owner continued performing the ROM exercises and walking. In addition, following suture removal, the owner would allow the dog to swim in a river daily. The length of time was gradually increased, so that he was swimming for 30 minutes daily by 1 month after surgery.

One month after surgery, Blackie returned for a recheck examination. It was noted that the stifle had improved ROM. The thigh muscles were increasing in size and the dog was using the leg quite well, although there was still an abnormal gait at faster speeds. Radiographically, there was continued but incomplete healing of the fracture site. Blackie was discharged with instructions to continue physical rehabilitation and increase the length of leash walks.

The swimming activity was continued, and the dog was exercised up and down hills by the owner. This activity was continued daily with the amount of hill activity increasing to 1 mile by 8 weeks after surgery.

Twelve weeks after surgery, Blackie returned for a recheck examination. At this time, Blackie had full flexion (35 degrees) and extension (170 degrees) of the stifle. There was a slight limp at a faster gait, but there were no signs of pain and there was increased musculature of the left rear limb. The fracture had reached union, and return to full activity was recommended.

Although several exercises were used in the management of this case, the early swimming activity was likely instrumental in the recovery of the dog. Because swimming was allowed very soon after surgery, the dog was able to actively flex and extend the stifle joint and contract and relax muscle groups with minimal weight-bearing activity. The gradual reintroduction of weight-bearing activity as the fracture site became more stable enhanced rehabilitation. In this case, the rehabilitation was primarily performed by the owner after careful instruction, and with minimal facilities.

REFERENCES

1. Haralson KM: Therapeutic pool programs, *J Clin Management* 5:510-513, 1988.
2. Hecox B, Mehreteab TA, Weisberg J: *Physical agents: a comprehensive text for physical therapists,* Norwalk, Conn, 1994, Appleton & Lange.
3. Bates A, Hanson N: *Aquatic exercise therapy,* Philadelphia, 1996, W.B. Saunders.
4. Edlich RF et al: Bioengineering principles of hydrotherapy, *J Burn Care Rehab* 8:579-584, 1987.
5. Skinner AT, Thompson AM, eds: *Duffield's exercise in water,* ed 3, London, 1983, Bailliere Tindall.
6. Jamison L, Ogden D: *Aquatic therapy using PNF patterns.* Tucson, Ariz, 1994, Therapy Skill Builders.
7. Geigle PR et al: Aquatic physical therapy for balance: the interaction of somatosensory and hydrodynamic principles, *J Aquat Phys Ther* 5:4-10, 1997.
8. Hay J: *The biomechanics of sports techniques,* Englewood Cliffs, NJ, 1978, Prentice-Hall.
9. Roberson JA, Crowe CT: *Engineering fluid mechanics,* Boston, 1985, Houghton Mifflin.
10. McLean SP, Hinrichs RN: Sex differences in the center of buoyancy location of competitive swimmers, *J Sports Sci* 16:373-383, 1998.
11. Harrison RA, Bulstrode S: Percentage weight-bearing during partial immersion in hydrotherapy pool, *Physiother Pract* 3:60-63, 1987.
12. Thein JM, Brody LT: Aquatic-based rehabilitation and training for the elite athlete, *J Orthop Sports Phys Ther* 27:32-41, 1998.
13. Levine D, Tragauer V, Millis DL: Percentage of normal weight bearing during partial immersion at various depths in dogs, Proceedings of the Second International Symposium on Rehabilitation and Physical Therapy in Veterinary Medicine, Knoxville, Tenn, 2002.
14. Johns KM: Aquatic therapy: therapeutic treatment for today's patient, *Phys Ther Prod,* May:24-25, 1993.
15. Bueche F: *Principles of physics,* ed 4, New York, 1982, McGraw-Hill.
16. Babb RW, Simelson-Warr A: Manual techniques of the lower extremities in aquatic physical therapy, *J Aquat Phys Ther* 14:7-15, 1996.
17. Bravo G et al: A weight-bearing, water-based exercise program for osteopenic women: its impact on bone, functional fitness, and well-being. *Arch Phys Med Rehab* 78:1375-1379, 1997.
18. Speer KP et al: A role for hydrotherapy in shoulder rehabilitation. *Am J Sports Med* 21:850-853, 1993.
19. Whitley JD, Schoene LL: Comparison of heart rate responses: water walking versus treadmill walking, *Phys Ther* 67:1501-1504, 1987.
20. Johnson BL et al: Comparison of oxygen uptake and heart rate during exercises on land and in water, *Phys Ther* 57:273-278, 1977.
21. Evans BW, Cureton KJ, Purvis JW: Metabolic and circulatory responses to walking and jogging in water, *Res Q* 49:442-449, 1978.
22. Hall J et al: Cardiorespiratory responses to underwater treadmill walking in healthy females. *Eur J Appl Physiol* 77:278-284, 1998.
23. Melton-Rogers S et al: Cardiorespiratory responses of patients with rheumatoid arthritis during bicycle riding and running in water, *Phys Ther* 76:1058-1065, 1996.
24. Tovin BJ et al: Comparison of the effects of exercise in water and on land on the rehabilitation of patients with intra-articular anterior cruciate ligament reconstructions, *Phys Ther* 74:710-719, 1994.
25. Kelsey DD, Tyson E: A new method of training for the lower extremity using unloading, *J Orthop Sports Phys Ther* 19:218-223, 1994.
26. Templeton MS, Booth DL, O'Kelly WD: Effects of aquatic therapy on joint flexibility and functional ability in subjects with rheumatic disease, *J Orthop Sports Phys Ther* 23:376-381, 1996.
27. Suomi R, Lindauer S: Effectiveness of arthritis foundation aquatic program on strength and range of motion in women with arthritis, *J Aging Phys Activity* 5:341-351, 1997.
28. Avellini BA, Shapiro Y, Pandolf KB: Cardio-respiratory physical training in water and on land, *Eur J Appl Physiol* 50:255-263, 1983.
29. Perk J, Perk L, Boden C: Cardiorespiratory adaptation of COPD patients to physical training on land and in water, *Eur Resp J* 9:248-252, 1996.
30. Choukroun ML, Varene P: Adjustments in oxygen transport during head-out immersion in water at different temperatures, *J Appl Physiol* 68:1475-1480, 1990.
31. Turner A, Higgens M, Craddock JC: Disinfection of immersion tanks (Hubbard) in a hospital burn unit, *Arch Environ Health* 28:101-104, 1974.
32. Millis DL et al: A preliminary study of early physical therapy following surgery for cranial cruciate ligament rupture in dogs. In *Proc 24th Annu Conf Vet Orthoped Soc,* 1997, p 39.
33. Taylor RA: Post-surgical physical therapy: the missing link, *Comp Contin Educ Pract Vet* 14:1583-1593, 1982.
34. Millis DL, Levine D: The role of exercise and physical modalities in the treatment of osteoarthritis, *Vet Clin North Am Small Anim Pract* 27:913-930, 1997.
35. Marsolais GS et al: Kinematic comparison of swimming and terrestrial motion in normal dogs and dogs stabilized for cranial cruciate ligament rupture. In *Proc 29th Annu Conf Vet Orthoped Soc* 2002, p 45.
36. Jackson A et al: Joint kinematics of dogs walking on ground and aquatic treadmills. In *Proc 2nd Int Symp Rehabil Phys Ther Vet Med,* Knoxville, Tenn, 2002, p 191.

C h a p t e r   1 6

Superficial Thermal Modalities

Kristinn Heinrichs

Superficial heat and cold have been used for centuries to manage soft tissue and joint injuries with specific goals of relieving pain, altering the physiologic processes underlying tissue healing, and affecting the plasticity of connective tissue, including muscle, tendon, ligament, and joint capsule. Superficial heat and cold may be delivered through hot or cold packs, hot or cold whirlpools, luminous or nonluminous infrared, ice massage, contrast baths, or cryokinetics. This chapter will focus on the physical principles governing the absorption of heat, the physiologic effects, and the clinical application of heat and cold. The primary goal of any thermal modality is to facilitate the ultimate therapeutic healing modality of exercise.

Electrophysical agents may be used for cryotherapy (the application of cold, using cold packs, ice massage, cold whirlpool, vapor coolant sprays, or cold compression units) or thermotherapy (the application of heat using moist heat or hydrocollator packs, paraffin baths, warm whirlpool, or infrared lamps). Cryotherapy is most effectively used immediately following trauma (accidental or intentional, as in surgical procedures) to provide analgesia, reduce inflammation and its sequelae, control bleeding, and reduce muscle spasm.

Cryokinetics combines cryotherapy with motion (passive, active-assisted, or active) to facilitate normal, pain-free movement, and to reduce edema through muscle pump action to return lymphatic fluid to the vascular system. The primary benefit of cryokinetics is to facilitate the patient's ability to perform pain-free exercise early in the rehabilitation process as long as the level of exercise remains below levels that cause further injury. As signs of acute inflammation begin to subside, the clinician may elect to transition to the use of heat. Contrast baths—alternating hot and cold baths—are most appropriate during the early subacute phase of tissue healing or in cases of chronic edema.

Superficial heat is best applied before performing flexibility exercises to take advantage of the benefits of tissue temperature elevation, including vasodilation that increases tissue oxygenation and transport of metabolites to exercising tissue, increased rate of enzymatic and biochemical reactions that may facilitate tissue healing, and altered viscoelastic properties leading to increased soft tissue extensibility, decreased joint stiffness, and increased range of motion. However, heat applied too early in the healing process may result in increased acute inflammation and possibly increase enzymatic activity detrimental to cartilage (e.g., collagenase and protease).

The Physics of Thermotherapy

Thermotherapy applications fall in the infrared portion of the electromagnetic spectrum just beyond the wavelength and frequency ranges for visible light.[1] The shorter the wavelength, the greater the frequency and depth of penetration. The thermal electrophysical modalities discussed in this chapter fall within the category of "near infrared" and possess shorter wavelengths than electrical stimulating currents. Therefore infrared electrophysical agents penetrate to a shallower depth compared to electrical stimulating currents. The biologic effects of electromagnetic radiation depend on the frequency used, duration of exposure, tissue characteristics, and power density.[1]

Electromagnetic energy and its transmission through the body are governed by several physical laws. The first law is the Arndt-Schultz Principle[2]: Tissue must absorb the energy produced by the thermal agent to stimulate the tissue's normal function. If the energy absorbed is insufficient to stimulate the tissue, there is no effect. If too much energy is absorbed, tissue damage may occur. The second law, related to the first, is the Law of Grotthus-Draper, which determines the fate of the energy. If a tissue does not absorb the energy, it is transmitted to deeper tissue layers. If the energy is absorbed more superficially, less energy will be transmitted to deeper layers and less penetration of the energy occurs. When electromagnetic energy encounters the body's tissues, it has three possible fates: it may be reflected (e.g., reflected from the skin's surface), it may be refracted (e.g., at the interface between the dermis and subcutaneous fat), or it may be absorbed (e.g., by muscle). The estimated depth of penetration for most infrared thermal modalities (cold or hot packs, whirlpools, paraffin baths, luminous infrared devices) is approximately 1 cm.

The application of superficial thermal modalities is governed by the physical laws of heat transfer, primarily conduction and radiation. Most thermal techniques transfer energy by conduction. Energy travels down a thermal gradient, with energy (heat) being removed from tissue, rather than cold being added. During cryotherapy, heat from body tissues is transferred to the cold modality via conduction provided there is direct contact between the two bodies. Heat always travels from the warmer object to the cooler.[3] According to Knight,[4] the rate at which heat transfer occurs depends on the following factors:

- *The temperature difference between the body and the modality:* The greater the difference, the more quickly the transfer of heat occurs.
- *Regeneration of body heat and modality cooling:* As the body tissue gives up heat, the heat lost is replaced by circulating blood and surrounding tissues. Cold penetrates more deeply than superficial heating modalities. For example, after a 20-minute ice pack application to the gastrocnemius muscle, the intramuscular temperature declined more slowly than the subcutaneous temperature (and never reached as cold a temperature as the subcutaneous tissue) (Figure 16-1). When the ice pack was removed, the subcutaneous tissue temperature rose steeply, whereas the intramuscular temperature continued to decline for a period of time until both tissues were within 2° to 3° C of each other.[5]

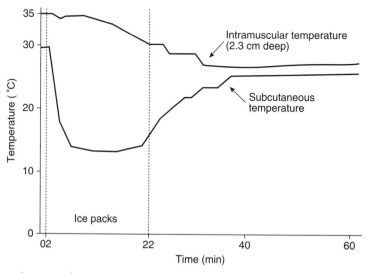

Figure 16-1   Intramuscular versus subcutaneous tissue temperature changes with cryotherapy. Intramuscular (gastrocnemius) and subcutaneous temperatures during and after a 20-min ice pack application. Note that intramuscular temperature declined much more slowly than subcutaneous temperature and continued to decrease after the ice pack was removed. (Redrawn from Hartviksen K: Ice therapy in spasticity, *Acta Neurol Scand* 38(suppl 3):79-84, 1962.)

- *The heat storage capacity of the cold modality:* The more energy it takes to convert a solid to a liquid (e.g., ice to water), the greater its latent heat of fusion and its capacity to remove heat from a tissue. For example, crushed ice packs require more energy for this conversion to occur as compared to semisolid gel packs. Therefore ice packs cool tissues for a longer time and to a greater extent than gel packs.
- *The size of the modality:* The larger the modality (e.g., cold pack), the greater the energy storage capacity.
- *The area of the body in contact with the modality:* For example, cold-water immersion results in the greatest temperature decline compared to other methods of cold delivery because a greater surface area is in contact with the cooling modality.[6] Ethyl chloride vapocoolant sprays result in the least temperature decline and provide only superficial cooling because of the relatively small surface area cooled.
- *The application duration:* The longer the contact time between the two surfaces, the more opportunity for energy exchange to occur and heat to be removed from the body.
- *Individual variability:* Individuals with lower body fat percentage exchange heat more quickly than those with greater amounts of subcutaneous fat.

Regardless of the cold pack type (ice versus commercially available cold packs), the surface temperature drops immediately after application of the cold pack and reaches its maximum effect in approximately 30 minutes in humans. Following removal, the surface temperature rises rapidly, although it may not reach preapplication levels for more than 60 minutes after removal from the skin.[4] Rewarming in animals follows a similar pattern, and it may take several hours after removal of the cold pack for complete rewarming to occur. A 30-minute cold gel pack application to the stifle joint of 10 healthy bulls decreased the intraarticular temperature 6.6° ± 1.0° C for 215 minutes.[7] Studies in dogs have reported similar decreases in intraarticular temperature.[6,8]

Physiologic Effects of Cryotherapy

Cryotherapy is used during the acute phase of tissue injury and healing to mitigate the effects and sequelae of tissue injury, and after exercise during rehabilitation to minimize adverse secondary inflammatory responses. The primary physiologic effects of cryotherapy include vasoconstriction, reduced blood flow, reduced cellular metabolism and permeability, decreased sensory and motor nerve conduction velocity, analgesia, prevention or reduction of trauma-induced edema, decreased muscle spasm, and temporary reduction of spasticity before exercise.[9,10]

During the inflammatory phase of tissue healing, increased permeability of the microvasculature occurs as a result of histamine and bradykinin release. In addition, these chemical mediators cause vasodilation and increased blood flow to the area. These events, coupled with hypoxic cellular changes, are primary factors in the formation of edema. (Centrally mediated sympathetic vasoconstriction helps to reduce edema as a result of decreased hydrostatic pressure.) The primary role of cryotherapy during the inflammatory phase is to reduce the metabolic rate of the injured tissue, which in turn results in decreased metabolite production and metabolic heat.[11] In addition, the decreased metabolic rate limits further injury and aids the tissue in surviving the cellular hypoxia that occurs after injury.[4]

The Hunting reaction, first described by Lewis in 1930, refers to the cyclical temperature oscillation of 2° to 6° C every 8 to 15 minutes after the tissue temperature approaches 2° C. This effect begins 20 to 40 minutes after cryotherapy application. He attributed these oscillations to cold-induced vasodilation (CIVD) as an attempt to protect tissues from cold-induced damage. However, his results have been incorrectly and widely applied to the sports medicine literature in an attempt to explain the success of cryokinetics.[2] Knight et al[12] replicated Lewis' experiment and concluded that Lewis' observation during cold immersion and subsequent rapid increase in temperature after cryotherapy are due to temperature effects, not CIVD and subsequent increased blood flow. Based on these studies, the primary benefits of cryotherapy are twofold: decrease in cellular metabolism and analgesic effects to permit cryoexercise to facilitate rehabilitation.[4,12]

The response to cryotherapy treatment is also mediated by the nervous system. Peripheral thermal receptors are categorized as cutaneous myelinated type III or A delta, which are sensitive to pricking or sharp pain and cold, unmyelinated type IV or C receptors for aching pain, and unmyelinated type IV or C cutaneous receptors for pain and temperature (Table 16-1).

The unmyelinated cutaneous receptors respond to absolute temperature and the rate of temperature change.[13] The cold-sensitive receptors begin firing at 36° C and increase their firing rate until reaching their maximum at approximately 25° C. The firing frequency drops sharply at temperatures below 20° C and is minimal by the time the receptors are cooled to 10° to 12° C. Conversely, the warm receptors also begin firing at 33° to 36° C, rapidly reach their maximum firing frequency at 43° C, and drop to a minimal firing rate at 45° C.[14] Both the hot and cold receptors rapidly adapt to temperature changes.

Central thermosensitive neurons in the preoptic and anterior hypothalamus respond to temperature changes with autonomic responses to stimulate heat retention by the body by altering cutaneous blood flow and thermoregulatory behavior such as panting. Figure 16-2 illustrates this central hypothalamic control of thermoregulation. The anterior hypothalamus also controls thermoinsensitive neurons, such as those that are sensitive to osmolarity and glucose concentration.[15,16] Stimulating the posterior hypothalamus by heating does not result in the autonomic responses characteristic of the anterior hypothalamus, but behavioral responses to the heat load occur. Local warming of the medulla increases respiratory frequency. Autonomic thermoregulatory responses also take place at the spinal cord level.[16] The sympathetic nervous system response to thermal load is also chemically mediated through the release of the neurotransmitters epinephrine and norepinephrine from the adrenal medulla to induce cutaneous vasoconstriction.[15]

A primary effect of cryotherapy is analgesia and the concomitant reduction of reflex muscle spasm. This may be due to the decreased nerve conduction velocity that occurs when nerves are cooled. This relationship, known as the Q10 effect, is thought to be linear until 10° C, when neural transmission is blocked.[17,18] Nerve cooling also increases the duration of the refractory period, the time when a nerve cannot be stimulated by a second impulse.[19]

■ ▨ ■ Table 16-1   Sensory Receptors: Anatomy, Location, and Function

Receptor	Type	Sensory Nerve Classification	Location	Diameter (μm)	Conduction Velocity (m/sec)	Sensory Function
Sensory (afferent) myelinated	A	Ia	Muscle	12-20	72-120	Muscle spindle primary ending (or 1-degree ending)
	A	Ib	Tendon	12-20	72-120	Golgi tendon organ Rate of muscle shortening
	A	II	Muscle	6-12	36-72	Muscle spindle, secondary ending (or 2-degree ending) muscle length changes
	A	II	Skin	6-12	36-72	Vibration, discriminatory touch, pacinian corpuscles
	A	III	Skin	1-6	6-36	Pricking, sharp pain, temperature (cold), light touch
Unmyelinated	C	IV	Muscle	~1	0.5-2.0	Aching pain
	C	IV	Skin	~1	0.5-2.0	Pain, temperature

From Guyton AC: Sensory receptors and their basic mechanisms of action. In *Textbook of medical physiology*, Philadelphia, 1986, WB Saunders, p 578.

Conversely, raising the subcutaneous tissue temperature increases sensory nerve conduction velocity, with the greatest effect occurring during the initial 2° C temperature elevation.[20] Another mechanism postulated for the analgesic effect afforded by cryotherapy is that the cold receptors are overstimulated by cryotherapy, resulting in pain control at the spinal level by preventing pain transmission to higher centers via the spinal gate control theory of pain transmission.

Cryotherapy may also decrease muscle spasm through a number of proposed mechanisms. Decreasing pain may decrease muscle guarding or spasm associated with an injury. The muscle spindle receptors and Golgi tendon organ receptors fire more slowly when cooled, although the effect is less pronounced on the Golgi tendon organs.[21] Sudden cooling has an excitatory effect on the muscle spindle, resulting in increased alpha motoneuron activity and increased muscle guarding. As the temperature continues to decrease, primary spindle afferent activity diminishes.[17] Muscle spasm, resulting from the pain–spasm–pain cycle, stimulates the static stretch response of the type II tissue afferents. Applying superficial heat until the temperature is above 42° C decreases the muscle spindle discharge rate while it increases the firing rate of the Golgi tendon organ.[21] This sequence of events results in a decrease in the firing rate of the alpha motor neuron. Thus cold may raise the threshold stimulus for muscle spindle activity, decreasing muscle spasm.[22]

Thermal effects on strength and endurance have also been observed by a number of authors. The force-velocity curve of muscle contraction shifts downward with decreasing temperature.[23] For a given concentric contraction velocity, cooler muscles have a lower force output. Interestingly, proprioception, joint position, and balance remain largely unaffected by cryotherapy.[24-26] Although most authors agree that changes in muscle torque production occur with cooling, it is less clear whether those effects are specific to a particular contraction mode (concentric acceleration or eccentric deceleration). One group of researchers reported that eccentric muscle action is augmented following cryotherapy,[27] while another group found increases in concentric, but not eccentric, torque.[28] Still others found no effects on peak torque, but increased muscle endurance following cooling.[29] Functionally, vertical jump performance, an indicator of lower-extremity explosive power, is adversely affected by cryotherapy.[30,31] These findings suggest that caution must be used in making recommendations for performance following cryotherapy. Clearly the literature on this subject is undecided as to the specific effects of cold (both immediate and delayed) on muscle strength. These findings have the most implication for dogs who are engaged in work or competitive athletic pursuits. It also

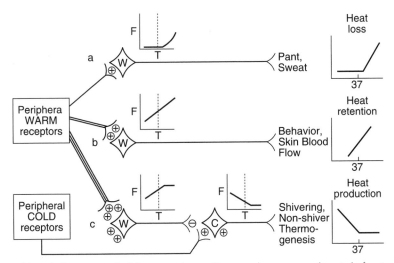

Figure 16-2 *Central hypothalamic control of thermoregulation. Diagram shows neuronal control of various thermoregulatory responses. +, Excitatory input; –, inhibitory control; dashed line, thermoneutral temperature; C, cold-sensitive neuron; F, neuronal firing rate; T, hypothalamic temperature; W, warm-sensitive neuron. (Redrawn from Boulant JA, Dean JB: Temperature receptors in the central nervous system, Ann Rev Physiol 48:639-654, 1986.)*

requires that the clinician understand the physiology and biomechanics of muscle actions and sport demands. Cold and exercise are an effective combination in the treatment of acute musculoskeletal dysfunction unless restrictions in flexibility are present.[32,33] Combining movement with cold allows for relatively greater pain-free exercise and assists in the muscle pump activity to reduce acute injury-related edema.

Cryotherapy Applications

A variety of methods are available for applying cryotherapy to dogs. Selection of the method depends on the desired effects and is influenced by the stage of tissue repair, physiologic goals (analgesia, edema reduction, lymphatic pumping, and so forth), depth of penetration desired, treatment area, and activity or exercise goals. Cryotherapy is particularly helpful in the management of acute inflammation (bursitis, tenosynovitis, tendinitis, and so forth) where application of heat causes additional pain and edema. Cryotherapy methods include ice packs (homemade, commercial cryogel packs, elastic wraps), cryomassage, ice bath immersion, contrast baths, and vapor coolant (ethyl chloride) spray (Figure 16-3). To prevent frostbite or cold-induced injuries, it is critical to observe the skin for response to cold. Near the end of a 20-minute treatment, the skin may normally be erythematous, but pale or white skin is an indication that cold-induced tissue damage may be occurring. The range of expected sensations during cryotherapy include an initial sensation of cold, followed by burn, sting, and ache, and finally a numb sensation.[12] For most injuries, application times of 20 to 30 minutes may not be sufficient to cool the injured tissues; the notion of "maximum benefit in 20 minutes" has not been substantiated with research.[4] Because animal patients cannot describe these sensations, careful observation of the animal's behavioral responses and skin condition every few minutes during the treatment session is critical.

Ice packs

Several methods may be used to apply superficial cold (see Figure 16-3). The simplest method of ice application is to wrap a freezer bag containing crushed ice in a thin damp cloth (such as a pillowcase) and apply directly over the affected area. Before sealing the bag, remove the excess air. The addition of a compression wrap to secure the bag to the body also insulates the body surface against air, resulting in additional reduction of surface temperature during cooling and slower rewarming following removal of the ice.[34] If crushed ice is not available, cold packs may be prepared by mixing 3 parts water to 1 part rubbing alcohol, double bagging with sealed bags, and placing in a freezer. The resulting slush may then be molded around irregular body parts. If the mixture freezes in a household freezer, more alcohol can be added to the mix. If it is too liquid, more water can be added. To prevent skin damage, apply a towel or cloth to prevent direct contact of the ice pack with the animal's skin. Apply the cryotherapy treatment for 15 to 25 minutes at a time, inspecting the tissue for its response after the first 5 to 10 minutes. Monitor closely for signs of frostbite.

The latent heat of fusion is lower for the alcohol-water mix than for water alone; therefore it performs similarly to crushed ice alone, but a lower temperature. Use caution with the water-alcohol mix because the potential for cold-induced injuries is greater. Never apply this mixture directly to the skin; instead apply using a layer of toweling, either wet or dry

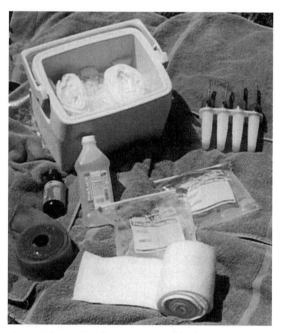

Figure 16-3   Cryotherapy options (clockwise starting top right): Popsicle-type molds for ice massage, alcohol-water slush plastic bags, cotton wraps, commercial cold wraps, flouromethane cold spray.

(wet conducts cold more rapidly). Commercial cold packs may also be applied. Packs that freeze solid (e.g., DuraKold) perform better than frozen gel packs, which contain gelatin or antifreeze to make them more pliable (Figure 16-4).[4] *Cold packs containing ethylene glycol antifreeze should not be used in animals because the contents are toxic if ingested.* As with the alcohol-water mixture, use caution because the risk for frostbite is greater than when using a crushed ice bag (Figure 16-4).

Artificial ice cubes (e.g., Cold Gold), manufactured by the sheet, may be trimmed to fit the body part and secured with elastic wrap or used with commercial custom-designed wraps (e.g., CanineIcer, www.canineicer.com) (Figures 16-5 and 16-6). They offer the advantage of ice cubes without the mess of melting ice. Used often in postoperative cryotherapy applications to minimize postoperative edema and pain, the sheets are somewhat pliable and may be refrozen.

Cold-Compression Units

Cold compression units, which are commercially available, combine compression with cryotherapy. Cold water circulates in a fabricated sleeve which is snugly applied to provide compression to the area. Combined with elevation, this method of treatment is highly effective during the acute phase of tissue inflammation and healing.

Cold Immersion and Contrast Baths

Cold immersion, because it exposes the greatest body surface area to cold, results in the greatest decreases in tissue temperature. The body part is immersed in an ice "slush" bath as part of the immediate first aid following injury (Figure 16-7). The analgesia from the immersion allows the animal to perform cryokinetics with relative ease. Contrast baths, in which the affected body part is immersed in cold water followed by immersion in hot water, have long been used as a method to induce cyclic vasodilation and vasoconstriction to facilitate flushing debris and inflam-

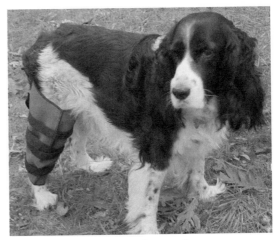

Figure 16-5   Canine stifle icer.

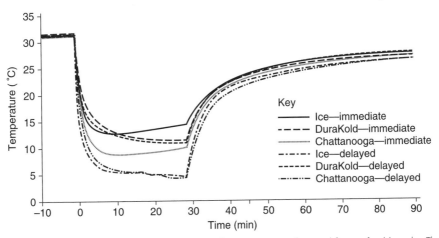

Figure 16-4   The effect of the heat of fusion can be seen in this comparison of several forms of cold packs. The crushed ice and DuraKold packs cool the skin more than the Chattanooga frozen gel pack. The effect is even greater when application is delayed for 20 min after the packs are removed from their cooling devices. (Knight KL et al: A re-examination of Lewis' cold-induced vasodilation in the finger and ankle, *Athletic Train* 15:238-250, 1980.)

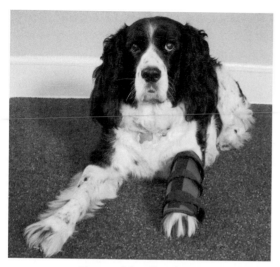

Figure 16-6   Carpal icer.

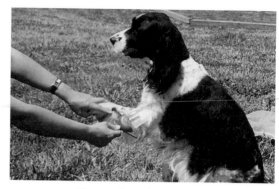

Figure 16-8   Ice massage.

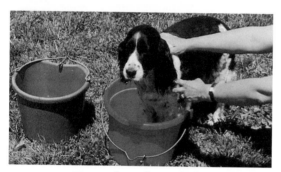

Figure 16-7   Contrast baths.

matory mediators from the injured area. However, some authors do not agree with this proposed mechanism.[4] Clinically, it may be appropriate to use contrast baths during the transition from acute to subacute injury management. The body part is immersed in alternating cold and hot baths, in a ratio anywhere from 4C:1H (4 minutes cold, 1 minute hot) near the end of the acute phase, to 2H:2C (2 minutes hot, 2 minutes cold). This cycle is repeated three to five times for a total of 15 to 30 minutes. If the injury is relatively acute, the final cycle should be in the cold bath to help reduce edema formation. If contrast baths are used before exercise in subacute or chronic conditions, then the final cycle should be in the hot bath. If used as a transition from the acute to subacute stages of tissue healing, the cold:hot ratio should be weighted more toward a cold emphasis (e.g., 4C:1H) progressing to 2H:2C and 3H:1C depending on

the clinical evaluation before treatment. Specific ratios of hot to cold depend on the clinical goals of the treatment.

Ice Massage

Ice massage is a very quick and effective method of applying cryotherapy to the affected area with the muscle in a position of gentle stretch (Figure 16-8). Molds to form a cylinder of ice with an application stick are commercially available. Placing tongue depressors in paper cups filled with water and freezing them is a low-cost alternative for making "ice Popsicles" to perform ice massage. Ice massage is applied parallel to the muscle fibers. The pressure from the ice massage stimulates the mechanoreceptors more than other forms of cryotherapy.[4] This technique is particularly useful for small, irregular areas. Treatment time is generally 5 to 10 minutes or until the affected area is erythematous and numb.

Vapocoolant Sprays

Vapocoolant sprays have long been used to treat trigger points in humans.[35] However, their ability to cool is the least effective of all the methods and results in cooling only of the superficial cutaneous tissue. To use the vapocoolant spray to treat trigger points, place the affected muscle in a position of slight stretch and spray from proximal to distal at a rate of 10 cm/sec from a distance of 30 cm (12 inches) (Figure 16-9). Repeat four or five times until the affected area has been covered. Because of the dog's hair, the effectiveness of this technique is questionable. These sprays can also be potentially dangerous if they accidentally get in the animal's eyes or are ingested.

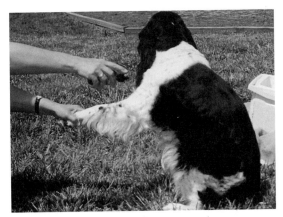

Figure 16-9 Flourimethane vapocoolant spray.

Indications for Cryotherapy

Cryotherapy is best applied during the acute inflammatory phase of tissue healing and after exercise to minimize any inflammatory response. Cryotherapy is effective in reducing pain, particularly acute postoperative pain. In addition, it is effective in reducing edema when combined with compression and elevation. Cold also decreases the metabolic rate of reactions involved in tissue injury and healing. At joint temperatures of 30° C (86° F) or lower, the activity of cartilage-degrading enzymes, including collagenase, elastase, hyaluronidase, and protease, is inhibited.[36] If cryotherapy is applied during the subacute or proliferative phase of tissue healing, recovery may be impaired. When there are minimal signs of inflammation and the patient tolerates simple range-of-motion and flexibility exercises without an increase in swelling or pain, the treatment may progress to heat.

Treatment Duration and Frequency

The duration and frequency of cryotherapy depend on the severity of the injury, the area of injury, and the desired outcome. Treatment times may be cycled to 30 to 45 minutes on, followed by an equal amount of time off. Practically, cryotherapy is typically administered three to six times daily. It should be continued until the healing tissue moves into the proliferative (subacute) phase of healing. Cryotherapy should be applied to support the goal of pain-free exercise and may also be applied following an exercise session to minimize reactive swelling and pain.

Precautions and Contraindications

Although the application of superficial cold and ice is relatively safe, there are conditions in which the use of cryotherapy is contraindicated. The clinician is cautioned to observe for signs of frostbite during and after cryotherapy application. If the individual has a history of frostbite to the area, further cold application is contraindicated. Cryotherapy should not be used in individuals who are cold-sensitive or demonstrate a response, such as cold urticaria, to the application of cold. Cold urticaria causes wheals and swelling on skin (due to a release of histamine) when the animal is exposed to a reduction in temperature. In dogs with cold sensitivites, care should be taken not to expose large areas of the skin to the cold and should not swim in cold temperatures.

Caution should be exercised when applying cryotherapy around superficial peripheral nerves because cases of cold-induced nerve palsy of the ulnar and superficial peroneal nerves have been reported in people. Knight estimates the incidence of cold-induced neuropathies to be less than 0.0011%.[4] Cold should also not be used in patients with generalized or localized vascular compromise or who possess an impaired thermoregulatory capacity. Use caution in applying cold over open wounds, areas of poor sensation, or in very young or old dogs.

Physiologic Effects of Heat

Heat is used in rehabilitation for its hemodynamic, neuromuscular, metabolic, and connective-tissue effects. Heat is most appropriately applied after the acute inflammatory phase of tissue healing has resolved. Premature application of heat may exacerbate swelling, pain, heat, and functional loss. If in doubt, apply cold or contrast baths until the dog is well into the subacute, or proliferative, stage of tissue healing.

Superficial heating agents such as hot packs or hot baths have the greatest effect on cutaneous blood vessels, resulting in the greatest temperature change within the first 1 cm of tissue depth. Increased superficial tissue temperature results in the release of chemical mediators, such as histamine and prostaglandins, which result in vasodilation. The second mechanism for vasodilation occurs with the stimulation of cutaneous thermoreceptors that synapse on the cutaneous blood vessels, causing the release of bradykinin to relax the smooth muscle walls, resulting in vasodilation. A third mechanism for vasodilation involves the reduction in sympathetic activation via spinal dorsal root ganglia to reduce smooth muscle contraction, resulting in vasodilation at the application site and indirectly to the cutaneous blood vessels of the extremities.[36] These vasodilatory mechanisms do not significantly affect blood flow in skeletal muscle since skeletal muscle blood flow is heavily influenced by other physiologic and metabolic factors. Exercise is the best means to increase blood flow to skeletal muscle.[37]

The neuromuscular effects of heat, in contrast to those of cold, include increased nerve conduction velocity and decreased latency time for both sensory and motor nerves. Nerve conduction velocity increases 2 m/sec for every 1° C (1.8° F) increase in temperature.[36] Muscle relaxation occurs as a result of a decreased firing rate of type II muscle spindle afferents and gamma efferents, and an increased firing rate of type II fibers of the Golgi tendon organs (see Table 16-1). These, in turn, contribute to a decrease in firing of the alpha motoneuron to the extrafusal muscle fiber, resulting in muscle relaxation. Heat lowers the stimulus threshold for muscle spindle activity.[22]

The pain threshold may be elevated with localized heat application. Stimulation of the cutaneous thermal receptors has been proposed to inhibit the transmission of pain at the dorsal horn of the spinal cord via the gate control mechanism. Second, vasodilatation increases the blood flow to reduce ischemia of injured tissue, resulting in decreased activity of the pain receptors. Decreased muscle spasm further relieves pressure of the muscles on blood vessels, reducing ischemia and promoting blood flow.

Heat accelerates biochemical reactions, both enzymatic and metabolic, up to a temperature of 45° C (113° F); increases above this result in decreased activity of these reactions. From 39° to 43° C (102° to 109° F), enzymatic activity increases 13% for every 1° C increase in temperature or doubles for every 10° C increase in temperature.[38] Although heat increases oxygen uptake and accelerates tissue healing, it also increases the activity of destructive enzymes, such as collagenase, and increases the catabolic rate. The oxygen-hemoglobin dissociation curve shifts to the right, making more oxygen available for tissue repair or exercise. Combined with the increased biochemical reaction rate, superficial heat may accelerate tissue healing if the tissue injury is superficial. For thermal effects in deeper tissues, ultrasound or diathermy are most appropriate. The patient's status and tolerance to treatment should be evaluated daily to determine the most appropriate treatment.

Heat causes increased connective tissue extensibility if the tendon, ligament, scar tissue, or joint capsule tissues are superficially located. Deeper musculotendinous or joint capsule structures should be heated using ultrasound or diathermy, which are capable of elevating tissue temperature at greater depths. For the maximum connective tissue plastic deformation to occur, the tissue temperature must be maintained at 40° to 45° C (104° to 113° F) for a minimum of 5 to 10 minutes while applying the stretch.[36] In cases where the viscoelastic properties of connective tissue are to be altered, the tissue must be subjected to adequate concurrent heat and stretch for a sufficiently long period of time to result in permanent tissue elongation.[39] Lower loads applied over a longer period of time during tissue heating and recooling result in less secondary tissue trauma.[40] Superficial heat may be successfully applied to reduce joint stiffness and increase the elasticity of superficial joint capsular structures to facilitate exercise.

Heat Application

Superficial thermal therapy may be applied using commercially available packs containing cornhusks, gel material that can be used for either hot or cold application, or packs containing iron filings (activation of such packs produces heat for several hours following a chemical reaction resulting in oxidation) (Figures 16-10, 16-11, and 16-12). Commercially available wraps may also be used for heat application by placing heat packs inside the wraps.

Treatment Duration and Frequency

The duration and frequency of thermal treatment depends on the severity of the injury, the stage of tissue healing, the area of the injured part, and the desired outcome. Treatment times may be cycled at 30 to 45 minutes on, followed by an equal amount of time off. Thermal modalities should be applied to support the goal of pain-free exercise, the ultimate therapeutic modality, to obtain the best results in the shortest period of time.

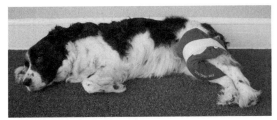

Figure 16-10 Superficial hot pack application with commercially available hot pack with straps.

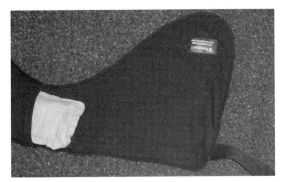

Figure 16-11 Shoulder heat pack with custom wrap (Courtesy CanineIcer, Charlottesville, VA, SofTouch hot/cold pack, PI Medical, Athens, TN).

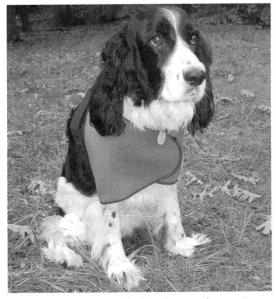

Figure 16-12 Canine shoulder heat application (www. canineicer.com).

Contraindications and Precautions for Superficial Heat Applications

Superficial heat is contraindicated during acute inflammation because it may exacerbate the inflammatory process, over an area of subcutaneous or cutaneous hemorrhage or thrombophlebitis, or over malignant tissue. Superficial heat should be used with caution in patients with poor thermoregulatory capacity, edema, impaired circulation, or over open wounds. Dogs should be monitored closely because they cannot verbalize their intolerance. A tissue burn may result if the patient is not able to dissipate the heat load via vasodilation or if too much heat (too hot or too long) is applied. Burns can be avoided by using materials that cool as the treatment progresses, by increasing the insulation layer between the patient and the hot pack, or by limiting the initial temperature increase. Monitor the skin condition before, during, and after treatment for any adverse effects.

Conclusion

Thermal heat therapy and cryotherapy are powerful adjuncts in the rehabilitation of musculoskeletal injuries in dogs. Successful management depends on an accurate assessment of the dog's presenting problems at the beginning of each treatment session. Cryotherapy and cryokinetics are most useful during the acute inflammatory stages of tissue healing. As tissue healing is established, with relatively weak hydrogen bonds it is susceptible to injury from exercise that is too aggressive or from changing from cold to heat too early, thus exacerbating the inflammatory response. After new tissue has been established and the tensile strength of the tissue continues to increase as the bonds strengthen into covalent bonds, the emphasis shifts to promoting a mobile scar, normal range of motion, and normal flexibility. In patients with limitations in these areas, concurrent application of superficial heat and flexibility exercises results in beneficial plastic changes to the tissue that may be relatively permanent. Superficial cold and heat modalities may be a very useful adjunct in a rehabilitation program to facilitate nature's ultimate therapeutic modality: controlled exercise. Selection of the appropriate modality depends largely on an understanding and accurate assessment of the stage (acute inflammatory, proliferative, or tissue remodeling) of tissue healing, an accurate clinical assessment of the dog's functional abilities, establishing appropriate treatment goals, and continued reevaluation when the patient status changes as tissue healing progresses. Any therapeutic modality (heat, cold, ultrasound, laser, etc.) should be used to facilitate the ability of the dog to participate with Mother Nature's ultimate therapeutic modality: exercise, first controlled, then free.

REFERENCES

1. Ritter HTM: Instrumentation considerations. In Michlovitz SL, editor: *Thermal agents in rehabilitation,* Philadelphia, 1996, FA Davis, pp 62-63.
2. Prentice WE: The science of therapeutic modalities. In Prentice WE, editor: *Therapeutic modalities in sports medicine,* New York, 1999, McGraw-Hill.
3. Palmer J. E, Knight KL: Ankle and thigh skin surface temperature changes with repeated ice pack application, *J Athletic Train* 31:319-323, 1996.
4. Knight KL: Temperature changes resulting from cold application. In *Cryotherapy in sport injury management,* Champaign, Ill, 1995, Human Kinetics Publishers.
5. Hartviksen K: Ice therapy in spasticity, *Acta Neurol Scand* 38(suppl 3):79-84, 1962.
6. Bocobo C et al: The effect of ice on intra-articular temperature in the knee of the dog, *Am J Phys Med Rehab* 70:181-185, 1991.
7. Kern H et al: Kryotherapie: das veralten der Gelenktemperatur unter Eisapplikation: Grundlage für die praktische Anwendung, *Wien Klin Wochenschr* 22:832-837, 1984.
8. Cobbold AF, Lewis OJ: Blood flow to the knee joint of the dog: effect of heating, cooling, and adrenaline, *J Physiol* 121:46-54, 1956.
9. McMaster W: A literary review on ice therapy in injuries, *Am J Sports Med* 5:124-126, 1977.
10. Olson J, Stravino V: A review of cryotherapy, *Phys Ther* 62:840-853, 1972.
11. Ho SSW et al: The effect of ice on blood flow and bone metabolism in knees, *Am J Sports Med* 22:537-540, 1994.
12. Knight KL et al: A re-examination of Lewis' cold-induced vasodilation in the finger and ankle, *Athletic Train* 15:238-250, 1980.
13. Yarnitsky D, Ochoa JL: Warm and cold specific somatosensory systems: psychophysical thresholds, reaction times, and peripheral conduction velocities, *Brain* 114:1819-1826, 1991.
14. Iggo A: Cutaneous thermoreceptors in primates and sub-primates, *J Physiol* 151:332-341, 1969.
15. Guyton AC: Sensory receptors and their basic mechanisms of action. In Guyton AC, editor: *Textbook of medical physiology,* Philadelphia, 1986, WB Saunders, p 578.
16. Boulant JA, Dean JB: Temperature receptors in the central nervous system, *Ann Rev Physiol* 48:639-654, 1986.
17. Lippold O, Nicholls J, Redfearn J: A study of the afferent discharge produced by cooling a mammalian muscle spindle, *J Physiol* 153:218-231, 1960.
18. Lowitzsch K, Hopf HC, Galland J: Changes of sensory conduction velocity and refractory periods with decreasing tissue temperature in man, *J Neurol* 216:218-231, 1977.
19. Evans T, Ingersoll C, Knight K: Agility following the application of cold therapy, *J Athletic Train* 30:231-234, 1995.
20. Lowdon B, Moore R: Determinants and nature of intramuscular temperature changes during cold therapy, *Am J Phys Med* 54:223-233, 1975.
21. Currier DP, Kramer JF: Sensory nerve conduction: heating effects of ultrasound and infrared, *Physiother Canada* 34:241, 1982.
22. Mense S: Effects of temperature on the discharges of muscle spindles and tendon organs, *Pflügers Arch* 374:159-166, 1978.
23. Ratanunga KW: Influence of temperature on the velocity of shortening and rate of tension development in mammalian skeletal muscle, *J Physiol* 316:35-36, 1981.
24. LaRiviere J, Osternig L: The effect of ice immersion on joint position sense, *J Sports Rehab* 3:58-67, 1994.
25. Pincivero D, Gieck J, Saliba E: Rehabilitation of a lateral ankle sprain with cryokinetic and functional progressive exercise, *J Sports Rehab* 2:200-207, 1993.
26. Thieme H, Ingersoll C, Knight K: Cooling does not affect knee proprioception, *J Athletic Train* 31:8-11, 1996.
27. Catlaw K, Arnold B, Perrin D: Effect of cold treatment on concentric and eccentric force-velocity relationship of the quadriceps femoris, *Isokinetics Evere Sci* 5:157-160, 1996.
28. Ruiz D, Myrer J, Durrant E: Cryotherapy and sequential exercise bouts following cryotherapy on concentric and eccentric strength in the quadriceps, *J Athletic Train* 28:320-323, 1993.
29. Kimura I, Gulick D, Thompson G: The effect of cryotherapy on eccentric plantar flexion peak torque and endurance, *J Athletic Train* 32:124-126, 1997.
30. Gallant S, Knight K, Ingersoll C: Cryotherapy effects on leg press and vertical jump force production, *J Athletic Train* 31:S18, 1996.
31. Grecier M, Kendrick Z, Kimura I: Immediate and delayed effects of cryotherapy on functional power and agility, *J Athletic Train* 31:S32, 1996.
32. Dufresne T, Jarzabaski K, Simmons D: Comparison of superficial and deep heating agents followed by a passive stretch on increasing the flexibility of the hamstring muscle group, *Phys Ther* 74:70, 1994.
33. Taylor B, Waring C, Brasher T: The effects of therapeutic application of heat or cold followed by static stretch on hamstring muscle length, *J Orthop Sports Phys Ther* 21:283-286, 1995.
34. Merrick MA et al: The effects of ice and compression wraps on intramuscular temperatures at various depths, *J Athletic Train* 28:236-245, 1993.
35. Travell JG, Simons DG: *Myofascial pain and dysfunction: the trigger point manual,* vols I and II, Baltimore, 1992, Williams & Wilkins.
36. Cameron MH: *Physical agents in rehabilitation: from research to practice,* Philadelphia, 1999, WB Saunders.
37. McArdle WD, Katch FI, Katch VL: *Exercise physiology: energy, nutrition, and human performance,* ed 5, Baltimore, 2001, Lippincott Williams and Wilkins.
38. Hocutt JE et al: Cryotherapy in ankle sprains, *Am J Sports Med* 10:316-319, 1992.
39. Lehmann JF: Effect of therapeutic temperatures on tendon extensibility, *Arch Phys Med Rehab* 51:481-487, 1970.
40. Sapega AA: Biophysical factors in range of motion exercises, *Phys Sports Med* 9:57, 1981.

■ C h a p t e r   1 7

Electrical Stimulation

Janna Johnson, David Levine

Terminology Used in Electrical Stimulation

Electrical stimulation (ES) is a commonly used modality in physical therapy, which is effective for many purposes, including increasing range of motion (ROM), increasing muscle strength, muscle reeducation, correction of structural abnormalities, improving muscle tone, enhancing function, pain control, accelerating wound healing, edema reduction, muscle spasm reduction, and enhancing transdermal administration of medication (iontophoresis).[1] Terminology associated with electrical stimulation can be confusing, and in 1990, a committee of the electrophysiologic section of the American Physical Therapy Association (APTA) developed the Standards of Electrotherapeutic Terminology, a document created to unify and standardize the terms and definitions used by biomedical engineers, researchers, educators, and clinicians. Historically, electrical stimulators and the terminology related to them have been referred to by their specific rehabilitative application, by the use of the inventor's name, or by the commercial companies that produced them. Examples include galvanic current, faradic current, diadynamic current, high voltage, low voltage, low frequency, medium frequency, transcutaneous electrical nerve stimulation (TENS), electrical muscle stimulation (EMS), functional electrical stimulation (FES), Russian stimulation, and interferential stimulation. Unfortunately, the multitude of names has created confusion regarding the physiologic effects and clinical results. TENS has been widely used to identify stimulators that modify pain, while neuromuscular electrical stimulators (NMESs) or electrical muscle stimulators (EMSs) have been identified with muscle reeducation, prevention of muscle atrophy, and enhanced joint movement. Accurate terminology dictates that almost all electrical stimulators are TENS units, as they work transcutaneously through surface electrodes to excite nerves. In the typical scenario where the muscle is innervated by a motor nerve, NMES is the appropriate terminology, and when a muscle is denervated and requires direct muscle fiber activation through electrical stimulation, the term EMS is used.

Neuromuscular electrical stimulation (NMES), the primary focus of this chapter, is a form of clinical electrotherapy used to treat a wide variety of physiologic disorders or injuries in humans and is beginning to be recognized as a promising treatment modality for similar disorders in veterinary patients. By definition, NMES is the administration of an electrical current generated by a stimulator that travels through leads to electrodes placed on the skin to depolarize the motor nerve and produce a skeletal muscle contraction. Stimulation of motor end plates with electrical current causes nerve depolarization and subsequent activation of muscle fibers.[2,3]

This chapter will describe the myriad potential clinical uses of electrical NMES, and therefore this term will be used throughout. In addition to the discussion of general uses of NMES, specific attention will be paid to ruptured anterior cruciate ligament (ACL)/cranial cruciate ligament (CrCL) rehabilitation because of the relatively high incidence in man and dogs and the amount of research information that is currently available on the use of NMES for knee/stifle rehabilitation. The emerging use of electrical stimulation to treat pain in the dog will also be examined.

History of Electrical Stimulation

Electricity has been used therapeutically since Scribonius Largus used an electric ray in a footbath to treat gout. Benjamin Franklin used electric shock to treat a frozen shoulder in 1757.[3] EMS has been specifically used in physical therapy since the mid-1700s, when electrostatic generators were used to treat patients with paralysis. In 1791, Galvani used galvanic current in in vitro experiments using neuromuscular preparations. By the early 1800s Faraday had invented the faradic current generator, which is the basis for most modern muscle stimulators. Documentation of NMES to reduce the loss of muscle weight and prevent atrophy in denervated muscles occurred in the early to mid twentieth century. Electrotherapy has since become commonplace in physical medicine for the restoration of muscle function after injuries, before patients are capable of voluntary exercise training.[4]

Basic Concepts of Electrical Stimulation

To understand the benefits that electrical stimulation may provide in veterinary practice, a basic explanation and definition of the electrical current parameters used is summarized in Box 17-1.

Electrical Current/Waveforms

Three types of currents are commonly used: (1) continuous direct current (Figure 17-1, A), (2) continuous alternating current (Figure 17-1, B), and (3) pulsed current (either AC or DC) (Figure 17-1, C). Continuous direct current is a unidirectional electrical current that flows for 1 second or longer; alternating current changes the direction of flow at least once every second. Continuous direct current (also called galvanic current) has been used for wound healing, iontophoresis, and in the treatment of denervated muscle. In current clinical practice it is used only for iontophoresis. Continuous alternating current is not used therapeutically, but is our typical line current. (See Box 17-2.)

■ ■ ■ BOX 17-1   Typical Parameters Available in NMES Devices

Waveform: The shape of the visual representation of pulsed current on a current/time plot or voltage/time plot. Can be symmetrical, asymmetrical, balanced, unbalanced, biphasic, monophasic, polyphasic, and so forth.

Amplitude: The current value in a monophasic pulse or for any single phase of a biphasic pulse.

Phase/pulse duration: The duration of a phase or a pulse, usually measured in microseconds.

Pulse rate or frequency: The rate of oscillation in cycles per second, expressed as pulses/sec (pps) or hertz (Hz). Often labeled as pulse rate or pulses/sec, or frequency on stimulators.

On/off time: The amount of time the stimulator is delivering current compared to the rest period between contractions, usually measured in seconds.

Ramp: The time from the leading edge of the phase at zero current to peak amplitude of one phase.

Polarity: Electrode may be either the anode (+) or cathode (−) (this is not relevant when using AC).

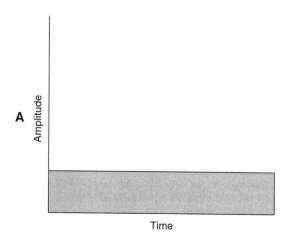

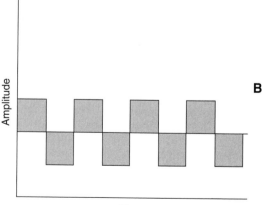

Figure 17-1   A, Continuous direct current. **B,** Continuous alternating current.

Pulsed current consists of a unidirectional or bidirectional flow of charges (AC or DC) that periodically stops for a finite time period. All NMES devices are pulsed current stimulators. Phase duration (also referred to as phase width) is defined as the time in which the current flows from the baseline in one direction and back to the baseline (Figure 17-2).

Pulse duration (also referred to as pulse width) is defined as the time during which charge flows in both directions (see Figure 17-2). In a monophasic current, the pulse duration and the phase duration are the same. In a biphasic current, two phases make up one pulse. Pulsed current consisting of a bidirectional flow of charge is called biphasic pulsed current.

When the flow in each direction is the same in time- and amplitude-dependent features, the biphasic current pulse is considered symmetrical (Figure 17-3, *A*). If the time-dependent and amplitude-dependent features differ, then the biphasic current is termed asymmetrical (Figure 17-3, *B*).

BOX 17-2 Current Parameters for Strengthening

Frequency: Generally between 25 and 50 Hz (these have been shown in humans to produce strong tetanic contractions while minimizing fatigue)
Waveforms: Many waveforms exist and any waveform capable of depolarizing the muscle is acceptable
Pulse or phase duration: Between 100 and 400 microseconds
Ramp up/down (rise and decay time): Adjust 2-4 seconds up to increase comfort, 1-2 seconds down
On/off time: A 1:4 or 1:5 ratio; 10 seconds on, 40 or 50 seconds off is commonly used. This may be decreased as muscle strength improves. A 1:1, 1:2, or 1:3 ratio is usually used for muscle endurance training.

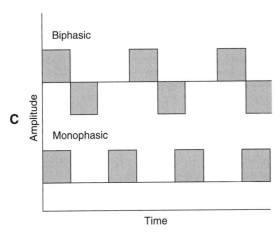

Figure 17-1 cont'd **C**, Pulsed current.

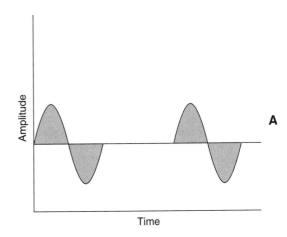

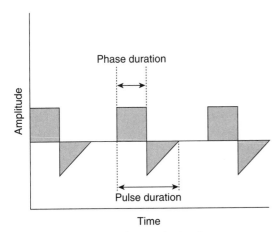

Figure 17-2 Phase and pulse duration.

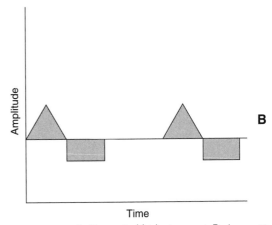

Figure 17-3 **A**, Symmetrical biphasic current. **B**, Asymmetrical biphasic current.

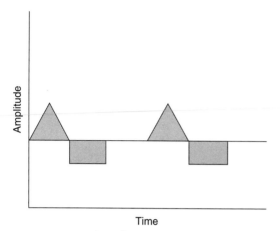

Figure 17-4   Balanced asymmetrical biphasic pulsed current.

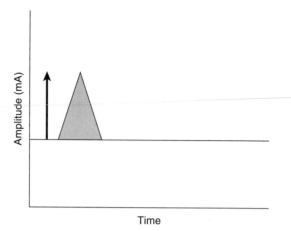

Figure 17-6   Amplitude.

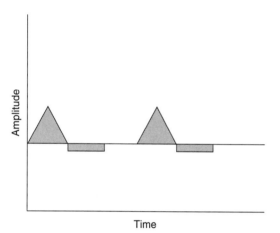

Figure 17-5   Unbalanced asymmetrical biphasic pulsed current.

Balanced asymmetrical biphasic pulsed current occurs when the total charge in one phase equals the total charge of the other phase (Figure 17-4). If the total charge in each phase is unequal, it is termed unbalanced (Figure 17-5). Both pulsed AC and DC current forms are commonly used in portable and clinical model NMES units.

Stimulator Parameters

Current amplitude (also called magnitude or intensity) is defined as the vertical distance from the highest to the lowest peak during one electrical wave and is typically measured in milliamperes (mA) (Figure 17-6). Increasing the amplitude induces a stronger force of muscle contraction by additional recruitment of muscle fibers at greater distances from the electrodes.[1,3]

Skin produces resistance to current flow by ohmic resistance and capacitive impedance. Capacitive impedance is patient dependent and cannot be modified. Clipping or shaving the coat hair and cleaning the skin with alcohol to wash away skin oils or other substances helps to lower ohmic resistance. Lowering the skin resistance diminishes the driving voltage that is necessary for current penetration of the skin, potentially making the treatment more comfortable.[1,3]

Increased current amplitude is required to produce a given amount of muscular force if the pulse or phase durations are short. Symmetrical or asymmetrical biphasic pulsed currents use intermediate current amplitude levels. Portable NMES units are not always capable of producing the current output that clinical models can produce; however, most units sold for electromedical purposes are usually adequate. Some bargain simulators possess a very low phase charge (<10 microcoulombs) and cannot create adequate contraction of large muscle groups.

Pulse durations of 200 to 400 microseconds produce powerful contractions while minimizing the likelihood of recruiting many pain fibers.[1,3] Some stimulators that are made only for NMES do not allow control of pulse duration, but will typically be set in this range. As the pulse duration increases, smaller diameter pain fibers are recruited.

Pulse rate (also called frequency and pulses per second, pps) is the number of pulses delivered per second and is measured in hertz (Hz). Tetanic muscle contractions may be produced with frequencies as low as 20 Hz, but only submaximal muscle contraction will typically be produced in this range. Maximal force of

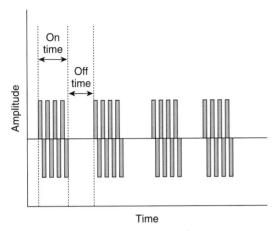

Figure 17-7 Duty cycle.

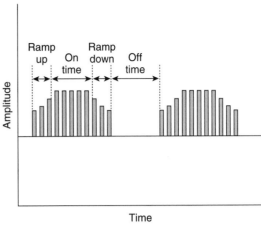

Figure 17-8 Ramp.

contraction generally occurs between 60 and 100 Hz. However, as frequency increases, the rate of fatigue also increases. Lower tetanic frequencies in the range of 35 to 50 pps reduce muscle fatigue while still providing strong muscle contractions.[1,3]

Duty cycle is the ratio of on-time to total cycle time, expressed as a percentage (Figure 17-7). On-time is the period of time in which a series of pulses or bursts is delivered to the patient. Off-time is the time between on-times. A single on-time duration plus a single off-time duration constitutes the total cycle time. For example, a stimulator that causes a muscle to contract for 10 seconds followed by a 30-second rest would have a 25% duty cycle, or a 1:4 ratio. As on-time increases, muscle fatigue increases.[2] Optimal duty cycles vary, depending on the patient. A patient with severe atrophy may require a longer off-time to recover between contractions. Many clinicians start with duty cycle ratios between 1:2 and 1:5 and watch for signs of fatigue, which indicates the need for a longer off-time.

Ramp is a feature of NMES that helps improve patient comfort. It involves a gradual increase or decrease in current amplitude such that the number of recruited motor units gradually increases the force of muscle contraction or gradually decreases the force of contraction (Figure 17-8). The ramp time is the period of time over which the pulse is increasing or decreasing. No data to date have identified the optimal ramp time. However, a ramp up of 2 to 4 seconds is commonly used to maximize comfort, with a 1- to 2-second ramp down.[1] Suggested current parameters for muscle strengthening are listed in Box 17.2.

Electrodes

Many types of surface electrodes are available. The main criteria in choosing electrodes are as follows:
1. Flexible enough to conform to the tissue
2. May be trimmed to a specific size
3. Have a low resistance (typically 100 ohms)
4. Are highly conductive
5. May be used many times
6. Are inexpensive

Some commercially available electrodes are effective for only a few uses, and some may be used 100 or more times (carbon-impregnated silicon rubber electrodes). Conductive performance of any electrode decreases over time. Electrodes require a medium to transmit current. Commonly used media include gels, sponges, or paper towels; some electrodes have the media already applied. Sponges and paper towels tend to dry out, and rewetting is necessary every 30 minutes. Electrodes should be of the appropriate size to stimulate the desired muscle without stimulating unwanted muscles in close proximity. The smaller the electrode, the higher the current density that enters the muscle, and the more painful the stimulus may be.

Recruitment

NMES recruits type II (fast twitch) fibers first, then type I (slow twitch), which is the reverse of the muscle recruitment pattern in a volitional contraction.[5-7] Increasing the pulse duration increases the recruitment of smaller diameter motor units at the same depth, but increasing the pulse duration too much may stimulate undesirable fibers (small-diameter pain fibers). Increasing either the amplitude or the pulse duration affects the strength of contraction because additional muscle fibers are recruited. Increasing the frequency results in the existing motor units firing at a faster rate and will increase the strength of contraction, but it also causes more rapid fatigue. Application of NMES at an optimal frequency results in an optimal physiological response while minimizing fatigue. In a healthy uninjured individual, a maximal voluntary muscle contraction produces a greater torque (more powerful contraction) than occurs in an electrically induced contraction. However, patients with injuries or immediately following surgery may be unable or unwilling to produce a maximum voluntary muscle contraction. In these patients, NMES may produce a stronger muscle contraction.

What to Look for When Buying a Unit for NMES

An acceptable NMES unit should allow flexibility in a number of parameters, including frequency (adjustable from at least 1 to 50 Hz), adjustable pulse duration, on/off times, ramp, phase charge of 30 microcoulombs or greater (avoid budget units), and multiple channels (at least two to allow cocontraction or alternating contraction of two different muscle groups). Acceptable clinical units may cost $500 or more.

Indications and Contraindications for NMES

NMES is commonly used in the rehabilitation of human patients who have had orthopedic or neurologic injury. A few examples are patients recovering from fracture repair, ACL reconstruction, and meniscal debridement or repair. Patients with neurological conditions, such as cerebrovascular accidents, closed head injuries, spinal cord injuries, or other neurologic disease involving paralysis or paresis, may also benefit from NMES. NMES has been used to increase joint mobility, decrease joint contracture, decrease edema, enhance circulation, minimize disuse atrophy, improve muscle strength, retard loss of volitional control, improve sensory awareness, decrease spasticity, diminish pain, and correct gait abnormalities.[8-11]

In human patients with low thoracic spinal cord injury, functional NMES has been used to produce knee extension with locking of the knees to allow weight-bearing. Within 3 weeks of spinal cord injury, up to 50% of quadriceps muscle loss may occur; in one study, NMES returned quadriceps muscle mass to near normal.[10] In a patient with an incomplete quadriplegic spinal cord injury, NMES was used to strengthen a paretic hand. Two weeks of NMES produced a 33% increase in muscle force with no loss of strength 4 weeks after the treatment was discontinued.[10] Children with mild cerebral palsy treated with NMES had statistically significant improvements in gross motor, locomotor, and receipt/propulsion skills.[9] NMES has also been used on tibial muscles of children with Duchenne and Becker muscular dystrophy. NMES resulted in mild, short-term increases in muscle strength, but it did not alter muscle fatigue. Whether chronic stimulation produces beneficial long-term effects has yet to be determined.[11]

In addition to the clinical use of NMES in people with neurologic and orthopedic disorders, it has been used in denervated muscle to retard atrophy and improve recovery after reinnervation in rats with surgically severed peroneal nerves. The use of NMES in improving reinnervation recovery in other species warrants further study, as it may be useful to those with denervation injuries.[12]

There are a number of circumstances in which electrical stimulation should not be used (contraindications), and other circumstances in which electrical stimulation should only be used with caution (precautions). Box 17-3 outlines these contraindications and precautions.

Effects of NMES in the Rehabilitation of Patients With Reconstructed ACLs

The specific physical effects of NMES on muscle enzymes, fibers, and perfusion has been examined experimentally in human patients with ACL injuries. The effects of NMES on dogs recovering from CrCL rupture are also beginning to be investigated.

Effect on Muscle Enzymes

In a study regarding the effects of low-frequency electrical stimulation on the metabolic profile of skeletal muscle, a portable NMES unit was used to stimulate the knee

BOX 17-3 Contraindications and Precautions for the Use of NMES

Contraindications
- High-intensity stimulation directly over the heart
- In animals with pacemakers
- In animals with seizure disorders
- Over areas of thrombosis or thrombophlebitis
- Over infected areas or neoplasms
- Over the carotid sinus
- Any time active motion is contraindicated
- Over the trunk during pregnancy

Precautions
- In areas with impaired sensation
- Over abdominal, lumbar, and pelvic regions during pregnancy
- In areas of skin irritation or damage
- Near electronic sensing devices such as ECG monitors (possible interference)

extensor muscles of sedentary men and women 6 days a week for 6 weeks.[13] No changes in creatine kinase and glutaraldehyde phosphatase concentrations were found in vastus lateralis muscle samples before or after NMES. There was a small decrease in phosphofructokinase, the rate-limiting enzyme of glycolysis in human muscle, which was only significant in men. Hexokinase, a regulatory enzyme of skeletal muscle glucose phosphorylation, was only significantly increased in the vastus lateralis of women. Krebs' cycle and electron transfer chain marker enzyme activity of fatty acid oxidation increased significantly in both sexes, with the greatest change occurring in women. The authors concluded that NMES can significantly increase the skeletal muscle aerobic-oxidative potential of sedentary subjects. In a study by Arvidsson et al,[14] there was no difference between a postoperative ACL reconstruction–NMES-treated group and an isometric exercise group in the activity of the oxidative enzyme citrate synthase or phosphofructokinase. Research by Wigerstad-Lossing et al[15] showed no significant reduction in the activity of the oxidative and glycolytic enzymes citrate synthase and triphosphate dehydrogenase in NMES patients following knee ligament surgery compared to control patients, which had decreased enzyme activity.

Effects on Muscle Fibers

The muscle fiber atrophy that occurs with disuse atrophy following cruciate injury and sur-

gery is significant. NMES may be more effective than volitional exercise in preventing atrophy and overcoming the effects of reflex inhibition in the first few days to weeks after surgery. Electrical stimulation also recruits type II muscle fibers first, thereby retarding their atrophy to a greater degree than type I muscle fibers.[5,6] As type II fiber augmentation occurs, the force of contraction increases and therefore strength increases. With volitional contraction in humans, a selective or preferential activation of fast-twitch motor units has not been demonstrated. Slow-twitch motor units with type I skeletal muscle fibers are recruited first, followed by the fast-twitch motor units with type II skeletal muscle fibers being recruited as the demand for force increases.[6]

NMES of the triceps brachialis muscle in monkeys did not affect the distribution of muscle fiber types but enhanced oxidative capacity and caused an increase in fiber size.[16] There was a preferential recruitment of large motor axons that innervate fast-twitch fibers. The activation of fast-twitch motor units was not exclusive. Motoneurons and muscle fibers were recruited primarily in the superficial portion of the muscle. The morphological and biochemical adaptations that occurred with NMES were similar to those occurring after voluntary heavy-resistance exercises.

Effect on Perfusion

NMES also induced capillary proliferation in monkeys in response to increased muscle blood flow. Because blood flow increased in capillaries around type II fibers to a greater degree than around type I fibers, there was a stimulus for proliferation of endothelial cells.[16]

Transcutaneous electrical stimulation was used on rat muscle to demonstrate that microvascular perfusion depends on evoked muscle contractions. This finding suggests that NMES should be applied at intensities that produce muscle contraction so that microvascular perfusion of stimulated skeletal muscle is enhanced.[17]

Overall Effects of NMES

The net physical effects of NMES are an increase in muscle strength, muscle mass, and oxidative capacity.[5,13,15,16,18,19] Another benefit of NMES is the ability to overcome the effects of reflex inhibition on the quadriceps muscles, and the potential enhanced effect of NMES on subsequent voluntary use of previously electrically activated motor units.[5] The negative effects of NMES include muscle fatigue and possibly increased pain. Muscle fatigue is the decrease in force-generating ability of a muscle due to recent activity. The rate of muscle fatigue during NMES is much greater than that which occurs during volitional exercises. The reverse recruitment order induced with NMES probably contributes to increased fatigue. However, stimulation intensity, stimulation frequency, and duty cycle may be altered to reduce muscle fatigue.[20] Increased current levels may recruit pain fibers and result in painful muscle contractions. In addition, discomfort is also associated with psychological factors in humans. Pain may be controlled by decreasing the current intensity to a level that elicits comfortable muscle contractions.[21]

Efficacy and Clinical Trials of NMES for the ACL Reconstructed Knee

Currier and Kellogg[18] used NMES to treat seven patients after ACL reconstruction. Treatment successfully reduced thigh girth loss compared to three control patients during the first 6 weeks.

Snyder-Mackler et al[5] studied the effects of clinical NMES on thigh muscle strength and gait in 10 patients undergoing ACL reconstructive surgery. Patients were randomly assigned to NMES and volitional exercise or volitional exercise alone for 4 weeks. Values obtained for cadence, walking velocity, stance time on the affected limb, flexion excursion of the knee during stance, thigh circumference, and extension and flexion torques were improved in patients receiving NMES. The knees of the patients receiving NMES were stronger in the eighth postoperative week than reported averages for non-NMES patients years after ACL reconstructive surgery. The authors concluded that NMES not only increased muscle strength but also improved functional use of the muscles at least in the immediate postoperative period. The increased muscle strength likely results in partial compensation for the loss of ACL receptors.

DeLitto et al[19] compared clinical NMES and isometric contraction to voluntary exercise and isometric contractions in 20 patients that had undergone ACL reconstructive surgery. Each group consisted of 10 patients. NMES patients received treatment for 3 weeks during the first 6 postoperative weeks. After their respective treatment period, bilateral maximal isometric measurements of gravity-corrected knee extension and flexion torque were obtained. Greater extension and flexion torque and higher individual thigh-muscle strength gains were reported when NMES was prescribed early in postoperative rehabilitation.

Lieber et al[22] compared maximal voluntary thigh muscle contraction after 4 weeks of treatment in 20 NMES patients and 20 voluntary contraction patients who had undergone ACL reconstruction within 2 to 6 weeks of the study. They compared the two groups under conditions where the total muscle tension in both groups was matched. When exercise intensity was matched between the two groups, the magnitude and time course of strength gains were identical. Given the variable intensity of maximal voluntary contraction that NMES patients tolerate, variability in outcomes may be expected between NMES strengthening and voluntary contraction groups. The authors concluded that when strong muscle contractions can be elicited with NMES, significant strengthening is possible.

Wigerstad-Lossing et al[15] compared NMES using a portable unit and voluntary muscle contractions to voluntary muscle contractions alone in patients immobilized in a cast following ACL surgery. Thirteen patients were randomly assigned to the treatment group and 10 to the control group. Electrical stimulation was applied to the quadriceps muscles only, through windows in the cast, and was initiated on the second postoperative day and continued until the sixth week after surgery. Preoperative data were compared to data obtained in the sixth postoperative week, and the authors concluded that NMES in combination with simultaneously performed voluntary muscle contractions can limit muscle weakness, muscle wasting, and reduction in oxidative and glycolytic muscle enzyme activity during immobilization after knee ligament surgery.

In another study, 18 male and 20 female patients undergoing ACL reconstruction were randomly assigned to one of two groups.[14] Individuals in an NMES group received a cast, isometric muscle training, and NMES with a portable unit. Individuals in the control group received a cast and isometric training alone. Transcutaneous electrical stimulation of the quadriceps was initiated during the first postoperative week and continued for a total of 5.5 weeks. Quadriceps muscle wasting was assessed with computed tomography (CT) before and 6 weeks after surgery. Percutaneous muscle biopsies were obtained from the vastus lateralis muscle before surgery, and 1 and 6 weeks after surgery. Electrical stimulation significantly reduced the amount of vastus medialis muscle wasting in female patients as measured by CT, but there was no significant difference in males. Muscle fiber area revealed that cross-sectional area of individual fibers decreased less in NMES patients than in controls, but the difference was not significant. The authors concluded that transcutaneous electrical stimulation was effective in significantly reducing vastus medialis atrophy as measured on CT, but had no significant effect on the vastus lateralis.

The results of clinical trials using NMES for postoperative rehabilitation of the ACL-deficient knee in people generally have demonstrated increased thigh girth, increased thigh muscle strength, improved cadence, improved walking velocity and stance time, and increased oxidative and glycolytic muscle enzyme activity.

Rehabilitation Programs for Treatment of ACL Deficiency

In human surgery, rehabilitation of patients after ACL reconstruction is necessary for an optimal outcome.[23-26] Controversy exists regarding what constitutes the ideal postoperative rehabilitation program for human patients. Current trends in volitional exercise regimens are geared toward accelerated rehabilitation programs. Typical accelerated programs involve ROM exercises and cryotherapy started immediately postoperatively, and crutch use for 2 to 10 days. Closed kinetic chain exercises in the form of exercises in which the foot is fixed and motion at the knee joint is accompanied by motion at the hip and ankle joint (such as squats) are initiated as early as 7 days postoperatively. Closed kinetic chain exercises appear to decrease knee joint compressive forces, thereby decreasing the anteroposterior translation of the tibia, as compared with open-chain knee extension exercises.[27] NMES is commonly used during the first 3 to 6 weeks of rehabilitation, depending on the ability of the patient to volitionally contract the quadriceps. In general, at approximately week 10, light jogging, Stairmaster, and agility drills may be attempted. From weeks 12 to 24, strengthening programs,

proprioceptive training, and increased running and agility programs are progressed as tolerated. Advancement from one level of activity to another is based on physical examination, knee laxity testing, and isokinetic and functional testing.[15,24,27-29]

Postoperative rehabilitation and the role of the quadriceps and hamstring muscles in improving stifle function have largely been ignored in veterinary medicine. Postoperative care of dogs, regardless of the surgical technique used, has traditionally included several days to weeks of external support to reduce postoperative swelling and provide joint immobilization. This is done to protect the surgical repair until pericapsular fibrosis occurs in the case of extracapsular repair, to provide protection of an intracapsular graft while it remodels and to protect the site of fixation of the graft, and to permit healing of the osteotomy and repair site with a tibial plateau leveling osteotomy (TPLO).[30-41] However, immobilization exacerbates muscle atrophy and weakness and produces deleterious effects on cartilage, bone, and ligaments.[4,14,15,23,25]

Veterinary surgeons should not make the error of using all aspects of the accelerated volitional rehabilitation protocols designed for human patients in their veterinary patients post-CrCL stabilization. The majority of human ACL surgical repairs involve using the bone–patellar tendon–bone technique, which is strongest the day of surgery and loses strength as tendon remodeling occurs. The majority of canine CrCL-deficient stifles are stabilized using the extracapsular lateral fabellar suture technique, which relies on collagen formation and scar tissue as the primary stabilizer of the joints.[42] This technique results in immediate strength following surgery because of the stabilization sutures, and the periarticular structures gain strength as tissue healing and collagen maturation occur over time. Intracapsular techniques are typically not as strong, and the graft weakens over several weeks before regaining some strength. Therefore rehabilitation protocols for canine patients must be based on the surgical stabilization technique used. However, NMES may be useful in the rehabilitation of the stifle without compromising the stability of the repair.

The negative effects of quadriceps reflex inhibition leading to quadriceps atrophy following ACL injury and the positive protective effects of hamstring muscle strengthening to enhance stability and constraint of the stifle following CrCL injury have not been adequately addressed in veterinary medicine. Clinicians may wish to consider adapting ACL-protective rehabilitation procedures to the dog, to protect the surgical repair. Improved postoperative functional outcome following ACL reconstruction in humans is positively correlated with return of quadriceps strength.[5,18,25] Although the hamstring muscles also atrophy following ACL injury and surgery, the atrophy is generally less than that found in the quadriceps muscles, probably because the hamstring muscles cross both the knee and hip joints, which results in continued function and muscle contraction, thereby diminishing the degree of atrophy.[25]

NMES Use and Clinical Recommendations in the Dog

The Use of NMES in Veterinary Medicine

In establishing a rehabilitation program, the cost-benefit ratio must be assessed. For a program to be cost and labor effective, there must be earlier or more protected return to function, increased joint ROM, increased muscle strength, and an overall improved outcome.[5] Although cost is a major concern in veterinary medicine, of equal importance is how the a rehabilitation program is applied to the dog. Obviously, the use of crutches, limb immobilization devices, and functional knee bracing are not directly applicable to the dog. However, external coaptation with soft padded bandages and cage rest appear to be practical alternatives. Bicycling, weightlifting, proprioceptive training, and jumping rope, which are the mainstays of rehabilitation of people, are generally not possible in dogs. A practical rehabilitation alternative to enhance operative outcome is needed for dogs. Electrical stimulation provides a cost and labor effective means of establishing early, protected return to function, as well as the possibility of decreased degenerative joint disease (DJD) and increased muscle mass.[43]

NMES is an effective means of rehabilitation of the ACL-deficient knee in people and is considered by some to be more effective than volitional exercise, especially during the early rehabilitation period. Since the CrCL-deficient dog has been used extensively as a model for ACL deficiency in humans, it would logically follow that post-ACL reconstruction rehabilitation methods in humans could be applied to the dog. Rehabilitation of the stabilized knee determines the success of surgical outcome, especially in the physically active human patient. Appropriate rehabilitation would seem especially important to enhancing surgical outcome in large working dogs used for hunting, obedience trials, service, tracking, or police work. Loss of function in the working dog not only affects the quality of life of the patient but may also lead to economic losses associated with an animal's inability to work. Surgical stabilization of the stifle is the treatment of choice in large-breed dogs, but all affected stifles appear to develop DJD and joint laxity regardless of the surgical intervention.

To date, only a few studies have reported the use of NMES in the rehabilitation of dogs. In a study by Johnson et al,[43] NMES was used following CrCL surgery in experimental dogs, and the portable units used in this study proved quite feasible for use in dogs. The affected thigh was clipped and scrubbed with isopropyl alcohol. A limb-positioning device was constructed to maintain the limb in a normal stance position during stimulation. The rationale for maintaining the limb in a normal stance position was that stimulating the muscles in this position would be more functional. Adhesive tape was used to fix the limb-positioning device to the lateral surface of the affected pelvic limb during the 30-minute treatment session.

Carbon electrodes (4.5 × 4.6 cm) were placed over the distal portion of the biceps femoris muscle, and the proximal portion of the semitendinosus muscle. Additional carbon electrodes (5.1 × 10.2 cm) were also positioned over the distal portion of the vastus medialis muscle and the proximal portion of the vastus lateralis muscle. Water-soluble electrode gel was applied as a coupling agent, and the electrodes were fixed in position with paper tape. Channel 1 was connected to the hamstring muscle electrodes, and channel 2 was connected to the quadriceps electrodes. The parameters for the program were as follows:
Channel 1: Ramp up—3 sec; ON: 12 sec; ramp down—2 sec; OFF: 25 sec
Channel 2: Ramp up—2 sec; ON: 12 sec; ramp down—1 sec; OFF: 25 sec
Channel 2 started 3 seconds after channel 1, automatically eliciting cyclic hamstring and quadriceps cocontraction. A symmetrical biphasic waveform of 35 pulses per second

was used. Amperage was increased to the tolerance level of the animal and was reduced if gross movement was noted at the stifle joint or if the animal displayed any signs of distress, including turning its head in recognition of the stimulus or becoming agitated. Amperage was reduced to a level below that which produced these signs. Each treatment session lasted 30 minutes once daily, five times per week, for 4 weeks. Outcome measures were assessed at weeks 0, 2, 5, 7, 9, 13, and 19. Outcome measures included radiographs, force plate analysis, subjective lameness scores, drawer sign, thigh circumference, ROM, palpable crepitation during ROM, and postmortem evaluation of stifle joints.

Radiograph results demonstrated that the NMES group had significantly fewer bony changes associated with osteoarthritis over time. Thigh circumference was significantly greater in the NMES group at weeks 9 and 13, and subjective lameness scores were also improved over time in the NMES group ($p <$ 0.001). The postmortem evaluation revealed that the NMES group had less cartilage damage ($p < 0.07$), less palpable crepitation during ROM, and less osteophyte formation. ROM, force plate analysis, and joint laxity were not significantly different between the groups. Meniscal damage was significantly greater in the NMES group, however.[43]

In a study by Millis et al[45] a clinical trial was designed to compare the outcomes of postoperative physical rehabilitation to traditional postoperative care in dogs surgically treated for cranial cruciate rupture. Ten dogs receiving treatment for cranial cruciate rupture were randomly assigned to either a treatment group for postoperative physical rehabilitation, or a control group. Lateral fabellar-tibial stabilization was performed in each dog by the same surgeon. Dogs in the control group were cage rested and walked on a leash for 20 minutes twice daily for 2 weeks. Dogs in the treatment group received passive ROM exercises, NMES, and walking exercises for the same 2-week period. Thigh girth measurements and maximum angles of flexion and extension were taken every other day during the 2-week period and 4, 8, and 12 weeks after surgery. The influence of other variables, such as meniscal injury and the degree of preexisting osteoarthritis, on outcome were also assessed.

By the end of the 2-week period, thigh girth was significantly larger in the rehabilitation group and remained greater throughout the rest of the study, but the difference late in the study was not statistically significant. Maximal extension of the stifle was significantly greater in the rehabilitation group beginning halfway through the initial 2-week period and remained greater throughout the rest of the study. Maximal flexion was not significantly different between the two groups. The presence of moderate to severe osteoarthritis at the time of surgery retarded recovery in both groups. Interestingly, meniscal injury at the time of surgery had no effects on any of the measured parameters in the short term. In this study, muscle mass and maximum range of stifle motion were improved with postoperative physical rehabilitation. The increased muscle mass in the dogs receiving rehabilitation may have been due, in part, to NMES.

NMES has been used clinically on dogs for many purposes, including to diminish joint contractures and to decrease muscle atrophy associated with a variety of disorders such as inherited Labrador myopathy, postoperative atrophy, and nerve injury. Other uses have included improving limb function, decreasing pain, decreasing muscle spasm (commonly associated with intervertebral disk disease), and decreasing edema.

NMES may be valuable as part of the treatment for postoperative rehabilitation of dogs undergoing femoral head and neck excision. It may also help to improve the outcome of surgically repaired chronic hip luxations, or any other surgical procedure where quick return of muscle mass is beneficial. NMES may also be used for the conservative treatment of shoulder instability[45] or iliopsoas muscle trauma.[46]

Animal Reaction and Safety

Precautions should be taken to avoid injury to the handler and animal. A muzzle should be applied and the animal placed in lateral recumbency during the initial treatment. In some cases, tranquilization may be necessary if the animal is anxious. We recommend that treatment only be given under the supervision of trained personnel.

Preparation and Electrode Placement

The hair over the area to which electrical stimulation will be applied must be clipped to lower impedance (Figure 17-9). The skin should be cleaned with alcohol before

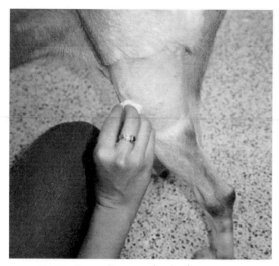

Figure 17-9 Preparing the skin for treatment.

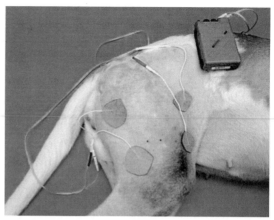

Figure 17-11 Application of electrical stimulation for cocontraction of the cranial and caudal thigh muscles. (Courtesy D. Millis.)

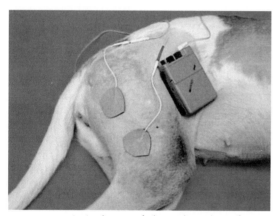

Figure 17-10 Application of electrical stimulation for contraction of the caudal thigh muscles. (Courtesy D. Millis.)

treatment. It will be necessary to locate the motor point (the area where the motor nerve enters the muscle), so that an adequate contraction is obtained with as low a current as possible to minimize discomfort to the patient. Electrodes may be placed solely on one muscle to cause a contraction and motion at the joint the muscle acts upon (Figure 17-10), or they may be placed on opposing muscle groups to cause a cocontraction (Figure 17-11) that may simulate an isometric contraction and result in little or no joint movement.

Motor point location is performed by first applying gel to the skin, and then placing the electrode over the general area of the motor point. With the unit on, the electrode may then be moved around until a good contraction is achieved. Setting the frequency at 1 Hz will help in motor point determination because the twitch contraction will be more obvious and will become stronger as the electrode moves closer to the motor point. An indelible marking pen is then used to draw a circle around the electrode. This allows the electrode to be placed in the same area during subsequent treatments, without having to repeat the process of motor point location. Remember to adjust the frequency to the desired setting (25 to 50 Hz) before beginning the actual treatment.

Treatment Time and Frequency

Although the optimum time and frequency of treatment are unknown, most clinicians believe that electrical stimulation should be applied to the desired area(s) for 15 to 20 minutes, three to seven times per week. Occasionally, a patient may experience muscle soreness early in the treatment program if electrical stimulation is used too frequently, for treatment periods that are too long, or with application of current that is too great (muscle contraction is too strong). In these cases, skipping treatment for a day or two and resuming treatment with reduced treatment time, frequency, or strength of contraction is usually adequate to resolve the problem. Cocontraction of opposing muscle groups should be considered if no joint motion is desired.

Electrical Stimulation for Pain Control

A recent study examined the effects of TENS on osteoarthritic pain in the stifle of dogs.[47]

Five dogs, which had chronic mild OA that was originally induced by CrCL transection and stifle stabilization, were treated. Pretreatment ground reaction forces were determined using a force plate before electrical stimulation to assess the functional use of the affected limb. Immediately following these measurements, premodulated electrical stimulation (70 Hz) was applied to the involved extremity around the stifle. After treatment, ground reaction forces were determined at 30-minute intervals over a 4-hour period. Each dog was also reevaluated 24 hours after treatment. Significant improvement in ground reaction forces was found 30 minutes after treatment. These differences persisted for 210 minutes after TENS application and were significant 30, 60, 120, 150, and 180 minutes after treatment. The greatest improvement was found immediately after treatment. Each of the dogs was reevaluated following a 4-day rest period and still exhibited an increase in weight-bearing on the affected extremity, but these differences were not significant. In this preliminary study, positive benefits of the application of TENS were apparent for dogs with osteoarthritic stifle joints.[47] Further study of TENS application in dogs, including different parameters and altered physical activity throughout the study, may reveal additional benefits.

Future Areas for Study

Electrical stimulation protocols for muscle strengthening and pain control have been minimally explored for clinical use in dogs. Given the similarities in neurologic and orthopedic conditions between dogs and people, it would seem that the indications for electrical stimulation are similar. Iontophoresis is another area that should be studied in dogs to investigate its possible use.

REFERENCES

1. Nelson RM, Currier DP: *Clinical electrotherapy,* ed 2, Norwalk, Conn, 1991, Appleton & Lange.
2. Krauspe R, Schmidt M, Schaible H: Sensory innervation of the anterior cruciate ligament, an electrophysiological study of the response properties of single identified mechanoreceptors in the cat, *J Bone Joint Surg* 74A:390-397, 1992.
3. Windsor RE, Lester JP, Herring SA: Electrical stimulation in clinical practice, *Phys Sportsmed* 21:85-93, 1993.
4. Hainaut K, Duchateau J: Neuromuscular electrical stimulation and voluntary exercise, *Sports Med* 14: 100-113, 1992.
5. Snyder-Mackler L, Ladin Z, Schepsis AA, Young JC: Electrical stimulation of the thigh muscles after reconstruction of the anterior cruciate ligament, *J Bone Joint Surg* 73A:1025-1036, 1991.
6. Sinacore DR et al: Type II fiber activation with electrical stimulation: a preliminary report, *Phys Ther* 70:416-420, 1990.
7. Knaflitz M, Merletti R, DeLuca DJ: Inference of motor unit recruitment order in voluntary and electrically elicited contractions, *J Appl Phys* 64:1657-1667, 1990.
8. Carroll SG, Bird SF, Brown DJ: Electrical stimulation of the lumbrical muscles in an incomplete quadriplegic patient: case report, *Paraplegia* 30:223-226, 1992.
9. Pape KE et al: Neuromuscular approach to the motor deficits of cerebral palsy: a pilot study, *J Pediatr Orthop* 13:628-633, 1993.
10. Taylor PN et al: Limb blood flow, cardiac output and quadriceps muscle bulk following spinal cord injury and the effect of training for the Odstock functional electrical stimulation standing system, *Paraplegia* 31:303-310, 1993.
11. Zupan A et al: Effects of electrical stimulation on muscles of children with Duchenne and Becker muscular dystrophy, *Neuropediatrics* 24:189-192, 1993.
12. Kanaya F, Tajima T: Effect of electrostimulation on denervated muscle, *Clin Orthop* 283:296-301, 1992.
13. Gauthier JM et al: Electrical stimulation-induced changes in skeletal muscle enzymes of men and women, *Med Sci Sports Exer* 24:1252-1256, 1992.
14. Arvidsson I et al: Prevention of quadriceps wasting after immobilization: an evaluation of the effect of electrical stimulation, *Electr Stim* 9:1519-1528, 1986.
15. Wigerstad-Lossing I et al: Effects of electrical muscle stimulation combined with voluntary contractions after knee ligament surgery, *Med Sci Sports Exer* 20: 93-98, 1988.
16. Bigard A: Effects of surface electrostimulation on the structure and metabolic properties in monkey skeletal muscle, *Med Sci Sports Exer* 25:355-362, 1993.
17. Clemente FR, Barron KW: The influence of muscle contraction on the degree of microvascular perfusion in rat skeletal muscle following transcutaneous neuromuscular electrical stimulation, *J Orthop Sports Phys Ther* 18:488-496, 1993.
18. Currier DP Kellogg R: Effects of electrical and electromagnetic stimulation after anterior cruciate ligament reconstruction, *J Orthop Sports Phys Ther* 17:177-184, 1993.
19. DeLitto A et al: Electrical stimulation versus voluntary exercise in strengthening thigh musculature after anterior cruciate ligament surgery, *Phys Ther* 68: 660-663, 1988.
20. Binder-Macleod SA, Snyder-Mackler L: Muscle fatigue: clinical implications for fatigue assessment and neuromuscular electrical stimulation, *Phys Ther* 73:902-910, 1993.
21. DeLitto A et al: A study of discomfort with electrical stimulation, *Phys Ther* 72:410-421, 1992.
22. Lieber RL, Silva PD, Daniel DM: Electrical and voluntary activation are equally effective in strengthening quadriceps muscles. In 1992 Orthopaedic Research Society Proceedings, Washington, D.C., February 17-20, 1992.
23. Anderson AF, Lipscomb AB: Analysis of rehabilitation techniques after anterior cruciate reconstruction, *Am J Sports Med* 17:154-160, 1989.
24. DeCarlo MS: Traditional versus accelerated rehabilitation following ACL reconstruction: a one-year follow-up, *J Orthop Sports Phys Ther* 15:309-316, 1992.

25. O'Meara PM: Rehabilitation following reconstruction of the anterior cruciate ligament, *Orthopedics* 16: 301-306, 1993.

26. Paulos L et al: Knee rehabilitation after anterior cruciate ligament reconstruction and repair, *Am J Sports Med* 9:140-149, 1981.

27. Lutz GE, Stuart MJ, Sim FH: Rehabilitative techniques for athletes: NMES after reconstruction of the anterior cruciate ligament, *Mayo Clin Proc* 65:1322-1329, 1990.

28. Fu FH, Woo SL, Irrgang JJ: Current concepts for rehabilitation following anterior cruciate ligament reconstruction, *J Orthop Sports Phys Ther* 15:270-278, 1992.

29. Shelbourne KD, Nitz P: Accelerated rehabilitation after anterior cruciate ligament reconstruction, *J Orthop Sports Phys Ther* 15:256-264, 1992.

30. Arnoczky SP et al: The over-the-top procedure: a technique for anterior cruciate ligament substitution in the dog, *J Am Anim Hosp Assoc* 15:283-290, 1979.

31. Bennett D, May C: An over-the top with tibial tunnel technique for repair of cranial cruciate ligament rupture in the dog, *J Small Anim Pract* 32:103-110, 1991.

32. Denny HR, Barr RS: An evaluation of two over the top techniques for anterior cruciate ligament replacement in the dog, *J Small Anim Pract* 25:759-769, 1984.

33. Dickinson CR, Nunamaker DM: Repair of ruptured anterior cruciate ligament in the dog: experience of 101 cases, using a modified fascia strip technique, *J Am Vet Med Assoc* 170:827-830, 1977.

34. Dupuis J, Harari J: Cruciate ligament and meniscal injuries in dogs, *Compend Contin Educ Pract Vet* 15: 215-233, 1993.

35. Elkins AD et al: A retrospective study evaluating the degree of degenerative joint disease in the stifle joint of dogs following surgical repair of anterior cruciate ligament rupture, *J Am Anim Hosp Assoc* 27:533-540, 1991.

36. Flo GL: Modification of the lateral retinacular imbrication technique for stabilizing cruciate ligament injuries, *J Am Anim Hosp Assoc* 11:570-576, 1975.

37. Hulse DA et al: Biomechanics of cranial cruciate ligament reconstruction in the dog. I. In vitro laxity testing, *Vet Surg* 12:109-112, 1983.

38. Paatsama S: Ligament injuries in the canine stifle joint a clinical and experimental study, *J Small Anim Med* 1:329-359, 1953.

39. Le DA, Liu W: The under- and over fascial replacement technique for anterior cruciate ligament rupture in dogs: a retrospective study, *J Am Anim Hosp Assoc* 20:69-77, 1984.

40. Smith GK, Torg JS: Fibular head transposition for repair of cruciate-deficient stifle in the dog, *J Am Vet Med Assoc* 187:375-382, 1985.

41. Tomlinson J, Constantinescu GM: Two methods for repairing ruptures of the cranial cruciate ligament in dogs, *Vet Med* 89:32-41, 1994.

42. Korvick, D, Johnson AL, Schaffer, D: The surgeons choice in treating CrCL ruptures in dogs, *J Am Vet Med Assoc* 25:1318-1324, 1994.

43. Johnson JM, Johnson AL, Pijanowski GJ: Rehabilitation of dogs with surgically treated cranial cruciate ligament deficient stifles by use of electrical stimulation of muscles, *Am J Vet Res* 58:1473-1478, 1997.

44. Millis DL, Levine D, Weigel JP: A preliminary study of early physical therapy following surgery for cranial cruciate ligament rupture in dogs. *Vet Surg* 26: 254, 1997.

45. Bardet JF: Diagnosis of shoulder instability in dogs and cats: a retrospective study, *J Am Anim Hosp Assoc* 34:42-54, 1998.

46. Breur G, Bkvins W: Traumatic injury of the canine iliopsoas muscle in three dogs, *J Am Vet Med Assoc* 210:1631-1634, 1997.

47. Levine D et al: The effect of TENS on osteoarthritic pain in the stifle of dogs. In *Proc 2nd Intl Symp Rehabil Phys Therap Vet Med*, 2002, p 199.

Chapter 18

Massage

Amanda Sutton

Biologic Basis

Massage has many definitions and is employed by many practitioners of various backgrounds. A working definition that will be used for this chapter is that massage is the manipulation of the soft tissues of the body. The use of massage has been well received in the human field and, despite a paucity of research, it has continued to be developed and explored.

The word *massage* is derived from the Arabic word *mass*, which means "to press." Many ancient civilizations developed a system of massage, which was used for various medical conditions. Just Lucas Championnies (1843-1913) used it in the management of fractures in the United States, and it was advanced by Mary McMillan, director of physical therapy at Harvard Medical School. Dr. J.B. Mennell described physical treatment by movement, manipulation, and massage, which was first published in 1917. There has been variable interest in massage by medical establishments in the twentieth century, but interest in complementary medicine has grown in the United States. The American Massage Therapy Association was founded in 1943 and had grown to 20,000 members by 1994.

Massage is now incorporated along with the medical management of human patients for pain relief and cases of decreased mobility. It is used as a prevention measure and in the management of competitive athletes. It is also incorporated into most chiropractic, physical therapist, and osteopathic manual therapy approaches.

Biomechanics of Connective Tissue

Massage must be directed toward a specific purpose and should be aimed at promoting physical and psychological change.

The main constituent of connective tissue is collagen. Its function is to resist axial tension, and it exhibits a stress-strain behavior (Box 18-1). Microscopically, collagen fibers are arranged in bundles and have a crimped appearance. Type I collagen is in the dermis and fascia and gives support and resistance to tension.

The basal lamina of epithelial tissue contains type IV collagen, which supports the epithelial cells. Hydrogen cross-links are formed between chains and between molecules, giving stability at fibril levels, assisting in the formation of collagen fibers. They allow the tissue to function under mechanical stress.

The orientation of the fibers depends on the stresses to which the fibers are subjected; connective tissue must be pliable, yet very strong. A stress-strain curve demonstrates the behavior of biological materials. When a longitudinal stress is applied to collagen, the tissue responds by elongation, which occurs in the toe region of the curve (Figure 18-1). Elongation occurs as a result of straightening of the crimped fibers, and probably also due to some interfibrillar sliding and shear of ground substance, which flows between the collagen fibers.

Massage produces most of its effects in the toe region of the stress-strain curve. Care should always be taken to not overstretch the tissues, to avoid damage to the internal structure of connective tissue fibers. Therefore the end feel of the tissues must be understood to avoid damage to connective tissues.

> ■ ■ ■ **BOX 18-1** Characteristics of Stress-Strain Behavior of Collagen
>
> ■ Stress and strain are linear up to the yield point. Elongation along this portion of the curve will not be permanent.
> ■ Elastic limit is the point to which maximum stress may be applied without permanent deformation.
> ■ Increased loading requires greater force to increase elongation of collagen because the tissue becomes stiffer.
> ■ Microfailure begins to occur in some of the fiber bundles in the linear region. However, the tissue retains its external appearance of continuity.
> ■ The end of the linear region is known as the yield point of the tissue. At this point, elongation of collagen occurs with a minimal increase in load. Beyond this point, major fiber bundle failure occurs, the external appearance changes, and the smooth outline is lost.
> ■ When maximum load point is reached (P_{max}), complete rupture occurs.

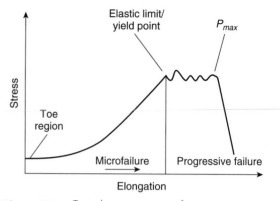

Figure 18-1 Typical stress-strain curve for connective tissue. *Stress,* Force applied per unit area; *strain,* proportional elongation; P_{max}, maximum load point.

Permanent deformation is termed plastic deformation, which occurs with microfailure and disruption of collagen cross-links. The undamaged fibers absorb a greater proportion of the load as a new length is established, which reflects the balance between elastic recoil and the resistance of the water and glycosaminoglycans to compression.

Biologic materials also have viscosity, a property of fluids of resistance to flow, and elasticity, a property of solids. Together, these result in the viscoelastic properties of tissues. The response of tissues to loading depends on how quickly the load is applied or removed. The faster the repetitive loading and unloading, the stiffer the material behaves. With rapid loading, friction results and tissue temperature rises. Energy is dissipated as heat when the tissue is returned to its original length. This is referred to as hysteresis.

This is relevant in the application of massage because it is important to be sensitive to the stiffness of tissues. If a low constant or repetitive load is maintained over a long period, the elongation of tissues that occurs is by creep. Conversely, if the tissue length is held constant, elongation occurs by relaxation. Massage produces low, repetitive loads over the medium term and may cause a nonpermanent creep response. Rapid loading of tissues during massage is undesirable because of increased tissue stiffness as a result of their viscoelastic properties. Also, dry tissue results in less compliance and elongates less readily. These are important facts for deciding the rate of massage application.

Lymphatics

In humans, one tenth of the tissue fluid is removed by the lymphatics. Understanding lymphatic anatomy, physiology, and function are necessary for successful massage. The rate of flow is determined by the interstitial fluid pressure and lymphatic pump activity.

Increased lymphatic flow is caused by the following:
■ Increased capillary pressure
■ Increased plasma osmotic pressure
■ Increased interstitial fluid pressure
■ Increased capillary permeability

It is believed that when tissues and fluid are compressed against the outer surfaces of the larger lymph vessels, lymph flow is impeded. This results in an increase in interstitial fluid pressure slightly above atmospheric pressure. Massaging increases interstitial fluid pressure and helps to move fluid into the lymphatic system. By massaging in a distal to proximal direction, fluid is moved from the extremity toward the central body core. This supports the practice of applying massage in a proximal direction.

Circulatory Effects

The pressure of the massage itself increases pressure within the tissues. Pressure gradients are created between the tissue spaces and vessels. As the hands are moved, changes in tissue pressure occur, creating fluctuating pressure differences between one area of tissue and another. It is believed that fluid moves constantly from tissues to vessels and back again, as it flows from areas of high pressure to areas of low pressure.

During an actual massage session, various massage manipulations are employed that are complex and involve a combination of squeezing, stretching, pulling, and traction forces, with movement occurring in different directions and in different tissue planes. Therefore there will be complex repetitive pressure changes occurring in varying directions and at different tissue depths. This is likely to have an effect on fluid interchange, whereby fluid is pushed from the tissue spaces into the vessels, toward the lymph nodes and heart, and new fluid is pushed or drawn into the spaces. Massage is believed to replenish the fluid in the spaces, producing a flushing effect, which brings in additional nutrients. There is evidence in humans that chemical irritants in the tissues (e.g., substance P, prostaglandins) and waste products of metabolism may decrease pain threshold by sensitizing free nerve endings. Replenishing tissue fluid and removing inflammatory products may reduce this effect, preventing or reducing some types of chronic pain. By removing metabolites and chemicals from muscles and "flushing" the muscle tissue with new circulation, muscle soreness following exercise may be reduced. However, controlled studies have not been able to demonstrate that massage reduces metabolites following exercise.

Tissue Movement

As the hands move along the superficial tissues, pressure to the tissues is increased, and layers of tissue are moved. A light glide causes movement of the epidermis. If friction is maintained between the therapist's hand and the patient's skin, the epidermis moves with the hand and is gently stretched. There will also be some movement of the dermis because of the traction between the two layers. More pressure with friction, although still very light, results in traction between the dermis and the subcutis. The end-feel of the stroke is when this traction reaches its limit and all layers are stretched.

Massage involves the interaction of energy between the person applying the massage and the dog, and the effects of touch to induce relaxation, communication, and a sense of general well-being. It also produces movement of the tissues in subsequent layers as a result of traction of the tissue interfaces. Sensory and autonomic nerves are stimulated, inducing changes in the nervous and circulatory systems, and movement may be affected in abnormal tissue, such as scar tissue or layers of adherent tissues.

Therapeutic Effects

Massage is generally enjoyed by small animal patients and helps to relieve distress, anxiety, and discomfort. There are many postulated effects of massage, which are indicated in literature regarding massage. Unfortunately, many of these have not been substantiated by systematic scientific investigations.

Stroking young animals results in a reduction in the animal's physiologic response to stress, demonstrated by a decreased output of adrenocorticotrophic hormone (ACTH).[1] Young animals that are handled also show greater development of the cortex and the subcortex of the brain. They learn faster and have a more advanced stage of neural development than nonhandled animals.[2] Resistance to infection later in life may also be beneficially influenced by cutaneous stimulation experienced by the infant animal.[3]

If a hand is placed over the surface of a dog's skin, heat is felt between the two surfaces. If the hand is placed on the skin and held still, this heat increases. Rubbing over the surface of the skin causes friction, and this results in an even greater increase in heat. Heat is a form of energy, and some schools of massage, particularly those grounded in Eastern practices, use the energy field that exists around the body. This is sometimes referred to as an electromagnetic radiation around the entire body. It is felt as heat and can be felt a small distance from the body. Some also believe that other forms of energy fields run through the body, along specific pathways known as medians. These are used in acupuncture and reflex therapy treatments

Most of the research on the effects of massage has been done in humans. Most studies have evaluated healthy individuals, which may be misleading because physiologic compensatory mechanisms are extremely efficient in healthy tissues and any alterations in local blood flow may be compensated for by autoregulatory processes. Most of the research studies have also been performed on small groups and often without control groups. One study by Hansen and Kirstensen[4] gave little detail concerning the massage itself, such as the amount of pressure applied. Although the research supported the concept that massage increases blood flow in muscles, the lack of information regarding the type of massage and length of treatment make interpretation of the results difficult.

Changes in blood constituents following massage have provided information regarding the mechanism of action of massage.[5] Ernst[6] found that a standard 20-minute massage treatment reduced the hematocrit and blood and plasma viscosity. It is believed that the fluid immediately surrounding poorly perfused vessels has low viscosity because of decreased cellularity and that the vasodilatation caused by massage aids in the recruitment of dormant vessels. It is desirable to increase local circulation to promote healing. The mechanical effect of the massage helps to remove low-viscosity tissue fluid into the circulation. The changes in blood detected within the vessels in this study support the belief that massage produces a flushing and mechanical effect on the circulation.

Effects on Muscle

Massage may also affect skeletal muscles. Muscles have a natural resting tone that may be increased in postural muscles by external influences, such as cold or stress. This occurs because of the interaction of the muscle spindle and the central nervous system. Stretching a muscle may stimulate the muscle spindle and cause a reflex muscle contraction, while reflex inhibition of the antagonist occurs. Massage may add an external stimulus to sensory organs and either increases muscle tone by stimulation or reduces it, probably by facilitating an accommodation of the spindle, causing it to reset at a lower threshold of excitability.

It is believed that the circulatory effect of massage will reduce muscle soreness and thus aid clinical signs associated with muscle injury or post exercise recovery. Danneskiold-Samsoe et al.[7] studied the effects of massage for shoulder and back pain in humans. Blood samples were evaluated for myoglobin concentrations. There was a statistically significant effect, with peak myoglobin concentrations occurring within 3 hours of the massage. Myoglobin concentrations gradually decreased, until after seven treatments, there was no difference.

Jacobs[8] advocated the use of massage for the relief of spasm of unknown cause but which resulted in a self-perpetuating muscle spasm cycle (Figure 18-2). Massage is also said to reduce tone in muscles that are tense or in spasm and to reduce the soreness and tender-

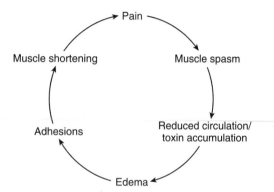

Figure 18-2   Self-perpetuating muscle spasm cycle.

ness of exercised muscles. It is also used to prepare muscles for exercise.

Jones and Round,[9] discussed the process by which an analgesic substance, possibly potassium, is released when muscles maintain excessive tone or static contraction for prolonged periods of time. Eccentric exercise of muscles, which generates high forces in muscles, produces delayed-onset soreness and a feeling of stiffness. Jones and Round[9] explained this by identifying swelling in muscles and inflammation of the connective tissue. Massage may help reduce or prevent the initial tenderness. It is also believed that massage may help to prevent subsequent postexercise pain. Regular massages may make the muscles softer and more pliable, and the stretching manipulations may increase extensibility and strength in the connective tissues.[7]

Pain experienced after exercising with the muscles in a lengthened position may also be due to inflammation of the connective tissue, rather than muscle damage. Massage may assist by increasing pliability in the connective tissue around the muscle fasciculi. Massage assists mobility between the interfaces within the muscle and also stretches any fibrous adhesions or scarring in the tissue.

The effects of massage on the H (Hoffman) reflex, which indicates the excitability in α motoneurons or anterior horn cells, has also generated interest. Goldberg et al[10] studied the effects of massage on healthy and spinal cord–injured human patients. They applied one-handed petrissage to deep and superficial tissues. There was a 49% reduction in H reflex activity with deep massage, and a 39% reduction with light massage. From this study, it was concluded that stimulating cutaneous mechanoreceptors and pressure receptors reduces H reflex activity. Sullivan et al.[11] also demonstrated a reduction in α motoneuron excitability of massaged muscles.

Effects on Pain and Sensation

The effects of massage on connective tissues, which helps to reduce muscle spasm and soft tissue discomfort, have already been discussed. Ueda et al[12] demonstrated that post-surgical massage has beneficial effects on sensation and analgesia. This study suggested that mild sensory stimulation may facilitate regression of sensory analgesia.

Carreck[13] evaluated the effect of massage on levels of pain perception in humans. She found that pain threshold was raised to significantly higher levels in the massage group and this work suggests that massage may be used to help manage pain and reduce treatment soreness.

Massage causes traction at tissue interfaces. Horizontal plexi lie at interfaces in the tissues and gentle pulling on these vessels may stimulate the accompanying sympathetic nerves, which supply the mechanoreceptors. These receptors may be distorted by the massage, possibly lowering of mechanoreceptor sensitivity and reducing pain and tenderness. If delayed-onset pain in the muscle is caused by connective tissue inflammation, the flushing effect in the surrounding fluids and removal of inflammatory mediators may increase the speed at which the inflammation resolves.

Effects of Massage on Connective Tissue

Following injury or disease, inflammation causes increased vascular permeability. The resulting edema contains fibrinogen, which may result in formation of fibrous tissue. Adhesions form within the tissues, binding tissue interfaces. These adhesions prevent normal sliding of fibers upon each other and also reduce the ability of the fibers to spread apart. Massage is described as being able to stretch tissues that have become short, tight, or adhered. Petrissage massage stretches and pulls the tissues in various directions and mobilizes the adjacent connective tissue fibrils. The molecular crossbridges between fibrils may be influenced and plastic changes may occur; their length may be maintained or increased because of elongation or creep. Mobility may also be increased at the fibrous crossbridges, between fibers and areas of adhesions, by stretching connections between the fibers. This facilitates spreading and sliding at tissue interfaces, and longitudinal elongation helps to increase flexibility.

Following surgery, scars may form with adhesions of various tissue layers to the underlying tissues. Massage helps mobilize and soften adhesions by elongation, creep, and increased fluid exchange of tissues. Collagen fibers align themselves along lines of stress. Techniques that stretch the fibers and adhesions in different directions eventually restore their mobility, promoting remodeling along the lines of normal stresses.

Following injury, it is important to maintain local flexibility of the involved structures to assist overall flexibility and to reduce the possibility of reinjury due to decreased extensibility of normal and scar tissues. Massage should be used to promote the functional recovery of a structure and prevent reinjury by maintaining mobility at the interfaces, both inside and outside the affected structures. Massage should be combined with controlled longitudinal stretching exercises.

One technique to mobilize scar tissue is deep friction.[14] It is applied at 90 degrees to the fibers and delivers a stretch and separation between individual fibers. Deep friction is believed to create movement and induce reactive hyperemia,[15] to stretch crossbridges between fibers, and to stretch adhesions within the structure. Fibrous scarring in tendons and their interfaces may become more pliable with massage. Although one researcher has suggested that deep friction application may result in some analgesia to the area,[16] there is little evidence to support this claim. Although many theoretical effects of massage have been put forth, there is little research evidence to support these claims.

How Massage Works

Massage may have immediate benefits to a patient, but it usually takes regular treatments to bring about significant improvements in a particular condition. Initially, massage may provide relief from pain, reduce tension, and help to sedate the nervous system. When pain has subsided, attempts to correct the underlying cause of the problem may begin. Healing is stimulated by both mechanical and reflex actions.

The mechanical effect of massage to the soft tissues may help to relieve tense muscles through relaxation, decreased pain, and increased mobility, and it may improve the circulation and lymphatic flow. The body, mind, and emotions all interact with the nervous system. It is possible that touching the skin sends messages, including reflex actions as the involuntary reaction of one part of the body to the stimulation of another part, to reduce the amount of stress hormones, which may lower blood pressure, slow breathing, improve digestion, and generate a sense of well-being. It is believed that massage also helps to release endorphins, the body's natural pain relievers, and to activate neuropeptides, the intercellular messages within the nervous system. These link the skin to the nervous system and the entire body, including the immune system. These actions as a result of massage are thought to have tremendous benefits.

Indications for Massage

Mechanical

If a dog has a chronic musculoskeletal problem, it may develop secondary problems, which lead to postural and gait adaptations. In time, these may also become primary problems in themselves due to changes in the soft tissues, which lead to unprotected joints, possible damage to the joints, and a painful response.

Surgical

If a dog has had surgery, massage may help to maintain mobility. If the dogs must be confined for a period of rest, or is on restricted exercise, it helps to maintain tone and muscle condition. Massage also helps psychologically by maintaining contact of the dog with the owner, and it may ease pain and discomfort. After resolution of the surgical condition, massage is indicated to maintain flexibility of all joints and soft tissues, and to prevent further loss of function.

Disease

For dogs suffering a permanent low-grade disease such as osteoarthritis, massage before exercise helps to encourage blood flow, delivery of nutrients and maintenance of soft tissue extensibility. For those that suffer chronic imbalances, which have caused structural changes of the soft tissues, massage helps to relax and ease discomfort and may have a significant effect on tension and muscular effort.

Massage for the Competitive Dog

Proper massage applied to competitive dogs may help to establish or reestablish full tissue function. Massage may be employed during the training period for treatment and rehabilitation, and to enhance athletic performance. It may also help to prepare the dog for competition or exercise, and to reduce stress and aid relaxation. After hard exercise or competition, it aids recovery.

At an amateur level, training may sometimes be somewhat neglected, and massage can play a significant role in maintaining tissue pliability, in hopes of preventing injury. At the other end of the scale, top canine athletes are more likely to be overtrained, and massage can assist in recovery from fatigue. In this case, 2 hours should be allowed to elapse before massage is started, for maximum effects. Care must be exercised to not massage too deep and induce mechanical trauma, which may be detrimental to fatigued muscles.

Massage for Performance

In order to perform properly, the body must be able to adapt to the extra stresses placed upon it. Requirements for excellence are power, agility, and coordination of the dog, and to attain this level of performance, the dog must cope with activity at the extremes of joint movement and muscle length. This places heavy demands on the strength and the endurance of the muscle, and the ability of the joints to move freely in all directions. The dog also needs freely mobile connective tissues. Inevitably, excess or repetitive stresses, or overwork, will increase the likelihood of other injuries, such as muscle strain. In all cases, this results in replacement of connective tissue with scar tissue, resulting in loss of power, flexibility, and movement in the tissues. Moreover, if the tissue is not rehabilitated before normal full activity is resumed, then it may never fully recover and return to normal limits. This in turn may overload the surrounding tissues, causing fatigue and hypertrophy of muscle groups.

Massage can be used to stretch and free this inelastic scar tissue and return tissue mobility to normal. It also helps to remodel and promote resorption of the scar and to reestablish full function of the tissues.

Fatigue

When a dog trains very hard, it may not fully recover between sessions, which may lead to general muscle soreness and increased likelihood of injury. Massage is used to decrease muscle tone and tension, thereby reducing muscular discomfort and promoting relaxation. There is also evidence to suggest that it helps recovery from fatigue, as compared with rest alone. It would therefore be very appropriate to use massage after competition, training, traveling, or any particularly stressful situation.

Muscle Soreness

Dogs suffer soreness in their muscles as a result of extreme exertion and adverse environmental conditions. Endurance dogs galloping over uneven terrain in wet weather conditions or in extreme heat and humidity are examples of extreme conditions. This form of soreness normally begins after completion of the event, and sometimes not until the next day. Less fit animals may also suffer discomfort during such exercises, but as a result of metabolic insufficiency. Well-conditioned muscles generally do not suffer from this problem because they have a well-functioning capillary bed and adequate oxygenation of the blood supply. Obviously, a dog will be at a disadvantage if it has not had an opportunity to fully recover from the previous competitive efforts. An inadequate rest period may result in very severe discomfort due to connective tissue inflammation, tenderness, and stiffness. Massage may delay the onset of soreness and reduce it.

Experience and some studies strongly suggest that the ideal time to massage is 1 to 3 hours after exercise to enhance athletic performance and for the best therapeutic benefit. Also, for certain muscles, massage may enhance tissue lengthening more than stretching alone.

There are also contraindications to massage (Box 18-2).

Planning a Massage

When planning a massage for a competitive animal, the stage of training, the fitness of the animal, and the purpose of the massage must be considered. The various purposes of massage include relaxation, toning, precompeti-

---

BOX 18-2 Contraindications to Massage

Do not massage if the dog is suffering from the following conditions:

- Shock (lowers blood pressure)
- Fever
- Acute inflammation (do not address area directly, but it would be acceptable to work elsewhere on the body)
- Skin problems (ringworm)
- Infectious diseases
- Acute stages of viral disease (herpes)

---

tion warmup, intercompetition treatment, aiding muscle soreness 1 to 3 hours after competition, improving healing, relief of acute or chronic injury and fatigue, muscle soreness, and preventing adhesion formation. A thorough patient evaluation is necessary to assess areas that might benefit the most from proper massage techniques.

Patient Evaluation

During the initial observation period, care should be taken to ensure that the dog is standing on a flat, even surface in an area with adequate lighting.

Caudal View

The patient is evaluated from a caudal view while standing. From this angle, the general posture is evaluated, looking for any skeletal abnormalities (e.g., scoliosis), areas of atrophy or hypertrophy, natural foot placement, weight-bearing tendencies of the limbs, head carriage, and the general appearance of the hindquarters and tail. The patient in Figure 18-3 has arthritis. Note that the dog has a clamped tail and decreased weight-bearing on the left hindlimb, with the limb held in slight flexion.

Cranial View

From this view it is important to note the symmetry of the head, eyes, ears, and paws, head carriage, forelimb weight-bearing tendencies, and the natural position of the forelimbs (e.g., neutral, rotation, adduction, abduction). Note in Figure 18-4 the deviation of the head to the left with slight rotation to the left and external rotation of the forelimbs. Also, the right paw is more splayed than the left.

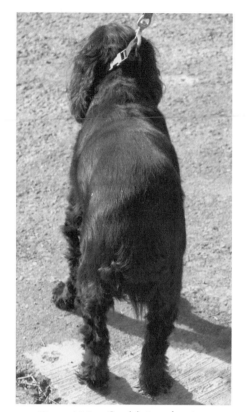

Figure 18-3   Caudal view of patient.

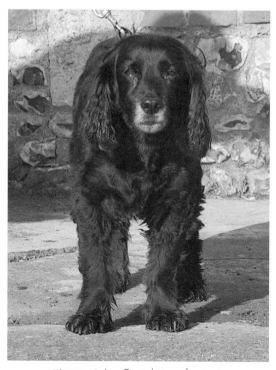

Figure 18-4   Cranial view of patient.

Lateral View

It is important to observe both sides of the patient. Important points to note are the general posture, appearance of the muscles, head carriage, tail position, and limb joint angles. In the dog in Figure 18-5, note the roached back and clamped tail. Also note that the limb angles cannot be truly assessed because the dog is not standing squarely and symmetrically.

Gait Assessment

WALK: CAUDAL VIEW

At this stage it is important to assess any hindlimb lameness. The ability of the dog to walk in a straight line should be assessed, along with the fluency of hindlimb movement (i.e., does the dog move forward in a straight line, or does it circumduct, abduct, adduct, and so forth). It is important that the dog handler move in a straight line and be educated in handling of dogs for evaluation purposes. Observations should be made of the lumbosacral rhythm, or the rise and fall of the tuber coxae and tuber sacrale, and the presence of any protective muscle splinting that may be occurring. In the dog in Figure 18-6, the tail is held low, the hindlimb toe off phase initiates in an adducted position, the dog appears to move toward the left, and the dog appears to be dragging the left hind toe.

WALK: CRANIAL VIEW

The cranial view should evaluate forelimb lameness and fluency of movement along with natural head carriage and foot placement. The nose, head, and neck deviate to the left, and foot placement appears close in the forelimbs in the dog depicted in Figure 18-7.

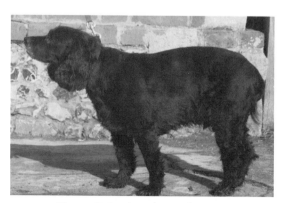

Figure 18-5   Lateral view of patient.

TROT: CAUDAL VIEW

Similar to assessing walking from a caudal position, it is also important to note any hindlimb lameness, symmetry, fluency of movement, protective splinting of muscle groups (e.g., hamstrings or gluteals), tail carriage, and limb carriage and placement at a trot (Figure 18-8).

TROT: CRANIAL VIEW

As with observation at a walk, observe the dog for any lameness, head and neck carriage, forelimb carriage and foot placement, and symmetry and fluency of movement. In Figure 18-9, note the low head carriage and the adducted position of the right forelimb.

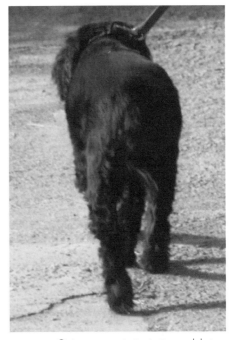

Figure 18-8   Gait assessment at a trot—caudal view.

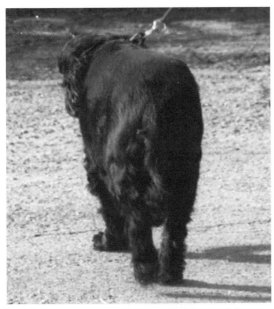

Figure 18-6   Gait assessment at a walk—caudal view.

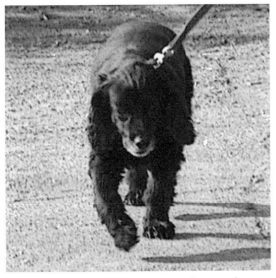

Figure 18-7   Gait assessment at a walk—cranial view.

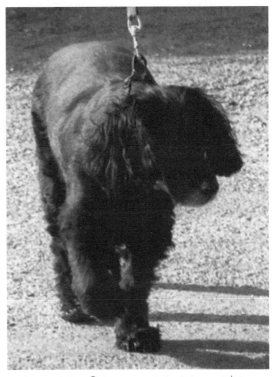

Figure 18-9   Gait assessment at a trot—cranial view.

SIDE VIEW

Both sides of the animal should be assessed. From this angle it is important to note the equality of the hindlimb and forelimb stride lengths, the ability of all limbs to retract and protract, head and tail carriage, protective muscle splinting, and general muscle interaction. In Figure 18-10, note the clamped appearance of the tail and possible guarding of the epaxial muscles.

Turning Short

It is important to evaluate the dog while turning in small circles in both directions, noting whether or not the bend follows through from nose to tail, whether the limbs cross over, and whether any areas look restricted. It is also important to recognize whether or not the dog actually understands what is being asked of him. In Figure 18-11 note the reluctance of the dog to perform the task: The dog appears to be braced from neck to tail, and the dog is also not crossing his legs.

Palpation

The dog's skeletal structure and muscle tone should be assessed after evaluation of the dog's gait. This is performed by palpating along the dog, from the wings of the atlas, along the spine and limbs, to the tail (Figure 18-12). Areas of irritability, spasm, atrophy, hypertrophy, and asymmetry are noted, along with any skeletal abnormalities.

By palpating on either side of the dorsal spinous processes with the thumbs, sensitive areas may be assessed (Figure 18-13). The surrounding areas are also palpated for any evidence of any other sensitive areas in the region, such as the withers and triceps region (Figure 18-14). Limb musculature is also assessed independently (e.g., shoulder girdle and pelvic girdle musculature), noting whether any tone or spasm are present. Bony landmarks are palpated bilaterally, noting the symmetry of position and surrounding musculature, for example, the tuber sacrale and tuber coxae (Figure 18-15).

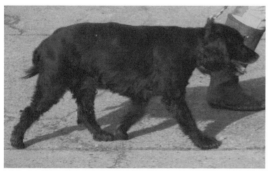

Figure 18-10   Gait assessment—side view.

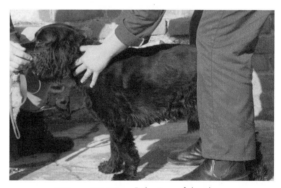

Figure 18-12   Palpation of the dog.

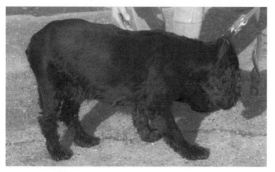

Figure 18-11   Turning short in small circles.

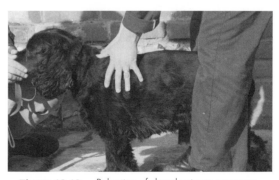

Figure 18-13   Palpation of dorsal spinous processes.

Passive Movements of the Cervical Spine

FLEXION

While standing above the dog, place one hand over the cervical spine to enable assessment of the muscles and joints as they move through a range of motion, then place the other hand over the dog's nose and guide the head down toward the forelimbs. Note the quality and range of movement and end feel, as well as the feel of the muscles and joints under the palpating hand. Although it is difficult to appreciate in the photograph, the dog in Figure 18-16 has restriction in flexion.

EXTENSION

Support the dog's head under its chin with one hand and palpate the cervical spine with the other. Using the supporting hand, guide the head dorsally into extension. Note the quality and range of movement, the end feel, and the characteristics of the muscles and

joints under the palpating hand. The dog in Figure 18-17 appears to resist this maneuver.

SIDE FLEXION

While placing one hand over one side of the dog's nose, use the other hand to stabilize the dog while palpating the cervical spine. First guide the dog's head to one direction, and then after changing positions of the hands, guide the head in the other direction. Note the range and quality of movement, end feel, and so forth for both sides. In Figure 18-18, left-side flexion appears restricted, and increased tone is palpated by the evaluator in the cervical musculature.

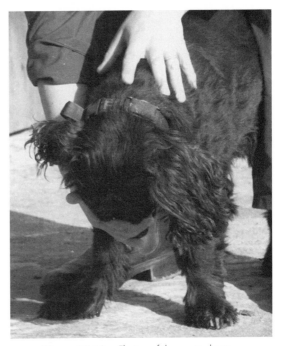

Figure 18-16   Flexion of the cervical spine.

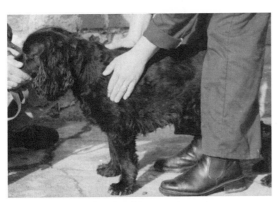

Figure 18-14   Palpation of the scapular and triceps region.

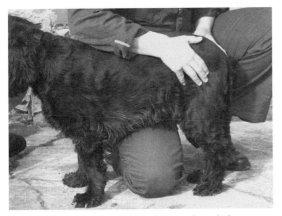

Figure 18-15   Palpation of the tuber sacrale and tuber coxae.

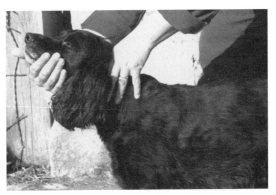

Figure 18-17   Extension of the cervical spine.

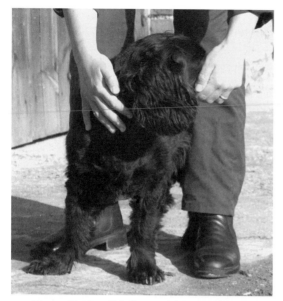

Figure 18-18   Side flexion of the cervical spine.

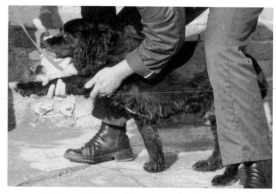

Figure 18-20   Protraction of a forelimb.

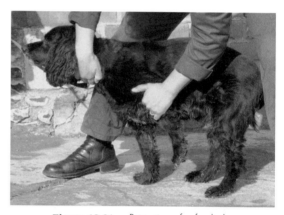

Figure 18-21   Retraction of a forelimb.

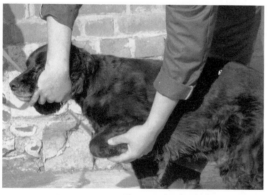

Figure 18-19   Flexion of a forelimb.

Forelimb

FLEXION

While ensuring that the dog is standing supported with the head pointing forward, flex the carpus and elbow. Note the range of movement, quality of movement, end feel, and scapular elevation. The dog in Figure 18-19 has good flexion in these joints.

PROTRACTION

After evaluating flexion, continue to guide the limb forward into full protraction. Again, note the range and quality of movement and the end feel. Any areas of increased muscle tone should be identified. Moving the limb across the midline into adduction tests the latissimus dorsi muscle. In this dog, protrac-

tion of the limb appears to be adequate (Figure 18-20).

RETRACTION

From the protracted position, guide the limb back into retraction, ensuring that the dog's neck is not tilted from midline. The range, quality, and end feel of movement are noted. The dog in Figure 18-21 appears to have restricted movement, possibly due to increased tone in the brachiocephalicus muscle, and the dog does not appear to be comfortable.

CERVICAL SPINE SIDE FLEXION
WITH FORELIMB RETRACTION

Support the dog between your legs and with one hand, flex the neck to the side. Hold this position, and use the other hand to gently retract the opposite forelimb to assess the range of movement (Figure 18-22).

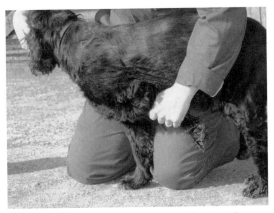

Figure 18-22   Side flexion of the cervical spine with retraction of the opposite forelimb.

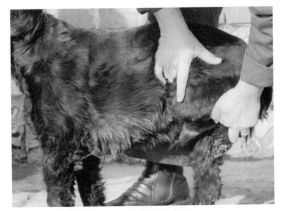

Figure 18-24   Flexion of a hindlimb.

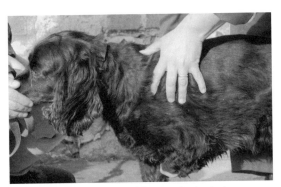

Figure 18-23   Adduction of a forelimb.

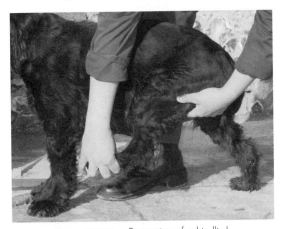

Figure 18-25   Protraction of a hindlimb.

ADDUCTION

From the neutral position, guide the limb across the chest toward the opposite leg. Note the range, quality, and end feel of the movement (Figure 18-23).

Hindlimb

FLEXION

With the dog supported, flex the hindlimb, obtaining full flexion of the hock and stifle. Assess the range and quality of movement, end feel, and the muscles. The dog in Figure 18-24 appears to have decreased limb flexion. Also note the dog's stance in the other limbs and overall level of comfort.

PROTRACTION

With one hand palpating the hindquarters and caudal thigh muscles, allow the other hand to guide the limb forward into protraction. Assess the range and quality of movement, end feel, and muscles. The dog in Figure 18-25 appears

to have full protraction, but may also have compensatory flexion of the lumbosacral area.

RETRACTION

With the dog in a standing position, use one hand to support the limb and guide it into retraction. Use the other hand to palpate the quadriceps and caudal thigh muscles. Again, note the range and quality of movement, end feel, and any fasciculation of the muscle. The dog in Figure 18-26 has very restricted retraction.

NOTE: All of the above passive limb movements can also be performed with the dog in lateral recumbency.

Tail

Tail movements may also be assessed, noting range of movement, quality of movement, and end feel. Elevation, depression, side flexion, and rotation movement of the tail can all be assessed (Figure 18-27).

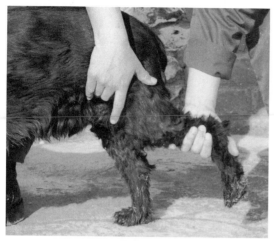

Figure 18-26   Retraction of a hindlimb.

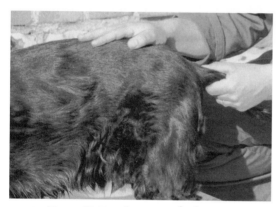

Figure 18-27   Assessment of tail motion.

Practical Application of Massage

Body Position and Comfort of the Clinician

Performing a massage can be quite tiring initially because you are concentrating on a new task and your body is learning new movements. If the clinician is not careful, this may lead to tension and fatigue. To prevent this from occurring, try to work in a systematic way. Also, be careful to maintain proper body posture and relax while learning the moves to help minimize these risks. Using your larger muscles such as the shoulder muscles instead of your hands helps to minimize fatigue. It is important that the dog feel confident in you, too. Dogs appear to be very good at picking up tension and any lack of confidence.

Maintaining good posture means greater comfort, and the clinician will not fatigue as

quickly. As a result, the massage will be more enjoyable for the clinician, resulting in greater relaxation for both parties. Altogether, the massage will be more effective, and a better result will be achieved.

Identification of Massage Areas and Application of Massage

When massaging, you may work on the entire dog, or selected areas. If the dog has a diagnosed condition, local massage may be appropriate on a regular basis. General massage helps with treatment of compensatory conditions and biomechanical changes.

Massage may be performed to isolated areas or to the entire limb and body. It may be used in conjunction with other therapies and veterinary treatments. It is also useful to be applied by the owner and may be successfully taught to the owner by the physical therapist.

Massage Techniques

Massage has many benefits for dogs, and there are many techniques that may be employed. Massage involves the use of a series of movements using the hands, which have an effect on the tissues. It is important to comfortably position the dog in lateral recumbency. It is also important to position yourself comfortably. The person performing the massage should be beside the dog on the floor, or place the dog on a raised surface, which may prevent you from stooping over or compromising your posture. It is best to start at one end, such as the head, and work along the dog in a sequenced manner (e.g., head, neck, shoulders, forelimbs, back, hindquarters, and tail). The following are techniques that may be used at any stage and over any muscle group.

Stroking

This is a good technique to start the treatment (Box 18-3). When the dog is positioned, run your hand over the dog from neck to tail and down the limbs with medium pressure. This technique aids relaxation of the dog and gives further opportunity to assess the tissues while the dog is not weight-bearing. Note the muscle tone and any swelling, masses, or temperature differences between body areas (Figure 18-28).

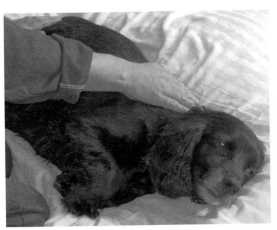

Figure 18-28 Stroking.

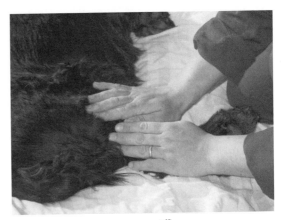

Figure 18-29 Effleurage.

■ ■ ■ **BOX 18-3** Stroking

This is often used initially in a massage and on most areas. Some consider this a form of effleurage.

Uses
- Relax the dog
- Introduce touch
- Sedate (slow stroking)
- Stimulate (brisk stroking)
- Decrease muscle tone (slow)

When to Use
- At the beginning or end of massage
- When only limited time is available, on a daily basis
- To calm and relax in a stressful situation
- Any time

Application
- Stroking is usually applied from the proximal limb toward the distal limb.
- Begin at the top of the area to be worked.
- Place the entire hand in contact with the skin.
- Maintain a gentle but firm pressure.

Effleurage

This is the opposite of stroking (Box 18-4). Beginning at a distal area, such as the paws, the hands move proximally, using medium pressure. This helps to move any toxins in the body toward the lymph nodes and aids drainage (Figure 18-29).

Compressions

When performing effleurage, an increase in muscle tone in certain muscles may be identified. The triceps and deltoideus muscles are

■ ■ ■ **BOX 18-4** Effleurage

This is often performed initially in a massage on most areas of the body, particularly on the limbs and when swelling is present. It is the most common type of massage used, and often it is used in an evaluative manner to assess for tissue tightness, presence of muscle spasm, and so forth.

Uses
- Increase venous and lymphatic return
- Aid removal of chemical irritants
- Improve mobility between tissues
- Stretch muscle fibers
- Decrease muscle tone
NOTE: If used deeply, it may be used to increase muscle tone.

When to Use
- At the start and end of a session, and often in between various techniques
- Should be performed toward the lymph nodes
- May be performed using one or both hands, fingers or thumbs

Application
- Begin at the distal part to be effleuraged.
- Make contact with the skin and apply even pressure to sink into the superficial tissues.
- Make a sweeping movement to the top of the area, molding to the contours and maintaining the same depth of pressure throughout the stroke.
- Finish the stroke over the lymph node, then remove the hands and reposition at the start of the next stroke. If the stroke is not to the lymph nodes, continue to the nearest body part.
- Bring the hands toward you as you work, using the heel of your hand.
- Watch that the fingers and palm of the hand do not lose contact with the patient.
- Maintain an even depth of pressure while the hands mold to the body.
- Overlapping strokes are used, continuing until the entire body region is covered.
NOTE: In a small area, use only one hand, finger or thumb.

■ ■ ■ **BOX 18-5** Compression and Wringing

Compressions can be used all over and are very effective on large muscles. Wringing is often very relaxing and has a great sedative effect.

Uses
- Aid venous and lymphatic return
- Help with removal of chemical irritants
- Increase the mobility and length of fibrous tissue
- Restore mobility between tissue surfaces
- Aid tissue fluid mobility
- Increase extensibility and strength of connective tissue
- May also trigger skin reflexes and others linked to it

Features
These techniques compress the soft tissues, then they squeeze or roll them (wringing), working to the tissue end.

When to Use
- Use on superficial tissue, ligaments or muscles to soften up large areas.

Application of Compressions
- Use one hand or both, or pads, fingers or thumbs.
- Begin at the proximal end of the tissue and move distally.
- Contact the skin and compress the tissue.
- Skin is moved on the underlying tissue; there is no glide.
- The hands or digits or back of fist are used in a circular motion; this will initiate a slight stretch behind, and skin wrinkling ahead.
- If using right and left hand, the right moves clockwise and the left counterclockwise.
- Pressure is applied to deeper tissues when tissues are compressed. It is a similar movement to that used to open a childproof medicine bottle: press down initially, twisting as you do so, then release.
- To go from one completed compression to the next, slide the hands across.

Application of Wringing
This is applied using two hands.
- One brings the tissue toward you, the other moves it away. Hold for 2-5 seconds, then slowly release.
- The hand then moves to take up position on the adjacent tissue.

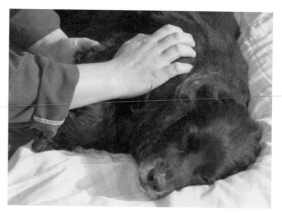

Figure 18-30 Compressions applied to tissues.

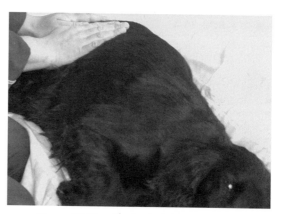

Figure 18-31 Placing technique over tissue.

Holding/Placing

An area of increased tone or spasm may be relaxed by placing a hand over the area. This technique traps heat in the area, increasing the local circulation and promoting local relaxation (Figure 18-31).

Percussion (Clapping, Hacking, Pounding)

If there is a general area of increased tone, such as in the caudal thigh or gluteal muscles, clapping and or hacking techniques may be employed (Box 18-6). This technique may also be used in areas of muscle weakness.

Clapping is performed by using a cupped hand. Gently but firmly, a clap is applied to the area (Figure 18-32). As the hands fall onto the muscle mass, a hollow sound should be heard. Hacking is performed by alternately using open hands, with the ulnar border of the

commonly affected. Compressions to the affected muscles may be easily administered and are often very effective (Box 18-5). The palm or heel of the hand is placed over the muscle and pressure is applied. This pressure is maintained for 15 seconds before moving on to another area. This maneuver should be repeated several times. By restricting blood flow and then releasing pressure, the circulation increases, and this is thought to help to decrease tone (Figure 18-30).

BOX 18-6   Percussion

Percussion consists of several techniques, the three most important being hacking, pounding and clapping.

Uses
- Stimulate local circulation
- Provoke muscle and tendon reflexes
- Provoke a general stimulatory effect
- Stimulate muscle tone
- Assistance in clearing airways (couppage)

Features
Light percussion has an effect on the superficial tissues; heavier application affects deeper layers and must not be used over organs.

Application of Clapping (Figure 18-32)
Hold the fingers and thumbs closed together to form a relaxed, cup shape. The elbows should be flexed and the arms abducted. The arms should be alternately flexed and extended so that the borders of the hands and fingers stroke the skin. The strokes are rapid, light, and brisk. Air is trapped between the hands and the skin, producing a hollow sound as contact is made. The entire treatment area should be covered.

Application of Hacking (Figure 18-33)
Hold the arms away from your sides, and flex the elbows approximately 90%, with the wrists fully stretched backward (extended) and fingers relaxed. The shoulders, where possible, should be over the area.
The border of the little finger and hand strike the skin alternately, lightly and rapidly. The movement comes from the wrist, and it involves a full side-to-side movement of the wrist in this position.
When doing very light hacking, only the fingers need strike the skin.

Application of Pounding
The arms should be held out, with elbows flexed to near 90 degrees. The wrists are extended with fingers flexed loosely into fists. The hips should be flexed to enable the shoulders to be over the area being treated. The medial borders of the fifth fingers strike the skin alternately and rapidly. The movement is at the radioulnar joint, which pronates and supinates.

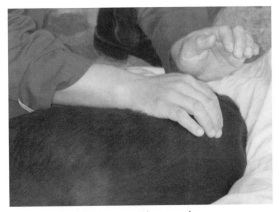

Figure 18-32   Clapping of tissue.

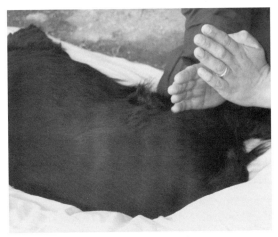

Figure 18-33   Hacking of tissue.

hands falling vertically on the muscle mass (Figure 18-33). In both cases the techniques are performed with light pressure initially, progressing to medium pressure. Both clapping and hacking improve general circulation in the areas treated, promoting relaxation.

Trigger Point Therapy

Often small areas of spasm may be felt within a muscle belly. Such nodules may be treated using trigger point therapy. The nodules are located and ischemic compression is applied using one or two fingers. The compression is held for approximately 20 seconds and released for 10 seconds before compression is reapplied. Generally three or four repetitions may be required (Figure 18-34).

Deep Transverse Friction

Scar tissue forms within muscles as a result of injury. Deep transverse frictions may be applied to help reduce the scarring (Box 18-7). These techniques were developed by Cyriax.[13] Using the index and middle fingers at a 90-degree angle to the muscle fibers, pressure is applied across the direction of the fibers. This is repeated 10 times and performed in sets of 3 to 10. It is a good practice to complete this technique with some gentle massage and stretching to relax the dog, as deep transverse friction may be uncomfortable (Figure 18-35).

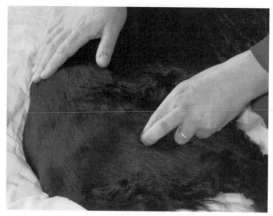

Figure 18-34   Compression of trigger point.

Passive Movements

To conclude the treatment session, when all the muscles are warm and relaxed, passive movements similar to those done in the weight-bearing position to evaluate the patient are performed. Again it is best to work in a sequence, such as from forelimbs to hindlimbs.

Forelimb and Scapular Mobilizations

Place one hand over the scapula and support the forelimb with the other. The scapula is mobilized from elevation to protraction, depression, and retraction. The limb is fully protracted and retracted (Figures 18-36 and 18-37).

Hindlimb

Similar movements are performed on the hindlimb. With one hand supporting the hindlimb and the other resting over the hip, the leg is elevated and depressed before it is protracted and retracted (Figures 18-38 and 18-39).

In some cases when passive movements are performed, areas of spasm may remain within the muscles, restricting full available range of movement. In these situations it is often useful to combine passive movements with trigger point therapy. The isolated muscle spasm is held by the therapist's finger and thumb while the other hand guides the limb through a range of motion (Figures 18-40 and 18-41). If restriction occurs again, the position should be held for a minimum of 15 seconds, then released before repeating. Following treat-

---

■ ■ ■ **BOX 18-7**   Friction Massage

Traditional Friction Massage
Uses
- Stimulate local circulation
- Aid in removal of chemical irritants
- Restore mobility between tissue interfaces
- Restore mobility to specific anatomical structures

Features
Performed with the tip of the thumb or fingers making small rotary movements, the pressure being appropriate to the desired tissue interface. Lubricants are not used as there is no glide on the skin.

Application of the Friction
The tip of the thumb or finger(s) should be placed on the skin, over the structure to be treated. The tissues are compressed to the depth of the structures being treated. Small rotary movements are performed on the structures while maintaining constant pressure, but there is no glide on the skin. The superficial tissues are moved on the underlying structures.

Deep Transverse (DT) Friction
Uses
- Stimulate local circulation
- Promote reactive hyperemia
- Restore mobility between tissue interfaces
- Restore mobility to specific anatomical structures

Features
Performed with the tip of the thumb or fingers making small rotary movements, the pressure being appropriate to the desired tissue interface. Lubricants are not used as there is no glide on the skin.

Application of Friction (Figure 18-35)
The tip of the thumb or finger(s) should be placed on the skin, over the structure to be treated. The tissues are compressed to the depth of the structures being treated. Small rotary movements are performed on the structures while maintaining constant pressure, but there is no glide on the skin. The superficial tissues are moved on the underlying structures.

---

ment, the dog should be very relaxed. The dog should be turned over and the massage should be repeated on the other side.

Alternative Methods

Several methods may be used as an alternative or adjunct to massage, including mechanical massagers, grooming the dog with a massager, and applying commercially available massage lubricant.

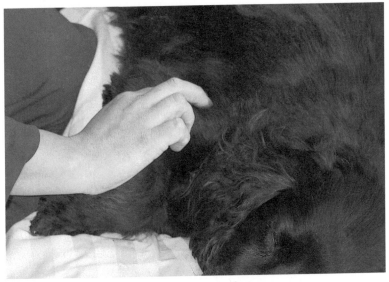

Figure 18-35   Deep transverse friction massage.

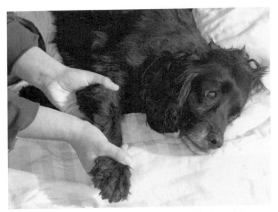

Figure 18-36   Forelimb mobilization with limb fully protracted.

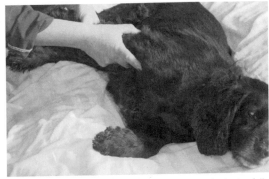

Figure 18-37   Forelimb mobilization with limb fully retracted.

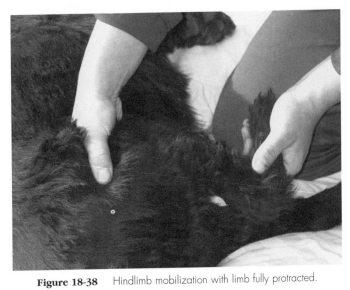

Figure 18-38   Hindlimb mobilization with limb fully protracted.

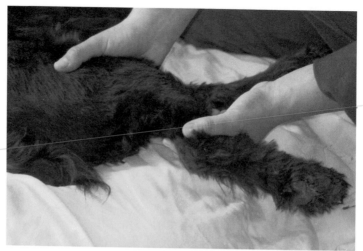

Figure 18-39 Hindlimb mobilization with limb fully retracted.

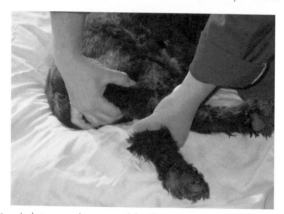

Figure 18-40 Isolating muscle spasm while placing rear limb through a range of motion.

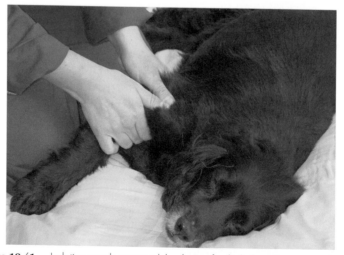

Figure 18-41 Isolating muscle spasm while placing forelimb through a range of motion.

REFERENCES

1. Seyle H: Stress and the general adaptation Synn Dme, *Jr J med* 1:1383,1950.
2. Ruegammer WR. et al: Growth food utilisation and thyroid activity in the albino rat as a function of extra handling, *Science* 120:134, 1954.
3. Soloman, GF, Moos, RH: Emotions, immunity and disease, *Arch Gen Psychiatry* 2: 657-674, 1964.
4. Hansen, TI, Kristensen, JH: Effect of massage, short-wave diathermy and ultrasound upon Xe disappearance rate from muscle and subcutaneous tissue in the human calf, *Scand J Rehab Med* 5:179-182, 1973.
5. Arkko, PJ, et al: Effects of whole body massage on serum protein, electrolyte and hormone concentrations, enzyme activities and haematological parameters. *Int J Sports Med* 4:265-267, 1983.
6. Ernst E et al: Massage cause changes in blood fluidity, *Physiotherapy* 73:43-45, 1987.

7. Danneskiold-Samsoe B et al: Regional muscle tension and pain (fibrositis); effect of massage on myoglobin in plasma. *Scand J Rehab Med* 15:17-20, 1982.

8. Jacobs M: Massage for the relief of pain: anatomical and physiological considerations, *Phys Ther Rev* 40:93-98, 1960.

9. Jones DA, Round JM: *Skeletal muscle in health and disease*, Manchester, England, 1990, Manchester University Press.

10. Goldberg J, et al: The effect of two intensities of massage on H-reflex amplitude, *Phys Ther* 72:449-457, 1992.

11. Sullivan SJ et al: Reduction of H-reflex amplitude during the application of effleurage to the triceps surae in neurologically healthy subjects. *Physiother Theory Pract* 9:25-31, 1993.

12. Ueda W et al: Effect of gentle massage on regression of sensory analgesia during epidural block, *Anesth Analg* 76:783-785, 1993.

13. Carreck A: The effect of massage on pain perception threshold, *Manipulative Physiotherapist* 26:10-16, 1994.

14. Cyriax J: *Textbook of orthopaedic medicine*, vol 2, London, 1984, Balliere Tindall.

15. Chamberlain GJ: Cyriax's friction massage; a review, *J Orthop Sports Phy Ther* 4:16-22, 1982.

16. Ombregt L et al: *A system of orthopaedic medicine*, London, 1995, WB Saunders.

SUGGESTED READINGS

Barnett K: A theoretical construct of the concepts of touch as they relate to nursing. *Nursing Res* 21:102-110, 1972.

Boigey M: *Manuel de massage*, 1955. Cited in Licht S, editor: *Massage, manipulation and traction*, Baltimore, 1960, Waverly Press.

Boni A, Walthard K: Massage et cinesterapie des rheumatismes abarticulaires, 1956. Cited in Licht S, editor: *Massage, manipulation and traction*, Baltimore, 1960, Waverly Press.

Bork K et al: Serum enzyme levels after a whole body massage, *Arch Dermatol Forsch* 240:342-348, 1971.

Carrier EB: Studies on the physiology of capillaries: reaction of human skin capillaries to drugs and other stimuli, *Am J Physiol* II:528-547, 1922.

Cassar MP, *Handbook of massage therapy*, Complete guide for the student and professional massage therapist, Oxford, 1999, Butterworth Heinemann.

Charman RA, editor: *Complementary therapies for physical therapists*, Oxford, 2000, Butterworth Heinemann.

De Bruijn R: Deep transverse friction; its analgesic effect, *Int J Sports Med* 5:35-36, 1984.

Ernst E, Fialka V: The clinical effectiveness of massage therapy: a critical review, *Forsch Komplementarmed* 1:226-232, 1994.

Field TM et al: Tactile/kinesthetic stimulation effects on preterm neonates, *Pediatrics* 77:654-658, 1986.

Flowers KR: String wrapping versus massage for reducing digital volume, *Phys Ther* 68:57-59, 1988.

Frank LK: Tactile communication, *Genet Psychol Monogr* 1957, pp 211-251

Goodhall-Copestake BM: *The theory and practice of massage*, London, 1926, Lewis.

Graham D: *Practical treatise on massage*, New York, 1884, Wood.

Guyton AC: *Textbook of medical physiology*, Philadelphia, 1991, WB Saunders.

Hack GD et al: Previously undescribed relation between muscle and dura, In *Proceedings of the Congress of Neurological Surgeons*, Phoenix, Arizona, February 14-18, 1995.

Hartelius I et al: How little you are? *Neonatal Netw* II(8):33-37, 1992.

Hoffa A: *Technik der Massage*, Stuttgart, 1897, Verlag Von Ferdinand Ernke.

Holey EA: *Therapeutic massage*, WB Saunders, 1997, Philadelphia.

Hourdeboight JP: *Canine massage*, New York, 1999, Howell Book House. Macmillan.

Hovind H, Nielson SL: Effect of massage on blood flow in skeletal muscle, *Scand J Rehab Med* 6:74-77, 1974.

Knight MTN, Dawson R: Effect of intermittent compression of the arms on deep vein thrombosis of the legs, *Lancet* ii:1265-1267, 1976.

Kubik ST, Manneston M: Anatomie der Lymphkapillaren and Prakollektoren der Haut. In Bonniger A, Partsch H, editors: *Intiale Lymphstrombahn, Internat. Symp. Zurich*, Stuttgart, 1984, G. Thieme.

Marin I et al: Postoperative pain after thoracotomy: a study of 116 patients, *Rev Maladies Resp* 8:213-218, 1991.

Mason A: Something to do with touch, *Physiotherapy* 71:167-169, 1985.

Mennell JB: *Physical treatment by movement, manipulation and massage*, ed 5, Philadelphia, 1945, Blakiston.

Montagu A: *Touching*, New York, 1978, Harper and Row.

Morelli M et al: Changes in H-reflex amplitude during massage of triceps surae in healthy subjects, *J Orthop Sports Phys Ther* 12:55-59, 1990.

Nordschow M, Bierman W: The influence of manual massage on muscle relaxation; effect on trunk flexion, *J Am Phys Ther Assoc* 42:653-657, 1962.

Pellechia GL et al: Treatment of infrapatella tendinitis; a combination of modalities and transverse friction massage versus iontophoresis, *J Sport Rehab* 3:135-145, 1994.

Poznick-Palewitz E: Cephalic spasm of head and neck muscles, *Headache* 15:261-266, 1976.

Prosser EM: *A manual of massage and movements*, ed 2, London, 1941, Faber and Faber.

Puustjarvi K et al: The effect of massage in patients with chronic tension headache, *Int J Acupuncture Electrotherapeut Res* 15:159-162, 1990.

Sabri S et al: Prevention of early deep vein thrombosis by intermittent compression of the leg during surgery, *Br Med J* 4:394, 1971.

Severini V, Venerando A: Effect of massage on peripheral circulation and physiological effects of massage, *Eur Medicophys* 3:165-183, 1967.

Troisier O: Les tendinities epicondyliennes, *Rev Prat* 41:1651-1655, 1991.

Wakim KG et al: Effects of massage on the circulation in normal and paralysed extremities, *Arch Phys Med* 30:135-144, 1949.

Walker JM: Deep transverse friction in ligament healing, *J Orthop Sports Phys Ther* 62:89-94, 1984.

Weber AS: *Traite de la massotherapie*, Paris, 1891.

Weinrich SP, Weinrich MC: The effect of massage on pain in cancer patients, *Appl Nursing Res* 3:140-145, 1990.

Westland G: Massage as a therapeutic tool, *Br J Occupat Ther* Part 1, 56:129-134; Part 2, 56:177-180, 1993

Williams PL et al, editors: *Gray's anatomy*, ed 37, Edinburgh, 1989, Churchill Livingstone.

Wood EC, Beckers PD: *Beard's massage*, Philadelphia, 1981, WB Saunders.

Yates J: *A physician's guide to massage therapy: its physiological effects and their application to treatment*, Vancouver, British Columbia, Canada, 1990, The Massage Therapist Association.

Ylinen J, Cash M: *Sports massage*, London, 1988, Stanley Paul.

Therapeutic Ultrasound

■ Janet E. Steiss and Laurie McCauley

The aim of physical rehabilitation is to reestablish normal function using modalities such as heat and electrical stimulation, mobilization, and therapeutic exercise.[1] Superficial heating agents penetrate to a depth of approximately 1 cm. Deep heating agents can elevate tissue temperatures at depths of 3 cm or more. Deep heating agents include ultrasound (US) and diathermy.

Therapeutic US is considered an effective treatment modality for rehabilitating musculoskeletal conditions such as restricted range of motion (ROM) resulting from joint contracture, pain and muscle spasm, and wound healing.[2] There are advantages and disadvantages of US therapy (Box 19-1). Many protocols for the administration of US are based on tradition or extrapolated from basic science research, and remain to be tested in controlled clinical trials.[3-6] This chapter is based on a review of current literature pertaining to the clinical application of US in humans, basic research findings, and available information published on US therapy in dogs with some reference to US therapy in horses.

Physical Principles

Energy within a sound beam decreases as it travels through tissue, because of scatter and absorption. Scattering is the deflection of sound out of the beam when it strikes a reflecting surface. Absorption is the transfer of energy from the sound beam to the tissues. Absorption is high in tissues with a high protein content,[7,8] and relatively low in adipose tissue.[7,9]

For more detailed information regarding the components of US machines, piezoelectric effects, sound generation, and sound propagation through tissues, the reader is referred to other sources.[10,11]

Coupling Techniques

The therapist must first consider the site of soft tissue involvement, such as muscle, joint capsule, tendon, bursa, and scar tissue and position the animal appropriately. Positioning is a compromise between patient comfort and access to the target tissue.

The US beam is attenuated in air and reflected at air–tissue interfaces. Consequently, a coupling medium must be placed between the sound head and the skin.[12] Methods for direct coupling, immersion, and use of coupling cushions have been described for dogs.[13]

Direct coupling is preferred when the surface to be treated is relatively flat and is larger than the applicator surface. A layer of water-soluble US gel is spread over the skin, and the sound head is placed in contact with the gel. Elimination of as much air as possible maximizes the US energy entering the tissues. If there are bony prominences in the treatment area or if the surface is very small, smaller applicators (transducer heads) are preferable.

Commercially prepared water-soluble US gels are the most practical. The gel may be preheated. Coupling agents that are not recommended include[1] substances that may irritate or penetrate through the skin[2]; electroconductive gels, such as for electrocardiography or electromyography, which contain salts that can damage the transducer face[3]; lanolin-based compounds, which would cause heating of the transducer head with poor transmission to tissue[8]; and[4] mineral oil, which is messy to remove.[13] Over-the-counter creams and lotions should not be used because they generally do not provide effective transmission of US.

Other methods of coupling have been used. However, research results on these indirect coupling methods are inconclusive, and further investigation is warranted.[14] The underwater method was popular before smaller transducer heads became available.[8] Immersion should be considered when the surface to be treated is so uneven that direct contact is too difficult. The part of the body to be treated, usually a distal limb, can be immersed in a container of tap water at room temperature. The water and the animal's skin must be clean.[15] Water in a whirlpool is not recommended if it has been agitated because air bubbles will have formed. Deionized, degassed water is not necessary, but the water may be boiled and cooled or allowed to stand to remove air bubbles. Even so, small air bubbles tend to accumulate on the transducer face and the skin during treatment. The therapist can wipe these off quickly, but should try to minimize his or her own exposure. With regard to container type, metal containers will reflect some of the US beam, which could increase the intensity in areas near the metal; rubber or plastic do not cause as much reflection. During treatment, the transducer should be held underwater 0.5 to 3.0 cm from the skin surface. The intensity may be increased by 0.5 W/cm^2 to compensate for absorption by water.[7]

Immersion has not compared favorably with direct coupling in several studies that examined the tissue temperatures achieved with these two methods. One study compared immersion to topical US gel on temperature rise at a depth of 3 cm in the gastrocnemius muscle of humans.[12] The treatment consisted of continuous US at 1.5 W/cm^2 for 10 minutes, with the sound head moved at a speed of 4 cm per second. With direct coupling, tissue temperature increased 4.8° C compared to 2.1° C with immersion. In another study, the lateral epicondyle of pigs was treated with the transducer in direct contact with the skin and with the limb immersed in a water bath with the applicator held 2 cm from the skin surface. The temperature in the tendons of the extensor muscles originating at the lateral epicondyle rose into the therapeutic range with direct coupling, but not with immersion.[16]

Another alternative to direct coupling is the use of a coupling cushion.[13] Placing a water-filled balloon between the transducer head and the skin, with coupling gel at the interfaces, has been described.[10] A recent in vitro study compared the transmission properties of commercial gel pads, bladder techniques, and water bath immersion, through pig skin from which the hair had been clipped.[14] Insufficient acoustic energy transmission occurred with degassed tap water in latex gloves, gel in a latex glove, degassed tap water baths, and gel-filled condoms. The authors recommended that if the direct method cannot be used because of the contour of the surface to be treated, clinicians should consider the use of commercially available gel pads. If other direct techniques are used, transmission is considerably less than with the direct coupling technique or with commercial gel pads.[14]

The Effect of the Hair Coat

Treating dogs with US presents a problem not encountered with human patients: the hair coat. Because US energy is absorbed by tissues with high protein content, and deflection of the US beam occurs at tissue interphases, it would be expected that US penetration through the hair coat into underlying tissues would be poor. For horses, one author has specifically recommended clipping the hair and using adequate coupling gel or having the horse stand in water to reduce any air interphase.[17]

A study has been conducted in dogs to determine temperatures in underlying tissues when delivering US through intact hair coats.[18] Despite application of a thick layer of gel on the skin, US delivered through short or long hair coats produced only minimal temperature increases in the underlying tissues, compared to therapy after the hair had been clipped, although there was considerable warming *within the hair coat* (Figures 19-1 and 19-2).

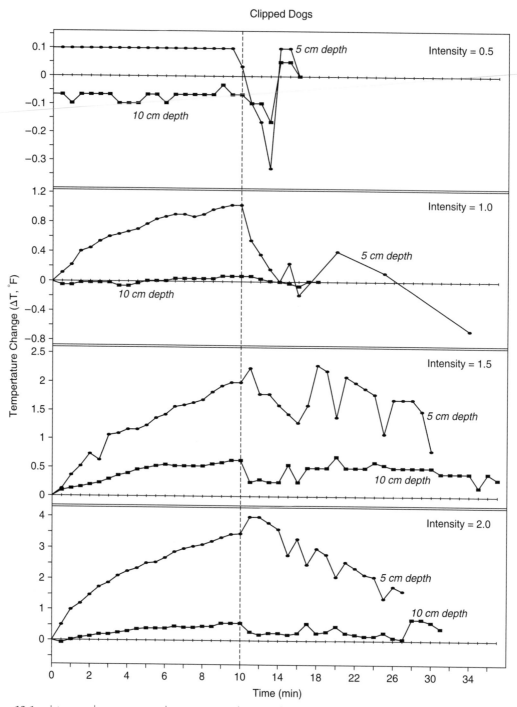

Figure 19-1   Intramuscular temperature changes measured at 5- and 10-cm depths during 1-MHz ultrasound at four intensities (W/cm²) applied to clipped skin over the caudal thigh in dogs. The vertical dashed line represents the end of 10 minutes of ultrasound exposure. The units on the y-axis differ for each intensity. (From Steiss JE, Adams CC: Rate of temperature increase in canine muscle during 1 MHz ultrasound therapy: deleterious effect of hair coat, *Am J Vet Res* 60:76-80, 1999.)

Short-Haired Dogs

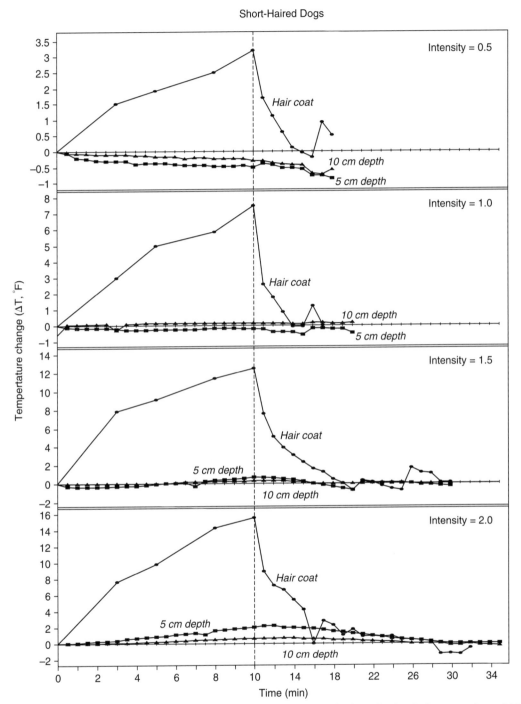

Figure 19-2   Temperature changes measured intramuscularly at 5- and 10-cm depths and within the hair coat, during 1-MHz ultrasound at four intensities (W/cm²) applied over the caudal thigh in dogs with short hair coats (Greyhounds). The vertical dashed line represents the end of 10 minutes of ultrasound exposure. The units on the y-axis differ for each intensity. (From Steiss JE, Adams CC: Rate of temperature increase in canine muscle during 1 MHz ultrasound therapy: deleterious effect of hair coat, *Am J Vet Res* 60:76-80, 1999.)

Treatment Variables

The following list contains treatment variables that must be considered for each patient. These items should be documented in the patient's record:

1. Frequency
2. Intensity
3. Duty cycle
4. Treatment area
5. Treatment duration
6. Speed of the sound head
7. Treatment schedule

Sound waves above a frequency of 20,000 hertz (20 kHz) exceed the upper range of human hearing and are termed *ultrasound* (US). The higher the frequency, the less divergent the sound beam. US beams are considered to be collimated, and frequencies in the megahertz (MHz) range expose a limited target area.

Frequency, not intensity, determines depth of penetration. The frequency most often used is 1 MHz because it represents a compromise between deep penetration and adequate heating. A frequency of 1 MHz frequency heats at depths between 2 and 5 cm.[19] As the frequency increases, penetration decreases. A frequency of 3 MHz heats at depths between 0.5 and 3 cm.[8,19,20] Therefore for superficial lesions, a frequency of 3 MHz is preferred; for deeper lesions, a setting of 1 MHz is needed.[8] If there is underlying bone, most of the US transmitted to that depth will hit the bone and may cause periosteal pain.[19,20,21] The intensity cannot be turned up very high to heat the underlying soft tissue if the bone is not adequately covered by soft tissues.[19] Recently, "long wave" machines have been investigated.[22] These units emit US at a lower frequency, around 45 kHz. In an in vitro study using fibroblasts, osteoblasts, and monocytes, 45 kHz and 1 MHz exposure both enhanced cell proliferation, protein synthesis, and cytokine production.[22]

Intensity refers to the rate of energy delivery per unit area. Most US machines indicate both watts (W) and watts per centimeter squared (W/cm^2). Available intensities typically range from 0.25 to 3.0 W/cm^2. Measurement of the total output (W) of the transducer divided by the transducer surface area (cm^2) is referred to as the *spatial average intensity*. The greatest intensity anywhere within the beam is termed the *spatial peak intensity*. The *beam nonuniformity ratio* (BNR) compares the maximal intensity from the transducer to the average intensity. This ratio should be low (between 2 and 6) to indicate that the energy distribution is relatively uniform, with minimal risk of tissue damage from areas of concentrated US energy ("hot spots"). This risk is minimized when the therapist keeps the US transducer moving during treatment.

The higher the intensity, the greater and faster the temperature increases. The depth of tissue penetration is not affected. Generally, intensities required to increase tissue temperature to a range of 40° to 45° C vary from 1.0 to 2.0 W/cm^2 continuous wave US for 5 to 10 minutes. To heat an area with much soft tissue, intensities as high as 2.0 W/cm^2 may be used. If there is less soft tissue, or if bone is close to the skin surface, lower intensity and higher frequency are appropriate. After selection of an initial intensity, the patient's tolerance to the heat produced by the US is the final determinant.[7] This may be difficult to determine in pets. Many dogs lie quietly during US treatment. However, some physical therapists have observed that dogs sometimes begin to whine or otherwise seem uncomfortable within 5 to 10 minutes after commencing US. It should be assumed that any distress demonstrated by a patient may indicate pain, and the intensity of the US should be reduced or the session interrupted or discontinued.

Most therapists tend to use intensities that produce no detectable sensation in human patients. However, some experts are currently advising that the intensity be increased until the person feels vigorous heating, after which time the intensity should be decreased if the patient experiences pain.[19] The US dosage that a patient is receiving cannot usually be monitored. In the past, in an effort to avoid tissue damage, the dosages have been low and the patient experiences no sensation. However, there is the possibility that the patient is not receiving a sufficient dose of US energy. These more recent recommendations seem to address this issue.

When the treatment goal is to heat periarticular structures, as is done when treating limited ROM, higher intensities are chosen. Lower intensities may be used for the relief of pain and muscle spasm, where the mechanism of action may be nonthermal.

Duty cycle refers to the fraction of time that the sound is emitted during one pulse period. With continuous mode, the US intensity is constant, whereas a pulsed wave is interrupted so that energy is delivered in an on/off manner.

$$\text{Duty cycle} = \frac{\text{Pulse duration (time on)}}{\text{Pulse period (time on + time off)}}$$

Typical duty cycles range from 0.05 (5%) to 0.5 (50%). For pulsed mode, the terms *temporal peak intensity* and *pulse average intensity* are used. Obviously, pulsing decreases the pulse average intensity and decreases the tissue heating. However, the spatial average intensity, which may be displayed on a meter, will be the same in pulsed and continuous mode. Pulsing may be used when the desired effect is based on a nonthermal mechanism or when minimal heating is desired, such as treating near bone.[8] Low-intensity continuous mode could also be chosen for these purposes.

The treatment area should be two to three times the size of the effective radiating area of the transducer head.[19] Increasing the total area beyond the recommended area decreases the dosage and the heating effect.

Experimental evidence indicates that a duration of 5 to 10 minutes is necessary to produce adequate tissue heating in an area equivalent to two to three times the diameter of the sound head.[21,23] For instance, when using direct coupling with topical US gel, continuous mode at 1.5 W/cm^2 for 10 minutes, and movement of the sound head at 4 cm per second, it took nearly 8 minutes for the temperature to reach therapeutic levels, when measured at a depth of 3 cm in the gastrocnemius muscle of humans.[12] For an intensity of 1.5 W/cm^2, Draper recommends a duration of 3 to 4 minutes at 3 MHz and at least 10 minutes at 1 MHz, assuming an area twice the size of the effective radiating area of the transducer.[19] The findings in dogs (see Figure 19-1) support these recommendations.

The speed at which the sound head is moved over the skin is generally recommended to be approximately 4 cm per second, or slower, to achieve uniform distribution of energy to the target tissues.[10] Moving the transducer too quickly diminishes the heating, and the therapist may have a tendency to cover too large an area. Various longitudinal and circular patterns may be used. The transducer should never be stationary when direct coupling is used. Because the US beam is nonuniform, some target areas within the beam could receive a large amount of energy. This predisposes to hot spots and tissue damage, including endothelial damage and platelet aggregation. Keeping the transducer moving is not as critical with underwater applications

because hot spots occur in the near field of the beam. Hot spots are situated in the water if a sufficient distance is maintained from the tissue. However, the distance might compromise the heating effect. Problems with achieving adequate tissue heating with the immersion technique have been previously described.

Treatment schedules may include daily treatment initially, followed by less frequent sessions as the condition improves.[7] Bromiley[8] states that treatment can be given daily for up to 10 days, but should not exceed two 10-day courses without a 3-week rest. Similar recommendations have been made for horses.[17]

Precautions and Contraindications

Tissue burns are a major concern.[13] These may occur if the intensity is too high or the transducer is held stationary, thereby concentrating energy in a small area. These same factors can put the patient at risk for cavitation, a phenomenon whereby bubbles of dissolved gas form and grow during each rarefaction phase.[10] Also, if the transducer is inadvertently held in the air while emitting US, the face of the transducer may overheat. The transducer may become damaged, and the animal could be burned if the overheated surface of the transducer contacts the skin. Some units have a built-in system to prevent the crystal from overheating. Regarding safety of the therapist, some US energy is unavoidably propagated through the housing of the sound head to the hand of the therapist, but the effects of this "parasitic" exposure are unknown.

Avoid direct US exposure to the following:
- Cardiac pacemakers.
- Carotid sinus or cervical ganglia. US could alter the normal pacing of the heart or stimulate baroreceptors.[7]
- Eyes. Because blood supply to the lens is poor, heat is poorly dissipated and could result in cataracts. Retinal damage could also result.[10]
- Gravid uterus.
- Heart. ECG changes have occurred in dogs.
- Injured areas immediately after exercise.[15,17]
- Malignancy. US applied to murine tumors resulted in larger tumors compared to controls.[24]
- Spinal cord if a laminectomy has been performed.[7] However, US therapy has been advocated in the area around the spinous processes in horses.[25]

- Testes. Temporary sterility could be associated with heating.
- Wounds that are contaminated. US could drive bacteria into the tissues[26]; infectious processes may be accelerated by heat.[7]
- Recent incision sites. It has been recommended not to treat incision sites for the first 14 days to avoid dehiscence.[17]

Exert precaution in the following situations:

- Bone fracture. This is controversial. Concern exists that high doses retard callus formation, delay calcification,[15] or cause pathologic fractures, subperiosteal damage, or demineralization.[26] Others think that US over fracture sites is acceptable unless sensation is impaired.[9] Experimentally, low-intensity pulsed US has accelerated fracture healing.[10]
- Bony prominences. Treat around bony prominences rather than directly over them, to avoid concentrating energy at the periosteum, or use an immersion technique. Treat bony areas with low dosage levels to avoid the danger of pathologic fractures.[8]
- Cold packs or ice before US. Cold alters pain and temperature perception, limiting the patient's ability to respond if the US intensity is too high.
- Decreased blood circulation. Normal blood flow dissipates the heat that is generated.
- Decreased pain and temperature sensation. Pain response serves as a sensitive monitor of excessively high intensities or faulty equipment[17] that could cause burns or other tissue damage.
- Animals that are overly sedated, restrained, or under local anesthesia.
- Physeal areas in immature animals.[8,10,15] High intensities could affect physes and bone growth.
- Injuries in the acute stage that should not receive heat therapy.[17]
- Acute inflammatory joint disease. Intracapsular heating may accelerate destruction of articular cartilage in acute inflammatory joint disease.[7]

Note that metal implants are *not* necessarily a contraindication for US therapy. The effects of US on cementing compounds such as methylmethacrylate are unknown.[10]

Equipment Safety

US equipment falls under the rules and regulations of the FDA's radiation safety performance standards.[15] Verification of such features as output accuracy and timer accuracy, as well as safety relating to the electrical components, is advised semiannually.[10] US power meters are available for testing. The manufacturer establishes the BNR of a transducer. Most equipment problems originate in the transducer or cable assembly. Recalibration is necessary when a transducer is replaced, and yearly calibration by the manufacturer is recommended even if the transducer is not replaced. Some machines feature self-calibration tests, output power control in response to tissue loading, and automatic shutoff in case of transducer overheating.

Thermal and Nonthermal Effects

Early applications of therapeutic US were those for which tissue heating was the goal.[26] More recently, attention also has been drawn to low-intensity US, which appears to stimulate physiologic processes, such as tissue repair, without biologically significant heating.[27]

The thermal effect is a major indication for the use of this modality. Increased tissue temperatures may increase collagen extensibility, blood flow, pain threshold, and enzyme activity, as well as mild inflammatory reactions, and changes in nerve conduction velocity. Heating is thought to alter the viscoelastic properties of collagen and collagen molecular bonding. Changes in blood flow in response to US have been measured with variable results.[28,29] It is likely that with treatment for 10 to 20 minutes at high intensities, skeletal muscle temperatures and blood flow increase.[10] With lesser intensities and durations, inconsistent changes have been found.

The degree of heat production depends on the intensity, frequency, duration, and size of the treatment area. In addition, the tissue type must be considered. US penetrates skin and subcutaneous fat relatively well, with little attenuation, whereas tissues with high collagen content absorb more of the US energy and are affected to a greater extent. The order of tissue attenuation, from least to most, is as follows: blood (approximately 3% attenuation), fat, muscle, blood vessels, skin, tendon, cartilage, and bone (approximately 96% attenuation).[10]

To achieve the thermal effects of US, the tissue temperature must be raised 1° to 4° C, depending on the desired outcome. Obviously, this is difficult to judge because thermistors are not inserted in clinical patients to monitor the temperature. Experimental studies in humans can provide guidelines. In healthy adult people, thermistors were inserted into muscle at depths of 2.5 and 5.0 cm for 1-MHz treatment, and at depths of 0.8 and 1.6 cm for 3-MHz treatment.[30] The rate of temperature increase per minute at the two depths for the 1 MHz frequency ranged from 0.04° C at 0.5 W/cm^2 to 0.38° C at 2.0 W/cm^2, whereas the corresponding values for the 3 MHz frequency ranged from 0.3° C at 0.5 W/cm^2 to 1.4° C at 2.0 W/cm^2. The 3-MHz frequency heated significantly faster than 1 MHz at all doses.

One protocol for treating humans consists of applying ice on the treatment area before US. Adding ice to the water for US delivered underwater has been recommended for horses, also.[25] However, if the aim is to increase tissue temperature, then it appears that US preceded by ice treatment yields little benefit. Experimentally, US alone increased tissue temperature an average of 4° C, whereas US preceded by 5 minutes of ice increased tissue temperature only 1.8° C.[2]

One prospective randomized experimental study examined the tissue temperature changes that occur at various depths during 3.3-MHz (US) treatments of the caudal thigh muscles in dogs.[30] Dogs received two US treatments (selected randomly), one at an intensity of 1.0 W/cm^2 and one at 1.5 W/cm^2. Needle thermistors were inserted in the caudal thigh muscles below the skin surface at depths of 1.0, 2.0, and 3.0 cm, directly under the US treatment area. Both intensities of US treatment were performed on each dog over a 10- cm^2 area for 10 minutes using a sound head with an effective radiating area of 5 cm^2. Tissue temperature was measured before, during, and after US treatment until tissue temperature returned to baseline. At the completion of the 10-minute US treatment the temperature rise at an intensity of 1.0 W/cm^2 was 3.0° C at the 1.0-cm depth, 2.3° C at 2.0 cm, and 1.6° C at 3.0 cm (Figure 19-3). At an intensity of 1.5 W/cm^2 tissue temperatures rose 4.6° C at the 1.0-cm depth, 3.6° C at 2.0 cm, and 2.4° C at 3.0 cm (Figure 19-4). Tissue temperatures returned to baseline within 10 minutes after treatment in all dogs. This study demonstrated that significant heating occurs in the superficial thigh muscles of dogs during 3.3-MHz US.

Clinical Conditions Treated With Ultrasound

The main indications for US therapy include the following:

■ Soft tissue shortening (such as contracture, scarring)

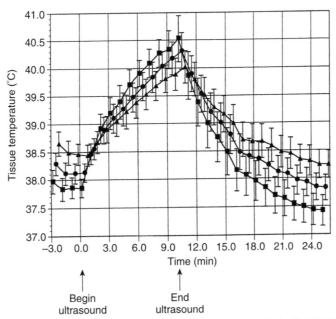

Figure 19-3 Baseline, US treatment, and posttreatment tissue temperatures for 1.0 W/cm^2, 3.3-MHz ultrasound at 1.0-, 2.0-, and 3.0-cm tissue depths. Values are means ± SEM. (From Levine D, Millis DL, Mynatt T: Effects of 3.3MHz Ultrasound on caudal thigh muscle temperature in dogs, *Vet Surg* 30:170, 2001.)

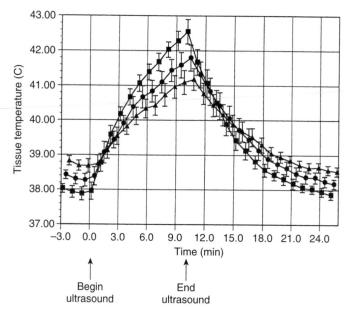

Figure 19-4   Baseline, US treatment, and posttreatment tissue temperatures for 1.5 W/cm², 3.3-MHz ultrasound at 1.0-, 2.0, and 3.0-cm tissue depths. Values are means ± SEM. (From Levine D, Millis DL, Mynatt T: Effects of 3.3MHz Ultrasound on caudal thigh muscle temperature in dogs, *Vet Surg* 30:170, 2001.)

- Subacute and chronic inflammation
- Pain (such as muscle guarding, trigger points)

In human athletes, some experts consider that the most beneficial results from US are in treating tendinitis.[19] In chronic tendinitis, recommended therapy includes heating with US, followed by cross-frictional massage, to eliminate scar tissue and increase ROM. Another indication is the treatment of limited ROM associated with joint contracture, for which patients receive US before passive ROM or joint mobilization. A third indication is for pain relief before activity, such as in athletes with tendinitis that is mild enough to allow the person to continue training. The US treatment is administered before activity to assist in the warm-up and provide some pain relief.

In horses, US therapy has been suggested for the treatment of similar conditions. These include tendinitis, desmitis, sprains, joint lesions, lacerations, reduction of scar tissue, edema, exostosis, and myositis.[17,25]

Tendinitis and Bursitis

Tendinitis and bursitis are treated with US because of the ability to increase blood flow to aid healing, increase tissue temperature to reduce pain, and drive antiinflammatory drugs across the skin by means of phonophoresis. In humans, lateral epicondylitis (tennis elbow),

subacromial bursitis, and bicipital tendinitis are typical conditions considered for US therapy. From animal studies, it appears that the stage at which US is given in the course of healing is important. Application of US in the early phase of tendon repair could be detrimental.[10]

Joint Contracture and Scar Tissue

US is often included in protocols for treating joint contractures and scar tissue.[10] Joint contracture typically results from immobilization or trauma. The periarticular connective tissues have high collagen content. The principle of "heat and stretch" can be applied in this situation in an effort to increase ROM. Tissues are heated to approximately 45° C, followed by gentle passive or active stretching. There tends to be a greater residual increase in tissue length with either preheating or simultaneous heating. The effects of heat on ligament extensibility were studied in humans.[31] Young adults underwent knee joint displacement tests before and after continuous-mode US (1 MHz, 1.5 W/cm² for 8 minutes). The investigators found small increases (1.3 degrees) in varus/valgus excursion at 0- and 20-degree knee flexion and in recurvatum excursion, but not in anterior-posterior drawer excursion. Their conclusion was that continuous mode US at commonly used intensities made some knee ligaments only slightly more extensible in normal subjects. Scar tissue is denser than surrounding tissues, so it can be selectively heated by US. However, more research is needed to determine which intensities and durations are most beneficial.

Pain and Muscle Spasm

Pain threshold is usually increased after US. The physiologic mechanism underlying pain reduction remains speculative. Diathermy and infrared therapy have a similar effect.[10] Therefore the probable mechanism is the ability of all three methods to elevate tissue temperature. Heating may elevate the activation threshold of free nerve endings, produce counter-irritation, or activate large-diameter nerve fibers.[10] Nonthermal mechanisms may also play a role in pain relief. For instance, peripheral nerve conduction velocities are either increased or decreased after US, partially depending on the intensity. Types A, B, and C nerve fibers have different sensitivities.[8] With intensities of 1 to 2 W/cm^2 US reduces the nerve conduction velocity of pain-carrying C fibers. This may help to reduce muscle spasm and reestablish circulation. US has also been used to treat pain associated with neuromas, low-back dysfunction, and skeletal muscle spasm. The mechanism of action for reduction of skeletal muscle spasm may be based on thermal effects that alter the skeletal muscle contractile process, reduce muscle spindle activity, or break the pain-spasm-pain cycle.[10]

Wound and Fracture Healing

The use of therapeutic US in wound healing has recently been reviewed.[32] Reher et al[33] suggested that the beneficial effects of US on wound healing, chronic ulcers, and fracture healing might be based on enhanced angiogenesis. Their experimental data indicated that therapeutic US stimulates production of angiogenesis factors such as interleukin-8, fibroblast growth factor, and vascular endothelial growth factor. These effects were noted with both 1-MHz and 45-kHz exposure. More research is needed to establish the mechanism of action of US at different stages of healing and with different treatment parameters to optimize its effects.

The results may depend on variables such as the intensity and duration of treatment and the time after injury. Low-intensity continuous- or pulsed-mode US has been used to treat acute and chronic wounds. Low intensities appear to enhance healing, whereas high intensities may have proinflammatory effects. Regarding the stage of healing, US therapy initiated within the first week may compromise repair, whereas US initiated after 2 weeks may be beneficial.

Dyson et al[34] reported that US enhanced growth of tissue in experimental wounds in rabbit ears. Because the temperature increases were small, the investigators suggested that the mechanism may have involved acoustic streaming. US has also been used to treat chronic skin ulcers. Rantanen et al[35] used a rat model of muscle contusion injury to study the effect of therapeutic US on muscle regeneration. They concluded that therapeutic US promoted the early phase of muscle regeneration, namely, the satellite cell proliferation phases, but US did not seem to significantly alter the final outcome. Low-intensity US may also have a role in the healing of fractures. Numerous animal studies and controlled clinical trials have shown that low-intensity US can promote the healing of fresh fractures; some evidence suggests efficacy in the treatment of delayed healing and nonunion fractures as well.[36,37]

Other Conditions

There was significant improvement after US treatment in people with mild to moderate idiopathic carpal tunnel syndrome.[38] They received 20 sessions (1 MHz, 1.0 W/cm^2, pulsed mode 1:4, 15 minutes per session) applied to the area over the carpal tunnel, with the first 10 treatments performed daily and 10 further treatments performed twice weekly for 5 weeks. Effects were sustained 6 months after treatment. It remains to be determined if any forms of nerve compression or entrapment in dogs would benefit from this protocol.

Claims have been made that US treatment causes calcium reabsorption. In a randomized, double-blind comparison of US and sham insonation of patients with symptomatic calcific tendinitis of the shoulder, US had a positive effect in resolving calcifications and was associated with short-term clinical improvement.[39] Patients in that study received 24 sessions of pulsed US over a 6-week period. The way in which US stimulates resorption of calcium deposits has not been established. Bromiley[8] has suggested that the excitation of calcium bound to proteins promotes the fragmentation and resorption of calcified masses within soft tissue. Ebenbichler et al[39] speculated that US may stimulate resorption of calcium deposits by (1) activating endothelial cells that subsequently release substances such as cytokines and interleukins, (2) increasing intracellular calcium levels, (3) at high intensities, causing disruption of apatite-like microcrystals, and (4) causing increased temperatures that may lead to increased blood flow and metabolism, thereby facilitating disintegration of calcium deposits.

US may also have a role in reduction of swelling. The mechanism has been attributed to acoustical streaming.[26] For this purpose, US may be combined with cold therapy.

Phonophoresis

The use of US to enhance the delivery of topically applied medications through intact skin is termed phonophoresis.[40] The target for the drug may be local (antiinflammatory or analgesic) or systemic. Some of the local conditions for which phonophoresis is used in humans and that parallel conditions in animals are tendinitis, bursitis, chronic sprains, rheumatoid arthritis, osteoarthritis (OA), and neuromas.[41] Systemic conditions that may be treated by phonophoresis include motion sickness and high blood pressure. Although many studies have been conducted on humans and research animals to evaluate the penetration of various drugs through the skin with the assistance of US, few studies have been performed on companion animals with clinical conditions. Therefore more research is needed to better define the benefits and limitations of this rehabilitation modality.

When a drug is applied topically, it transfers through the skin by passive diffusion.[42,43] This may be hastened by denuding the epidermis to create minor abrasions, such as in shaving. Phonophoresis enhances transdermal drug delivery by altering the stratum corneum, which is the major barrier to drug penetration.[44,45] The mechanism of action may be that US denatures the structural keratin proteins in the stratum corneum, strips or delaminates the cornified layers of the stratum corneum, changes cell permeability, or alters the lipid-enriched intercellular structures between the cells.[40] After the stratum corneum is crossed, the molecules penetrate the dermis, are absorbed into the tissues and capillaries, and travel throughout the circulatory system.[42] In animals, shaving and scrubbing the skin with alcohol increases the rate of diffusion.[40] Drug penetration may occur transcellularly or intercellularly, but it occurs most readily through the hair follicles and sebaceous glands.[46] Though heating the skin before treatment dilates the hair follicles to enhance penetration, it also causes vasodilatation that enhances systemic delivery and decreases local delivery. Low-intensity, longer duration US appears to be more effective at transferring medication than high-intensity, shorter duration doses.[47] Higher concentrations of drugs applied topically may also increase tissue concentrations.[41,48]

Another variable to consider is the transmission of US energy through the drug and coupling agent. Some compounds (with such active ingredients as diethylamine salicylate, hydrocortisone, alclometasone dipropionate, and fluclorolone acetonide) are used to decrease soft tissue inflammation and had no transmission at three different frequencies (0.75 MHz, 1.5 MHz, and 3.0 MHz) in one study.[49] Because the sound waves were unable to penetrate the drug, they were also unable to penetrate the skin. Not only could using a drug that has poor transmission properties decrease the success of phonophoresis, it may also negate the effectiveness of the US therapy. Intensity, frequency, time, drug, and coupling agent transmission may have played a role in some studies of phonophoresis that were unsuccessful.[50,51]

Several studies have been performed using steroidal antiinflammatory drugs (hydrocortisone and dexamethasone) and have shown a decrease in pain and increase in ROM for human patients with OA, periarticular arthritis, and joint or muscle pathology.[52] In a human study using hydrocortisone phonophoresis (100 mg/g of ointment) on patients with OA, tendinitis, or bursitis, there was improvement (marked decrease in pain and a substantial gain in active ROM) in 68% of patients and partial improvement (decrease in pain but some pain remaining, and a gain in active ROM with limitations still present) in 18% of patients as compared to 27% improvement and 16% partial improvement when treated with US alone.[52] In one study using dexamethasone sodium phosphate (7 g of 0.33% dexamethasone using 1 MHz at 1.5 W/cm^2) in humans, the amount of dexamethasone delivered systemically did not alter adrenal function.[53] Another study of phonophoresis in humans showed detectable blood levels of dexamethasone sodium phosphate 30 and 60 minutes after treatment, while none was detected in the blood of patients that had the drug applied topically with no US.[54]

When using phonophoresis on small animals, the skin should be shaved and scrubbed. The drug may be either applied topically with a gel over it or compounded in glycerol, cream, oil, gel, or water.[47] Pulsed US is most commonly used because continuous US increases blood flow to the area and may exacerbate inflammatory conditions.

One of the key benefits of phonophoresis is that it can deliver higher drug levels to the target area, decreasing systemic side effects as compared with parenteral or oral medications.[55] Additionally, US is relaxing and may have analgesic properties.

REFERENCES

1. Taylor RA: Applications of physiotherapy to sporting dogs, *Rec Med Vet* 167:799-805, 1991.
2. Draper DO et al: Temperature changes in deep muscles of humans during ice and ultrasound therapies: An *in vivo* study, *J Orthop Sports Phys Ther* 21:153-157, 1995.
3. Ebenbichler G: Critical evaluation of ultrasound therapy, *Wien Med Wochenschr* 144:51-53, 1994.
4. Gam AN, Johannsen F: Ultrasound therapy in musculoskeletal disorders: a meta-analysis, *Pain* 63:85-91, 1995.
5. Fedorczyk J: The role of physical agents in modulating pain, *J Hand Ther* 10:110-121, 1997.
6. Feine JS, Lund JP: An assessment of the efficacy of physical therapy and physical modalities for the control of chronic musculoskeletal pain, *Pain* 71:15-23, 1997.
7. Hayes KW: *Physical agents*, ed 4, Norwalk, Conn, 1993, Appleton & Lange.
8. Bromiley MW: *Physiotherapy in veterinary medicine*, Oxford, 1991, Blackwell Scientific.
9. Draper DO, Sunderland MS: Examination of the law of Grotthus-Draper: does ultrasound penetrate subcutaneous fat in humans? *J Athlete Train* 28:246-250, 1993.
10. Michlovitz SL: *Thermal agents in rehabilitation*, ed 2, Philadelphia, 1990, FA Davis.
11. Ter Haar G: Basic physics of therapeutic ultrasound, *Physiotherapy* 64:100-103, 1978.
12. Draper DO et al: A comparison of temperature rise in human calf muscles following applications of underwater and topical gel ultrasound, *J Orthop Sports Phys Ther* 17:247-251, 1993.
13. Downer AH: *Physical therapy for animals. Selected techniques*, Springfield, Ill, 1978, Charles C Thomas.
14. Klucinec B et al: Transmissivity of coupling agents used to deliver ultrasound through indirect methods, *J Orthop Sports Phys Ther* 30:263-269, 2000.
15. Porter M: *Equine sports therapy*. Wildomar, Calif, 1990, Veterinary Data.
16. Forrest G, Rosen K: Ultrasound: effectiveness of treatments given under water, *Arch Phys Med Rehab* 70:28-29, 1989.
17. Grant BD. In McIlwraith CW, Trotter G, editors: *Joint disease in the horse*, Philadelphia, 1996, WB Saunders.
18. Steiss JE, Adams CC: Rate of temperature increase in canine muscle during 1 MHz ultrasound therapy: deleterious effect of hair coat, *Am J Vet Res* 60:76-80, 1999.
19. Schulthies SS: Interview with Dr David O Draper, *Sports Phys Ther Sect Newslett, Am Phys Ther Assoc*, Winter 1995, pp 12-13.
20. Levine D, Millis DL, Mynatt T: Effects of 3.3 MHz ultrasound on caudal thigh muscle temperature in dogs, *Vet Surg* 30:170-174, 2001.
21. Lehmann JF et al: Therapeutic temperature distribution produced by ultrasound as modified by dosage and volume of tissue exposed, *Arch Phys Med Rehab* 48:662-666, 1967.
22. Doan N et al: In vitro effects of therapeutic ultrasound on cell proliferation, protein synthesis, and cytokine production by human fibroblasts, osteoblasts, and monocytes, *J Oral Maxillofacial Surg* 57:409-419, 1999.
23. Kimura IF et al: Effects of two ultrasound devices and angles of application on the temperature of tissue phantom, *J Orthop Sports Phys Ther* 27:27-31, 1998.
24. Sicard-Rosenbaum L et al: Effects of energy-matched pulsed and continuous ultrasound on tumor growth in mice, *Phys Ther* 78:271-277, 1998.
25. Denoix J, Pailloux J: *Physical therapy and massage for the horse*. North Pomfret, Vt, 1996, Trafalgar Square Publishing.
26. Loving NS: *Veterinary manual for the performance horse*, Grand Prairie, Tex, 1993, Equine Research.
27. ter Haar G: Therapeutic ultrasound, *Eur J Ultrasound* 9:3-9, 1999 (Review).
28. Robinson SE, Buono MJ: Effect of continuous-wave ultrasound on blood flow in skeletal muscle, *Phys Ther* 75:145-151, 1995.
29. Fabrizio PA et al: Acute effects of therapeutic ultrasound delivered at varying parameters on the blood flow velocity in a muscular distribution artery, *J Orthop Sports Phys Ther* 24:294-302, 1996.
30. Draper DO, Castel JC, Castel D: Rate of temperature increase in human muscle during 1 MHz and 3 MHz continuous ultrasound, *J Orthop Sports Phys Ther* 22:142-150, 1995.
31. Reed B, Ashikaga T: The effects of heating with ultrasound on knee joint displacement, *J Orthop Sports Phys Ther* 26:131-137, 1997.
32. Hart J: The use of ultrasound therapy in wound healing, *J Wound Care* 7:25-28, 1998 (review).
33. Reher P et al: Effect of ultrasound on the production of IL-8, basic FGF and VEGF, *Cytokine* 11:416-423, 1999.
34. Dyson M et al: The stimulation of tissue regeneration by means of ultrasound, *Clin Sci* 35:273-285, 1968.
35. Rantanen J et al: Effects of therapeutic ultrasound on the regeneration of skeletal myofibers after experimental muscle injury, *Am J Sports Med* 27:54-59, 1999.
36. Hadjiargyrou M et al: Enhancement of fracture healing by low intensity ultrasound, *Clin Orthop Rel Res* 355(suppl):S216-S229, 1998.
37. Mayr E, Frankel V, Rueter A: Ultrasound: an alternative healing method for nonunions? *Arch Orthop Trauma Surg* 120:1-8, 2000.
38. Ebenbichler GR: Ultrasound treatment for treating the carpal tunnel syndrome: randomised "sham" controlled trial, *Br Med J* 316:731-735, 1998.
39. Ebenbichler GR et al: Ultrasound therapy for calcific tendinitis of the shoulder, *New Engl J Med* 340:1533-1538, 1999.

40. Byl NN: The use of ultrasound as an enhancer for transcutaneous drug delivery: phonophoresis, *Phys Ther* 75:539-551, 1995.

41. Kleinkort JA, Wood F: Phonophoresis with 1 percent versus 10 percent hydrocortisone, *Phys Ther* 55:1320-1324, 1975.

42. Webster RC, Maibach HI: Individual and regional variation with in vitro percutaneous absorption. In Bronaugh RL, Maibach HI, editors: *In vitro percutaneous absorption: principles, fundamentals, and applications,* Ann Arbor, Mich, 1991, CRC Press.

43. Scott R: In vitro absorption through damaged skin. In Bronaugh RL, Maibach HI, editors: *In vitro percutaneous absorption: principles, fundamentals, and applications,* Ann Arbor, Mich, 1991, CRC Press.

44. MacKie RM: *Clinical dermatology: an illustrated textbook,* ed 3, New York, 1991, Oxford University Press.

45. Cooper E: Alterations in skin permeability. In Chien YW, editor: *Transdermal controlled systemic medications,* vol 31, New York, 1987, Marcel Dekker.

46. Bronaugh RL: A flow-through diffusion cell. In Bronaugh RL, Maibach HI, editors: *In vitro percutaneous absorption: principles, fundamentals, and applications,* Ann Arbor, Mich, 1991, CRC Press.

47. Shim SM, Choi JK: Effect of indomethacin phonophoresis on the relief of temporomandibular joint pain, *Cranio* 15:345-348, 1997.

48. Davick JP, Martin RK, Albright JP: Distribution and deposition of tritiated cortisol using phonophoresis, *Phys Ther* 68:1672-1675, 1998.

49. Benson HAE, McElnay JC: Transmission of ultrasound energy through topical pharmaceutical products, *Physiotherapy* 74:587-589, 1998.

50. Holdsworth LK, Anderson DM: Effectiveness of ultrasound used with a hydrocortisone coupling medium or epicondylitis clasp to treat lateral epicondylitis: pilot study, *Physiotherapy* 79:19-25, 1993.

51. Bare AC et al: Phonophoretic delivery of 10% hydrocortisone through the epidermis of humans as determined by serum cortisol concentrations, *Phys Ther* 76:738-749, 1996.

52. Griffin JE et al: Patients treated with ultrasonic driven hydrocortisone and ultrasound alone, *Phys Ther* 47:594-601, 1967.

53. Franklin ME et al: Effect of phonophoresis with dexamethasone on adrenal function, *J Orthop Sports Phys Ther* 22:103-107, 1995.

54. Conner-Kerr TA et al: Efficacy of utilizing phonophoresis for the delivery of dexamethasone to human transdermal tissues, *J Orthop Sports Phys Ther* 23:79, 1996.

55. McNeill SC, Potts RO, Francoeur ML: Local enhanced topical delivery (LETD) of drugs: does it truly exist? *Pharmaceut Res* 9:1422-1427, 1992.

Chapter 20

Acupuncture for Veterinary Rehabilitation

Laurie McCauley and Maria H. Glinski

Acupuncture has been used for over 4000 years as one medical method within traditional Chinese medicine (TCM). Early Chinese veterinary applications of acupuncture, coinciding with the domestication of animals, concentrated on horses, but eventually included cattle, swine, camels, fowl, sheep, goats, dogs, and cats. The practice fell into disfavor in the nineteenth century but was revived during the next 100 years. Current veterinary practice may include a combination of TCM and Western approaches. The International Veterinary Acupuncture Society (IVAS) was founded in 1974 with the aims of fully integrating acupuncture into Western veterinary science and standardizing training. IVAS is now active in the United States, Europe, Canada, and Australia, publishes the *International Journal of Veterinary Acupuncture,* and holds annual meetings.[1]

In 1998 the American Veterinary Medical Association adopted a resolution to change the practice of veterinary acupuncture from an experimental to a surgical or medical procedure, and to recommend educational programs for veterinarians who practice acupuncture.[2] In the United States, acupuncture is increasingly used to treat musculoskeletal disorders, including osteoarthritis, intervertebral disk disease, hip dysplasia, and rheumatoid arthritis. Medication and surgery are frequently effective in treating musculoskeletal conditions, but there are some cases in which medications produce serious side effects and surgical intervention entails considerable risk, particularly in geriatric animals. Owners may seriously consider euthanasia because a pet is in pain, and medication and surgery cannot sufficiently resolve the painful condition. In these cases, acupuncture may be indicated.[3]

In contemporary practice acupuncture may be used alone to treat musculoskeletal pain, or in conjunction with more conventional modalities to obtain a synergistic effect. Acupuncture may provide chronic stimulation of peripheral nerves as a result of the microinjury that needling produces. Acupuncture can be used to relieve pain, cause an autonomic nerve response, and effect surgical analgesia.[4] This chapter will review the neurophysiology of how acupuncture is believed to affect the body and will present a strategy for incorporating this tool into a rehabilitation treatment plan.

Terminology Specific to Acupuncture

Acupuncture Point

An acupuncture point is a specific body area that is pierced with a fine needle for therapeutic purposes. Acupuncture points, or acupoints, are specific foci along a meridian that have increased local conductivity and an increased density of capillaries, arterioles, venules, and fine lymphatics.[4] There is also a higher concentration of mast cells in the connective tissue and along the blood vessels. Electrical resistance, which is increased compared to the surrounding tissue, is found at an acupuncture point, and this resistance is measurable in cadavers for several hours after death.[5]

Acupuncture points are associated with four different anatomical entities[6]:

Type I acupuncture points correspond to the motor point of a muscle. The motor point is a region on a muscle that requires the least stimulation for the muscle to relax.

Type II acupuncture points correspond to the focal meeting of superficial nerves in the sagittal plane.

Type III acupuncture points lie over a superficial nerve or plexus.

Type IV acupuncture points are at a muscle-tendon junction over the Golgi tendon organ.

In humans undergoing an acupuncture treatment, there is a feeling of heaviness, distention, cramping, soreness, warmth, or occasionally discomfort when an acupuncture point is stimulated with a needle. This may be predominantly caused by stimulation of A delta fibers and C fibers.[7] The sensation requires an intact somatic nervous system and is not reproducible at placebo sites.[8] The feeling of warmth is secondary to vasodilation, and there is a consistent, measurable change in skin temperature.[9] The needle stimulates a muscle reflex that causes muscle contraction directly around the needle, a contraction that the acupuncturist can feel as the needle is "grabbed." This microtrauma activates the complement system and the coagulation cascade, causing release of plasminogen, histamine, heparin, kinins, and kinin protease.[6] These substances cause vasodilation and increased vascular permeability, creating a local inflammatory reaction. Local effects include improved local tissue perfusion and muscle relaxation.

Meridian

Acupuncture points are connected through pathways that are called meridians or channels. The body's vital energy or life force (which some Western practitioners call bioelectricity) circulates in a cyclic predetermined course through the meridians. In humans and dogs, there are 14 classical meridians. Twelve are associated with specific organ systems on which they have a primary influence, and two run on the midlines of the body. The organ-related meridians are named lung (LU), large intestine (LI), stomach (ST), spleen (SP), heart (HT), small intestine (SI), bladder (BL), kidney (KI), pericardium (PC), triple heater (TH), gallbladder (GB), and liver (LI). The conception vessel (CV) runs on the ventral midline, and the governing vessel (GV) runs on the dorsal midline.

Individual acupuncture points are named by pairing the meridian and a number (for example, LV3 or SP6). In dogs (and cats) there are 360 named permanent points that lie on the meridians, of which 150 are commonly used for therapeutic purposes. In addition, there are "extra" points that do not lie on meridians, and trigger points, temporary tender areas that can move on and off the meridians in episodes of pathology.

According to TCM theory, energy circulates through each meridian every 24 hours. The meridians run on the surface of the body, where acupuncture points can be accessed and manipulated. Blockage of energy circulation manifests as dysfunction or disease. Medical conditions that can be helped by rehabilitation may also have stagnant energy circulation or lack of sufficient energy for optimal function. Stagnant energy manifests as painful spasms or swelling, while deficient energy manifests as atrophy or weakness. To bring the body into balance and to facilitate healing, it is necessary to stimulate or sedate energy levels at acupuncture points (Figure 20-1).

Review of Literature in Humans

The relevant acupuncture literature in human patients concerns the neurophysiology of how acupuncture is believed to work in the body. Since the 1950s, when reports from China showed that acupuncture alone could produce a surgical plane of analgesia, scientific interest has been piqued. Since then, there has been an abundance of research attempting to determine the exact mechanisms of how and why acupuncture works. To date there are several theories, but no single theory explains all the effects of acupuncture. The most current theories discussed in the human literature are: (1) the gate theory, (2) the endogenous opioid theory, (3) the autonomic nervous system input theory, (4) the humoral theory, and (5) the bioelectric theory.

The Gate Theory

The gate theory may explain the analgesic effects of acupuncture.[4] To understand this proposed mechanism, it is essential to have an understanding of pain receptors and of nerve fibers of the central and peripheral nervous system. Pain results from a noxious stimulus applied to pain receptors in the skin, musculoskeletal structures, or visceral structures. Pain receptors are free nerve endings that transmit information regarding mechanical, chemical, or thermal stimuli.[10]

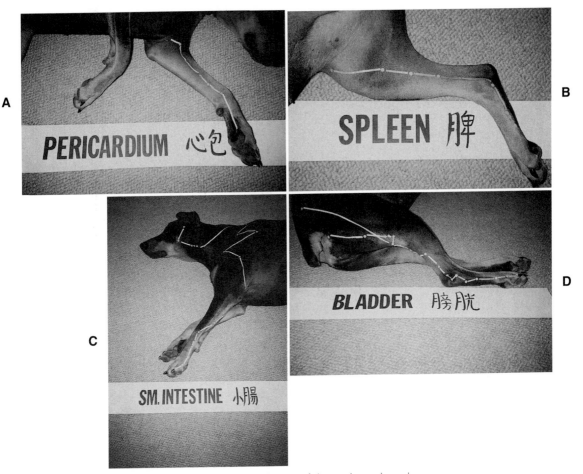

Figure 20-1 Schematic diagram of dog, with meridians shown.

Different types of neurons transmit pain. A-delta fibers are thin and poorly myelinated and transmit pain rapidly. C fibers are one-tenth the diameter of A-delta fibers, are unmyelinated, and transmit impulses 10 times more slowly than A-delta fibers. A-alpha and A-beta sensory neurons transmit sensory, non-painful information much faster than do A-delta or C fibers and may play a role in acupuncture. C fibers have a high threshold for stimulation and transmit an unpleasant pain sensation.[11] Stimulation of A-delta fibers and C fibers transmit pain sensation along the peripheral nerve to the spinal cord. Somatic and visceral sensory neurons enter the dorso-lateral funiculus and Lissauer's tract, from which impulses can be transmitted to spinal segments cranial and caudal to the point of entry.[12] Sensory neurons then synapse with projection neurons and excitatory and inhibitory interneurons in the substantia gelatinosa of the dorsal horn gray matter of the spinal cord. Excitatory interneurons are believed to release glutamate or substance P, and inhibitory interneurons release endorphins.[11]

In the gate theory, many fast A-beta or A-delta fibers are stimulated and carry sensory information to the substantia gelatinosa, synapse on inhibitory interneurons, and close the "gate" to ascending pain transmission before the impulses of the slower C fibers arrive.[12,13] As a result the pain impulses cannot be transmitted to the brain, and no pain is perceived. This may also explain regional analgesia that may occur because the sensory afferent signals are transmitted several spinal segments cranially and caudally in the dorso-lateral fasciculus before entering the dorsal horn gray matter.[14] It has been suggested that the small myelinated fibers are essential for acupuncture effects.[7] Though the gate theory accounts for some of the effects of acupuncture, it does not explain the delayed onset (30 to 60 minutes) of surgical analgesia, the results of cross-circulation studies (humoral effects), or why chronic pain may be controlled after several treatments (Figure 20-2).

Endogenous Opioid Theory

Segmental analgesia has been well documented and was originally thought to be unrelated to the endogenous opiate system. It was then found that acupuncture analgesia could be reversed by naloxone. It was also determined that a cross-tolerance can develop between acupuncture and morphine.[15] Levels of the opiate peptide NAGA and beta-endorphin were shown to increase in the brain

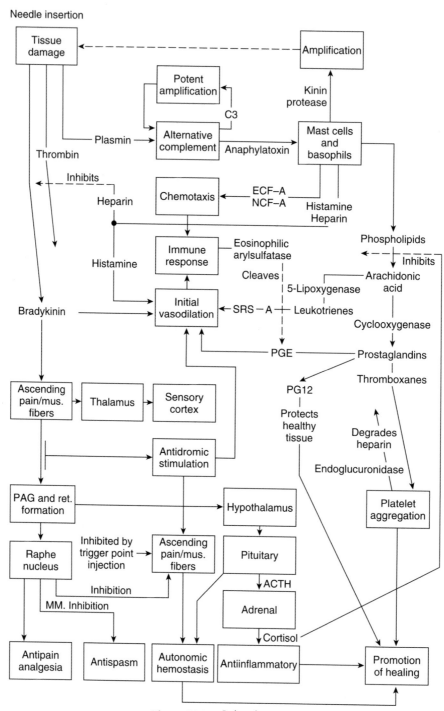

Figure 20-2   Dekes diagram.

and cerebrospinal fluid (CSF) after acupuncture.[16] A correlation between an increase in beta-endorphin levels in CSF and pain threshold or pain tolerance has been demonstrated.[17] It has also been shown that levels of met- and leu-enkephalins significantly increase in the brain after electrical acupuncture.[18] Opiates are also known to have systemic effects that may also be produced by acupuncture. For example, opioid drugs have an effect in the gastrointestinal tract by decreasing peristalsis and increasing segmental contractions, helping to control diarrhea.

Autonomic Nervous System Theory

Numerous viscerosomatic relationships have been studied. Type A-delta visceral and somatic fibers have a similar distribution in the dorsal gray matter and tract of Lissauer. Inputs from both converge in the spinothalamic tract. Visceral A-delta fibers form reflex arcs with propriospinal afferents and may cause muscle cramping secondary to visceral inflammation. Conditions of somatic pain can also cause visceral manifestations of disease. These interactions may explain the phenomenon of "referred pain." Stimulation of acupuncture points may cause a reflex arc, resulting in sympathetically induced segmental superficial and visceral vasodilation.[12] This could explain how acupuncture may be useful in treating internal organ dysfunction. Studies in rabbits have indicated that the ability of acupuncture to produce analgesia is lost if sympathetic chains are surgically interrupted.[18] Acupuncture increases cAMP levels by stimulating the CNS and releasing catecholamines from the adrenal medulla.[19] The cAMP also increases catecholamine binding to its target receptors and affects many cellular functions, including vasodilation and bronchodilation.[20]

Humoral Theory

This theory was first postulated after studies demonstrated that transferring blood, CSF, or brain tissue from an animal under acupuncture analgesia to an animal not receiving acupuncture resulted in analgesia in the recipient.[21-23] This analgesia was generalized and reversed by naloxone.[21,24] The analgesia level required for surgery took 20 to 30 minutes of stimulation to reach its peak and lasted hours after stimulation of the points had ceased.[24] Beta-endorphins are released by acupuncture

and may contribute to analgesia, but it is not the only component. Serotonin is also important and increases 30% to 40% in the systemic circulation after acupuncture.[9] Studies have shown that if brain levels of serotonin decrease by using pCPA, an inhibitor of serotonin synthesis, systemic endorphin levels increase.[24] Conversely, inhibiting the effects of endorphins with naloxone increases brain serotonin levels.[24] Further studies have shown that decreasing brain levels of endorphins or serotonin have no effect on acupuncture analgesia, but decreasing both has a profound inhibitory effect.[25] Acupuncture has also been shown to cause systemic increases in growth hormone, prolactin, oxytocin, luteinizing hormone, white blood cells, immunoglobulins, antibodies, and interferons, depending on which points are stimulated.[26,27]

Bioelectric Theory

Becker and Reichmanis, proposed a theory that the healing and analgesic properties of acupuncture are based on a DC current system.[28,29] In this system, electric signals are generated and propagated by Schwann cells, satellite cells, and glial cells.[5] Acupuncture points, like amplifiers, may boost the DC signal along the nerve pathways. Insertion of a metal acupuncture needle may short-circuit the system and block pain perception. In this system, acupuncture points boost the DC signal along the meridian, comparable to an amplifier boosting electricity along a high-power tension wire.[29] Reichmanis et al[29] studied the electrical properties of two meridians and found that half the acupuncture points did act as DC power sources and the current flowed toward the CNS. They postulated a complete control system separate from, but working with, the nervous system. Its function is to detect injury and help regulate the healing process. Acupuncture points are positively charged in relation to the surrounding tissue.

Review of Literature in Dogs

The literature indicates that acupuncture treatment is most commonly used in canine practice for the following conditions[4]:

- Paralysis, paresis, or pain, usually resulting from trauma or intervertebral disk disease in small dogs
- In large dogs, paresis or paralysis from compression of nerves caused by type II

disk protrusion, spinal instability, spondylosis, and degenerative myelopathy
- Pain from hip dysplasia
- Arthritis
- Miscellaneous conditions that have not responded to conventional therapy

An extensive bibliography of acupuncture articles has been compiled and is available online.[30] A medical acupuncture Web page is also available.[31]

Conditions Treated With Acupuncture

Acupuncture has been used in the management of chronic musculoskeletal pain and in treatment following injury or surgery.

Arthritis

Acupuncture may improve mobility and ambulation, and therefore strengthen muscles around arthritic joints. Acupuncture may reduce pain, so that muscles near arthritic joints can be strengthened and the animal taught to walk in a more balanced, less compensatory, fashion. In a study of 65 dogs that had stopped responding to conventional therapy and were recommended for euthanasia, 70% showed a 50% or greater improvement in mobility and ambulation with the use of acupuncture in this manner.[32]

Intervertebral Disk Disease

In studies of dogs with intervertebral disk disease (IVDD), acupuncture, surgery, and conservative measures may be compared.[33,34] The results suggest that acupuncture may be success rates similar to those of surgery. In studying cervical IVDD, dogs were divided into three grades, depending on clinical severity. In grade I (only neck pain present), the success rate for surgery was 90% and the success rate for acupuncture was 80%. For grade II (neck pain and proprioceptive deficits), the success rate for surgery was 85% and the success rate for acupuncture was 67%. There were too few grade III patients (neck pain and paralysis) for determination of a success rate. Conservative treatment of dogs resulted in a success rate between 30% and 50% for all three grades.

In a thoracolumbar IVDD study, success rates for surgery and acupuncture were similar for four grades of clinical severity. Dogs with grades I (dogs with back pain, reluctant to jump or climb stairs, occasionally crying when moved) and II (similar to grade I but also paretic, ataxic, and loss of conscious proprioception in hind legs) injuries had a 90% success rate for both interventions. Grade III (paralytic, unable to bear weight on back legs, bowel and bladder control varied, reflexes normal if lesion cranial to L3) patients had an 80% success rate, and grade IV (paralyzed, no deep pain in hind toes) dogs had a 25% success rate with both therapies. For grade IV thoracolumbar IVDD, early decompression surgery is the treatment of choice, and acupuncture is recommended only if more than 36 hours have elapsed since the onset of clinical signs.

Spondylosis and Fibrocartilaginous Emboli

Spondylosis and fibrocartilaginous emboli may be treated in similar fashion to IVDD.

Degenerative Myelopathy

In treating degenerative myelopathy with acupuncture, it is not possible to change the progression of the nerve dysfunction, but it is possible to relieve pain of other conditions of the back, hips, or both, so that the muscles of the hind legs may be maximally strengthened. In the course of the disease, decreased innervation may result in secondary muscle atrophy. As the dog becomes weaker in the rear, it is less able to compensate for diseases of the hips, stifles, or back. As the animal compensates by shifting its weight forward, further atrophy occurs, resulting in fewer muscle fibers to respond to nerve stimulation. The goal of acupuncture treatment in this case is to decrease pain so that the dog may walk in a balanced fashion (e.g., with an aquatic treadmill or an inclined land-based treadmill). With a more balanced gait, it is possible to increase muscle tone and slow the effects of this debilitating disease.

Open Wounds

Acupuncture or electroacupuncture with needles around the edge of ulcers may cause vasodilation, and perhaps speed healing time. Acupuncture is also used to treat pressure sores.

Technique, Equipment, and Instrumentation

Acupuncture management of musculoskeletal pain is an exercise in palpation skills, segmental neuroanatomy, and knowledge of the techniques and instrumentation available to the practitioner. Acupuncture points can be stimulated in various ways including pressure, needles, moxibustion, aquapuncture, electroacupuncture, implants, laser, cold, ultrasound, and microcurrent.

Acupressure, a form of massage using digital pressure on acupuncture points, is an important method used to relieve muscle spasms. Dry needling is performed using stainless steel acupuncture needles (Figure 20-3). These filiform needles are 25 to 36 gauge, and the needles used on companion animals are usually ½ to 2 inches long The smaller needles are used in small breeds, over bony prominences, or where body cavities are at risk of penetration. Medium-size needles are best used in upper thighs and the paravertebral muscles. Long needles are useful for stimulating points around the hip or in the popliteal fossa of larger dogs. The needles themselves are solid, flexible, and have a rounded point

like a pencil tip. Because of their unique structure, they are able to glide through tissue and gently push structures apart, compared to the traumatic nature of a hollow, cutting hypodermic needle. They are presterilized and come packaged individually or in groups of 10. Depending on the location, they can be inserted perpendicularly, obliquely (30 to 60 degress), or horizontally (10 to 20 degress) (Figure 20-4).

Moxibustion is the burning of dried leaves of the *Artemesia vulgaris* or mugwort plant. The plant material is most commonly rolled into a stick that, when ignited, burns at approximately 450° F and can be moved slowly over an acupuncture point, or inserted needle, until the skin becomes slightly red or the animal is perceived to feel slight discomfort. This technique has been used for chronic pain and arthritis, especially when the animal seems worse in cold damp weather.

Aquapuncture is the injection of a solution into an acupuncture point. A 25- to 30-gauge needle is used to inject 0.25 to 2 ml of a solution, depending on the size of the animal. The most commonly used substance is vitamin B_{12}, although electrolyte solutions, saline, DMSO, vitamin C, antibiotics, herbal extracts, homeopathics, and local anesthetics can be used. It is

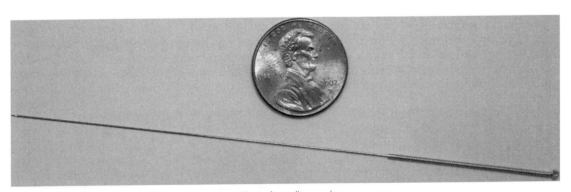

Figure 20-3 Typical needles used in acupuncture.

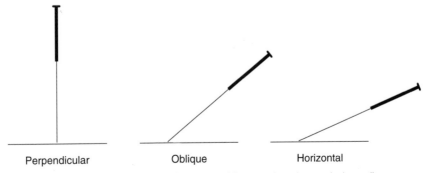

Perpendicular   Oblique   Horizontal

Figure 20-4 Diagram of perpendicular oblique, and horizontal angles at which needles are inserted.

thought that the pressure on the point or the solution itself may stimulate nerve fibers. The advantages are that the materials needed are readily available, the patient needs less restraint, and the needle is removed immediately so treatment time is shorter. The disadvantage is that because the needles are sharper they cause more tissue damage and there may be added discomfort.

Electroacupuncture is the passing of electrical energy through acupuncture points. Stimulation is accomplished by connecting an electronic device to needles or, in some cases, saline-soaked gauze surrounding a painful area. Indications include paralysis or paresis, severe and chronic painful conditions, or painful conditions not responsive to dry needling. Research regarding peripheral nerve injuries in animals has shown an increase in electrical muscle potential in animals treated with electroacupuncture as compared to a control group.[35] This increase in electrical muscle potential has been hypothesized to be due to changes in electrical potential at the wounded nerve fiber bud or the release of an unknown substance that stimulates the growth of the bud. Research on toad sciatic nerves, using electroacupuncture, has shown that as electrical stimulation increased, the nerve's electrical potential rose.[35]

Contraindications for electroacupuncture include fractures (unless it is a nonunion fracture), cardiac arrhythmias, epilepsy, shock, fever, active infections or malignancies, generalized weakness, hypotension, and pregnancy.[36] Electrical current should not be passed across the cardiac area. Current is conducted parallel to the spine rather that across the midline of the body. For chronic pain without trigger points, a low frequency (less than 15 Hz) is used to release beta-endorphins and met-enkephalins into the CNS.[37] This low-frequency technique reduces pain slowly, but the analgesic effects are longer lasting. To treat acutely painful problems and chronically painful problems with distinct trigger points, a higher frequency (usually 25 to 150 Hz) is used. In rats, this was shown to accelerate the release of dynorphin in the spinal cord.[37] This high-frequency technique eliminates pain quickly, but the analgesic effects are not as long lasting.[37] By using a dense-disperse mode (alternating between high and low frequency) there is less chance of the body developing tolerance to electrical stimulation, and the benefits of both high and low frequencies are obtained (Figure 20-5).

Implantation

To achieve continuous stimulation of an acupuncture point, various materials may be surgically implanted. Though catgut, stainless steel, and silver can be used, the most common implant is gold in the form of solid beads or wires.[38] This technique is most commonly used for young dogs with painful hip dysplasia or older dogs with coxofemoral arthritis that have been helped with acupuncture.* The main advantage is that it negates the need for fre-

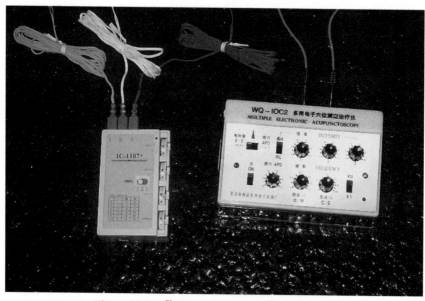

Figure 20-5 Electroacupuncture stimulation devices.

quent lifelong needling sessions. There is also preliminary evidence that implantation has successfully been used to treat spondylosis.[4] Disadvantages include (1) possible migration of the implant, (2) increased cost (this is done as a sterile surgical procedure), (3) necessity of special training, and (4) potential scar tissue decreasing effectiveness.

Laser Puncture

Low-intensity or "cold" lasers have been used to stimulate acupuncture points. Laser puncture is a noninvasive form of stimulation that has not gained universal acceptance by acupuncturists. It is considered to be a form of intense light therapy using various frequencies and wavelengths that promote positive physiologic changes within cells that support healing and reduce or eliminate pain.[39] Laser puncture has been used to (1) stimulate acupuncture points, (2) enhance healing of wounds and burns, and (3) treat acutely inflamed joints. The advantages are that it is safe and painless, treatment time is short, and minimal animal restraint is required. The disadvantages are cost and the inability to obtain the same physiologic effects as needling. Therefore laser-puncture is considered a useful adjunct to traditional acupuncture, but cannot replace needling.

Two types of laser units are commonly used in veterinary acupuncture[20]:
- The helium-neon gas tube (a red light emitter) has a wavelength of 632 to 650 nm and penetrates 0.8 to 15 mm deep.
- The gallium arsenate diode (an infrared light emitter) has a wavelength of 902 nm and penetrates 10 mm to 5 cm deep.

Cold, in the form of ice or chemical coolants, may be applied to acupuncture or trigger points. Cold is not commonly used and is contraindicated in chronic conditions.

Ultrasound may be used to stimulate an acupuncture point when a 0.35-inch-diameter sound head is used on each point for 10 to 30 seconds.[4] This is also not commonly per-

formed, perhaps because of the cost and the necessity of shaving hair at each acupuncture point that is treated.

Microcurrent therapy, which is the use of an acuscope, is gaining popularity with human sports physicians and chiropractors. It generates a microcurrent of electricity that is used on acupuncture points or directly over areas of pain or muscle spasm. The primary advantage is rapid pain relief, especially to spastic muscles. Disadvantages include cost of the equipment and long treatment duration.

Clinical Applications

Acupuncture may be used immediately after surgery or injury as well as in chronic, painful conditions. It can be used in conjunction with many medications, although it may be less beneficial and require more treatments when the animal is concurrently on corticosteroids. This may be due to the inhibition of endogenous corticosteroid and endorphin release by exogenous corticosteroids.

The most common indications for veterinary acupuncture with rehabilitation include the following:
- Pain arising from muscle spasm or trigger points
- Paresis
- Paralysis
- Wound healing

These conditions may be associated with osteoarthritis, rheumatoid arthritis, intervertebral disk disease, fibrocartilaginous emboli, spondylosis, spinal stenosis, vertebral instabilities, degenerative myelopathy, postsurgical pain and inflammation, open wounds, trauma, soft-tissue injuries, joint injuries, tendinitis, bursitis, circulatory insufficiencies, and pain or injuries associated with compensatory body mechanics.

Acupuncture Point Selection

Several techniques for combining acupuncture points should be considered when deciding on a treatment plan. Although these methods need not be followed for every treatment, the following guidelines should be considered[4]:
- Treating points bilaterally
- Treating points cranial and caudal to the lesion
- Treating local and distal points

Editor's note: Two prospective studies have been conducted that have shown no benefit of gold bead implantation for the treatment of hip dysplasia of dogs: Hielm-Bjorkman A et al: Double-blind evaluation of implants of gold wire at acupuncture points in the dog as a treatment for osteoarthritis induced by hip dysplasia, *Vet Rec* 149:452-456, 2001; and DeCamp CE et al: Double blind study to evaluate the clinical response to gold bead acupuncture as a treatment in dogs with naturally occurring hip dysplasia, *Proc Vet Orthop Soc* Snowmass, Color, 1998, p46.

All points on the 12 main meridians are located bilaterally. Therefore when points are chosen, both sides can be treated. To strengthen an acupuncture formula, points from the forelimb and the hindlimb can be combined, even if the injury affects only one limb. When treating a painful area, points should be selected distal to the area (distal to the elbow or stifle), proximal to the area, and in local areas (Figure 20-6). Another consideration is that it is believed that too many needles will dilute a formula and make it less effective. The average patient should be treated with 20 or fewer needles per session. When starting acupuncture on a geriatric dog or a puppy under 6 weeks old, the first session should consist of even fewer needles. Additionally, electroacupuncture is generally not used the first treatment session. The acupuncture points that are used for treating various conditions are described in the following section.

Treating Arthritis

The goals when treating arthritis are to eliminate pain, to strengthen the muscles around the joints, and to reeducate the animal to walk in a more balanced, less compensatory fashion.

Chronic osteoarthritis responds favorably to acupuncture. Dry needles or electroacupuncture are usually tried first. A formula combining local and distal points can be used with the needles left in place 15 to 20 minutes.[4]

Vertebral column: Bladder meridian points cranial and caudal to the lesion are often needled and then attached to an electrostimulator.

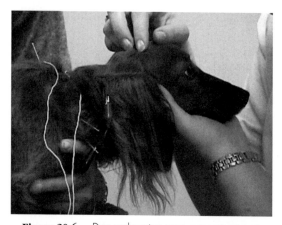

Figure 20-6   Dog undergoing acupuncture treatment.

Rheumatoid arthritis is immune-mediated and therefore points should be added with immunoregulatory effects. These include LI-4, LI-11, GV-14, and ST-36. Another technique, especially if a distal joint is too painful to needle locally, is to soak cotton gauze in saline and use electroacupuncture, hooking the alligator clips directly to the soaked gauze rather than the needle.

Treating by Joint

Joints commonly treated in rehabilitation are the hip, stifle, hock, and shoulder.

Hip Pain

Pain in the coxofemoral joint is often treated by needling three points of the "hip triangle" that work synergistically: GB-29, GB-30, and BL-54. The effects may be amplified with electroacupuncture, by connecting GB-29 to GB-30 and using a low- to medium-frequency current. Points that complement the local hip triangle may include the following:

- B-11 if arthritis is present
- BL-23 if there is concurrent pain or weakness in the caudal spine
- BL-28 if caudal back pain or urinary incontinence is present
- GB-31 if pain is present in the caudal spine or pelvic area or if the hindlimb is paralyzed
- GB-34 if there is paresis, weakness, swelling, or pain at, or distal to, the stifle
- ST-36 if there is pain in the hindlimb
- BL-40 if there is pain in the caudal spine, contracture of the tendons in the popliteal fossa, rear-limb muscle atrophy, or motor impairment of the rear limb
- BL-60 if there is pain or swelling in the hock (BL-40 and BL-60 are not usually used together, unless an electrical current is being used)

Stifle Pain

Pain in the stifle can be treated by needling Heding, Xiyan (this is actually two points), GB-34, ST-36, and SP-9. Two to four of these points are commonly used together. Complementary point selection is determined by other complicating factors in the body. If one needle can alleviate pain in two places or effectively alleviate two or more problems, this is preferable to using two or three needles to accomplish the same purpose. Complementary points for the stifle can include local hip points: ST-40 if there is muscle atrophy, motor impairment, pain, or swelling of the rear limb; and ST-41 if there is muscle atrophy, motor impairment, or pain of the rear limb.

Tarsal Pain

Pain at the hock can be treated with the BL-60 and KI-3 combination, where one needle activates two points when it is inserted in one side of the webbing of the hock and protrudes from the other side. ST-41 is needled when pain in the hock is combined with muscle atrophy and motor impairment of the rear limb. BL-62 can also be needled for pain associated with the hock.

Shoulder Pain

Pain in the shoulder can be associated with forelimb lameness, but may also be a common sequel to pain in the rear limbs. As dogs shift their weight forward to relieve the pain in the rear limbs, they tend to hyperextend the carpal joint, causing pain and ligament laxity, and to push the shoulders forward, preventing normal extension of the forelimbs and causing pain at this joint. Triceps muscle knots and trigger points, commonly seen in this instance, should not be overlooked. Local points for pain and motor impairment of the shoulder include SI-9, LI-15, and TH-14. GB-21 and BL-11 are needled if pain is also found in the cervical region. Points that complement the local shoulder points may include the following:

- LI-4 and LI-11 if weakness or motor impairment of the forelimb are present
- SI-3 if there is pain in the cervical or lumbar regions or contracture of the digits
- TH-4 if carpal pain is present

Elbow Pain

Local points for the elbow may include LI-10 and LI-11 if motor impairment of the forelimb is evident, or LU-5 and PC-3 if elbow pain is the primary presenting complaint.

Treating Neurologic and Vertebral Diseases

The mechanism of action of acupuncture for thoracolumbar and cervical IVDD is not fully understood. It may relieve trigger points, muscle spasms, and pain. Acupuncture may stimulate regeneration of axons in the spinal cord.[35] It is also believed to decrease local inflammation, and therefore may decrease spinal cord compression and scar tissue formation. It is thought that acupuncture does not decrease healing time just by causing vasodilation.[40]

Local and distal points are used to treat IVDD. When treating lesions in the thoracolumbar area, BL-14 to BL-28 are used as local points. Points on the governing vessel and tip of tail may also be incorporated as local points. Distal points vary with each case but most are on the bladder (BL), stomach (ST), and gallbladder (GB) meridians.[4] BL-40, BL-60, GB-34, GB-39, SP-10, ST-36, and ST-41 are commonly used distal points.[4] Some practitioners use as few as four needles, and some use as many as 20. Needles are usually left in place 10 to 20 minutes and may be stimulated by hand, moxibustion, or electrical stimulation.

When electroacupuncture is used for nerve regeneration, a frequency of 40 to 200 Hz is thought to be beneficial.[20] This current can be run through the inner or outer bladder meridian from points cranial to caudal of the injured area. Aquapuncture may also be implemented. Treatments can be given daily in acute cases where pain is evident, weekly or every other week if the case is chronic. Supportive treatments of rest and maintaining healthy bladder function are also important.

When treating cervical IVDD, local and distal points are also used. Local points that can be used include GV-14, GB-20, GB-21, BL-10, BL-11, and painful trigger points. Distal points commonly used include LI-4, LI-11, SI-3, and TH-5.[4,41] When urinary incontinence is present, CV-3 and SP-6 can be added. BL-25 and BL-32 can be added when fecal incontinence is present.[41] Huatojiaji points are a set of extra points medial to the bladder meridian along the vertebral column. These points correspond to the intervertebral spaces from T1 to L5 and can be used for paresis or paralysis.[41,42] When the lesion is causing forelimb paralysis, T1–T3 is stimulated. When hindlimb paralysis is evident, L1–L5 is stimulated.[42] These points are stimulated by placing a needle, stimulating it by twirling the needle with the fingers, and removing it once the muscle around the needle has released. Placing a needle in the tip of the tail has also been suggested as a point for treating paralysis.

■ ■ ■ **Table 20-1**   Proportional Measurements

Body part	Distance	Proportional measurement
Upper forelimb	Between the axilla and the transverse cubital crease of the elbow	9 units
Lower forelimb	Between the transverse cubital crease of the elbow and the transverse cubital crease of the carpus	12 units
Upper (outer) hindlimb	From the prominence of the greater trochanter to the lateral aspect of the popliteal crease	19 units
Lower (outer) hindlimb	From the lateral aspect of the popliteal crease to the prominence of the lateral malleolus	16 units
Upper (inner) hindlimb	From the level of the upper border of the symphysis pubis to the medial epicondyle of the femur	18 units
Lower (inner) hindlimb	From the lower border of the medial condyle of the tibia to the prominence of the medial malleolus	13 units

Treating Peripheral Neuropathy

The peripheral neuropathies commonly seen in rehabilitation include those associated with trauma (i.e., brachial plexus injuries or concussion), nerve entrapment following surgery, idiopathic neuropathies, and degenerative myelopathy. When a specific nerve is affected, as in trauma or nerve entrapment, needles are placed in points along the meridian that runs close to the affected nerve starting proximal to the injured area and ending distal to the injured area, or at the toes if the entire limb is affected. High-frequency electroacupuncture is used to stimulate nerve regeneration. In brachial plexus injuries it is important to remember that the trauma affects the nerve roots and should be treated with electroacupuncture from the Huatuojiaji points or inner bladder points to points distal on the forelimb. An electromyogram may be performed to assess nerve function 6 to 12 weeks after trauma. Without the aid of acupuncture, the rate of nerve regeneration is approximately 1 to 4 mm per day.[43] At this time, the accelerated rate by applying electroacupuncture has not been documented.

Idiopathic neuropathies can be treated locally but should be monitored closely to rule out malignancies, because acupuncture increases perfusion to the area. Malignancies pressing directly on a nerve or on the nerve sheath may not become evident for months after clinical neurologic signs have become apparent. Presenting clinical signs may include lameness, muscle atrophy, and decreased reflexes or conscious proprioception.

Point Information

This section addresses the location and individual action of each of the previously mentioned points. The location of these points are adapted from "Official location of points, 1997" according to the International Veterinary Acupuncture Society. The functions of the points will only be described as they pertain to the musculoskeletal and neurologic system. It is important to keep in mind that these points may have many other functions.

All of the points are needled perpendicularly unless otherwise indicated. In human acupuncture, there are three methods for locating acupuncture points.

Proportional Measurements

For proportional measurements, various portions of the body are divided into equal units. These units (known as body or proportional inches) are used as proportional standards of measurement. These standards can then be applied to any patient, regardless of species, sex, or body size (Table 20-1). For example, it has been established that there are 12 proportional units from the transverse cubital crease

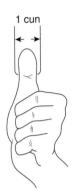

Figure 20-7   Finger-measurement equivalent of one unit.

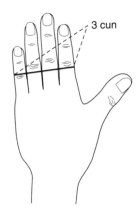

Figure 20-8   Finger-measurement equivalent of three units.

of the elbow to the transverse cubital crease of the carpus. The point TH-5 is described as two units proximal to the carpus. Thus it is one-sixth (2 units/12 units) the distance from the carpus to the elbow.

Anatomic Landmarks

These landmarks can be fixed or moving. In other words, sometimes the animal's body must be moved in a certain way to create a landmark, such as flexing a joint to create a transverse crease. For example, SI-3 is located just proximal to the metacarpophalangeal joint on the lateral aspect of the fifth metacarpal bone.

Finger Measurement of the Patient

In humans, one unit is equivalent to the width of the thumb across the knuckle (Figure 20-7) and three units are equivalent to the width of four fingers close together at the level of the dorsal skin crease of the proximal interphalangeal joint of the middle finger (Figure 20-8). Obviously, in dogs there are differences in unit size depending on the size of the dog. Large dogs are similar to humans, and smaller dogs are proportionately smaller. Some authors have compared the width of the 12th

rib to one unit. However, it is more practical to use the proportional measurements and anatomical landmarks when treating animal patients, rather than attempting to estimate units.

Acupuncture points in animals have been transposed from those in humans, and confusion may arise when traditional descriptions are used. To aid in point location, acupuncture points are identified by both traditional and proportional descriptions (Table 20-2).

Summary

The preceding information is an overview of canine acupuncture and is not intended to take the place of a full training program. Acupuncture has been applied to animals for pain relief for more than 4000 years. It may be useful for pain relief so atrophied muscles can be strengthened and animals can be reeducated to walk in a balanced fashion. Further, it may increase nerve regeneration for quicker return to optimal function. Acupuncture can be performed using several different techniques and can be combined with conventional Western medicine for possible improved outcomes and healing. Although much information is known, research is still needed to fully understand the science of acupuncture and to realize its full potential.

■ ■ Table 20-2 Point Locations, Indications, and Methods

Point	Location	Indications	Method
Lung (LU) 5	On the transverse cubital crease, on the lateral side of the tendon of the biceps brachii muscle, found with the elbow in flexion	Pain in the humerus, elbow, neck	Puncture obliquely upward
Lung (LU) 7	Proximal to the styloid process of the radius, 1.5 units above the transverse crease of the carpus (one-eighth the distance from the carpus to the elbow)	Stiff cervical muscles and pain or weakness of the carpus	
Large intestine (LI) 4	Between the first and second metacarpal bones, approximately in the middle of the second metacarpal bone on the radial side	Pain in the neck, general pain, weakness and motor impairment of the forelimb	
Large intestine (LI) 10	Two units distal to LI-11, between the extensor carpi radialis muscle and the common digital extensor muscle (one-sixth the distance from the elbow to the carpus)	Motor impairment of the forelimb and pain in the shoulder and back	
Large intestine (LI) 11	At the end of the lateral cubital crease, halfway between the biceps tendon and the lateral epicondyle of the humerus. Found with the elbow in flexion	Motor impairment in the forelimb	
Large intestine (LI) 15	Cranial and distal to the acromion, on the cranial margin of the acromial head of the deltoid muscle	Pain and motor impairment of the forelimb	Puncture periodically or obliquely
Stomach (ST) 35	In the depression below the patella and lateral to the patella ligament	Numbness, soreness, and motor impairment of the hindlimb and stifle	
Stomach (ST) 36	Three units below ST 35, one finger width from the cranial crest of the tibia, in the belly of the cranial tibial muscle (three-sixteenth, or slightly less than one-fourth, the distance from the middle of the patella to the lateral malleolus)	Pain in the stifle and hindlimb	
Stomach (ST) 40	Eight units proximal to the lateral malleolus, cranial to the fibula, two units lateral from the tibial midline, between the cranial tibial muscle and the long digital extensor (halfway between the patella and the lateral malleolus)	Muscle atrophy, motor impairment, and pain and swelling or paralysis of the hindlimbs	
Stomach (ST) 41	On the dorsum of the rear foot at the level of the hock, between the tendons of the long digital extensor muscle and the cranial tibial muscle, approximately at the level of the tip of the malleolus	Pain in the hock, muscle atrophy, motor impairment, and pain and paralysis of the lower extremities	
Stomach (ST) 44	Proximal to the web margin between the second and third toes, in the depression distal and lateral to the second metatarso-phalangeal joint	Pain of the dorsum of the hind paw	
Spleen (SP) 6	Three units directly above the tip of the medial malleolus, on the caudal border of the tibia, on the line drawn from the medial sophamalleolus to SP-9	Muscle atrophy, motor impairment, and paralysis and pain of the lower extremities	
Spleen (SP) 9	On the lower border of the medial condyle of the tibia, in the depression between the caudal border of the tibia and gastrocnemius muscle	Pain in the stifle	

Point	Location	Indication
Spleen (SP) 10	When the stifle is flexed, the point 2 units above the craniomedial border of the patella, on the bulge of the cranial portion of the sartorius muscle (two-nineteenths, or slightly greater than one-tenth, the distance from the patella to the prominence of the greater trochanter)	Pain in the medial aspect of the upper hindlimb
Heart (HT) 3	On the medial side of the elbow, between the end of the transverse cubital crease and the medial epicondyle of the humerus when the elbow is flexed	Pain and numbness of the paw and forelimb, tremors of the paw, and pain in the axilla
Small intestine (SI) 3	Proximal to the metacarpophalangeal joint on the lateral aspect of the fifth metacarpal	Pain and rigidity of the neck, acute lumbar sprain, contracture and numbness of the digits, and pain in the shoulder and elbow
Small intestine (SI) 9	In a depression between the long head and lateral head of the triceps muscle and the caudal border of the deltoid muscle	Pain in the scapular region and motor impairment of the forelimb
Bladder (BL) 10	On the lateral side of the origin of the trapezius muscle between C-1 and C-2	Neck rigidity and pain in the shoulder and cranial back
Bladder (BL) 11	Midway from the spinous process of the first thoracic vertebra to the medial border of the scapula	Pain in the neck, back, and scapula
Bladder (BL) 23	1.5 units lateral to the caudal border of the spinous process of the second lumbar vertebra (midway between the dorsal midline and the lateral border of the paravertebral musculature)	Pain and weakness of the caudal spine and stifle
Bladder (BL) 25	1.5 units lateral to the caudal border of the spinous process of the fifth lumbar vertebra (midway between the dorsal midline and the lateral border and the lateral border of the paravertebral musculature)	Caudal back pain, muscle atrophy, sciatica, fecal incontinence, and pain, numbness, and motor impairment of the hindlimbs
Bladder (BL) 28	Lateral to the second sacral foramen, in the depression between the medial border of the dorsal iliac spine and the sacrum	Stiffness and pain of the caudal back and urinary incontinence
Bladder (BL) 32	In the second posterior sacral foramen	Caudal back pain, muscle atrophy, pain, numbness and motor impairment of the hindlimbs, and fecal incontinence
Bladder (BL) 40	In the center of the popliteal crease	Caudal back pain, contracture of the tendons in the popliteal fossa, muscular atrophy and pain, numbness, and motor impairment of hindlimbs
Bladder (BL) 54	Dorsal to the greater trochanter. Midway between the greater trochanter and the hiatus of the sacrum	Pain in the lumbosacral region, muscle atrophy, and motor impairment of the hindlimbs
Bladder (BL) 60	In the depression between the lateral malleolus and the calcaneal tendon, level with the tip of the lateral malleolus	Neck rigidity, pain in the shoulder, back and forelimb, and swelling and pain in the hock
Bladder (BL) 62	In the depression directly distal to the lateral malleolus, when the hock is flexed at a 90-degree angle	Pain in the back and hindlimb, especially the hock

Continued

Table 20-2   Point Locations, Indications, and Methods—Cont'd

Point	Location	Indications	Method
Kidney (KI) 3	In the depression between the medial malleolus and calcaneal tendon level with the tip of the medial malleolus	Pain and/or weakness in the caudal back	
Pericardium (PC) 3	In the cubital crease, on the medial side of the biceps tendon	Pain in the elbow and forelimb and tremors of the forelimb	
Triple Heater (TH) 4	On the dorsum of the forepaw, at the junction of the forelimb and the radial and ulnar carpal bones, lateral to the tendon of the common digital extensor	Pain in the shoulder and carpus	
Triple Heater (TH) 5	Two units above the carpus, on the dorsal aspect of the interosseous space between the radius and ulna (one-sixteenth the distance from the transverse crease of the carpus to the transverse crease of the elbow)	Strained cervical muscles, motor impairment of the forelimb, and pain in the carpus and digits	
Triple Heater (TH) 14	Caudal and distal to the acromion, on the caudal margin of the acromial head of the deltoid muscle	Pain and motor impairment of the shoulder and upper forelimb	
Gallbladder (GB) 20	In the dorsocranial aspect of the neck, caudal to the occipital bone, in the depression medial to the jugular process of the occipital bone, in the depression between the sternomastoideus and the sternooccipital muscles	Pain and stiffness of the cervical muscles	
Gallbladder (GB) 21	Midway between GV 14 and the acromion	Pain in the neck, shoulder and back, and motor impairment of the forelimb	
Gallbladder (GB) 29	One-third the distance between the greater trochanter and the cranial dorsal iliac spine	Pain and numbness of the upper hindlimb and lumbar region, paralysis and muscle atrophy of the lower hindlimb	
Gallbladder (GB) 30	Midway between the greater trochanter and the tuber ischii	Pain in the lumbar region and upper hindlimb, and muscle atrophy of the lower hindlimbs	
Gallbladder (GB) 31	On the midline of the lateral aspect of the thigh, seven units above the transverse popliteal crease (seven-ninths, or slightly more than one-third the distance from the transverse popliteal crease to the prominence of the greater trochanter)	Pain in the lumbar area and upper hindlimb, and paralysis of the lower hindlimbs	
Gallbladder (GB) 34	In the depression cranial and distal to the head of the fibula	Hemiplegia, weakness, numbness and pain of the lower hindlimbs, and swelling and pain in the stifle	
Gallbladder (GB) 39	Three units above the tip of the lateral malleolus, in the depression between the caudal border of the fibula and the tendons of the peroneus longus and brevis muscles(three sixteenths, or slightly less than one-fourth, the distance from the lateral malleolus to the transverse popliteal crease)	Hemiplegia, pain in the neck, muscle atrophy and spastic pain of the hindlimbs	

Point	Location	Indication	Technique
Gallbladder (GB) 41	In the depression distal to the junction of the fourth and fifth metatarsal bones, on the lateral aspect of the tendon of the extensor digitorum longus muscle	Pain and swelling of the hind paw and toes	
Liver (LV) 3	On the medial aspect of the second metatarsal, proximal to the metatarsal phalangeal joint, midway between the dorsal and medial aspect of the bone. (NOTE: Some authors place this point on the medial aspect of the third metatarsal)	Pain in the hock, back, and local pain of the hind paw	
Conception vessel (CV) 1	In the depression between the anus and scrotum or vulva	Urinary retention or incontinence	
Conception vessel (CV) 3	Four units caudal to the umbilicus on midline one-fifth the distance from the cranial border of the symphysis pubis to the umbilicus)	Urinary retention, incontinence, or increased frequency of urination	
Governing vessel (GV) 4	On midline, between the dorsal spinous process of the second and third lumbar vertebrae	Stiffness of the back and weakness of the back and stifles	
Governing vessel (GV) 14	On midline, between the dorsal spinous processes of the seventh cervical and first thoracic vertebrae	Neck and back pain and stiffness	
Extra points			
Huatuojiaji	A group of 40 points on both sides of the spinal column 0.5 units lateral to the lower border of each spinous process from the first thoracic vertebra to the seventh lumbar vertebra one-sixth the distance from the dorsal midline to the lateral border of the paravertebral musculature)	T1 to T3 is used for diseases of the forelimbs, T1 to T8 is used for diseases of the chest region, T6 to L7 is used for diseases in the abdominal region, and L1 to L7 is used for diseases in the hindlimbs. These points are commonly used locally for IVDD dogs, often with remarkable results.	
Shiqizhui (in people); called lumbar Bai hui in animals	In the lumbosacral space	Lumbar, sacral, and thigh pain, and paralysis of the hindquarters	
Baxie	In the web between the toes of the forelimbs	Numbness, spasm, and contracture of the forelimb toes	Puncture obliquely and slightly upward
Bafeng	In the web between the toes of the hindlimbs	Numbness, spasm, and contracture of the hindlimb toes	Puncture obliquely and slightly upward
Xiyan	The pair of points on both sides of the patella ligament distal to the patella with the stifle slightly flexed. ST-35 is the lateral point	Stifle pain and weakness of the hindlimbs	
Heding	In the depression of the midpoint of the superior patella ligament just proximal to the patella	Stifle pain, weakness of the hind leg and paw, and paralysis	

REFERENCES

1. Jagger DH: History and concepts of veterinary acupuncture. In Schoen AM, editor: *Veterinary acupuncture: ancient art to modern medicine*, St Louis, 1994, Mosby.
2. LaFrana JE. Schaumburg, IL, 1990, American Veterinary Medical Association.
3. Schoen AM: Acupuncture for musculoskeletal disorders. In Schoen AM, editor: *Veterinary acupuncture: ancient art to modern medicine*, St Louis, 1994, Mosby.
4. Schoen AM, Wynn SG: *Complementary and alternative veterinary medicine: principles and practice*, St Louis, 1998, Mosby.
5. Reichmanis M et al: DC skin conductance variation at acupuncture loci, *Am J Chinese Med* 4:69-72, 1976.
6. Gunn CC: Type IV acupuncture points, *Am J Acupunct* 5: 51-52, 1977.
7. German Acupuncture Society, Dusseldorf: *Dusseldorf acupuncture symposium report: the basis of acupuncture* 198; 164: 362-365
8. Bressler DE, Kroening RJ: Three essential factors in effective acupuncture therapy, *Am J Chinese Med* 4: 81-86, 1976.
9. Omura Y: Patho-physiology of acupuncture treatment: effects of acupuncture on cardiovascular and nervous systems, *Acupunct Electrother Res* 1:51-140, 1975.
10. Smith, FWK Jr: The neurologic basis of acupuncture. In Schoen AM, editor: *Veterinary acupuncture: ancient art to modern medicine*, St Louis, 1994, Mosby.
11. Hyman SE et al: *Pain*. New York, 1989, Scientific American.
12. Kendall DE: A scientific model of acupuncture, *Am J Acupunct* 17:251-268, 1989.
13. Melzack R, Wall PD: Pain mechanisms: a new theory, *Science* 150:971, 1965.
14. Latshaw WK: Current theories of pain perception related to acupuncture, *J Am Acupunct Holistic Assoc* 11:449-450, 1975.
15. Pert A: Mechanisms of opiate analgesia and role of endorphins in pain suppression, *Adv Neurol* 33: 107-122, 1982.
16. Pan XP et al: Electro-acupuncture analgesia and analgesic action of NAGA, *J Trad Chinese Med* 4:273-278, 1984.
17. Han JS: *The neurochemical basis of pain relief by acupuncture: a collection of papers (1973-1987)*, Beijing, 1973-1987, Beijing Medical University.
18. Loony GL: Autonomic theory of acupuncture. In Proceedings oft the Second World Symposium on Acupuncture and Chinese Medicine, *Am J Chinese Med* 2:232, 1974.
19. Sun SM et al: The effects of electro acupuncture on the function of sympatheo-adrenal medulla, *J Trad Chinese Med* 4:11-14, 1984.
20. Schoen AM, editor: *Veterinary acupuncture: ancient art to modern medicine*, St Louis, 1994, Mosby.
21. Cheng RS, Pomeranz BH: Electroacupuncture is mediated by stereoscopic opiate receptors and is reversed by antagonists of type I receptors, *Life Sci* 26:631, 1980.
22. Levine D: Acupuncture in review: a mechanistic perspective, *Am J Acupunct* 8:5-17, 1980.
23. Yang MMP, Kik SH: Further study of the neurohumoral factor, endorphin, in the mechanism of acupuncture analgesia, *Am J Chinese Med* 7:143-148, 1979.
24. Han J: The role of some central neurotransmitters in acupuncture analgesia. In *Proceedings of the National Symposium of Acupuncture, Moxibustion and Acupuncture Anesthesia*, Beijing, People's Republic of China, 1979.
25. Han JS, Terenius I: Neurochemical basis of acupuncture analgesia, *Ann Rev Pharmacol Toxicol* 22:193-220, 1982.
26. Xie QW: Endocrinological basis of acupuncture, *Am J Chinese Med* 9:298-304, 1982.
27. Chao WK, Loh JWP: The immunologic responses of acupuncture stimulation, *Acupunct Electrother Res* 12: 229, 1987.
28. Becker RO, Seldon G: *The body electric*, New York, 1985, William Morrow.
29. Reichmanis M et al: Electrical correlates of acupuncture points, *IEEE Trans Biomed Electrother* Nov, 1975, p 553.
30. Rogers PAM: Acupuncture in pain and painful conditions. Section F in *Acupuncture and homeostasis of body adaptive systems: acupuncture bibliography*. Available at http://users.med.auth.gr/~karanik/english/hels/helsframe.html, Dec 3, 2001; and veterinary acupuncture: canine and feline in *Veterinary acupuncture: a bibliography from the veterinary library, University of Montreal*. Available at http://users.med.auth.gr/~karanik/english/articles/vetbibl.html, No. 6, Dec 3, 2001.
31. The medical acupuncture web page. Available at http://users.med.auth.gr/~karnik/english/main.htm, Dec 3, 2001.
32. Batra A, Negi O: Therapeutic electroacupuncture in the treatment of cervical spine syndrome, *Am J Acupunct* 15:49-51, 1987.
33. Janssens LA: Treatment of canine cervical disc disease by means of acupuncture: a review of 32 cases, *J Small Animal Pract* 26:206-210, 1985.
34. Seim H, Prata R: Ventral decompression for the treatment of cervical disc disease in the dog: a review of 54 cases, *J Am Animal Hosp Assoc* 18:233-240, 1982.
35. O'Connor J, Bensky D: *Acupuncture: a comprehensive text*. Shanghai, 1985, Shanghai College of Traditional Medicine.
36. Ellis A: *Fundamentals of Chinese acupuncture*, Brookline, MA, 1988, Paradigm.
37. Han J, Si S: Differential release of enkephalin and dynorphin by low and high frequency electroacupuncture in the central nervous system, *Acupuncture* 190:19-27.
38. Dukes T: Gold bead implantation in small animals. Presented at the International Veterinary Acupuncture Society 25th annual conference. Available at http://users.med.auth.gr/~karanik/english/articles/darkgold.html, Dec 3, 2001.
39. Basko IJ: A new frontier: laser therapy, *Calif Vet* 37: 17-18, 1983.
40. Griffiths RC: Spinal cord blood flow after acute experimental cord injury in dogs, *J Neurological Sci* 27: 247-259, 1976.
41. Xinnong C: *Chinese acupuncture and moxibustion*, ed 1, Beijing, 1987, Foreign Language Press.
42. Maciocia G: *The foundations of Chinese medicine: a comprehensive text for acupuncturists and herbalists*, ed 1, Churchill Livingstone, 1989.
43. DeLahunta A: *Veterinary neuroanatomy and clinical neurology*, ed 2, Philadelphia, 1983, WB Saunders.

PHYSICAL THERAPY FOR SPECIFIC DIAGNOSES

■ C h a p t e r   2 1

Common Orthopedic Conditions and Their Physical Rehabilitation

David Levine, Robert A. Taylor, and Darryl L. Millis

Shoulder Conditions

Bicipital Tenosynovitis

Bicipital tenosynovitis is a degenerative process of the tendon and tendon sheath of the biceps brachii muscle.[1] This condition is commonly seen in middle- to older-age large-breed dogs. These animals present with a variable weight-bearing lameness. Flexion of the shoulder joint with simultaneous extension of the elbow joint increases the tension on the biceps tendon as it crosses over the bicipital groove, resulting in discomfort. In addition, there may be pain on direct palpation of the bicipital groove of the proximal craniomedial aspect of the humerus. Bicipital tenosynovitis may occur in conjunction with osteoarthritis (OA) of the shoulder or glenohumeral ligament damage.

Conservative management involves rest and injection of corticosteroids into the shoulder joint, which communicates with the biceps tendon sheath. Pulsed-mode 3-MHz therapeutic ultrasound may also be used over the tendon. Because of the close proximity to bone, the intensity must be carefully monitored for any signs of pain. Pulsed-mode ultrasound should not result in significant tissue temperature increase. The ultrasound treatment must

extend down the tendon to the musculotendinous junction, because the inflammation commonly extends to this point. Oral nonsteroidal antiinflammatory drugs (NSAIDs) and cryotherapy are also prescribed. Continued improvement may be seen with up to three injections of corticosteroids at 2- to 4-week intervals. There is up to a 50% response rate with conservative therapy, but the condition is often nonresponsive to conservative treatment or recurs with active exercise or work.

In cases that fail to respond to conservative measures, surgical release of the biceps tendon and reattachment to the proximal humerus with a bone screw and spiked washer is done. An arthroscopic bicipital tendon release procedure without reattachment of the tendon has been recently reported and has good results.[2] With this procedure, postsurgical physical rehabilitation is important. Cryotherapy, passive range of motion (PROM), and short leash walks (preferably with a harness) are used for the first 3 weeks. After this initial phase, treatment involves gradual strengthening exercises, especially to the brachialis muscle to help improve the animal's ability to flex the elbow joint. Neuromuscular electrical stimulation to the brachialis muscle, aquatic therapy, and treadmill activity may all be used. Cryotherapy may be continued after bouts of exercise to minimize postexercise soreness or inflammation.

Mineralization of the Supraspinatus Tendon

This is an overuse condition that is observed in active medium- to large-breed dogs. It is characterized by point tenderness at the insertion of the supraspinatus into the humeral greater tubercle of the humerus. This condition often exists with generalized scapulohumeral OA, medial glenohumeral ligament damage, and bicipital tenosynovitis. Radiographs of the scapulohumeral joint are used to confirm the presence of diffuse mineralization of the point of insertion.[3] Conservative treatment is most commonly employed and involves use of rest, NSAIDs, cryotherapy, and PROM exercises. In humans, therapeutic ultrasound has been successfully used to treat the deposits and may have promise for treating this condition in dogs.

Medial Glenohumeral Instability

Medial glenohumeral instability results in degenerative joint changes and loss of ligament integrity. This may manifest as an acute medial luxation of the humeral head in severe cases or as a chronic weight-bearing lameness with mild instability.[4] In cases of acute luxation, patients are most commonly treated conservatively by immobilizing the shoulder joint with a sling. Following a period of immobilization, the sling is removed and PROM is initiated but is limited to the sagittal plane to avoid motions that stress the medial capsule such as abduction. Weight-bearing exercises are also limited. Surgical repair involves imbricating the medial glenohumeral ligament and joint capsule, and possible transfer of the tendon of the biceps brachii tendon to a more medial position to assist in stabilizing the shoulder joint. Postoperative physical rehabilitation following this repair consists of rest, NSAIDs, cryotherapy, and PROM exercises for the first 3 weeks, followed by gradual resumption of weight-bearing exercises.

Osteochondritis Dissecans of the Caudal Head of the Humerus

This is a developmental disease that occurs in rapidly growing medium- to large-breed dogs

typically between 6 and 8 months of age.[5,6] This disease is more common in dogs receiving too much energy (calories) and calcium in the diet. Studies have shown that limiting dietary intake reduces the incidence of this condition, as well as other developmental orthopedic conditions. There is a failure of appropriate endochondral ossification, making the cartilage more susceptible to damage. This condition is termed osteochondrosis. When cracks occur in the surface of the articular cartilage and a flap forms, it is referred to as osteochondritis dissecans (OCD). The most common location for OCD in the dog is the shoulder. This condition produces a mild to moderate weight-bearing lameness. A diagnosis is commonly made by physical examination, plain or contrast radiography, and arthroscopy (Figure 21-1). Conservative therapy of osteochondrosis lesions involves the use of oral NSAIDs, glucosamine and chondroitin sulfate therapy, rest, cryotherapy, and PROM exercises to maintain range of motion (ROM) and provide joint nutrition and stress along normal lines of movement. OCD of the humeral head is best managed surgically and includes debridement of the defective cartilage, creation of vascular access channels, and, in partial-thickness cartilage injuries, removal of the osteochondral fragment and debridement of the cartilage bed. These procedures may be performed either through an arthrotomy or, less invasively, through an arthroscope. Postoperative treatment consists of NSAIDs, cryotherapy, PROM exercises, and short controlled leash walks. Three weeks postoperatively, swimming may be initiated, as well as ground treadmill walking, gradually

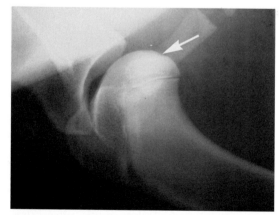

Figure 21-1   Osteochondritis dissecans of the caudal aspect of the head of the humerus. The *arrow* indicates an area of lucency where a flap of cartilage has broken off.

increasing the duration of walks. At approximately 6 weeks postoperatively, light jogging may be initiated and increased as tolerated.

Fibrotic Contracture of the Infraspinatus Muscle

This condition is commonly seen in active dogs following a period of strenuous activity.[7] Patients may initially be presented with a mild weight-bearing lameness the day of injury, but over a period of several days to weeks there is a breakdown of muscle fibers, with replacement by fibrous tissue and resulting contracture of the muscle, limiting normal ROM. The infraspinatus muscle is a major lateral supporting structure of the shoulder, and when it undergoes contracture it causes the limb to be held in an abducted position. Dogs with infraspinatus contracture hold their distal extremity in abduction, tend to paddle the leg when they walk, and are unable to fully extend the scapulohumeral joint.

If this condition is identified very early, physical rehabilitation may possibly prevent it. Conservative physical rehabilitation is not commonly performed because the surgical procedure is so successful. Continuous ultrasound coupled with stretching exercises may help to lengthen the contracted tissues preoperatively, but because the contracture is usually so severe that the shoulder is maintained in abduction almost 100% of the time, it is difficult to achieve any progress. Maintaining the limb in shoulder adduction using a splint or bandage is difficult to achieve, and there are no reports in the literature to support this as an efficacious treatment.

Surgical management involves transecting the fibrous tissue and muscle to release the affected tissue. Postoperatively, the dog should be allowed full weight-bearing as soon as possible and given gentle, pain-free PROM exercises to the shoulder, elbow, and carpus several times daily to maintain ROM and to promote normal alignment of the healing tissues. Cryotherapy may be used after exercise if indicated. Excessive activity such as unrestricted running or playing should be avoided in the first several weeks to avoid tissue damage and recurrence of fibrous tissue. If the contracture has been present for more then a few weeks before the surgery is performed, atrophy of the other forelimb muscles may be present, and a prominent scapular spine may be present. In these cases, general conditioning exercises for the limb, such as progressive

walking, wheelbarrowing, and aquatic therapy, should be used to gradually return the muscle to normal size and strength. The use of neuromuscular electrical stimulation may also be indicated if the atrophy is severe and the dog is having difficulty using the limb because of weakness.

Articular Fractures

It is critical that articular fractures be treated surgically with anatomic reduction of the articular surfaces. This is generally achieved using implants such as screws, wires, and pins. Analgesics such as NSAIDs, PROM exercises, and short leash walks are used for the first few weeks after surgery. The goal of the early postoperative period is to maintain joint ROM, limit periarticular fibrous tissue, and allow time for adequate bone healing to support more active weight-bearing exercises. After adequate healing has occurred, physical rehabilitation consists of continued ROM exercises with stretching if needed, and active weight-bearing exercises such as progressive leash walking and aquatic therapy.

Avulsion of the supraglenoid tubercle is an injury that occurs in immature dogs and results in displacement of the tubercle.[7] This injury may be classified as a traction physeal injury. Affected dogs have an acute non–weight-bearing lameness and pain on palpation of the distal scapula. Surgical repair of this injury involves reduction and stabilization of the supraglenoid tubercle with pins, wires, or screws. Alternatively, the fragment may be removed and the biceps tendon left unattached. Physical rehabilitation includes NSAIDs, cryotherapy, leash walks, and PROM for the first 3 weeks. After this initial healing period, limb strengthening, especially of the biceps brachii and brachialis muscles, is begun.

Scapular fractures may occur in any breed of dog as a result of trauma. If the neck of the scapula, articular surface of the glenoid, or scapular spine is involved, open reduction and internal fixation are usually indicated.[7] Alternatively, many nondisplaced comminuted scapular fractures are best treated conservatively. In either case it is important to maintain or regain normal scapular motion in all three planes. Postoperative physical rehabilitation includes NSAIDs, cryotherapy, and PROM exercises to the glenohumeral joint for the first several weeks. As healing progresses, scapular PROM is performed in increasing amounts in all planes to prevent fibrosis and decreased ROM. Superficial heat applied with hot packs may be used before exercise to allow increased tissue extensibility, and cross-fiber frictional massage may help to prevent or break down adhesions. Joint mobilization using scapular glides is also effective for increasing ROM. Aquatic therapy and gait activities such as treadmill walking may also be incorporated to regain muscle strength.

Pectoral Muscle Tears

Athletic dogs may tear or avulse the deep or superficial pectoral muscle. These injuries become apparent after strenuous activity and are characterized by pendulant edema, bruising, and ecchymosis of the affected muscle and local area, and variable lameness. Conservative treatment involves NSAIDs, cryotherapy, and controlled leash walking. The dog should be walking within a week after injury and be back to jogging in approximately 1 month.

Elbow Conditions

The triad of fragmented medial coronoid process (FCP), OCD of the medial condyle of the humerus, and ununited anconeal process (UAP) is commonly referred to as elbow dysplasia. Dogs with elbow dysplasia typically have only one of the three conditions, and it is rare for a single dog to have all three components of elbow dysplasia. Elbow dysplasia occurs most commonly in large or giant breeds of dogs, such as Bernese Mountain dogs, Golden Retrievers, Labrador Retrievers, and Rottweilers, and has also been associated with too much energy and calcium intake. Males are more commonly affected, and it is likely that there are genetic components to the condition. It is relatively common that dogs have elbow dysplasia in both elbows, although it is typically worse on one side than the other.

Fragmented Medial Coronoid Process (FCP) of the Ulna

This condition may occur as a result of elbow incongruity or may occur in a relatively congruent joint. A genetic component is likely involved.[8] Many believe that this condition is another manifestation of OCD. Dogs will typically be presented between 5 and 11 months

of age with lameness of the forelimb.[9] Physical examination findings usually include a mild to moderate weight-bearing lameness, reduced ROM of the elbow, joint effusion and swelling of the craniomedial compartment of the elbow, and pain when the region of the medial coronoid process is palpated.[10] A diagnosis may be made relatively early in the course of the condition using computerized tomography. Radiographs are helpful, but the FCP may not be seen on standard radiographs (Figure 21-2). Rather, secondary signs associated with OA are typically seen, including sclerosis of the subchondral bone and osteophyte development, especially in the areas of the medial coronoid process, medial epicondyle of the humerus, and the dorsal aspect of the anconeal process.

Depending on the specific case, either medical or surgical treatments may be recommended. Medical therapy includes maintaining an appropriate body weight, controlled low-impact exercise, aquatic exercise, monitoring pain, NSAIDs, and chondroprotective agents. Surgical therapy is aimed at removing any abnormal cartilage or bone and attempting to return the joint to more normal function. Arthroscopic removal may have advantages over an open arthrotomy because the supporting structures such as the joint capsule and medial collateral ligament are left relatively undisturbed. With either medical or surgical treatment, OA will progress. It is important to provide rehabilitation as with other forms of OA to maintain an acceptable quality of life for the patient.

Osteochondritis Dissecans (OCD) of the Medial Humeral Condyle

Dogs with OCD of the medial condyle of the humerus develop a weight-bearing lameness by 5 to 9 months of age.[10] There is usually swelling of the craniomedial joint compartment with pain on complete ROM. The diagnosis is confirmed by finding a radiolucent defect in the articular surface of the medial condyle on an anterior-posterior radiograph of the elbow (Figure 21-3).

OCD of the elbow joint is usually treated surgically with either an open arthrotomy or arthroscopically. Following surgery, NSAIDs, cryotherapy, PROM, and controlled leash walks are the focus of rehabilitation for the first several weeks. Weight control is important to avoid unnecessary force on the joint. The prognosis for OCD of the elbow joint is

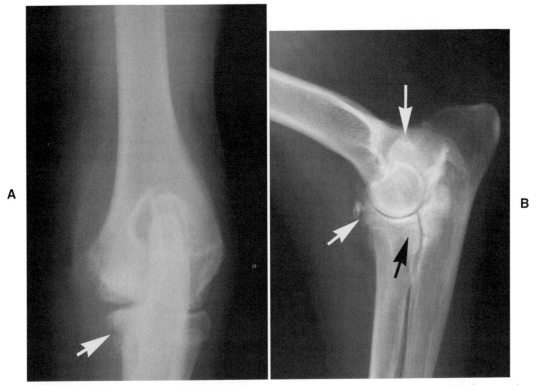

Figure 21-2 Fragmented medial coronoid process of the ulna. The *dark arrow* indicates the region of the fragmented coronoid process (not clearly seen). The *white arrows* indicate secondary arthritic changes in the elbow joint.

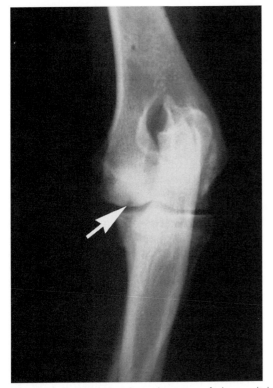

Figure 21-3 Osteochondritis dissecans of the medial condyle of the humerus. Note the dark defect indicated by the *arrow*, which corresponds with the area of defective ossification.

much more guarded than for OCD of the caudal head of the humerus in the shoulder joint. In addition, caution must be used in interpreting changes of the medial humeral condyle in cases with a concurrent FCP. This area of the medial humeral condyle may undergo erosion and ulceration as a result of contact with the FCP, and may not be an OCD lesion at all. It is sometimes called a "kissing lesion."

Ununited Anconeal Process (UAP)

The anconeal process has a physis that normally closes at 5 months of age.[7,10] If it remains open at 6 months of age, it is generally a pathologic condition and will not close without intervention. Most people believe that UAP is a manifestation of OCD. It is most common in German shepherd dogs, which are usually presented with a weight-bearing lameness of the affected limb. Typically, there is moderate to severe effusion of the caudolateral compartment of the elbow, with restricted ROM.

A lateral radiograph with the elbow in a flexed position confirms the diagnosis (Figure 21-4). The traditional treatment is removal of the UAP. Recently, other surgical

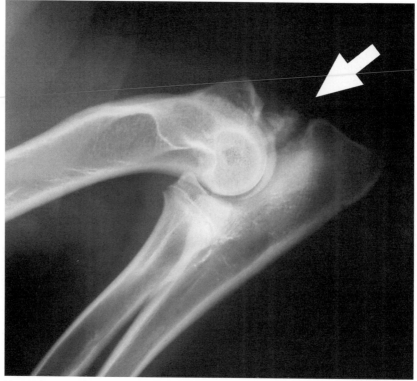

Figure 21-4   Ununited anconeal process. The anconeal process has not fused with the ulna, and many secondary arthritic changes have occurred.

approaches have included lag screw fixation of the UAP with the main segment of the anconeal process. Another treatment that is sometimes used separately or in combination with screw fixation is an ostectomy of the proximal ulna, in hopes that any incongruity will be relieved and allow the UAP to successfully fuse. If the condition is chronic, the fragment edges do not match well because of the erosion of bone and cartilage, and the piece may not be easily fixed in place. Also, because there is a defect in endochondral ossification, healing may be delayed. With any treatment, OA progresses and further treatment revolves around management of the pain and OA.

If an attempt is made to attach the UAP to the ulna with a screw, a rehabilitation program should have a slower progression of weight-bearing activities until healing is complete. This may take up to 8 to 12 weeks in some cases. Cryotherapy, ROM, aquatic therapy, and light leash walks are encouraged. If the UAP has been removed, the progress of the rehabilitation program may be accelerated according to the tolerance of the patient.

Attention should be paid to control of joint effusion, improving ROM, pain control, and weight-bearing. Aquatic activity can be very beneficial because of the active ROM while weight-bearing in a buoyant environment.

Elbow Incongruity

This is a congenital disorder of the bones and articular surfaces of the elbow joint. This problem typically manifests between 4 and 8 months of age, is commonly seen in chondrodystrophic breeds such as Bassett hounds, and may result in generalized osteochondral destruction as a result of incongruency of the various components of the elbow joint. In addition, UAP and FCP have been associated with elbow incongruity, although these conditions may occur without any apparent incongruity. This condition is most effectively treated with surgery, which may involve removal of loose osteochondral fragments and attempts to improve elbow congruity, such as corrective osteotomy or ostectomy of the radius or ulna, removal of the medial coronoid process of the ulna, or forage or curettage of

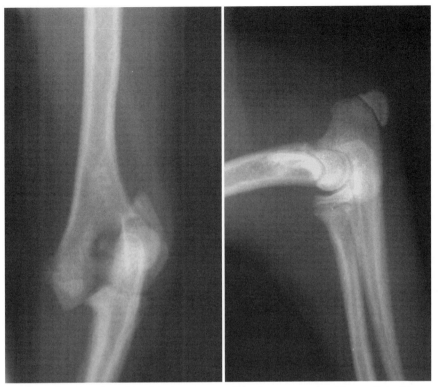

Figure 21-5 Fracture of the lateral condyle of the humerus in a skeletally immature dog. This is a Salter-Harris type IV fracture.

subchondral bone to enhance the formation of fibrocartilage in those areas devoid of articular hyaline cartilage.

With either conservative or surgical intervention, elbow incongruity invariably results in OA of the elbow. Physical rehabilitation for this condition includes NSAIDs, chondroprotective agents, cryotherapy, PROM, and progressive leash walking. Dogs with end-stage OA of the elbow often present for some form of rehabilitation. These dogs often have chronic synovial effusion, reduced ROM, crepitus of the joint, pain on manipulation of the elbow, muscle atrophy, and lameness. Physical rehabilitation cannot correct the underlying problem, but efforts to improve joint health, increase ROM, reduce weight, and rebuild atrophied muscles may significantly improve the patient's quality of life. Physical rehabilitation considerations would include PROM and stretching, active ROM activities, redeveloping muscle strength with exercise or neuromuscular electrical stimulation, low-impact exercises, and aquatic therapy. Careful monitoring of ROM is important with a home program to avoid permanent losses in ROM.

Articular Fractures

Fractures of the articular surface of the humerus are common and typically result from trauma. Articular fractures of the radius and ulna are much less common. In the young dog, Salter-Harris type IV fractures of the lateral condyle of the humerus are commonly seen in skeletally immature dogs, and fractures of the lateral humeral condyle are also seen in older dogs that have jumped from a height (Figure 21-5).[11] In spaniel breeds, such as Cocker spaniels, it is not uncommon for mature animals to present with articular fractures with minimal evidence or history of trauma. These individuals appear to have incomplete ossification of the humeral condyles.[12] As with any articular fracture, decreased ROM and destruction of articular cartilage may be sequelae of an articular fracture. In addition, Salter-Harris fractures in immature dogs may have alteration in bone growth that is necessary for a congruent elbow joint. Repair is accomplished with placement of a transcondylar screw with compression of the fracture site and placement of a small antirotational pin driven up the lateral epicondyle (Figure 21-6). The principles of articular fracture rehabilitation described for articular fractures of the scapula apply here. It is imperative that ROM exercises continue for 3 to 4 weeks after surgery to be certain that ROM is maintained. Normal ROM may return 10 to 14 days after surgery, but fibrous tissue and other healing periarticular tissues are not yet mature. If ROM exercises are discontinued too soon, it is possible that some maturation and contracture of tissues may occur with some loss of normal joint motion.

A more challenging fracture to repair and rehabilitate is a bicondylar (sometimes referred to as a T or Y) fracture, in which both the medial and lateral condyles of the humerus are fractured from the main shaft of the humerus and from each other. It is fairly common for several additional fragments to be separated from the shaft of the humerus. Repair involves stabilization and fixation of the condyles, and then stabilizing them to the main shaft of the humerus with plates, intramedullary pins, or an external fixator. In many instances, an osteotomy of the olecranon is necessary to repair this type of fracture.

The olecranon osteotomy is then repaired with a pin and tension band or screw technique. Decreased ROM is very common, especially after an olecranon osteotomy, along with OA development after surgery. Newer techniques that use separate medial and lateral approaches to the joint to avoid an olecranon osteotomy seem to result in maintenance of greater ROM. It is critical that rehabilitation be performed following repair of bicondylar fractures of the humerus. Particular attention is paid to achieving as complete ROM as possible, using passive and active ROM exercises. Control of periarticular swelling and edema with cryotherapy, NSAIDs, and bandages helps to improve motion and reduce postoperative pain. Swimming or walking in an underwater treadmill has the additional benefit of limb usage in a buoyant environment. As weight-bearing improves, other activities, such as walking over cavaletti rails may be initiated. Daily rehabilitation for at least 2 to 3 weeks is recommended.

Avulsion fractures of the olecranon may also occur. In immature dogs, there may be an avulsion fracture of the olecranon with sepa-

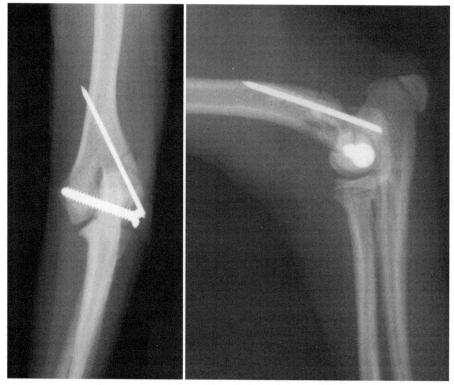

Figure 21-6 Repair of the fracture shown in Figure 21-5 with a transcondylar screw placed in lag fashion to allow some compression at the fracture site, and a small pin placed up the lateral epicondyle to counteract rotation of the fragments.

ration across the physis. Olecranon fractures prevent extension of the elbow which is necessary for normal weight-bearing and ambulation. This condition is treated by surgically replacing and stabilizing the avulsed fragment with a screw or pin and tension band technique, or if the fragment is large enough, a bone plate. Physical rehabilitation is important to achieve optimal elbow extension, and gentle PROM in the first 3 weeks, NSAIDs, and cryotherapy are used. Following adequate healing, more vigorous ROM and stretching exercises may be initiated, along with active exercises to rebuild atrophied muscles.

Elbow Luxation

Luxation of the elbow joint is usually the result of trauma and most commonly occurs in a lateral direction at the elbow.[7] In some instances the luxation can be manually reduced and, in spite of collateral ligament damage, the elbow joint is usually quite stable after the luxation is reduced. In cases of recurrent luxation, if the instability persists after closed reduction, or if closed reduction is unsuccessful, primary repair of the collateral ligaments may be necessary. The limb is generally immobilized in extension in a cast or spica splint for up to 2 weeks after reduction to allow for adequate healing. Following splint removal, it is important to regain elbow ROM, while being careful not to reluxate the joint. It is important to remember that the elbow is a hinge joint, and ROM activities should be limited to the sagittal plane and to minimize varus and valgus stresses that could destabilize the joint. After adequate healing, active exercises are gradually increased, but uncontrolled play is limited until the joint is deemed stable, usually in 8 to 12 weeks. OA frequently occurs following elbow luxation. Failure to reduce an elbow luxation results in a nonfunctional joint.

Forearm Conditions

Fractures of the Antebrachium

Fractures of the radius and ulna commonly occur.[7,13] These injuries may be treated by closed reduction and immobilization in a cast, or they may be repaired by open reduction and fixation with wires, plates, screws, or external skeletal fixation (Figure 21-7). In small dogs, distal radius and ulnar fractures

have a high incidence of delayed or nonunion fracture healing when treated with external coaptation. These fractures require anatomic reduction and rigid internal fixation to have optimal healing. In addition to problems with bone healing, prolonged immobilization by splinting or casting leads to disuse atrophy of bone and muscle in the affected limb. In some cases there is frank loss of bone distally in response to disuse of the leg. Following the first few weeks of physical rehabilitation, which involves reduction of pain and swelling, rehabilitation efforts can be undertaken to increase weight-bearing activities to load the bone during fracture healing and help stimulate normal healing. One of the main impediments to limb use is decreased ROM of the carpus as a result of flexural contracture of the soft tissues. Assisted extension of the carpus to a normal position is often painful and results in a non–weight-bearing lameness, despite healing of the fracture in many cases. Therefore it is essential, if a coaptation device is used, that particular attention be paid to stretching and ROM exercises. In some cases, an extension splint molded to the normal contralateral side may be placed on the affected limb, applying some tension to pull the digits and metacarpals to a more normal position in between rehabilitation sessions. It may take 10 to 14 days to achieve a normal angle of the carpus for weight-bearing.

Angular Limb Deformities

Angular limb deformities that occur as a result of congenital or traumatically induced growth abnormalities of the physes of the radius or ulna are common in young dogs.[7] If untreated these deformities produce significant carpal valgus, deformity of the radius and ulna, and subluxation of the carpus and elbow joints. Angular limb deformities also commonly result in OA. Correction of angular limb deformities involves a corrective osteotomy of the affected bone(s) and stabilization of the bones with plates or external fixation. In some severe cases, treatment with a circular external fixation device is necessary to correct the angular deformity and elongate the bones through distraction osteogenesis. During recovery, it is important to maintain normal ROM of the joints proximal and distal to the repair and provide pain relief and edema reduction with NSAIDs and cryotherapy. In particular, dogs receiving distraction osteogenesis must be monitored very carefully because soft tissue

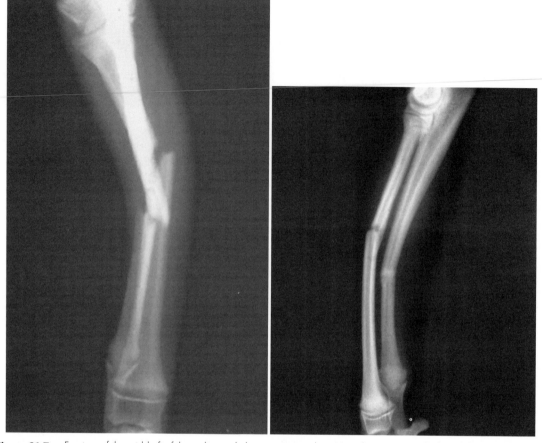

Figure 21-7   Fracture of the midshaft of the radius and ulna in a young dog. Note the open growth plates (physes) at the ends of the long bones. These are susceptible to premature closure as a result of the trauma.

elongation may not keep pace with continued elongation of the bones. This may result in reduced joint ROM, stiffness, and lameness. Stretching and ROM activities with simultaneous application of therapeutic ultrasound may be beneficial. As bone healing progresses, more aggressive activities such as aquatic therapy and weight-bearing therapeutic exercises may be initiated.

Carpal, Metacarpal, and Phalangeal Conditions

Fractures

Fractures of the carpal bones are rare but may involve the accessory carpal bone or the radial carpal bone in race athletes such as Greyhounds. In other breeds carpal fractures are invariably the result of automobile or other traumatic insults.[14] Some carpal fractures may

result in medial or lateral instability if the fracture involves the origin or insertion of the respective collateral ligament. A relatively common injury is a shearing injury, in which the dog's limb becomes trapped beneath a skidding automobile tire. The soft tissues, including skin, subcutaneous tissues, tendons, ligaments, and in severe cases, bone and tendon are eroded away, leaving the joint unstable. Many of these injuries cannot be primarily repaired, and an arthrodesis is performed in these cases. Fortunately, function is usually very acceptable after bony fusion has occurred.

Metacarpal and phalangeal fractures usually occur as a result of trauma, and phalangeal fractures are often open fractures. Carpal, metacarpal, and phalangeal fractures may be treated using closed reduction and immobilization in a coaptation device, or with variety of implants, including intramedullary pins, wires, and plates and screws (Figure 21-8).[14] A splint or light cast is usually applied

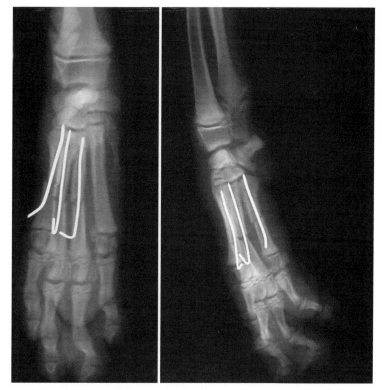

Figure 21-8   Metacarpal fractures that have been stabilized with an intramedullary pin in each metacarpal bone. (From Probst CW, Millis DL: Carpus and digits. In Slatter DH, editor: *Textbook of small animal surgery,* ed 3, Philadelphia, 2002, WB Saunders.)

to the limb after internal fixation to protect the relatively small implants that must be used. If a cast or splint is used, elbow ROM must be preserved during the time of coaptation application, and after coaptation removal. Sagittal plane ROM exercises and joint mobilization work well to restore ROM to the area. In cases of fracture and carpal instability, splinting is often used to protect the repair. If possible, removing the splint on a weekly basis to perform ROM exercises to maintain joint and tendon mobility is advised. The splint is reapplied to protect the fracture following ROM exercises.

Carpal Hyperextension Injury and Carpal Joint Luxations

Carpal hyperextension injuries occur as a result of damage to the palmar fibrocartilage and the carpal ligaments, which usually occur as a result of jumping of falling from a height, placing all of the body weight on the limb.[14] The antebrachiocarpal, middle carpal, carpometacarpal, or any combination of joints may be involved. Affected dogs are lame and

walk with overextension of the carpus; in severe cases, the carpus may touch the ground during weight-bearing. It is important to obtain stress radiographs to delineate which joint(s) is(are) involved because this information helps to guide the surgical treatment, which usually involves surgical fusion (arthrodesis) of one or more of the joints (see carpal arthrodesis). If the antebrachiocarpal joint is involved, fusion of all carpal joints (pancarpal arthrodesis) is performed. If the middle carpal or carpometacarpal joint(s) is (are) involved, a partial carpal arthrodesis is performed, sparing the antebrachiocarpal joint, which is the major motion joint of the carpus. The arthrodesis is performed by removing the articular cartilage, placing a bone graft to help speed bony union, and stabilizing the area with a bone plate (Figure 21-9). A coaptation device is placed after surgery until early bony union occurs to help reduce the stress on the implants. Treatment of a carpal hyperextension injury with a coaptation device alone is generally unsuccessful; a quicker return to function is achieved by fusing the offending joints.

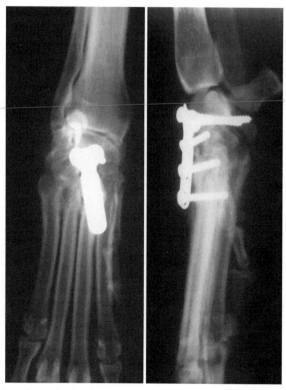

Figure 21-9   Partial carpal arthrodesis performed in a patient with carpal hyperextension injury.

Luxations of an individual carpal bone as a result of an acute traumatic event or luxation of multiple bones as a result of progressive OA or rheumatoid arthritis with ligamentous instability may cause carpal instability. If a single bone is involved, reduction of the bone with stabilization of surrounding soft tissues or an implant may result in a successful outcome. If the luxation results from arthritic changes, carpal arthrodesis generally results in a more favorable outcome. However, if rheumatoid arthritis is the cause of the luxation, this condition affects multiple joints in a progressive fashion and eventually results in severe, crippling lameness.

Metacarpophalangeal luxations and phalangeal luxations are uncommon injuries that are most often treated with open repair of the collateral ligaments. Following open reduction and ligament repair, a period of immobilization is required. During the period of immobilization it is helpful to remove the splint on a weekly basis and cycle the distal joints though their ROM. This is followed by reapplication of the splint. Following 3 weeks of immobilization, the joints are reassessed for

stability and if satisfactory, the splint is removed, and limited weight-bearing activities, continued ROM exercises, and protective bandaging are used.

Tendon and Ligament Conditions

Tendinitis of the insertion of the ulnaris lateralis on the accessory carpal bone may occur in athletic dogs. This is evident by painful swelling in the soft tissues just proximal to the insertion. These cases usually respond to NSAIDs and cryotherapy to minimize inflammation, followed by 3-MHz, pulsed therapeutic ultrasound to stimulate collagen fiber formation and alignment.

Laceration or avulsion of the superficial and deep digital flexor tendons are also relatively common traumatic injuries in dogs. Avulsion of the superficial and deep digital flexor tendons from their insertions on P2 and P3 result in abnormal toe carriage. Although this is not a career-ending injury, these tendons may be reattached for improved cosmesis and function. Lacerations of these tendons are common and may result in the same physical appearance. Following repair of the laceration with standard tendon repair techniques, or attempted reattachment of the avulsed fragment, the distal extremity is immobilized in a splint for 2 to 3 weeks. When possible the splint should be removed on a weekly basis and the neighboring joints subjected to ROM exercises, followed by replacement of the splint. In general, it is important to remove the coaptation splint within 3 weeks of the injury. Research has suggested that prolonged coaptation periods may actually slow healing and weaken the repaired tissue. It is equally important, however, that decreased activity be strictly enforced, so that no running, jumping, or playing occurs and places catastrophic stress on the healing tissues, resulting in failure. After a period of initial healing, restoring ROM and strength is the focus of the physical rehabilitation program. If contracture of the muscles or tendons has occurred, 3-MHz continuous-mode therapeutic ultrasound or hot packs immediately followed by stretching is indicated.

Flexor Tendon Contractures

The flexor tendons may undergo contracture following prolonged immobilization of any portion of the forelimb, or after a forelimb injury in which the dog does not use the limb for a period of time (Figure 21-10). These patients have shortened (tight) flexor tendon-muscle units and limited ability to extend the joints distal to the carpus during gait, which may impede rehabilitation of the involved limb because it precludes normal weight-bearing. Interventions to lengthen and stretch the tendon-muscle units include 3-MHz therapeutic ultrasound or hot packs, manual stretching exercises, and massage. This condition may be a difficult and challenging problem and requires careful management. The therapist may occasionally feel adhesions give way during stretching; it is also possible to produce fractures if the stretching is too aggressive, so caution is advised. The key is to stretch and realign tissues without ripping or tearing them.

Hip and Pelvis Conditions

There are a number of important orthopedic problems that occur in the pelvis of dogs. In addition, traumatic injuries of this region, such as those obtained from an automobile accident, are very common.

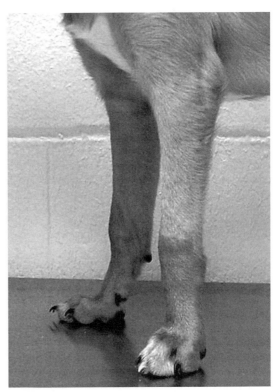

Figure 21-10   Tendon and muscle contracture after treatment of a left radius and ulna fracture with a cast.

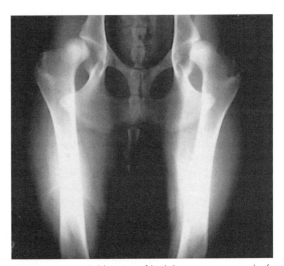

Figure 21-11   Subluxation of both hip joints as a result of hip dysplasia.

Hip Dysplasia

Hip dysplasia is a condition of the coxofemoral joint with multifactorial genetic and environmental components.[15-19] Hip dysplasia is essentially failure of the hip joint (acetabulum, femoral head and neck) to develop into a well-seated and congruent joint (Figure 21-11).

With time, the instability and incongruency result in progressive OA. It has variable genetic expression and is influenced by dietary intake, especially excess energy and calcium. In several studies, young large-breed puppies with genetic tendencies toward hip dysplasia failed to develop hip dysplasia when fed a calorie-restricted diet, as compared to littermates that were allowed ad libitum feeding.

Physical rehabilitation of chronic OA of the coxofemoral joint involves NSAID therapy, oral chondroprotective agents such as glucosamine and chondroitin sulfate, ROM exercises, limb-strengthening activities such as sit-to-stand exercises, and aquatic therapy, especially underwater treadmill walking. Weight reduction is critical if the patient is overweight. Surgical treatment of hip dysplasia most commonly involves triple pelvic osteotomy (TPO), total hip replacement (THR), or a femoral head and neck ostectomy (FHO), sometimes also called an excision arthroplasty.

Immature dogs with clinical signs of hip dysplasia and hip laxity, but no radiographic evidence of OA, may benefit from a TPO, which allows rotation of the acetabulum to provide better coverage and stability of the femoral head (Figure 21-12). In properly selected patents, this procedure has successfully reduced the severity of hip dysplasia and the progression of OA. Postoperatively, NSAIDs, cryotherapy, PROM, and assisted ambulation, followed by controlled therapeutic exercises, are indicated. After adequate healing has occurred, physical rehabilitation efforts are directed to strengthening activities, which should parallel appropriate tissue healing and tissue strength.

Total hip replacement or total hip arthroplasty is performed to provide a pain-free biomechanically adequate hip in dogs suffering from OA. OA of the hip is most commonly the result of hip dysplasia or trauma. THR surgery involves removing the femoral head and neck and securing a polypropylene acetabular component and stainless steel femoral stem and head into place (Figure 21-13). The implants are most often fixed in place with polymethylmethacrylate, but cementless total hip prostheses are available that allow for bony ingrowth to secure the components in place. Following THR, NSAIDs, cryotherapy, PROM, and controlled activities are indicated. It is important during early ambulation efforts that the patient be supported with a sling and

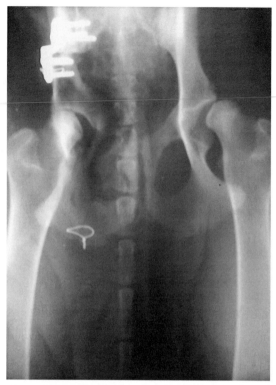

Figure 21-12 Triple pelvic osteotomy has been performed to improve coverage of the head of the femur by the acetabulum.

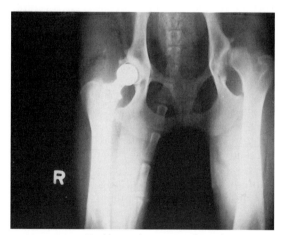

Figure 21-13 Total hip replacement performed in a patient with severe osteoarthritis secondary to hip dysplasia.

that abduction of the hindlimb be prevented to avoid dislocation of the prosthesis. Following anesthesia recovery, most dogs typically begin limited to full weight-bearing almost immediately; it is important to restrict animals to leash walks only with no running, jumping, or playing for 10 to 12 weeks to reduce the chances of implant loosening or dislocation. Because of preexisting muscle

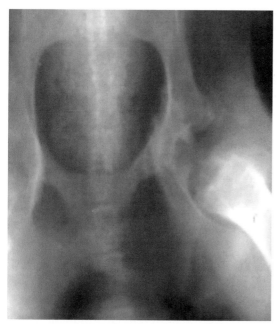

Figure 21-14 Femoral head and neck excision performed in a patient with severe osteoarthritis. Note the complete removal of the femoral head and neck.

atrophy in most cases, it is important to focus on muscle strengthening. Controlled walking, treadmill activity, and balance and proprioception reeducation are all important parts of the physical rehabilitation program.

An FHO is a salvage procedure in which the femoral head and neck are removed in severe cases of OA, or sometimes as a result of severe acetabular or femoral head fractures (Figure 21-14). In spite of the nature of this procedure, many dogs with appropriate surgical and postsurgical management can resume a near-normal activity level. Smaller dogs that are not obese tend to recover faster and have better use of the limb as compared with larger, less active, obese patients. When the femoral head and neck are removed, the supporting hip muscles (the gluteal, internal obturator, and gemelli muscles) and a pad of fibrous tissue provide support for the coxofemoral joint. With appropriate case selection, the joint is usually less painful following surgery and rehabilitation and the dog is more willing to use the leg.

Postoperatively, periarticular fibrosis provides some cushioning between the remaining bones of the hip. Rehabilitation is important to prevent excessive fibrosis and loss of motion of the pseudoarthrosis (Appendix 4C). Physical rehabilitation begins the day of surgery with PROM while the patient is recovering from anesthesia, opioid analgesic medications in the immediate postoperative period, NSAIDs, and cryotherapy. The day after surgery, PROM and controlled activities that encourage active limb use are initiated. Weight-bearing activities begin immediately and progress to higher levels as tolerated. With full recovery, the animal should have a near-normal walking and trotting gait, but these dogs rarely achieve full and powerful ROM, with hip extension being the most limited.

Legg-Calvé-Perthes Disease

Legg-Calvé-Perthes disease is also sometimes called avascular necrosis of the femoral head, and it occurs in miniature and small-breed dogs.[7] It is most commonly treated by performing an FHO. Immediate postoperative physical rehabilitation is crucial to obtain near-normal ROM of the pseudoarthrosis to ensure as complete a recovery as possible. In fact, it is beneficial to slowly place the limb through a ROM while the animal is awakening from anesthesia. This is similar to a person recovering from anesthesia on a PROM machine and may be continued until the patient indicates that it feels some discomfort. Following surgery, an aggressive analgesic and antiinflammatory protocol consisting of cryotherapy, opioid medications, and NSAIDs may begin. PROM and assisted weight-bearing is initiated the day after surgery, and cryotherapy and NSAID administration are continued. Aquatic exercise, including underwater treadmill walking and swimming, is very beneficial. As the patient tolerates more active weight-bearing, therapeutic exercise and limb movement activities may become more vigorous. A desirable endpoint at 4 weeks is a near-normal gait at the walk and the ability to trot comfortably. Small dogs with this condition generally do very well if appropriate rehabilitation is started immediately after surgery.

Pelvic Fractures

Pelvic fractures account for a large percentage of fractures seen in veterinary practice. Because of the anatomic structure of the canine pelvis, there are usually two or more fractures or injuries to the pelvis as a result of trauma, usually from an automobile injury.[7] In general, surgical repair is recommended for injuries that are part of the weight-bearing axis of the pelvis, including sacroiliac

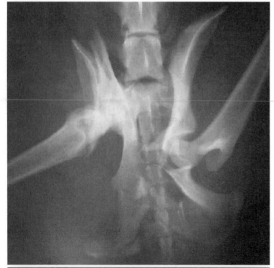

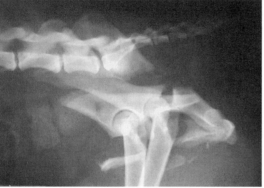

Figure 21-15 Multiple pelvic fractures may occur in dogs because the pelvis is in the form of a box, so that injury to one portion of the pelvis frequently results in injuries to other portions of the pelvis.

luxations, fractures of the body of the ilium, and acetabular fractures (Figure 21-15). Surgical repair results in a quicker return to function with fewer changes secondary to tissue disuse, and the level of function will generally be superior. It is important that surgical repair be undertaken within the first 7 to 10 days after injury to avoid damage to soft tissues and nerves during reduction of the fractures. In some instances, conservative treatment in the form of cage rest may be adequate to allow healing. Examples of injuries amenable to conservative treatment include greenstick fractures of the body of the ilium, mild displacement of the sacroiliac joint with minimal pain or lameness, and fractures of the caudal 20% of the acetabulum in small dogs. Although pubic and ischial fractures may appear quite severe on a radiograph, these injuries are rarely repaired because they are not part of the weight-bearing axis of the pelvic limb. Repair of the injuries to the sacroiliac joint, ilium, and acetabulum generally results in adequate reduction and realignment of pubic and ischial fractures for healing if the animal is rested.

It is important to identify any concurrent injuries with pelvic fractures. Trauma to the spinal cord or peripheral nerves is relatively common, especially with fractures of the sacrum (not necessarily with sacroiliac luxation, but with fractures of the sacrum), fractures of the body of the ilium with medial displacement of the caudal fracture fragment, and fractures of the cranial ischium in the region traversed by the sciatic nerve. It is important to perform a thorough neurologic examination, checking for pain sensation and reflexes. Because injuries to the pelvis tend to involve both pelvic limbs and other injuries to the distal limbs are frequently present, evaluation of the patient while ambulating or performing proprioceptive tests may not be possible. In addition, urinary tract trauma, liver trauma, and thoracic trauma are relatively common in animals with pelvic injuries.

Sacroiliac joint luxations are surgically managed by placing one or more screws in lag fashion to compress the joint. The screw(s) should engage the body of the sacrum and be deeply seated into the bone, so that the screw engages at least 60% of the width of the sacrum. Fractures of the sacral body or wing can be challenging to repair, and concurrent nerve injuries are quite common.

Fractures of the body of the ilium are usually repaired with a bone plate and screws (Figure 21-16). It is important that the plate be properly contoured to pull the caudal half of the pelvis out to avoid future problems of constipation and obstipation. Caution should be exercised during the reduction of fragments that have severe medial displacement because of the proximity to the lumbosacral plexus just medial to the body of the ilium.

Fractures of the acetabulum secondary to automobile trauma are very common in dogs. While the principles of fracture repair and management are the same as for other joint fractures, some additional commentary is useful. Most acetabular fractures should be treated with open reduction and internal fixation. Depending on the size of the patient and the nature of the fracture, repair may involve plates, screws, wires, or polymethylmethacry-

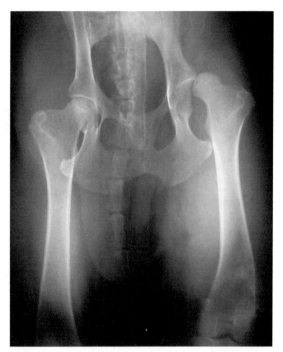

Figure 21-17   Craniodorsal hip luxation in a patient that had been hit by a car.

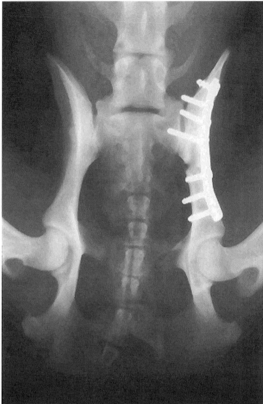

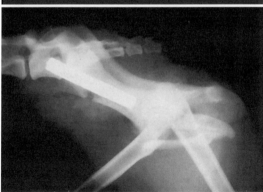

Figure 21-16   Plate fixation of the body of the ilium.

late. In many acetabular fractures, anatomic reduction is difficult to achieve, and many animals with these fractures develop OA.

Coxofemoral Luxation

Coxofemoral or hip luxations are very common and usually occur in a craniodorsal direction as a result of automobile trauma (Figure 21-17).[7] Depending on the severity of trauma, the coxofemoral anatomy, and time since the

injury, many coxofemoral luxations can be successfully reduced and immobilized with an Ehmer sling for approximately 2 weeks. The sling provides non–weight-bearing immobilization of the hip in a flexed and internally rotated position, which helps to keep the hip joint reduced while the soft tissues begin to heal. In one study, 50% of dogs with traumatically luxated normal hips were successfully treated with closed reduction, the use of an Ehmer sling, and immobilization. In cases of recurrent luxation, these patients are candidates for surgical reduction and stabilization, or an FHO or THR.

Procedures for surgical stabilization vary and are largely chosen based on surgeon preference and experience. Common techniques include open reduction of the coxofemoral luxation and suture repair of the joint capsule tear (capsulorrhaphy), relocation of the greater trochanter distally and caudally to redirect forces on the hip and provide additional stability, prosthetic capsule using screws and suture, toggle pin fixation, or flexible external skeletal fixation (Figure 21-18). A combination of techniques is often used. In cases requiring surgical reduction, an Ehmer sling is also placed postoperatively.

Some cases of hip luxation occur as a result of relatively minor trauma, such as falling or

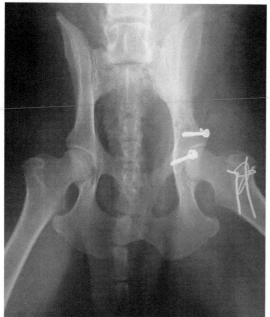

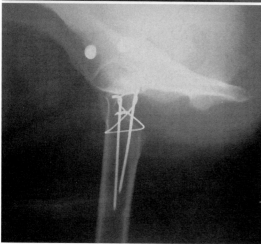

Figure 21-18   Stabilization of a hip luxation with a prosthetic capsule technique. Note the screws located in the dorsal acetabulum. These serve as anchor points for strong suture material, which is placed in figure-of-eight fashion around the screws and through a tunnel drilled in the femoral neck.

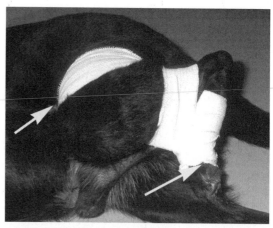

Figure 21-19   An Ehmer sling has been applied to manage a hip luxation that has been reduced. Note the areas to inspect on a daily basis to detect irritation of the skin (arrows).

bumping into a doorway or furniture. Invariably, these dogs also have severe hip dysplasia. Conservative or surgical reduction of the coxofemoral joint in these situations is uniformly unsuccessful, and treatment is generally restricted to an FHO or THR.

Important postreduction considerations include monitoring the Ehmer sling (Figure 21-19) and underlying tissues for signs of skin irritation or excessive compression of the tissues, which may result in skin necrosis. Following removal of the Ehmer sling, muscle strengthening and reeducation may begin with walking on level surfaces or downhill if the joint is stable. Depending on the nature of the luxation, certain motions should be avoided. For example, external rotation of the hip should be avoided with a closed reduction of a craniodorsal luxation, and abduction should be avoided following reduction of a ventral luxation. Controlled walking exercises are useful, but aggressive exercises such as jogging or swimming are limited until 4 to 6 weeks after reduction.

Femoral Fractures

Proximal femoral fractures may occur through the capital femoral physis of immature dogs or across the femoral neck of skeletally mature dogs.[7] Rarely do fractures of the articular surface of the femoral head occur. The most serious of the fractures of the proximal femur is the capital femoral physeal fracture, especially in dogs less than 5 months of age (Figure 21-20). In this fracture, the physis closes prematurely, causing a short femoral neck and a small femoral head which result in an incongruent hip joint (Figure 21-21). In spite of anatomic reduction and internal fixation, many of these fractures result in OA because of this incongruity.

Fractures of the shaft of the femur are probably the most common fractures seen in veterinary practice. As such, they also have the highest incidence of complications, including delayed or nonunion fracture healing and osteomyelitis. Most complications are related

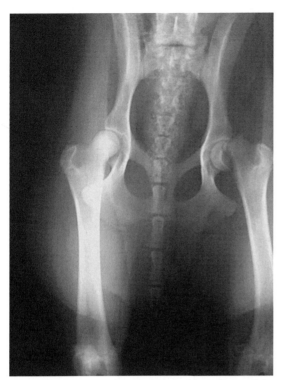

Figure 21-20   Capital femoral physeal fracture in a skeletally immature dog.

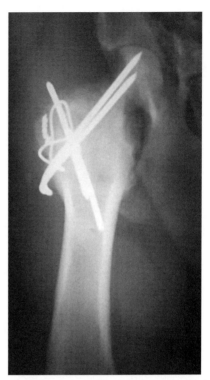

Figure 21-21   Incongruent hip joint in a puppy that has sustained a fracture of the proximal capital femoral physis. Although the fracture has reached clinical union, there is significant loss of bone in the femoral neck, and the femoral head is small in relation to the acetabulum because of differences in growth between the two components of the hip joint.

to inadequate fixation or errors in the application of the implants. The possible configurations of femoral fractures vary widely, from a two-piece spiral fracture to a highly comminuted fracture resulting from a gunshot injury. Most of the implants that are available for fracture repair in veterinary medicine may be used to stabilize fractures of the femur, including plates, screws (Figure 21-22), wires, pins, interlocking nails, and external skeletal fixators (Figure 21-22). External coaptation with splints or casts is contraindicated for stabilization of femur fractures, however, because they cannot be placed high enough to immobilize the joint above and below the fracture.

Based on the nature of the injury(ies) and fixation method(s) used, a specific postoperative rehabilitation program must be developed, considering the type of injury and repair. It is vital that the therapist understand the nature of the fracture and the type of repair that has been applied to know how much activity the dog should have, and what types of complications may occur. For example, if a puppy with a two-piece spiral fracture that has been stabilized with an intramedullary pin and cerclage wires has a sudden loss of limb use with knuckling on the dorsum of

the paw and severe pain, the therapist should realize that the pin may have migrated and entrapped the sciatic nerve. This patient must be treated immediately if there is hope of preventing permanent nerve damage.

In general, NSAIDs, cryotherapy, PROM, and controlled activities are initiated following surgery. More active forms of rehabilitation such as treadmill walking, leash walking, stairs, and swimming are added according to the nature of the injury, method used for fixation, stability of the repair, and temporal aspects of wound and fracture healing. The ROM achieved by the coxofemoral joint is affected by the severity of the fracture and the amount of periarticular fibrosis that occurs. Although most dogs will develop some degree of OA with acetabular fractures, most dogs will do reasonably well, although some will be candidates for total hip replacement THR or FHO. In addition, if concurrent neurological injuries are present, appropriate balancing, proprioceptive, and strengthening activities should be initiated.

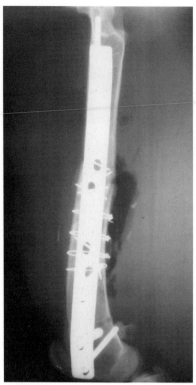

Figure 21-22   Repair of a comminuted fracture of the femur with a bone plate, screws, and cerclage wire.

Muscle Injuries

Tears of the tensor fasciae latae and gluteal muscles have been reported. These injuries most commonly appear in sprinting athletes and involve tears of the muscle sheath and fibers. In many cases, these injuries are treated conservatively with NSAIDs and cryotherapy. In addition, pulsed therapeutic ultrasound beginning within the first week after injury may be initiated for its nonthermal effects on tissue repair. Surgical repair, when undertaken, involves attempted repair of the muscle sheath and reapproximation of torn muscle fibers. This repair is followed by a period of immobilization for 3 weeks in a Spica splint. NSAIDs, PROM of joints neighboring the affected area, and cryotherapy are indicated. Following healing, continuous-mode therapeutic ultrasound in combination with stretching, and active exercises, such as swimming, may be introduced.

Stifle Conditions

The stifle is the joint most commonly afflicted with orthopedic conditions in the dog. The causes include trauma and degenerative, congenital, and developmental conditions.

Cranial Cruciate Ligament Rupture

Frank rupture or gradual loss of fiber integrity of the cranial cruciate ligament (CCL) is a common occurrence in dogs. While acute rupture may occur as a result of trauma, nearly all cases of cranial cruciate ligament rupture (CCLR) occur as a result of a slow degenerative process of the fibers of the ligament. Degenerative changes of the CCL are most commonly reported in medium- to large-breed dogs and in spayed females 4 to 8 years of age.[7,20] Loss of CCL support invariably leads to progressive OA (Figure 21-23).[21] In small dogs (less than 25 kg), conservative therapy may suffice, although surgical treatment is preferred to reduce the atrophic and degenerative changes that invariably occur with conservative treatment. In larger dogs, some form of stifle stabilization is nearly always advocated to prevent or minimize the progression of OA. To date, more than 50 different techniques have been devised to treat CCLR.[22] These techniques range from simple forms of extracapsular stabilization using wire, nylon bands, or suture material to sophisticated arthroscopic prosthetic ligament replacement. In addition to the stabilization procedure, it is important to debride loose and torn ligament remnants and to inspect and debride damaged portions of the menisci, especially the caudal horn of the medial meniscus, which is frequently damaged in dogs with CCLR. Arthroscopic debridement results in earlier use of limb and return to function as compared with an open arthrotomy.[23] In addition, there is less postoperative inflammation and swelling, and patients seem to experience less pain.

Several studies have indicated a positive benefit to various forms of postoperative physical rehabilitation for patients with CCLR.[24-26] In summary, rehabilitation has been documented to improve muscle mass and attenuate muscle atrophy that occurs following surgery, increase joint ROM, especially stifle extension, improve weight-bearing as measured by force plate analysis of gait, and reduce the progression of OA. To provide the therapist with a basic understanding of CCL surgery in dogs, an explanation of the most commonly performed procedures is beneficial.

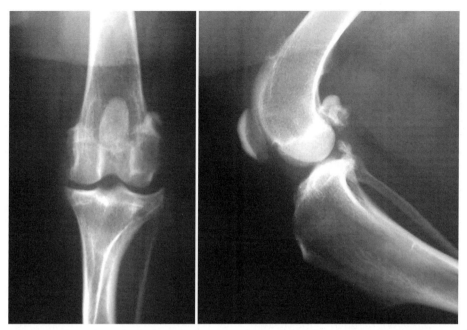

Figure 21-23 Secondary arthritic changes in the stifle as a result of rupture of the cranial cruciate ligament. Note the osteophytes along the trochlear ridges, subchondral sclerosis of bone, and the enthesiophytes on the fabellae.

EXTRACAPSULAR STABILIZATION

In this form of stabilization, nylon suture or stainless steel suture material is used to provide extracapsular (outside the joint capsule) support, mimicking the support provided by the intact CCL (Figure 21-24). Most commonly, the suture is passed around the lateral (and sometimes medial) fabella (sesamoid bone located in the origin of the gastrocnemius muscle) and through a tunnel drilled into the proximal tibial crest.[7] This procedure minimizes cranial drawer and provides immediate extracapsular stabilization of the stifle, allowing early rehabilitation to be initiated. At some point, the prosthetic material fatigues and breaks. However, the periarticular fibrosis that develops over 8 to 10 weeks provides the ultimate stabilizing factor for the stifle. Nevertheless, it is common for some degree of cranial drawer motion to be present weeks to months after surgery. Rehabilitation after surgery seems to reduce the amount of postoperative drawer motion and may result in a more stable joint.

Another form of extracapsular stabilization is the fibular head transposition. This procedure takes advantage of the fact that the lateral collateral ligament inserts on the fibular head. The fibular head is detached from its normal position and is displaced cranially and held in place with a pin and tension band. With this new position, the lateral collateral ligament

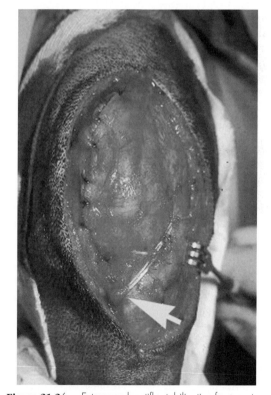

Figure 21-24 Extracapsular stifle stabilization for a rupture of the cranial cruciate ligament. The suture is passed around the lateral fabella and through a hole that has been drilled into the tibial crest *(arrow)*. (From Probst CW, Millis DL: Carpus and digits. In Slatter DH, editor: *Textbook of small animal surgery,* ed 3, Philadelphia, 2002, WB Saunders.)

essentially provides the same function as the CCL, namely limiting cranial drawer and internal rotation of the limb. Again, the repair provides immediate stability to the stifle joint, but over time, some drawer motion may return.

Physical rehabilitation starts the day of surgery with cryotherapy, NSAIDs, and gentle PROM (Appendix 4A). Controlled leash walks are started within 24 hours, and active use of the limb is encouraged. Treadmill walking may be useful to encourage weight-bearing, and aquatic therapy may be started approximately 1 week postoperatively if the incision is sealed and there is no gaping of the wound edges or drainage or discharge from the incision. PROM is continued with an emphasis on regaining preoperative levels of stifle joint extension by 10 days after surgery. Rear-limb strengthening can be facilitated by stair climbing, uphill walking, pulling a cart, or slow dancing. Jumping up on the hindlimbs is prevented for the first 10 to 12 weeks to prevent damage to the repair.

INTRACAPSULAR STABILIZATION METHODS

These procedures use fascial strips, a portion of the patellar ligament, or prosthetic materials placed in an intraarticular fashion via arthrotomy or arthroscopy to mimic the anatomic path of the original CCL and allow more normal stifle joint kinematics.[7] Most procedures using a graft leave one end of the graft attached to the tibial crest and have the free end of the tissue pass through the stifle joint, going caudally and proximally through the joint capsule; the tissue is then secured to the lateral femoral condyle. Other procedures have the free end of the graft pass under the intermeniscal ligament before traversing caudally and proximally through the joint (Figure 21-25). If the placement is not isometric, stretching and tearing of the implant may occur. In addition, biological tissues undergo a prolonged period of weakness until the tissue revascularizes and gains additional strength. This process may take months, and the tissue may not regain sufficient strength to function in the same fashion as a normal CCL. To combat this process, some surgeons also use an extracapsular fabella-tibial suture to augment the repair and reduce the stress on the graft. To date, prosthetic material used in veterinary medicine has been unsuccessful in providing permanent stability to the stifle. Invariably, the material degenerates, often resulting in chronic intraarticular inflammation.

Postoperative physical rehabilitation includes reducing pain and the inflammatory

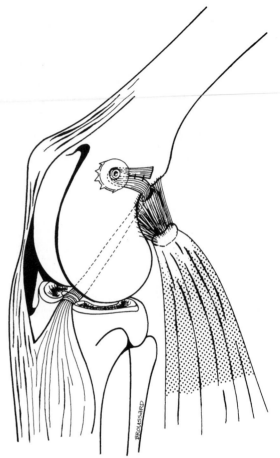

Figure 21-25   Under and over technique in which a strip of fascia latae is passed under the intermeniscal ligament, through the stifle joint, and over the top of the lateral femoral condyle, where it is secured with a screw and washer. (From Hulse DA, Shires PK: The stifle joint. Carpus and digits. In Slatter DH, editor: *Textbook of small animal surgery*, Philadelphia, 1985, WB Saunders.)

response through the use of NSAIDs and cryotherapy. Depending on the material used, the rehabilitation efforts must follow changes in tissue strength. For example, in cases with an autograft or allograft of fascia, rehabilitation efforts must conform to changes in the strength of the implant over a period of time. In particular, autografts and allografts are generally strong when initially put in place, but when put under tension, they stretch. Also, the tissue becomes much weaker over the next 2 to 20 weeks while revascularization and incorporation occur. If graft incorporation is augmented with an extracapsular suture, a rehabilitation program similar to that for extracapsular repair may be initiated, although attention to controlling inflammation is particularly important to prevent a hostile environment for the graft. Ultimate tissue

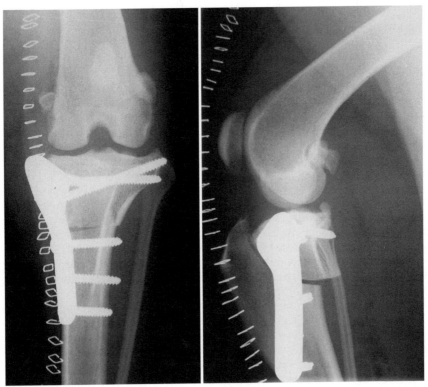

Figure 21-26 A dog with a cranial cruciate ligament injury has had the stifle stabilized with a tibial plateau leveling osteotomy.

strength is only achieved following bio-integration of the graft.

TIBIAL PLATEAU LEVELING OSTEOTOMY
(TPLO)

This is a relatively new procedure that has a completely different concept for providing stability to the stifle joint. The main concept behind the previously described procedures is to limit cranial drawer motion by physically restraining the tibia from shifting cranially in relation to the femur during weight-bearing or non–weight-bearing activities. The TPLO is based on the principle that cranial drawer motion during weight-bearing is prevented using a combination of altered biomechanical forces and active muscle contraction acting on the stifle during weight-bearing to stabilize the joint.[27]

The principles of this procedure are most easily understood if one considers that in the normal stifle, the weight-bearing surface of the tibial plateau slopes caudally. With CCLR, the femoral condyle is not restrained by the CCL and the femoral condyles roll down this slope during weight-bearing, resulting in a net cranial displacement of the tibia in relation to the femur. This overall concept is sim-ilar to performing a cranial tibial thrust maneuver, in which forces and muscle tension acting on the stifle result in cranial displacement of the tibia in the CCL-deficient stifle. With the TPLO, an osteotomy of the proximal tibia is performed, allowing the tibial plateau to be rotated to a nearly level position. The osteotomy is then stabilized using screws and a specially designed bone plate (Figure 21-26). This reduces the shear forces acting at the articular surfaces of the femur and tibia, resulting in more compressive forces and eliminating the cranial tibial thrust during weight-bearing. The periarticular muscles provide additional stability to the stifle during weight-bearing.

The postoperative complications associated with this procedure are primarily related to the altered biomechanics of the stifle. In particular, patellar ligament desmitis is very common during the first month. Clinically, patients may demonstrate more lameness during the postoperative period than is normally expected, the patellar ligament is wider, and there is pain on palpation of the ligament, especially at its insertion to the tibial crest. Also associated with the altered biomechanical stresses placed on the joint is the occurrence of avulsion of a portion of the tibial crest in some patients. Postoperative rehabilitation protocols must consider these possible complications, and the therapist must be diligent in monitoring these areas and altering the treatment protocol if they occur. Fortunately, the vast majority of the patients with these complications may be managed with enforced rest, NSAIDs, and cryotherapy. The problems are usually self-limiting as tissue remodeling and healing progress. Early detection and treatment of complications should result in an earlier return to function and an improved outcome as compared with allowing the conditions to progress to the point of clinical lameness and pain. Preventive strategies, centered on preventing excessive stresses of the patellar ligament on the tibial crest, may be useful in the early postoperative period. Specifically, preventing excessive flexion of the stifle while weight-bearing should reduce the tensile forces at the ligament insertion point. Preventing jumping, running, stair climbing, and walking while crouching should help to keep the quadriceps muscle-patellar ligament unit in a relatively shortened position, reducing the tensile forces on the tibial crest and patellar ligament. In some situations, using a hinged knee brace to limit flexion of the stifle may be beneficial. If patellar ligament desmitis occurs despite these preventive measures, treatment in the form of severely restricting exercise, cryotherapy, and NSAIDs should help to resolve the problem before it becomes more serious. A more gradual increase in activity level should be instituted after the tissues have healed adequately to resume activity.

Cryotherapy, NSAIDs, and PROM exercises, along with limited activity in the form of progressively longer leash walks, are provided in the initial postoperative period (Appendix 4B). As healing of the osteotomy site progresses, a gradually increasing protocol of limb use is prescribed. It is important to realize that in addition to healing joint capsule and altering stresses on the cartilage and bone of the joint, the osteotomy must have adequate time to heal to prevent complications related to bone healing and implant failure. In this regard, aquatic therapy may be particularly useful to reduce weight-bearing stresses on structures.

Caudal Cruciate Ligament (CdCL) Injuries

Isolated tears of the caudal cruciate ligament (CdCL) are very rare. CdCL injuries occur most commonly with severe traumatic stifle injuries, either alone or in combination with damage to other stifle structures, or they may occur as a sequela of the TPLO procedure as a result of overrotation of the tibial plateau, which places additional stresses on the CdCL. In most dogs, surgical stabilization using an extracapsular technique is required. With extracapsular repair, the sutures are passed around or through the head of the fibula to the patella region in an effort to provide stability by mimicking the course and function of the CdCL.[7] As with CCL extracapsular repairs, ultimate stability is provided by the resultant periarticular fibrosis. Physical rehabilitation starts the day of surgery with cryotherapy, NSAIDs, and gentle PROM. Controlled leash walks are started within 24 hours, and active use of the limb is encouraged. Treadmill walking may be useful to encourage weight-bearing, and aquatic therapy may be started approximately 1 week postoperatively if the incision is sealed and there are no gaping wound edges or drainage from the incision. PROM is continued with an emphasis on regaining extension. Rear-limb strengthening may be facilitated by stair climbing, uphill walking, pulling a cart, or dancing.

Collateral Ligament Injuries

The most common collateral ligament injury of the stifle in dogs is disruption of the medial collateral ligament (MCL), usually in conjunction with CCLR and medial meniscal damage as a result of severe trauma. Collateral ligament injuries in the dog are most commonly treated with surgical repair. The repair may involve reapproximating the torn ligament with suture material if adequate ligament tissue is available, or the use of bone screws or tissue anchors, and prosthetic material to provide joint stability. Postoperatively many of the patients undergo a period of joint immobilization with a Robert Jones bandage or light cast; other practitioners advocate immediate postoperative ROM to prevent joint contracture, promote cartilage homeostasis, and stimulate scar formation along normal lines of stress, which results in a stronger scar. The ultimate decision of coaptation or immediate rehabilitation depends, in part, on other concurrent injuries to the stifle and the severity of those injuries. A reasonable approach is to provide coaptation for no more than 2 to 4 weeks, followed by initial rehabilitation. Following this period of protection, some joint stiffness is expected. Therefore the initial goal should be to reestablish ROM through passive and active ROM exercises and gentle stretching, which may be facilitated by therapeutic ultrasound. Encouraging weight-bearing activities through weight shifting, slow leash walks, and treadmill walking is beneficial. Aquatic therapy may also be initiated at this time. Appropriate challenges to the healing tissues help enhance the process of tissue remodeling and strengthening. Therapeutic exercises may progress so that some endurance and strengthening activities are performed beginning between 4 and 6 weeks, with progression to near full return to activities by 12 to 16 weeks.

Meniscal Injuries

Isolated meniscal injuries in the absence of CCLR are rare in dogs. Meniscal damage is nearly always related to partial or complete rupture of the CCL, and the caudal aspect of the medial meniscus is most commonly affected (Figure 21-27).[7] The reason that this region is preferentially damaged is related to the anatomic attachment of the medial meniscus to the proximal tibia. When the femur is displaced caudally in relation to the tibia during weight-bearing, the femoral condyle creates abnormal compressive and shearing forces on the meniscus, eventually causing gross damage to the tissue.

Approximately 50% of the patients that are presented with CCLR have concurrent medial meniscal damage. Meniscal damage is most commonly treated with either arthrotomy or arthroscopic debridement of the damaged portion. Cases with damage to the entire meniscus are treated with a complete meniscectomy, but whenever possible, it is preferable to remove only the damaged portion with a partial meniscectomy. It is also possible that, even if the meniscus is normal at the time of stifle stabilization for a CCLR, the medial meniscus will become damaged at some time in the future. In fact, this probably occurs more commonly than is reported, and it may explain why some dogs do well initially and then perform poorly several months to years after surgery. In these situations, if a clicking of the stifle is palpated or heard during joint manipulation or walking, joint exploration is recommended. Removal of the damaged meniscus often results in significant improvement. Of late, several reports have identified damage to the lateral meniscus in association with CCLR during careful arthroscopic examination.[28] Following partial meniscectomy and stifle stabilization, NSAIDs, cryotherapy, and controlled ROM are indicated followed by progressive leash walks starting the day after surgery.

Patella Luxation

Patella luxation is common in dogs and is often the result of femoropatella alignment discrepancies. Medial luxation of the patella is most common in both small and large breeds of dogs (Figure 21-28).[7,29] However, if a lateral patella luxation is diagnosed, it will most likely be a large-breed dog. Some breeds, such as Bassett hounds, may have a patella that luxates both laterally and medially, although luxation in one direction is usually more common. Torsional deformities and malalignment of the femur and tibia result in patella luxation. The severity of patella luxation is graded from I to IV, with I indicating a patella that can be luxated but remains reduced in most circumstances and IV indicating a patella that is luxated and cannot be reduced. Grades II and III fall between these two extremes. It is also interesting to note that dogs with chronic patella luxation may also be predisposed to developing a CCLR, which is a more serious problem to treat.

When gait abnormalities, lameness, or disuse of the affected limb result from the luxation, surgery is indicated. Depending on the severity of luxation and malalignment,

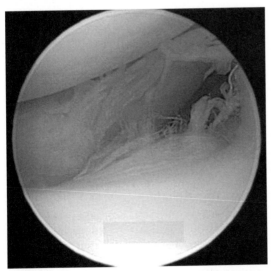

Figure 21-27 The caudal aspect of the medial meniscus is commonly damaged because of stifle instability as a result of cranial cruciate ligament rupture.

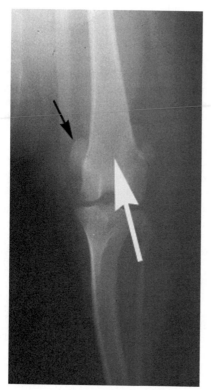

Figure 21-28 Medial luxation of the patella. The small *black arrow* indicates the patella. The *white arrow* shows the location where the patella should be.

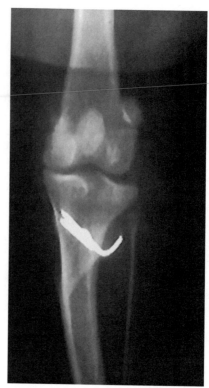

Figure 21-29 A transposition of the tibial crest has been performed to realign the quadriceps mechanism.

surgical procedures may include tibial crest transposition, capsular release, trochleoplasty, relocation of the rectus femoris muscle, transection of muscle tendons, corrective osteotomies, and other surgical procedures (Figure 21-29). Following surgical repair it is important to allow adequate tissue healing before vigorous physical rehabilitation begins. Short leash walks, cryotherapy, and NSAID therapy are used as needed for the first 3 weeks. Strengthening may be started after that, but exercises should be limited to sagittal-plane motion to avoid stress on the repair and possible recurrence of patella luxation.

Osteochondritis Dissecans

The pathophysiology and risk factors are the same for OCD of the distal femur as for those sites in the forelimb.[30] In the hindlimb, this condition generally involves the axial aspect of the lateral femoral condyle (Figure 21-30) and is usually treated through an arthrotomy or arthroscopically to remove the osteochondral fragment(s), and to curette, forage, or micropik the cartilage bed to create an opportunity for vascular ingrowth and fibrocarti-

lage formation. NSAIDs cryotherapy, gentle PROM, and leash walks are advocated for the first 2 to 4 weeks, depending on the severity of the lesion. After that, if the lameness is improving, leash walking is increased and more aggressive activities are added after 4 to 6 weeks.

Quadriceps Contracture or Fracture Disease of the Rear Limb

Quadriceps contracture, also sometimes called quadriceps tie down or fracture disease of the rear limb, is an unfortunate sequela to limb immobilization or limb disuse following treatment of a distal femoral physeal fracture in a puppy, typically a Salter-Harris type I or II configuration.[31] The fracture line is at the function of the bone and articular cartilage, in the region of the joint capsule. Delayed surgical treatment or poor attention to postoperative rehabilitation predispose patients to this condition. In some cases, the limb is inappropriately splinted or immobilized in extension as the primary treatment or following surgical stabilization. Splinting in extension for as little as 5 to 7 days may result in quadriceps contracture. The

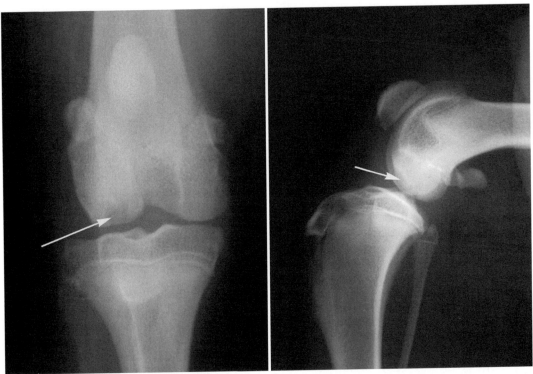

Figure 21-30 Osteochondritis dissecans of the medial aspect of the lateral femoral condyle. Note the large lucency, indicating the affected area.

combination of muscle trauma, rapid bone callus formation, joint capsule thickening and fibrosis, and immobilization cause joint stiffness, fibrosis of the quadriceps muscle to the underlying fracture callus, the loss of quadriceps muscle fibers, and loss of muscle function. As the collagen fibers organize and mature, contracture of the joint and loss of ROM develop. The end result is a stifle that remains in the extended position or one in which very limited flexion is possible. When seen in its late stages, this problem is also associated with atrophy of bone, disuse atrophy of the articular surfaces of the stifle, intraarticular fibrosis, and eventually fusion of the stifle joint.

This problem is best treated by preventing its occurrence (Appendix 4D). Stable fixation performed with minimally invasive techniques will result in less postoperative pain and early use of the limb. The most common repair technique is to use two pins placed in cross-pin fashion across the fracture site, paying attention to minimal dissection of tissues and gentle tissue handling. For any distal physeal fracture in a puppy or fracture of the distal femur in an adult dog, rehabilitation must begin the day of or the day after surgery. In some instances, the limb is bandaged in a flexed position to maintain the quadriceps muscle in a stretched position during the acute postoperative inflammatory phase. The sling should remain in place no longer than 72 hours, and if feasible, the bandage should be removed on a daily basis and PROM and stretching exercises performed.

It is also important to provide cryotherapy, NSAIDs, and massage for edema reduction to reduce swelling and pain as soon as possible. Patella mobilization and tissue mobilization techniques may be useful to help prevent fibrosis of the various tissue layers to one another. If the patient is not actively toe-touching by the third postoperative day, measures should be employed to encourage active contraction and relaxation of muscles and flexion and extension of the stifle. Slow leash walks with weight-shifting activities may be employed. Gentle tug-of-war may take the puppy's mind off of the injury and result in limb use, but caution is used to be certain that excessive force is not placed on the limb. If the puppy is leash trained, treadmill walking may cautiously be attempted. It is recommended that an attendant help support the patient and be immediately available in case of resistance on the part of the patient. A syringe cap placed under the contralateral rear foot is also useful to encourage limb use. Finally, swimming is useful to encourage active flexion and extension of the stifle joint, but the incision should be sealed with no drainage or discharge. If the process of quadriceps contracture has already begun or if rehabilitation is initiated too late, surgery may be performed to release tissues and relieve the contracture, but it is rarely successful if mature fibrosis of the tissues, intraarticular fibrosis, or permanent cartilage damage have occurred. If surgical release procedures are performed, excellent postoperative analgesia and early, diligent rehabilitation are essential to any type of successful outcome.

Articular Fractures of the Stifle

Fractures of the femoral condyles occur relatively rarely. Fractures of the patella may occur as a result of falling on the stifle on a hard surface, or as avulsion fractures of the quadriceps muscle. Physeal fractures of the proximal tibial physis sometimes occur. Salter-Harris type III and IV fractures are more serious because the fracture line involves the articular surface. As with any articular fracture anatomic reduction, rigid fixation with pins or screws (Figure 21-31) and early, gentle, diligent joint mobilization are necessary for success. Surgical fixation of articular fractures must be strong enough to withstand early PROM exercises. Rehabilitation of fractures of the stifle is similar to that of fractures of the elbow.

Avulsion of the Long Digital Extensor Tendon

This is a very rare injury that occurs in young dogs and results in a loose osseous body in the stifle joint. It is treated by surgical reattachment of the fragment to the femur. In chronic cases it may be impossible to reattach the fragment, necessitating removal of the fragment and reattachment of the extensor tendon to the proximal tibia. If the fragment is reattached, it is important to allow bony union to occur before aggressive rehabilitation is done. Initial efforts are aimed at resolving pain and inflammation, allowing limited weight-bearing, and muscle reeducation and proprioceptive training as the fracture heals.

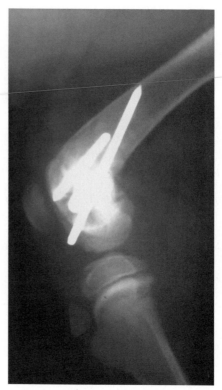

Figure 21-31   A Y fracture of the distal femur, in which the condyles have been fractured from the femoral shaft. Repair has been performed with a transcondylar screw and pins placed in a crosspin fashion.

With excision of the fragment and reattachment of the tendon, leash weight-bearing exercises are appropriate following recovery from surgery.

Rupture of the Patellar Ligament

Rupture of the patellar ligament rarely occurs, but is usually the result of direct trauma delivered to the stifle or is associated with forceful quadriceps contraction with concurrent forced flexion of the stifle. This condition is treated by repairing the patellar ligament. Because of the tension that exists across this repair, the repair must be protected. This is usually accomplished with a transarticular external fixator or splint for 2 to 3 weeks, followed by careful and protected remobilization. During the period of immobilization and immediately following, 3-MHz pulsed therapeutic ultrasound applied directly over the tendon is appropriate to help stimulate collagen production.

Crus Conditions

Avulsion of the Tibial Tuberosity

This condition most often occurs in immature dogs before fusion of the crest with the main shaft of the tibia. Avulsion results in proximal and cranial displacement of distal portion of the tibial crest, or of the entire crest. In addition, patella alta results and the dog is unable to fully extend the stifle. This fracture is best treated with a pin and tension band technique to reattach the bony fragment. Following surgery, cryotherapy, NSAIDs, and limited weight-bearing are initiated. Follow-up radiographs are made 3 to 4 weeks after surgery to monitor the progress of fracture healing and to guide the initiation of a more aggressive weight-bearing and muscle reeducation program.

Fractures of the Tibia and Fibula

Fractures of the tibia and fibula are common in the dog. Depending on the fracture type and configuration, they may be treated with closed reduction and external coaptation, or open reduction with internal or external fixation.[7] NSAIDs, cryotherapy, massage to help resolve edema, and PROM are used to decrease pain and inflammation and maintain ROM for the first 2 to 3 weeks. Active weight-bearing exercises are then initiated, with the rate and progression of increased activity dictated by the severity of the fracture and stability of repair. Because relatively little soft tissue covers the medial surface of the tibia, open fractures are quite common, and bandaging with care of open wounds is also necessary until the wound heals. Osteomyelitis tends to occur in the tibia more commonly than other bones and is probably related to the high incidence of open fractures. Of course, aquatic therapy is contraindicated in patients with open wounds and open fractures until wound healing is complete.

Fibrotic Myopathy

Fibrotic myopathy is a pathologic condition in which the muscle fibers are replaced with dense fibrous connective tissue, resulting in a fibrous band within the muscle. Lameness, which appears not to be painful, is the most common clinical sign. Clinical examination usually reveals some degree of lameness and decreased ROM in the hip and stifle joints. Fibrous band(s) may be palpated in the affected muscles, ranging from small longitudinal bands to large bands several centimeters in diameter. On gait evaluation, there is a characteristic external rotation of the hock and internal rotation of the stifle during the swing phase of gait. The most commonly affected muscles are the hamstring muscles (semimembranosus, semitendinosus, and biceps femoris) and the gracilis. Reports have indicated that there is bilateral involvement in 39% to 61% of cases, and the most commonly affected breed is the German shepherd. Muscle trauma has been suggested as one cause of fibrotic myopathy, especially the repetitive type of trauma that occurs in physically active dogs. There may also be a history of blunt trauma. Little has been written about the early detection of this type of muscle injury in German shepherds; however, the diagnosis and treatment of gracilis muscle injuries in the racing Greyhound have been discussed.[32] If the condition is diagnosed in the acute stage immediately after muscle injury, then intermittent rest and ice (15 minutes on, 15 minutes off) would seem appropriate. Later during recovery, stretching and strengthening programs may be initiated, being careful to avoid recurrence of muscle trauma and being vigilant with regular examination and assessment of the area. Incorporating basic physical rehabilitation principles such as proper warmup and cooldown might help to prevent recurrence of this condition.

Although surgical release of the fibrotic tissue either through tenotomy or excision of the fibrotic muscle usually yields temporary improvement of the lameness and ROM deficits, some degree of fibrosis almost always recurs within a few months. The key is to apply aggressive, long-term rehabilitation, especially during the period of wound maturation when fibrous tissue is strengthening and contracture is at its peak, usually between 3 and 6 weeks. It is essential that evaluation and assessment of the condition, including palpation of the area and joint flexion and extension measurements, be performed twice weekly to allow early detection and intervention of problems. The therapist should not be complacent if the early outcome appears successful and the condition seems static, because deleterious changes often do not occur until 1 or 2 months after surgery. If contracture begins to occur despite a good ROM, stretching, and therapeutic and aquatic exercise program, placing the limb in a device, such as a cast or sling, to allow chronic passive stretch with the tissues in an elongated position and some tension on the tissues for 8 to 12 hours per day, should help to prevent or delay the progress of contracture until the fibrous tissue matures in an elongated position. Long-term, diligent monitoring and aggressive intervention greatly improve the chances for a successful outcome in an otherwise difficult condition with traditionally poor outcomes.

Tarsal, Metatarsal, and Phalangeal Conditions

Fractures

Fractures of the distal fibula, tibia, or tarsal bones may occur as a result of trauma, athletic injury, or automobile accidents. Repair of medial or lateral fractures of the malleolus are important because these are the origins of the collateral ligaments. Metatarsal and phalangeal fractures usually occur as a result of trauma, and phalangeal fractures are often open fractures. Tarsal, metatarsal, and phalangeal fractures may be treated using closed reduction and immobilization in a coaptation device, or with a variety of implants, including intramedullary pins, wires, and plates and screws. A splint or light cast is usually applied to the limb for 2 to 3 weeks after internal fixation to protect the relatively small implants that must be used.

As is the case for all articular fractures, early ROM is important following open reduction, anatomic reduction, and rigid fixation with screws, pins, or small bone plates. If a cast or splint is used, stifle ROM must be preserved during the time of coaptation application, and after coaptation removal. If possible, removing the splint on a weekly basis to perform ROM exercises to maintain joint and tendon mobility is advised. The splint is reapplied to protect the fracture following ROM exercises. Following permanent removal of the splint or cast, remobilization of the joints is important, along with weight-bearing therapeutic exercises and muscle reconditioning. Sagittal-plane ROM exercises and joint mobilization work well to restore ROM to the area.

Luxations of the Tarsus, Metatarsus, and Phalanges

Luxations of the various levels of the tarsus may occur with severe damage to the tarsocrural collateral ligaments, the plantar intertarsal ligament, or the dorsal intertarsal ligaments.[7] Following primary repair of the ligaments or repair using a prosthetic collateral ligament technique, most injuries are immobilized for 3 weeks in a coaptation device and treated as above. It is especially important to avoid therapeutic exercises or ROM exercises that might place varus or valgus stresses on the healing site.

Similar to the analogous condition of the carpus, a relatively common injury is a shearing injury to the medial aspect of the tarsus, in which the dog's limb becomes trapped beneath a skidding automobile tire. The soft tissues, including skin, subcutaneous tissues, tendons, ligaments, and in severe cases, bone, are eroded away, leaving the joint unstable. If adequate articular cartilage remains, repair of the damaged ligaments with a prosthetic collateral ligament technique using screws and sutures can be a valuable treatment to maintain some joint function. For severe injuries with major destruction to the articular surfaces, pantarsal arthrodesis may be the only option to salvage a functional limb (Figure 21-32). Fortunately, function is generally very acceptable after bony fusion has occurred. Skin grafts are frequently required to provide

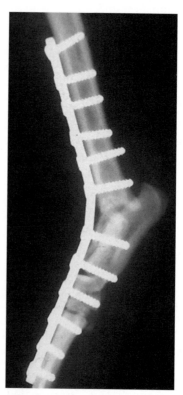

Figure 21-32 Pantarsal arthrodesis as a treatment for a severe shearing injury of the hock.

soft tissue coverage over the area, requiring excellent wound care while the graft is undergoing incorporation.

Metatarsophalangeal luxations and phalangeal luxations are reasonably common injuries that most often are treated with surgical repair of the collateral ligaments. Following repair of the ligament, a coaptation device is placed for 2 to 3 weeks to immobilize the area. During the period of immobilization it is helpful to remove the splint on a weekly basis and cycle the distal joints though their ROM. The splint is then reapplied. Following immobilization, the joints are reassessed for stability and if satisfactory, limited weight-bearing activities and ROM exercises are continued. A soft protective bandage may be applied to help support tissues and limit swelling.

Tendon Conditions

Rupture of the superficial digital flexor tendon retinaculum may occur during strenuous athletic activity, resulting in medial displacement of the superficial digital flexor tendon as it passes over the tuber calcis.[7] The clinical signs may be subtle and include a mild weight-bearing lameness. Careful palpation of the tuber calcis while the hock is flexed and extended is necessary to detect luxation of the superficial digital flexor tendon. Return of the ligament to its normal position and surgical repair of the torn retinaculum are necessary to correct this condition. The repair is protected with a coaptation device for 2 to 3 weeks to immobilize the healing tissues. Following removal of the splint, the joints are remobilized, and ROM and weight-bearing exercises are begun. It is especially beneficial to apply gentle tissue mobilization techniques to the area to prevent fibrosis and tie-down of the tendons to each other, which might limit motion of the digits.

Injuries to the common calcanean (Achilles) tendon can be catastrophic. These injuries may result from chronic repetitive use or sharp penetrating trauma. Chronic degeneration of both common calcanean tendons is relatively common in Doberman Pinschers. In veterinary medicine, rupture of the Achilles tendon is treated surgically. In some cases, primary repair by suturing the ligament is possible. The hock joint is immobilized in relative extension to prevent tension on the healing tendon. A splint or transarticular external fixator is placed for 3 weeks. In some large

dogs, a screw is placed from the calcaneus to the distal tibia to provide additional stability to the coaptation device (Figure 21-33). If the hole in the calcaneus is overdrilled at the time of surgery, the screw is able to glide easily back and forth in the calcaneus without restriction. The screw acts as a safety stop following removal of the coaptation device, allowing the dog to extend the hock (because the screw is able to glide in the hole), but preventing flexion beyond the point at which the screw head contacts the surface of the calcaneus. During the time of immobilization, pulsed 3-MHz therapeutic ultrasound may be used to stimulate collagen repair. Ultrasound or hot packs may also be used following removal of the fixation device to warm the tissues before stretching and to help with tissue healing.[33] Regaining adequate tendon strength and flexion ROM may take several months to a year. It is important to avoid explosive movements that place large extension forces on the hock, which damages the repair. Examples of activities to avoid include jumping up on the rear limbs and bounding up stairs or onto furniture.

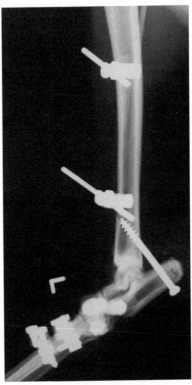

Figure 21-33 A screw placed from the calcaneus to the distal tibia and a transarticular external fixator help to stabilize a repaired common calcanean tendon.

General Physical Rehabilitation Management of Joint Arthrodesis

Surgical fusion of joints is considered a salvage procedure to improve function of a limb as a result of a severe joint condition. The more distal the fusion, the better the expected function of the limb and prognosis. Bone grafting in combination with pins, wires, plates, and screws is performed to fuse the joint in a functional position. Having the dog in a standing position with all four limbs squarely and symmetrically placed under the body while examining the contralateral joint is the best method to determine the optimal angle of fusion. In general, the shoulder is fused at approximately 105 to 110 degrees, the elbow at 110 degrees, and the carpus 105 to 110 degrees. In the rear limb, the hip is never fused; the stifle is fused at approximately 135 degrees, and the tarsus at 120 to 135 degrees.

Immediately postoperatively, a pressure bandage is applied to help limit edema and swelling of the distal limb and digits, which can be quite profound. Pretreating with an injection of dexamethasone before surgery and placement of a wrap immediately following surgery are important strategies to help limit swelling. Massage may also be helpful in the first few days, along with cryotherapy and NSAID administration. When the edema begins to resolve between 3 and 5 days, a cast is placed to help augment stability during early bone healing. In the first few weeks, PROM to the joints above and below the affected area is performed along with wound care. Gait training, starting with assisted standing and progressing to treadmill walking, should be performed to restore as normal a gait pattern as possible. Muscle strengthening exercises are prescribed if atrophy is present.

General Physical Rehabilitation Management of Amputation

In general, dogs do well after amputation, whether it is a forelimb or hindlimb. Given the fact that dogs bear 60% of their weight on their forelimbs, a forelimb amputation subjects the remaining forelimb to greater forces. Therefore weight reduction is an important part of treatment if the dog is overweight. It is also important to examine the other limbs and

joints before amputation for conditions such as elbow and hip dysplasia to be certain that they will be able to accommodate the additional loads placed on the remaining limbs. In general, most dogs are already bearing weight on just three limbs as a result of their injury or condition in the affected limb, but it may be useful to place the proposed amputated limb in a sling for several hours to assess how the dog will do postoperatively, and to begin some rehabilitation training. Most forelimb and hindlimb amputations are the result of cancer such as osteosarcoma, or trauma such as brachial plexus or sciatic nerve injuries.

Many postamputation patients may be assisted to a standing position the day of surgery. It is important to use some type of supportive sling to accomplish this. Care must also be given to the surgical wound site. Patients must regain their sense of balance with a new center of gravity, regain proprioception, and relearn many tasks. Physical rehabilitation begins with standing, progressing to walking and more challenging activities such as varied terrains, therapeutic balls, and the use of devices such as balance boards. As the dog undergoes rehabilitation activities, muscle soreness caused by overuse may require treatment such as heat, cryotherapy, and massage.

REFERENCES

1. Stobie D et al: Chronic bicipital tenosynovitis in dogs: 29 cases (1985-1992), *J Am Vet Med Assoc* 207:201-207, 1995.
2. Wall CR, Taylor R: Arthroscopic biceps brachii tenotomy as a treatment for canine bicipital tenosynovitis, *J Am Anim Hosp Assoc* 38:169-175, 2002.
3. Flo GL, Middleton D: Mineralization of the supraspinatus tendon in dogs, *J Am Vet Med Assoc* 197:95-97, 1990.
4. Puglisi TA: Canine humeral Joint instability. I. *Compend Contin Educ Pract Vet* 8:593-601, 1986.
5. Whitehair JG, Rudd RG: Osteochondritis dissecans of the humeral head in dogs, *Compend Contin Educ Pract Vet* 12:195-204, 1990.
6. Rudd RG, Whitehair JG, Margolis JH: Results of management of osteochondritis dissecans of the humeral head in dogs: 44 cases (1982 to 1987), *J Am Anim Hosp Assoc* 26:173-178, 1990.
7. Piermattei DL, Flo GL: *Brinker, Piermattei, and Flo's handbook of small animal orthopedics and fracture repair,* ed 3, Philadelphia, 1997, WB Saunders.
8. Padgett GA et al: The inheritance of osteochondritis dissecans and fragmented coronoid process of the elbow joint in Labrador retrievers, *J Am Anim Hosp Assoc* 31:327-330, 1995.
9. Read RA et al: Fragmentation of the medial coronoid process of the ulna in dogs: a study of 109 cases, *J Small Anim Pract* 31:330-334, 1990.

10. Lewis DD, McCarthy RJ, Pechman RD: Diagnosis of common developmental orthopedic conditions in canine pediatric patients, *Compend Contin Educ Pract Vet* 14:287-301, 1992.

11. Rorvik AM: Risk factors for humeral condylar fractures in the dog: a retrospective study, *J Small Anim Pract* 34:277-282, 1993.

12. Macias C, Marcellin-Little DJ: Incomplete humeral condylar fractures in the dog, *J Small Anim Pract* 43:93, 2002.

13. Muir P: Distal antebrachial fractures in toy-breed dogs, *Compend Contin Educ Pract Vet* 19:137-145, 1997.

14. Probst CW, Millis DL: Carpus and digits. In Slatter DH, editor: *Textbook of small animal surgery,* ed 3, Philadelphia, 2002, WB Saunders.

15. Kealy RD et al: Five-year longitudinal study on limited food consumption and development of osteoarthritis in coxofemoral joints of dogs, *J Am Vet Med Assoc* 210:222-225, 1997.

16. Lust G, Williams AJ, Wurster-Burton N, et al: Joint laxity and its association with hip dysplasia in Labrador retrievers, *Am J Vet Res* 54:1990-1999, 1993.

17. Lust G: An overview of the pathogenesis of canine hip dysplasia, *J Am Vet Med Assoc* 210:1443-1445, 1997.

18. Cook JL, Tomlinson JL, Constantinescu GM: Pathophysiology, diagnosis, and treatment of canine hip dysplasia, *Compend Contin Educ Pract Vet* 18:853-867, 1996.

19. Smith GK et al: Evaluation of risk factors for degenerative joint disease associated with hip dysplasia in German shepherd dogs, golden retrievers, Labrador retrievers, and Rottweilers, *J Am Vet Med Assoc* 219:1719-1724, 2001.

20. Moore KW, Read RA: Rupture of the cranial cruciate ligament in dogs. I. *Compend Contin Educ Pract Vet* 18:223-234, 1996.

21. Visco DM et al: Experimental osteoarthritis in dogs: a comparison of the Pond-Nuki and medial arthrotomy methods, *Osteoarthr Cart* 4:9-22, 1996.

22. Moore KW, Read RA: Rupture of the cranial cruciate ligament in dogs. II. Diagnosis and management, *Compend Contin Educ Pract Vet* 18:381-391, 405, 1996.

23. Hoelzler MG, Millis DL, Francis DA: Outcome assessment following arthroscopic and arthrotomy techniques for extracapsular stifle stabilization in dogs, *Vet Surg* 31:502, 2002.

24. Johnson JM et al: Rehabilitation of dogs with surgically treated cranial cruciate ligament–deficient stifles by use of electrical stimulation of muscles, *Am J Vet Res* 58:1473-1478, 1997.

25. Millis DL et al: A preliminary study of early physical therapy following surgery for cranial cruciate ligament rupture in dogs, *Vet Surg* 26:434, 1997.

26. Marsolais GS, Dvorak G, Conzemius MG: Effects of postoperative rehabilitation on limb function after cranial cruciate ligament repair in dogs, *J Am Vet Med Assoc* 220:1325-1330, 2002.

27. Slocum B, Devine T: Cranial tibial wedge osteotomy: a technique for eliminating cranial tibial thrust in cranial cruciate ligament repair, *J Am Vet Med Assoc* 184:564-569, 1984.

28. Ralphs SC, Whitney WO: Arthroscopic evaluation of menisci in dogs with cranial cruciate ligament injuries: 100 cases (1999-2000), *J Am Vet Med Assoc* 221:1601-1604, 2002.

29. Tomlinson J, Constantinescu GM: Repair of medial patella luxation, *Vet Med* 89:48-56, 1994.

30. Montgomery RD, Milton JL, Henderson RA: Osteochondritis dissecans of the canine stifle, *Compend Contin Educ Pract Vet* 11:1199-1208, 1989.

31. Bardet JF: Quadriceps contracture and fracture disease, *Vet Clin North Am Small Anim Pract* 17:957-973, 1987.

32. Blythe LL, Gannon JR, Craig AM: *Care of the racing greyhound: a guide for trainers, breeders and veterinarians,* ed 1, Portland, Ore, 1994, American Greyhound Council.

33. Saini NS et al: A preliminary study on the effect of ultrasound therapy on the healing of surgically severed Achilles tendons in five dogs, *J Vet Med A Physiol Pathol Clin Med* 49:321-328, 2002.

Neurologic Conditions and Physical Rehabilitation of the Neurologic Patient

Paul Shealy, William B. Thomas, and Loretta Immel

Intervertebral Disk Disease

Protrusion or extrusion of an intervertebral disk is a common cause of pain and weakness in dogs.[1,2] Although a normal disk can extrude as a consequence of major trauma, most disk extrusions and protrusions are secondary to underlying degeneration of the disk. There are two types of disk degeneration. Chondroid degeneration is most common in chondrodystrophic breeds (Dachshund, Pekingese, French bulldog, Cocker Spaniel) and is characterized by a decrease in water and glycosaminoglycan content in the disk, often culminating in calcification of the disk. This process starts as early as 2 months of age in affected breeds. This type of degeneration predisposes to sudden extrusion of a large volume of the nucleus pulposus through a complete tear of the annulus fibrosis (type I extrusion).

Fibroid degeneration is the second type of disk degeneration and is characterized by replacement of the disk with fibrous tissue. This is most common in older, large-breed dogs and predisposes to slowly progressive protrusion of the annulus fibrosis without a complete tear (type II protrusion). The clinical signs are typically less severe with a slower onset compared to type I extrusions.

Cervical Disk Disease

Cervical disk disease commonly affects small, middle-age to older chondrodystrophic breeds and is usually classified as a type I extrusion. Beagles, Dachshunds, Pekingese, and Poodles tend to be overrepresented. The C2-C3 disk space is most commonly affected, with the frequency decreasing at progressively more caudal disk spaces. Cervical disk disease in large-breed dogs is usually associated with type II protrusion of the caudal disks and is often secondary to cervical spondylomyelopathy. Breeds commonly affected are Doberman pinschers and Great Danes.

Neck pain is the most common and often the only sign of cervical disk disease. This is manifested as low head carriage, stiffness or decreased motion of the neck, vocalizing, and spasms of the neck muscles. Some dogs exhibit lameness of one or both thoracic limbs, due to nerve root or spinal nerve compression (root signature). In severe cases, there may be ataxia, conscious proprioceptive deficits, weakness, or rarely, paralysis of all limbs. Spinal reflexes are usually normal to exaggerated, although reflexes may be weak or absent in the thoracic limbs with caudal cervical disk extrusions. Other causes of neck pain include trauma, neoplasia, meningitis, discospondylitis, cervical spondylomyelopathy, and atlantoaxial instability.

Diagnosis is based on the clinical features, neurological examination, spinal radiography, myelography, and advanced imaging techniques, including computed tomography (CT) and magnetic resonance imaging (MRI).[3] Cerebrospinal fluid (CSF) analysis is helpful in identifying or ruling out meningitis.

Treatment options include surgery and nonsurgical therapy, with the decision based on the duration and severity of clinical signs. The cervical spinal canal is relatively spacious and can accommodate a bulging disk and small amounts of herniated disk material without accompanying neurological deficits. Nonsurgical therapy is indicated as the initial treatment in patients with no or mild neurologic deficits. The most important aspect of treatment is strict cage confinement to minimize stress on the damaged disk to allow the disk time to heal. A short course of antiinflammatory doses of corticosteroids or nonsteroidal antiinflammatory drugs is administered if necessary for pain control. Muscle relaxants may be beneficial to some patients with spasm of the cervical muscles. Analgesic drugs without cage confinement are contraindicated, because they may lead to increased patient activity and risk further disk extrusion. If the patient does well, cage confinement is continued for at least 2 to 3 weeks. About 65% of dogs with neck pain due to disk disease will recover with nonsurgical therapy. Recurrence of signs occurs in about one third of patients.

Surgery is indicated for patients with substantial neurologic deficits, neck pain unresponsive to appropriate nonsurgical therapy, or recurrent bouts of neck pain. Removal of extruded disk material by a ventral slot to decompress the spinal cord and nerve roots is the procedure of choice in most patients. Dorsal hemilaminectomy may be necessary for lateral or far-lateral extrusions. In chondrodystrophic dogs, prophylactic fenestration of the other disk spaces at the time of ventral slot is indicated to decrease the risk of extrusion of another disk. Fenestration alone of the affected disk is not indicated because it does not allow removal of extruded disk material. In dogs with neck pain and mild neurologic deficits, the success rate with surgery is about 95%.[1,2] Preoperative, intraoperative, and postoperative management may include drugs described for medical management. Postoperative physical rehabilitation is an integral part of the overall care of the patient.

Physical Rehabilitation for Cervical Disk Disease

Physical rehabilitation as part of medical management includes massage, heat therapy, and electrical stimulation (ES) and therapeutic ultrasound (US) for muscle spasms and pain relief. Whirlpool therapy may also be cautiously used in patients carefully supported in a sling (Figure 22-1).

Postoperative therapy is staged and begins immediately or within 48 hours of surgery to relieve pain and muscle spasms. Modalities such as cryotherapy, ES, carefully administered US, and massage may be used based on the clinical needs of the patient. In ambulatory patients, neck leashes are not advised, and

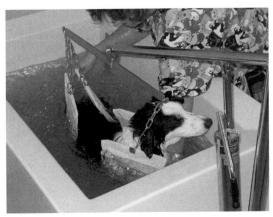

Figure 22-1 Whirlpool with hydraulic hoist and sling.

leashes should be attached to a harness or across the chest and under one forelimb.

Methods of actively eliciting cervical motion may begin in the first few days after comfort is achieved. Active range of motion can be achieved using toys or treats to motivate the patient to turn the head and neck in all directions. Begin with smaller movements and progress to the point that the patient is able to take a toy or treat from near the rear limbs for lateral excursion, between the forelimbs for cervical flexion, and high above the head for extension. Pain-free passive range of motion and stretching are used to help treat muscle spasms.

Resistive exercises can be used in tetraparetic and hemiparetic patients. Pushing on the bottom of the foot of an extended extremity stimulates muscles, tendons, ligaments, joints, and bones of the limb. While maintaining limb extension and force on the foot, move the limb slightly in all directions. Careful use of a sling and hoist may be useful in larger nonambulatory patients.

Assistance should be provided to patients that are able to stand and support weight to attain correct limb placement. Necessary support through the chest is provided as needed to invoke as much independent weight-bearing as possible. Patients are assisted in slow ambulation by placing and moving any limbs with motor deficits. Assisted walking (tail, sling), proprioception stimulation, and limb placement exercises facilitate neuromuscular reeducation and proprioceptive functioning, as well as muscle strengthening.

To help achieve strengthening, swimming may be initiated after the incision site is healed. The time of suture removal is generally a safe time to initiate hydrotherapy. Some therapists may initiate some form of aquatic

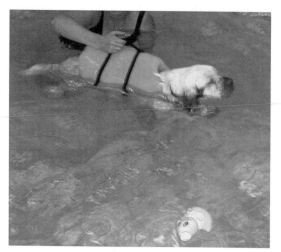

Figure 22-2   Life preserver used for flotation.

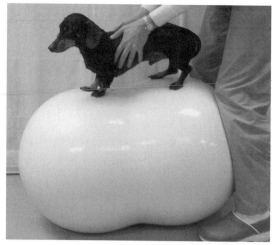

Figure 22-3   Therapy roll used for improving conscious proprioception.

therapy earlier, with caution to avoid submersion of the incision. In any case, the incision should be sealed, with apposed edges, no discharge or drainage, and no separation of the incision with gentle manipulation of the edges. In small dogs, a whirlpool may be used for aquatic therapy. The duration of swimming depends on the fitness, endurance, and ability of each patient. Assistance or life preservers are provided as required (Figure 22-2). If the patient does not actively move its limbs through an adequate range of motion, assistance is given either by passively moving the limb(s) or by providing resistance to motion to stimulate the patient to engage the limb against the applied resistance.

Patients can be placed on exercise rolls to strengthen proprioception and joint stability. They may be further challenged with mild bouncing and slight movements of the ball to create an unstable surface (Figure 22-3). Requiring patients to walk on foam, bubble wrap, or an inflatable object or challenging them with a rocker board (Figure 22-4) will also help them to develop stability and proprioception. To assist in regaining kinesthetic awareness, patients can be challenged to step over objects of varying shape and size (Figure 22-5). Small objects are initially used; the height and width are increased as the patient progresses. Strengthening the forelimbs can be achieved by ambulating on land, a dry treadmill (Figure 22-6), and deep water and underwater treadmill hydrotherapy. Additional strengthening exercises include walking down inclines with variable pitch, wheelbarrowing (Figure 22-7), and increased weight-bearing with an exercise roll beneath the hindlimbs (Figure 22-8).

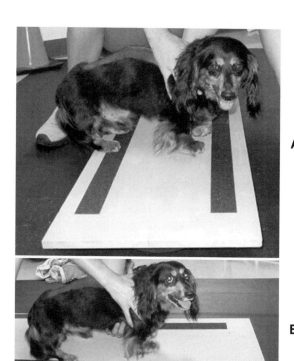

A

B

Figure 22-4   Rocker boards for rehabilitation. **A,** Side-to-side motion. **B,** Forward and backward motion.

Therapeutic modalities are provided for a minimum of 3 weeks. Owners are instructed further in performing strengthening exercises after discharge. Continued rehabilitation modalities are often prescribed after discharge on a recommended weekly schedule.

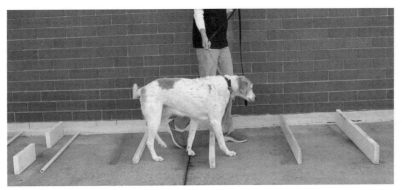

Figure 22-5   Various sized rails used as obstacles.

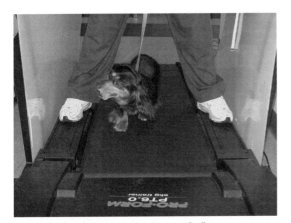

Figure 22-6   Dry treadmill.

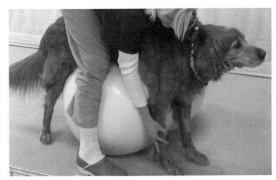

Figure 22-8   Facilitating patient standing using a therapy roll.

Thoracolumbar Disk Disease

Disk disease most commonly occurs near the thoracolumbar region (T12-T13 to L1-L2 are the most commonly afflicted sites, although other areas may also be affected) and primarily affects young adult to middle-aged chondro-dystrophic breeds. Dachshunds seem to be overrepresented, but Poodles, Cocker Spaniels, Beagles, Pugs, and Basset hounds are other breeds commonly afflicted with this condition. Type I extrusions are most common in these breeds. Type II protrusions are more common in large, nonchondrodystrophic dogs, but large dogs can also suffer acute, type I extrusions.

Onset of signs can be sudden or gradual and depend on the force, quantity, and location of the disk material, and the duration of disk herniation. About 10% of affected dogs have back pain with no neurologic deficits. They are often reluctant to run, jump, or climb stairs and may have kyphosis. Neurologic deficits range from ambulation with mild ataxia of the pelvic limbs to complete paralysis

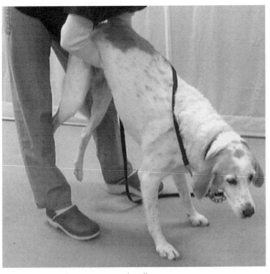

Figure 22-7   Wheelbarrow exercises.

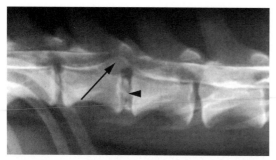

Figure 22-9   Intervertebral disk extrusion. Myelography showing compression of the spinal cord *(arrow)* caused by extrusion of the L2-L3 disk. There is still some calcified disk material in the disk space *(arrowhead)*.

of the pelvic limbs with urinary and fecal incontinence and absent deep-pain perception. The neurologic deficits may be symmetric or worse on one side. Spinal reflexes are usually normal to exaggerated, but are weak to absent if the extrusion occurs caudal to L2-L3. In severe or prolonged compression, progressive ascending-descending myelomalacia of the spinal cord may result. This is a rare, serious condition that the therapist should be aware of if deterioration of the patient is noted. Other diagnostic considerations include trauma, fibrocartilaginous embolism, degenerative myelopathy, discospondylitis, degenerative lumbosacral stenosis, neoplasia, meningitis, and orthopedic conditions such as severe hip dysplasia or bilateral cranial cruciate ligament insufficiency.

Diagnosis is based on clinical features and neurological examination, spinal radiography, myelography, and CT or MRI (Figure 22-9). Myelography is generally satisfactory in small chondrodystrophic breeds; however, advanced imaging may be necessary to assess whether multiple disk spaces are involved, to evaluate a wide area of contrast attenuation, to rule out coexisting discospondylitis, or to evaluate suspicious areas of the spinal cord for neoplasia. Advanced imaging may be especially useful to confirm the diagnosis in large, nonchondrodystrophic breeds.

About 85% of dogs with back pain and no neurologic deficits will improve with nonsurgical therapy, as described for cervical disk disease.[1,2] Surgery is indicated in patients with substantial neurologic deficits, or back pain refractory to nonsurgical therapy. Patients with a sudden onset of severe neurologic deficits need urgent surgery. Removal of extruded disk material via hemilaminectomy is the procedure of choice in most cases. A dor-

sal laminectomy is also sometimes used for decompression. Fenestration of the affected intervertebral disk space is routinely performed. Some surgeons and neurologists believe that prophylactic fenestration of other thoracolumbar disk spaces may reduce recurrence. Prognosis depends in large part on the severity and duration of the neurologic deficits. About 95% of dogs that are still walking before surgery have a good outcome.[1,2] The recovery rate is about 80% in dogs with complete paralysis and intact deep pain perception.[1,2] In dogs with loss of deep pain perception, the recovery rate is about 50% if surgery is performed within 48 hours of loss of pain perception. The prognosis is worse if surgery is delayed beyond 48 hours.

Physical Rehabilitation for Thoracolumbar Disk Disease

Although physical rehabilitation has been used with pharmacological intervention in the conservative management of acute and recurrent thoracolumbar disk disease with some success, the major application of therapeutic modalities is in the postoperative period. The initiation of therapy and protocols used are similar to those used for cervical disk patients, but the focus is on the rear limbs. Patients with thoracolumbar disk disease are more likely to have proprioceptive and motor deficits, requiring greater attention to balancing and strengthening activities. Additional nursing care is required more often in postoperative thoracolumbar disk patients, such as bladder management, extending the skills of the veterinary therapist and dictating close interaction between the therapist and veterinarian.

Therapeutic modalities and exercises prescribed depend on the stage of the postoperative period and the neurological status of the patient. Control of pain and swelling and the beginning of exercise are the focus of the initial postoperative period. Swelling of the surgical site is addressed with cryotherapy. ES is applied for pain relief using interferential or premodulated interferential waveforms. Therapeutic US must be used with care over the thoracic and lumbar epaxial musculature to avoid generating excess heat over the laminectomy site and possibly damaging nerves and the spinal cord.

Depending on the neurological deficits, the patient may be unable to sit, stand, ambulate, or urinate independently. Appropriate supportive care, including bladder management, must be carefully performed, and there must be close communication between the therapist and veterinarian. Occasionally, patients will have significant hyperesthesia along the thoracolumbar areas. In these cases, light massage and desensitization procedures may be useful. Patients with significant paraparesis or paraplegia may benefit from therapeutic exercises designed to help gain trunk control. One exercise is to assist patients to a sitting position with decreasing amounts of support until they are able to sit independently. After this is achieved, balance can be challenged using perturbation exercises on firm surfaces initially, and then progressing to unstable surfaces such as an exercise roll, foam mats, bubble wrap, or pillows. Russian or biphasic ES to the muscles of the hindlimbs may be used to induce stifle and hock extension and flexion, as tolerated by the patient.

Standing exercises may begin as soon as treatment is initiated. Appropriate support is provided while placing the patient in a standing posture to ensure some loading of the hindlimbs and correct positioning of the feet. After the patient is able to maintain a standing position, pressure is applied to the hindlimbs by pressing on the dorsal aspect of the pelvis. This joint approximation fosters continued extension of the limbs by the proprioceptive neuromuscular facilitation theory and allows the patient to remain in the standing position for a longer period of time. This can be performed on a firm surface or with the patient standing on an exercise roll. Gentle perturbations are applied from all angles while the patient is standing so that it is challenged to maintain stability and a standing position. Early ambulation may be assisted by moving the hindlimbs in a reciprocal walking pattern.

Ambulation is allowed at controlled paces in patients with motor control. Assisted tail walking, sling or towel walking, and underwater treadmill hydrotherapy may be used to unload weight before attaining complete ambulatory independence. Strengthening exercises are initiated as independent ambulation improves (Figures 22-10 to 22-14). Activities include ascending and descending inclines, walking in circles or figure-eights, walking on terrain with varying textures, stepping over objects of varying size to regain proprioceptive awareness, and practicing sit-to-stand activities for coordination.

After the incision has healed, deep water hydrotherapy may be initiated. Before active movement of the hindlimbs, swimming bene-

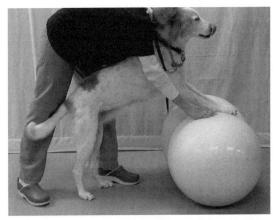

Figure 22-10 Facilitation of weight-bearing on rear limbs using a therapy roll.

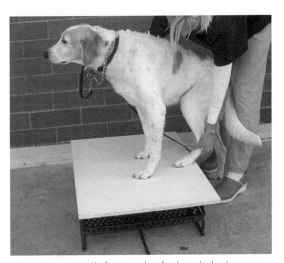

Figure 22-11 Platform used to facilitate limb placement.

fits the trunk muscles, aiding the patient's overall stability. Active movement of the rear limbs may be elicited by applying resistance to the paw, stimulating the medial aspect of the stifle, or flexing the hock.

A minimum of 3 weeks of physical rehabilitation is recommended. Frequently, the standard 3-week duration of physical therapy is extended to continue facilitating recovery. The degree of success in rehabilitation of thoracolumbar disk disease varies greatly and may take several months of dedicated treatment by the therapist and owner.

Degenerative Lumbosacral Stenosis

The lumbosacral region is characterized by unique anatomical features and considerable

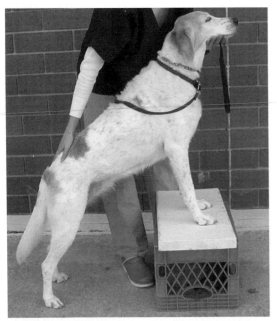

Figure 22-12   Platform used to facilitate weight-bearing and limb strengthening.

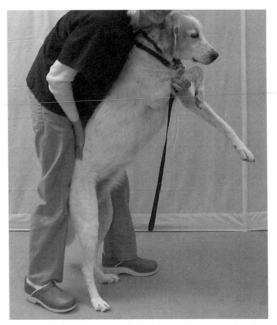

Figure 22-14   Dancing exercise.

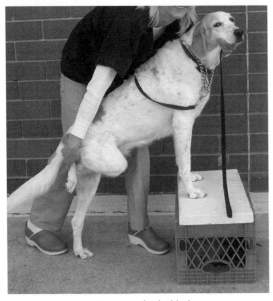

Figure 22-13   An individual limb exercise.

movement, especially flexion and some rotation. Motion is normally limited by the vertebrae and their articulations, ligaments, and intervertebral disks. Degenerative lumbosacral stenosis occurs when soft tissue and bony changes, possibly in conjunction with abnormal motion of the lumbosacral joint, impinge on the nerve roots of the cauda equina.[4,5] The most common change is protrusion of the L7-S1 disk, but osteophytes of the articular facets and hypertrophy of the interarcuate ligament and articular facet joint capsule may also cause nerve root compression. Spondylosis deformans also commonly occurs in conjunction with this condition.

Degenerative lumbosacral stenosis is most common in middle-age, large-breed dogs. German shepherd dogs are the most commonly affected breed, possibly because of the conformation of the lumbosacral angle. Working dogs and other large-breed dogs, including Dalmatians, and retriever breeds may also be at increased risk. Alternatively, congenital abnormalities may alter the forces placed on the lumbosacral region, resulting in compression and pathologic changes to the nerve roots. Instability, malalignment of the vertebrae, or congenital stenosis of the spinal canal may create secondary changes with the same clinical consequences.

The most common sign is lumbosacral pain, characterized by reluctance to work or participate in normal activity, run, jump, or climb stairs. Affected dogs often maintain a characteristic posture, keeping their lumbosacral region flexed, which decreases nerve root compression. Tail weakness, urinary or fecal incontinence, and pelvic limb lameness or weakness can also occur. On examination, palpation or extension of the lumbosacral joint and elevation of the tail usually induce pain. Other findings may include a weak perineal reflex, proprioceptive positioning deficits in one or both pelvic

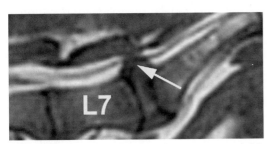

Figure 22-15 Sagittal plane MRI showing protrusion of the L7-S1 disk *(arrow)* with compression of the cauda equina. *L7,* The L7 vertebral body.

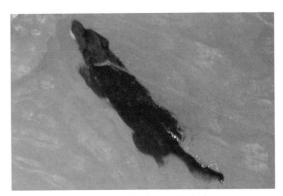

Figure 22-16 Deep-water hydrotherapy.

limbs, and decreased hock flexion when eliciting a withdrawal reflex. The differential diagnosis includes other lesions of the lumbosacral region (discospondylitis, neoplasia), degenerative myelopathy, fibrocartilaginous embolic myelopathy, orthopedic diseases (hip arthritis, cruciate rupture), trauma, and urogenital diseases, such as prostatic disease.

Diagnosis is based on clinical features and imaging. Survey radiographs may be normal or reveal chronic nonspecific changes to the lumbosacral region, including sclerosis of the vertebral end plates, ventral spondylosis deformans, and arthritis of the articular facets. Myelography is useful in assessing the caudal region of the lumbar spine, but will not identify lumbosacral stenosis when the dural sac ends cranial to the lumbosacral junction, which happens in about 25% of large-breed dogs. Although contrast radiography may provide evidence of static and dynamic compression, definitive diagnosis and localization of the lesions is most consistent when CT and MRI are used (Figure 22-15).

Nonsurgical treatment is appropriate for initial treatment of mild pain and entails strict rest, antiinflammatory or analgesic medications, and weight loss if necessary. Muscle relaxants may be beneficial if the dog has painful muscle spasms. Physical rehabilitation may also be useful in the medical management of lumbosacral disease. About 35% of these patients will recover with nonsurgical therapy. Surgery is indicated when there is persistent pain or neurologic deficits. The most common procedure is dorsal laminectomy of L7-S1 with excision of the protruded disk and foramenotomy if necessary. Some surgeons also include fusion of the L7-S1, but it is unclear in which patients this is necessary.

Most dogs recover with surgery, but those with urinary or fecal incontinence for more than a few weeks before surgery have a poor prognosis for recovery of continence.

Physical Rehabilitation for Degenerative Lumbosacral Stenosis

Physical rehabilitation is beneficial as part of the medical and postoperative management of lumbosacral disease. In combination with medications, therapeutic modalities focusing on pain management, such as ES protocols and therapeutic US, massage therapy, and aquatic therapy, are prescribed. Surgical patients are provided routine care of the incision site with icing and limited ES for pain management while hospitalized. Therapists should be informed of the type and location of any implants. The protocol for continued care consists of cage or crate confinement with assisted walking for 3 weeks after discharge. Physical rehabilitation then resumes following reassessment of the patient and radiographs if fusion was performed. Standard protocols are prescribed for strengthening and muscle reeducation including ES, passive range of motion, standing exercises, leash walking, proprioceptive and gait training, and aquatic therapy (Figure 22-16). As with most protocols, therapy continues for a 3- to 6-week period and is lengthened if necessary.

Cervical Spondylomyelopathy

Cervical spondylomyelopathy, also called caudal cervical stenotic myelopathy or wobbler syndrome, is a disorder caused by abnormal development of the cervical vertebrae resulting in compression of the spinal cord.[2]

Middle-aged Doberman pinschers and young Great Danes are most commonly affected, but the condition occurs in many large breeds. The specific changes vary, but may include stenosis of the vertebral canal, malformation of the articular facets, disk protrusion, capsular and ligament proliferation, synovial cysts, and vertebral instability. The C5-C6 and C6-C7 vertebrae and disk spaces are most commonly affected. Younger dogs are more likely to have stenosis, whereas disk protrusion and chronic instability are the most common changes in older dogs. Both compressive myelopathy and radiculoneuropathy are possible.

Clinical signs may be acute or slowly progressive. Mild cases are characterized by subtle ataxia of all limbs, often evident as long, protracted strides in the pelvic limbs, with a short-strided "floating gait" in the thoracic limbs. Because of the anatomical arrangement of the long spinal tracts to the rear limbs, the clinical signs are usually more pronounced in the rear limbs. Additional signs vary and may include low head carriage, a stiff neck, proprioceptive deficits, and paraparesis. In severe cases there is paresis or paralysis of all limbs. Neck pain is variable, but is more likely in acute cases. The differential diagnosis includes congenital anomalies, trauma, meningomyelitis, discospondylitis, neoplasia, and degenerative, ischemic, and embolic conditions.

A thorough history, physical examination, gait evaluation, and neurological examination are helpful to localize the lesion. A definitive diagnosis is based on spinal imaging. Survey radiographs may be normal or show abnormally shaped vertebra, narrowed disk space(s), and osteoarthritis of the articular facets. Myelography or MRI is necessary to fully characterize the specific changes and is essential if surgery is a consideration (Figure 22-17). Hypothyroidism, von Willebrand's disease, and cardiomyopathy are relatively common in middle-age Dobermans, so thyroid testing, buccal mucosal bleeding time, and chest radiographs should be considered in affected Dobermans.

Treatment is based on the severity of the neurological signs, the results of diagnostic imaging, quality-of-life issues, and the wishes of the owner. Nonsurgical treatment consists primarily of exercise restriction, antiinflammatory doses of corticosteroids such as prednisone, and, in some cases, a neck brace that immobilizes the caudal cervical region. Many patients will temporarily improve, but the underlying disease often progresses over time,

leading to deterioration in neurologic function. Surgery is indicated in patients with substantial neurologic deficits and patients that do not adequately respond to nonsurgical treatment. The goals of surgery are to relieve any spinal cord compression and stabilize vertebral instability. The particular technique chosen is based on the specific changes evident on myelography or MRI and surgeon preference, but may include ventral slot decompression, dorsal laminectomy, or distraction and fusion of affected vertebrae. Overall, about 75% of patients do well with surgery.[2] Patients that respond may do so over a prolonged period of time. The prognosis is worse for those patients with long-term paralysis, nonambulatory tetraparesis, or multiple lesions. Aftercare is a major part of the treatment, requiring significant intervention and effort of the caregiver.

Physical Rehabilitation for Cervical Spondylomyelopathy

Physical rehabilitation plays a significant role in patient care. Modalities directed toward decreasing muscle spasms, such as US and ES, passive range of motion of limbs, and support with a soft sling to provide assisted standing and weight-bearing, may be used in nonambulatory tetraparetic patients. Assisted sling walking and assisted aquatic therapy are useful to help patients regain unassisted ambulation. Neuromuscular ES for muscle building and reeducation may be performed in selected cases. As ambulation improves and strength is gained, unassisted deep-water and underwater treadmill therapy may be initiated. Gait training and strengthening exercises are incrementally implemented. Modalities used must be compatible with the patient's current neurological status and the stage of wound healing in the postoperative period if surgery was performed. Extended time in rehabilitation is

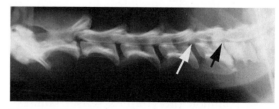

Figure 22-17 Myelography of cervical spondylomyelopathy. There is compression of the spinal segments dorsal to the C5-C6 disk space *(white arrow)*. There is a second, less severe lesion dorsal to the *C6-C7* disk space *(black arrow)*, which is narrowed.

often necessary for proper management of these cases because of the difficulties in managing large and giant breeds in a home environment.

Fibrocartilaginous Embolic Myelopathy

Fibrocartilaginous embolic myelopathy (FCEM) is an acute infarction of the spinal cord caused by a vascular embolus of fibrocartilage, probably originating from the intervertebral disk (Figure 22-18).[2] Adult large- or giant-breed dogs, miniature schnauzers, and Shetland sheepdogs are most commonly affected. This disease is rare in small dogs, chondrodystrophic dogs, and cats.

The onset is invariably acute and often associated with vigorous activity or mild trauma. Neurologic deficits rarely progress beyond the first few hours. Although patients sometimes appear painful at the onset of signs, spinal pain is rarely evident by the time of examination. This lack of focal spinal pain is helpful in ruling out other causes of acute spinal diseases, such as fracture/luxation and disk extrusion. Any region of the spinal cord may be affected, and the spinal cord segment(s) involved dictate the specific neurologic deficits. Ataxia, paresis, or paralysis may affect the pelvic limbs or all limbs. Asymmetrical or unilateral deficits are fairly common. Lower or upper motor neuron deficits may result. In severe cases, there is loss of deep pain perception caudal to the lesion. The severity of clinical signs, and the rate and

extent of recovery depend on the insult to the white or gray matter of the spinal cord. More severe gray matter pathology is often associated with slower recovery and residual neurologic deficits.

Diagnosis is based on the clinical features and exclusion of other causes. The differential diagnosis includes intervertebral disk disease, trauma, neoplasia, and inflammatory disease. Radiographs and myelography are typically normal, although myelography occasionally shows focal spinal cord swelling. Cerebrospinal fluid analysis is nonspecific. MRI usually shows a focal region of spinal cord edema, sometimes with hemorrhage.

There is no specific treatment for this condition. Many veterinarians administer corticosteroids, although there is little evidence that any drug is beneficial. The absence of deep pain perception indicates a very poor prognosis. Most patients that improve show some signs of improvement within 2 weeks. Further improvement is less likely beyond this period. Treatment consists of intensive and supportive care.

Physical Rehabilitation for Fibrocartilaginous Embolic Myelopathy

Physical rehabilitation may be beneficial for patients with FCEM. Modalities and techniques used are similar to those used to rehabilitate patients with intervertebral disk disease. Rehabilitation techniques vary depending on the location of the lesion and the degree of damage to the spinal cord. Depending on the severity of the condition, the patient may have increased muscle tone and spasticity, or decreased muscle tone and flaccidity. In general, ES, passive range of motion of affected joints, aquatic therapy, and assisted ambulation are early modalities that may be used. Continued ES, assisted sling walking, deep-water aquatic therapy, and gait and strength training are performed as the patient improves.

Nonambulatory patients require increased nursing care, including appropriate bladder care, assistance with adequate nutrition and fluid intake, and appropriate monitoring to ensure cleanliness and comfort. Patients should be repositioned every 4 to 6 hours to prevent decubital sores. A positioning protocol should be initiated immediately. If increased tone to the limb(s) is present, at-risk muscles are placed in elongated positions.

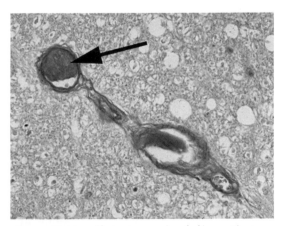

Figure 22-18   Photomicrograph of fibrocartilaginous embolic myelopathy. There is a piece of fibrocartilage *(arrow)* occluding one of the vessels in the spinal cord. There is necrosis of the adjacent portion of the spinal cord (hematoxylin-eosin with PAS stain).

Passive range of motion to joints and muscles at risk of developing contracture and adaptive shortening is performed regularly, typically three to six times daily. Passive range of motion or active assisted range of motion and stretching using the body weight and movement of the body in closed-chain activities can be effective. Slow rhythmic bouncing on a therapy ball assists in decreasing hypertonia and allows for more effective muscle stretch and more normal movement patterns.

If the patient is unable to sit or stand independently, assistance to these positions, with proper joint alignment, should be promptly initiated. Placing the patient over a small therapy ball with the feet still in contact with the floor assists in maintaining a standing position (see Figure 22-8). It is important to provide weight-bearing on the affected limbs while maintaining a standing position. Weight shifting in functional planes of movement may also be initiated in this position. If working only with the hindlimbs, the torso and front limbs may be placed on the ball while the hindlimbs are worked in a weight-bearing position.

Firm, deep pressure through manual contacts activates the tactile receptors, neuromuscular proprioceptive pathways, and sensory awareness. Proper hand placement provides security and support to unstable body segments and may stimulate contraction of the muscles under the hands of the therapist (Figure 22-19). Applying techniques of approximation and compression facilitates postural extensors and stabilizers and enhances body awareness. Approximation of the affected joints can be achieved by bouncing the patient while it is sitting on a therapy ball or weight-bearing over a ball, and through manual compression of the joint. Providing intermittent pressure through the pelvis and legs (bouncing) stimulates approximation of affected joints in patients with hindlimb pathology that are able to assume a standing position.

Deep-water hydrotherapy is another modality that is used to stimulate muscle activity and motor learning (see Figure 22-16). Depending on the functional level of the patient, life preservers or manual assistance in the pool may be necessary to ensure safety (see Figure 22-2). This assistance also allows the therapist to more easily provide reciprocal movements to the affected limbs. Assisting the patient to stand in shallow water or weight-bearing on the hindlimbs with the forelimbs elevated are also useful treatments in the pool.

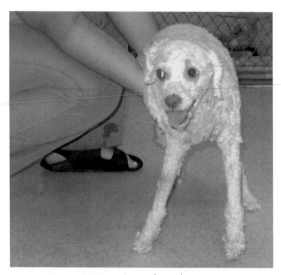

Figure 22-19 Assisted standing exercise.

Assisted ambulation with manual reciprocal placement of the patient's feet may stimulate motor memories and initiate motor learning. Sling or tail walking aids ambulation. As the patient improves, the use of an underwater treadmill or land treadmill further benefits strengthening and gait training.

Standard 3-week rehabilitation protocols may be lengthened in those patients experiencing a slower recovery. Occasionally, patients have a relapse of the condition, necessitating changes in the protocol to meet the needs of the patient.

Neoplasia

Spinal tumors are classified by their location as extradural, subarachnoid (intradural-extramedullary), and intramedullary.[6] Extradural neoplasia is most common and includes osteosarcoma, multiple myeloma, fibrosarcoma, chondrosarcoma, hemangiosarcoma, and lymphosarcoma. Vertebral involvement is relatively common. Extradural lymphosarcoma is the most common spinal tumor in cats and is usually secondary to infection with the feline leukemia virus. Subarachnoid tumors include nerve sheath tumors, meningioma, lymphosarcoma, and neuroepithelioma. Intramedullary tumors include glioma, lymphosarcoma, and hemangiosarcoma. Metastatic tumors, including metastatic carcinomas and sarcomas, may occur in any location. Spinal neoplasia is more common in middle-age or older animals. However, neuroepithelioma

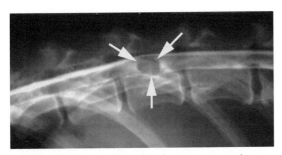

Figure 22-20 *Myelography showing a spinal tumor (meningioma) at the level of L1. There is a well-defined filling defect (arrows) outlining the mass.*

affects young, large-breed dogs, and lymphoma may affect a cat at any age.

Clinical signs are typically insidious and progressive but can be acute. Focal spinal pain is the most common initial sign. Later ataxia and paresis may develop as the spinal cord becomes progressively affected. Systemic signs, such as weight loss, may occur with metastatic cancer.

The history reflects the accommodating nature of the spinal cord to increasing pressure until deterioration of white and gray matter occurs. Acute exacerbation of neurologic signs and pain may be seen with vertebral involvement or with vascular insults. Intramedullary tumors may present with deteriorating neurologic signs without evidence of pain or discomfort.

Diagnosis is based on the history, physical and neurologic examinations, and diagnostic imaging. If neoplasia is suspected, chest radiographs are indicated to screen for metastasis. Spinal radiographs may show abnormalities in cases of vertebral tumors, although initial changes may be subtle. Myelography is helpful in identifying spinal cord compression (Figure 22-20). CT, CT-myelography, and MRI are more sensitive. Definitive diagnosis often requires surgical exploration and biopsy.

Medical management may provide temporary relief of pain and weakness to maintain a reasonable quality of life for a short period of time. Generally this consists of judicious activity, analgesics, and corticosteroids. Chemotherapy may be appropriate for specific tumor types. Definitive treatment usually consists of surgical excision or debulking. Surgical exploration and debulking (dorsal laminectomy, durotomy, dorsal myelotomy, and so forth) are generally not curative but can provide decompression and prolonged quality of life. Radiation therapy may be used as a primary treatment or as an adjunct to surgery, depending on tumor type. The prognosis depends on the tumor type.

Physical Rehabilitation for Neoplasia of the Spinal Column

Postoperative physical rehabilitation protocols are generally similar to those used in the rehabilitation of patients after intervertebral disk decompression. One key difference, however, is that protocols must generally be stepped down rather than stepped up as the disease progresses and the condition and ability of the patient diminish.

Trauma

Major traumatic insults may result in various head and spinal lesions, depending on the anatomical location.[7] A thorough history usually documents the type of trauma the patient has sustained, although the cause is sometimes unknown or surmised by concurrent findings if the accident is not witnessed. Automobile accidents, gunshot wounds, falls, and dog-fight injuries are common. Spinal injuries may consist of vertebral subluxation or luxation, vertebral fracture, vertebral fracture/luxation, or trauma-induced intervertebral disk herniation. The forces acting on the vertebral column must be considered when injuries to the spinal column are present. These include rotational, dorsoventral, and lateral bending, axial loading, and shearing forces. To estimate which of these biomechanical forces are creating instability, anatomical features of the spine are classified into the dorsal and ventral compartments of the vertebral body. Additionally, the integrity of the vertebral body and articular facets is evaluated to further define the ability of the vertebral column to resist these biomechanical forces.

As with any trauma patient, full assessment of all body systems is essential to diagnose and treat shock and any other life-threatening or concurrent injuries. Following or concurrently with a complete patient assessment, a neurologic examination is performed to localize the injury and to determine the severity of the deficits. It is vital that the examination be carefully performed, minimizing movement of the patient to avoid further damage to the spinal cord as a result of instability of the spinal column. Assessment of mentation, cranial nerves, voluntary movement, and spinal reflexes, as well as head and spine palpation, is performed, but moving the patient to test gait and postural reactions is avoided until unstable spinal injuries are ruled out with radiographs. The presence or absence of deep pain caudal to the injury is the most important prognostic sign; lack of deep pain sensation after spinal trauma carries a grave prognosis for neurologic recovery.

Following initial assessment and stabilization, appropriate analgesics are administered. Methylprednisolone (30 mg/kg IV, then 1 hour later 5.4 mg/kg/hr IV infusion for 24 to 48 hours) may improve the chance of recovery from severe spinal cord injury if started within 8 hours of injury. A lateral-view radiograph of the affected region of the spine is obtained when the patient is stable. If dorsoventral views are necessary, a horizontal beam view is safest. The purpose of radiography is to confirm the localization, classify any fracture/luxation as stable or unstable, and try to determine if there is any persistent spinal cord compression that may require surgery. The two components of the spine that maintain stability are (1) the dorsal compartment, consisting of the articular facets and lamina, and (2) the ventral compartment, consisting of the vertebral bodies and intervertebral disk. Damage to one of these components usually does not result in severe instability, whereas damage to both the dorsal and ventral components may require internal fixation to prevent further displacement. Myelography or CT may be indicated if survey radiographs are normal or inconclusive. Routine chest and abdominal films may also be indicated to determine other body systems affected by the trauma.

The decision to treat the patient is based on the severity of the neurologic deficits, the type of vertebral injury, the severity of any concurrent injuries, and the owner's understanding of the risk, prognosis, and expense of the injury and treatment. Animals with mild neurologic deficits caused by cervical injuries or stable thoracolumbar injuries often recover with nonsurgical therapy. This consists of 4 to 6 weeks of complete cage rest, with very cautious movement of the animal to assist it with posturing to urinate and defecate. Weight-bearing is generally not encouraged, unless the vertebral column is stable. Sometimes an external splint is used in conjunction with cage rest.

Indications for surgery include (1) unstable fracture/luxation, usually evident on radiographs by disruption of the dorsal and ventral components of the vertebrae, (2) persistent compression of the vertebral canal, evident as a substantially displaced fracture/luxation or a myelographic pattern of extradural compression, and (3) progressive deterioration in neurological status despite conservative treatment, usually due to an unstable fracture/luxation or progressive spinal cord compression from hemorrhage or disk extrusion. Surgery is generally contraindicated in patients with unstable associated injuries or absent deep pain perception.

Surgery usually involves decompression of the spinal cord and fixation of unstable vertebrae. The choice of fixation technique depends on the size of the animal, the type and location of the injury, and the surgeon's preference and experience. In general, dorsal techniques (spinal staples, dorsal spinal plates, and modified spinal instrumentation) are indicated if the ventral components of the vertebrae are intact. Ventral techniques (vertebral body plates, pins/screws, and bone cement) are stronger and can be used with dorsal and ventral component injuries (Figure 22-21). A laminectomy to decompress the spinal cord from intervertebral disk material, ligament, or bone may be necessary before fixation, but further destabilization of the vertebral column associated with the decompression procedure may result. Most surgeons believe that careful reduction and stabilization of the spinal column provide adequate decompression without causing further destabilization of the spinal column as a result of hemilaminectomy. External splints of light casting material or moldable thermoplastic materials provide some stability and are most applicable to midthoracic and lumbar areas. Splints may be applied to the cervical area but require more creativity. Splints may create sores and have the potential for creating complicated wounds that necessitate additional nursing care. Splints may also be used as an adjunct to internal fixation.

Physical Rehabilitation for Traumatic Injuries

Physical rehabilitation protocols and modalities are similar to those used for rehabilitation of lumbosacral decompression/stabilization and cervical spondylomyelopathy patients. ES

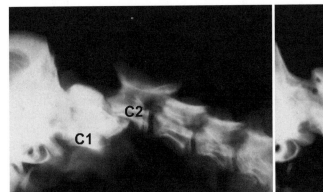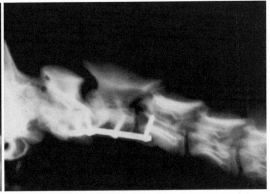

Figure 22-21   Surgery for a spinal fracture/luxation. **A,** There is a fracture of C2 with dorsal displacement of C2 relative to C1. **B,** Postoperative view. The injury has been repaired with a plate and screws affixed to the ventral aspect of C1, C2, and C3.

protocols to enhance wound healing may be useful in those patients that develop cast wounds. Extended care and therapy beyond the standard 3-week rehabilitation protocol may be required in some cases.

Discospondylitis

Discospondylitis is an infection of the intervertebral disk and adjacent vertebral bodies, resulting in an inflammatory response surrounding the associated spinal cord or nerve roots.[8] It is usually caused by hematogenous spread of organisms from infected sites elsewhere in the body, such as the urinary tract, skin, or mouth. Penetrating wounds, surgery, or plant material migration can cause direct infection of the disk space or vertebra. In certain geographic regions, migrating plant material such as grass awns is a relatively common cause of vertebral osteomyelitis and discospondylitis of the L2-L4 vertebrae. *Staphylococcus intermedius* is the most common etiological agent identified in dogs with discospondylitis. Other frequently documented pathogens include *Streptococcus* spp, *Brucella canis*, and *Escherichia coli*, but virtually any bacterial agent can be causative. Some infections are caused by fungal organisms, including *Aspergillus, Paecilomyces* and *Coccidioides immitis*. Vertebral infections due to grass awn migration are often associated with mixed infections, with *Actinomyces* being a common isolate.

Discospondylitis most commonly affects large, middle-age dogs. Small dogs and chondrodystrophic breeds are uncommonly af-

fected, and the disease is rare in cats. The most common initial sign is pain and discomfort of the affected region of the spinal column, which varies in intensity from mild to extreme. The duration of signs noticed by the client usually ranges from several days to several weeks. Neurologic deficits ranging from ataxia to paralysis are seen in some patients, although usually not as the initial abnormality. Signs suggestive of systemic illness, such as fever, lethargy, depression, anorexia, and weight loss, occur in about 30% of affected dogs. Concurrent prostatitis in male dogs and lower urinary tract infection in either gender are common.

Diagnosis is based on clinical features and diagnostic imaging. Radiographs of the involved region are usually diagnostic, although they may be normal early in the course of disease. The earliest radiographic sign is subtle irregularity of the vertebral end plates. As the infection progresses, the erosion of the end plate becomes more pronounced, and there are osteolytic and osteoproductive changes of the intervertebral disk space, vertebral end plates, and in severe cases, the entire vertebral body (Figure 22-22). CT and MRI are more sensitive and are helpful when radiographs are normal or inconclusive. Myelography is indicated only in patients with substantial neurologic deficits when decompressive surgery is considered. Complete blood count, urine culture and sensitivity, blood cultures, and serology for brucellosis are performed in all dogs with radiographic evidence of vertebral infection. The differential diagnosis includes chronic intervertebral disk disease, inflammatory disease, and neoplasia.

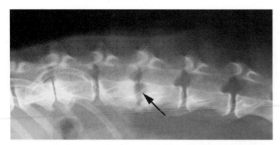

Figure 22-22   Discospondylitis. The radiograph shows lysis of the vertebral end plates *(arrow)* adjacent to the L2-L3 disk space.

Initial treatment consists of antibiotics, cage rest, and analgesics. Selection of antibiotics is based on culture and sensitivity of blood and urine and serology for *B. canis*. Pending these results or if these tests are negative, treatment is started with a bactericidal antibiotic effective against β-lactamase–producing *Staphylococcus*. First-generation cephalosporins are effective against the majority of isolates from affected dogs and are a good choice for initial therapy. Clindamycin and amoxicillin with clavulanic acid are also usually effective. Patients with fever, neurologic deficits, or rapidly progressing signs are treated with intravenous antibiotics for 3 to 5 days, followed by a course of oral antibiotics. Initial oral therapy is appropriate in patients with mild, slowly progressing spinal pain.

Clinical signs such as spinal pain and fever usually resolve within 5 days of starting effective therapy, although neurologic deficits usually resolve more slowly. Patients should be treated for at least 8 weeks in an attempt to completely clear the infection and prevent relapse. Patients that fail to improve within 5 days of starting treatment are reassessed. Options include treating with a different antibiotic or culture of the affected disk space by needle aspiration. Most animals recover with appropriate medical treatment. Surgery is rarely indicated to obtain biopsy when there is no response to initial therapy, or to decompress the spinal cord in patients with substantial neurologic deficits, evidence of spinal cord compression on imaging, and no response to medical therapy.

Physical Rehabilitation for Discospondylitis

Physical rehabilitation is indicated in more severely affected patients after a positive response to medical management is achieved.

Protocols used are similar to those for conservative intervertebral disk disease management, specifically aquatic therapy, and strength and gait training. Postoperative patients are managed similar to those following lumbosacral decompression procedures with or without stabilization. Particular care should be exercised because affected patients generally have significant weakness of the affected bones of the vertebral column.

Atlantoaxial Luxation

The anatomy of the atlas (C1) and the axis (C2) is distinctly different from the rest of the vertebral column. There is no intervertebral disk and very little flexion. The anatomical relationship between C1 and C2 is primarily maintained by ligaments. Atlantoaxial luxation occurs when instability of the joint allows C2 to luxate dorsally, relative to C1, and compress the spinal cord. Pathology leading to secondary neurological disease includes congenital absence of the dens, fracture of the dens, and loss of ligament integrity either from absence or rupture.[9] Atlantoaxial luxation is most common in toy-breed dogs with malformation of the dens or ligaments that maintain normal stability. It can occur in any animal as a consequence of trauma.

In dogs with congenital instability of the atlantoaxial joint, clinical signs usually occur within the first few years of life and are often precipitated by relatively minor trauma. Yorkshire terriers, Chihuahuas, miniature and toy Poodles, Pomeranians, and Pekingese dogs are most commonly affected. Clinical signs include neck pain and gait dysfunction, ranging from ataxia to tetraplegia, with normal or exaggerated reflexes. Cases with severe spinal cord trauma may be fatal due to respiratory paralysis. It is critical to avoid flexion of the neck during examination, as this exacerbates spinal cord compression. The differential diagnosis includes vertebral fracture or luxation, intervertebral disk disease, discospondylitis, neoplasia, and meningomyelitis.

The diagnosis is based on a history, physical and neurologic examination, and radiographs. Typical radiographic findings include dorsal displacement of C2 relative to C1 and an increased space between the arch of C1 and spine of C2 on the lateral view (Figure 22-23). The size and shape of the dens of C2 is best evaluated on a ventrodorsal view. The dens

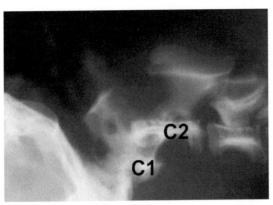

Figure 22-23 Atlantoaxial luxation. The radiograph shows dorsal displacement of C2 relative to C1.

may be normal, hypoplastic, aplastic, or dorsally angulated. If survey radiographs are equivocal, the atlantoaxial joint may be slightly flexed during fluoroscopy to assess stability. CT or MRI is also useful if the diagnosis is uncertain. Cerebrospinal fluid analysis may be useful to differentiate structural from inflammatory disease. Lumbar puncture for fluid collection or radiographic contrast injection avoids flexion of the cervical spine.

Nonsurgical treatment is indicated in patients with mild signs. This consists of cage rest and application of a neck brace that prevents neck flexion for 6 weeks. Steroidal antiinflammatory agents may be useful in some cases. Conservative treatment may be successful in patients with traumatic luxations, but dogs with congenital instability often suffer relapse because of the inherent instability. Surgery to reduce and stabilize the atlantoaxial joint is the definitive treatment. Techniques include ventral stabilization using pins or screws and dorsal fixation using suture or wire. Potential complications include implant failure, worsening of neurologic deficits, and upper respiratory problems associated with the ventral surgical approach.

Physical Rehabilitation for Atlantoaxial Subluxation

Postoperatively, a cervical splint fashioned from light casting material is applied. Periodic removal allows assessment of underlying tissues. External coaptation is continued for 4 weeks along with strict confinement. Physical

rehabilitation begins after cast removal, and it is important to match the rehabilitation plan to the neurologic status of the patient. Whirlpool aquatic therapy combined with ES and therapeutic US is appropriate in the early phases of rehabilitation. Assisted aquatic therapy is beneficial until ambulation begins. Strengthening and gait training exercises and underwater treadmill aquatic therapy may be incrementally added.

Miscellaneous Conditions

Miscellaneous diseases creating neurologic dysfunction that are treatable and have a reasonable prognosis may benefit from physical rehabilitation. These include congenital vertebral anomalies and arachnoid cysts. Because of the uncommon clinical presentation of these conditions and the lack of experience in rehabilitating these conditions, the use and success of specific protocols are unknown. Adherence to therapeutic principles and selecting protocols used for similar diseases should provide a sound basis for rehabilitation of these patients.

REFERENCES

1. Toombs JP, Bauer MS: Intervertebral disk disease. In Slatter D, editor: *Textbook of small animal surgery,* ed 2, Philadelphia, 1993, WB Saunders.
2. Wheeler SJ, Sharp NJH: *Small animal spinal disorder, diagnosis and surgery.* London, 1994, Mosby-Wolfe.
3. Shores A, Braund KG: Neurological examination and localization. In Slatter D, editor: *Textbook of small animal surgery,* ed 2, Philadelphia, 1993, WB Saunders.
4. Prata RG: Cauda equina syndrome. Overview. In Slatter D, editor: *Textbook of small animal surgery,* ed 2, Philadelphia, 1993, WB Saunders.
5. Slocum B, Slocum TD: Cauda equina syndrome. L7(S1 fixation-fusion for cauda equina compression: an alternative view. In Slatter D, editor: *Textbook of small animal surgery,* ed 2, Philadelphia, 1993, WB Saunders.
6. Seim, HB III: Nervous system. In Slatter D, editor: *Textbook of small animal surgery,* ed 2, Philadelphia, 1993, WB Saunders.
7. Bruecker KA, Seim HB III: Spinal fractures and luxations. In Slatter D, editor: *Textbook of small animal surgery,* ed 2, Philadelphia, 1993, WB Saunders.
8. Kornegay JN: Discospondylitis. In Slatter D, editor: *Textbook of small animal surgery,* ed 2, Philadelphia, 1993, WB Saunders.
9. Shires PK: Atlantoaxial instability. In Slatter D, editor: *Textbook of small animal surgery,* ed 2, Philadelphia, 1993, WB Saunders.

Physical Rehabilitation for the Critically Injured Veterinary Patient

Anne Marie Manning

The critically injured veterinary patient can present a daunting challenge to the clinician trying to provide physical rehabilitation. Types of injuries sustained may range from single or multiple orthopedic and soft tissue trauma to the chest, abdomine, or head or a combination of these injuries. The common thread in all of these patients is a debilitating injury that renders them partially or completely immobile for prolonged periods. Although bed rest is important to the recovery from critical injuries, prolonged inactivity can have deleterious effects on both injured and healthy body systems. The goals of providing physical rehabilitation to critically injured patients are to prevent complications stemming from injuries, prevent complications secondary to prolonged inactivity, maintain body condition, improve patient comfort, and hasten recovery. The purpose of this chapter is to discuss the effects of prolonged inactivity on traumatized and healthy body systems and to describe the application of basic physical rehabilitation techniques for specific critical injuries.

The Musculoskeletal System

Rarely do traumatized animals escape injury to the musculoskeletal system. Injuries can include single or multiple fractures of the appendicular or axial skeleton, hemorrhage into skin, muscle, and joint spaces, or injury to nerves supplying these structures. Patients with head, chest, or abdominal trauma may be unable to move because of decreased consciousness or pain. Disuse or injury to the musculoskeletal system may result in muscle weakness and muscle atrophy; skin, muscle

and joint contractures; and, eventually, may limit an animal's ability to move, groom, eat, and ambulate. With these global implications, maintenance of this body system is paramount.

The balance between collagen synthesis and degradation is abnormal in immobile patients. Trauma with bleeding into soft tissue and muscle and subsequent inflammation and degeneration can trigger increased collagen synthesis. Increased collagen synthesis in an inactive patient leads to tighter packing of collagen fibers and contributes to the development of contractures.

Muscle contracture is shortening of the muscle due to either intrinsic or extrinsic causes. Intrinsic changes are structural and can result from inflammatory or traumatic processes. Trauma, inflammation, ischemia, and hemorrhage in injured patients can restructure muscle tissue components and result in fibrosis and the development of adhesions. Following hemorrhage into a muscle, fibrin deposition occurs. Within 2 to 3 days, fibrin is replaced with reticular fibers that form a loose connective tissue network. If the affected muscle is kept immobile, the network becomes more dense and resistant to stretch.[1]

Extrinsic muscle contracture is secondary to neurologic abnormalities or mechanical factors and is commonly associated with prolonged immobilization. Causes of extrinsic muscle contracture include paralytic or spastic muscle conditions. Paralyzed muscles cannot provide adequate resistance to opposing muscles across a joint. Eventually, the antagonistic muscle will shorten. Carpal contracture in brachial plexus injuries illustrates this type of extrinsic contracture. To prevent contracture of the carpus in this situation, stretch must be applied to the normal muscle. Spastic muscle, which may exist in the pelvic limb musculature following trauma to the spinal cord between T3-L3, results from imbalance of muscle control. Increased muscle tone reduces the resting length of the spastic muscle and results in abnormal joint positioning. Treatment is aimed at stretching the abnormal muscle. *Joint contracture* is defined as an inability to move a joint through its full range of motion (ROM). Conditions that contribute to joint contracture include absence of mobility at the joint, immobilization of a joint in an inappropriate position, joint pain, paralysis, and muscle damage.

The position in which limbs are immobilized also contributes to the development of contractures. Muscle fibers lose up to 40% of sarcomeres when immobilized in a shortened position. Therefore, whenever possible, joints should be kept in a neutral position to keep muscle fibers at equal length and tension to minimize contracture.[2] Additional factors that affect the rate of contracture development include the precipitating cause, duration and degree of immobilization, and preexisting joint restrictions. Edema, ischemia, and bleeding accelerate the development of muscle and joint contracture. Immobile, injured patients therefore require efforts directed at prevention and treatment of contracture development following soft tissue injuries (Table 23-1).

Respiratory System

The respiratory complications of prolonged immobility and those resulting from primary injuries are numerous and potentially catastrophic in critically injured patients. Injuries to the head, chest, and abdomen often result in reduced respiratory function due to pain, inability to move, altered consciousness, or damage to thoracic structures. Impaired consciousness from head injury may lead to altered breathing patterns, diminished ability to cough, and inability to change body position. Rib fractures, pneumothorax, pulmonary contusions, and painful soft tissue injuries to the chest and abdomen may result in a restrictive breathing pattern characterized by shallow, rapid ventilation. This type of breathing pattern causes a reduction in tidal volume, functional residual capacity, and lung compliance. Altered respiratory patterns in conjunction with immobility may lead to atelectasis, accumulation of respiratory secretions, and pneumonia. It is important for the clinician to note any injuries that may compromise respiratory function and devise a physical rehabilitation plan to address those concerns. The goals of chest physical rehabilitation are to maintain bronchial hygiene, eliminate secretions from the airways, reexpand atelectatic lung segments, improve oxygenation, and reduce the incidence of pneumonia (Table 23-2). These

■ ▣ ▤ **Table 23-1**   Treatment of Musculoskeletal Injuries

Technique	Benefits	Frequency
Cryotherapy	Reduces inflammation, swelling, and pain	Every 4 hr (after initial 24-72 hr)
Superficial or deep heating	Improves circulation, reduces muscle spasm, provides pain relief	Every 4-6 hr (after initial 72 hr)
Massage	Increases circulation to paralyzed musculature, reduces/breaks down adhesions, provides pain relief, reduces edema	4-6 times/day
Range-of-motion (ROM) exercises		
Passive	Maintains existing mobility of joints and soft tissue, minimizes contracture formation, prevents loss of ROM, maintains muscle elasticity, improves circulation, reduces edema	4-6 times/day
Active	Same as passive ROM exercises plus maintains physiologic muscle elasticity, maintains bone integrity	4-6 times/day
Serial splinting and casting	Corrects severe muscle and joint contracture by providing prolonged stretch to muscle and joint structures	

Table 23-2   Goals of Chest Physical
Rehabilitation

Technique	Goals
Positioning	Reduce risk of atelectasis, improve ventilation/perfusion, improve gas exchange, reduce risk of pressure sores, minimize muscle and joint stiffness
Cough	Remove secretions from trachea to fourth-generation bronchi
Postural drainage	Increase mobilization and elimination of secretions from upper airways
Percussion	Dislodge bronchial secretions
Vibration	Move secretions into larger airways

goals can be achieved through techniques such as stimulating the animal to cough, frequent repositioning, postural drainage, percussion, vibration, and exercise. Each of these techniques will be reviewed in detail.

Cough

Coughing is the most important defense mechanism to eliminate retained secretions. A cough can eliminate secretions from the trachea to the level of the fourth-generation segmental bronchi.[3] An effective cough is initiated by a deep inspiration, followed by closure of the glottis and contraction of the chest wall and abdominal musculature to generate high intrathoracic pressure. After high intrathoracic pressure is attained, the glottis opens and is followed by rapid expulsion of air during exhalation. Critically injured patients may not be able to initiate a cough because of impaired consciousness, pain, weakness, or injuries to the chest or abdominal wall. These animals can be assisted to cough by applying gentle pressure to the trachea at the level of the third tracheal ring. Placing an animal in sternal recumbency may also improve an animal's ability to cough. Animals should be assisted to cough after postural drainage, percussion, and vibration and before changes are made in the patient's position.

Positioning

Injured animals are often unable to move or change position within their cage. Alternating right, sternal, and left lateral recumbency every 4 hours is recommended for immobile

patients. Frequent repositioning helps prevent atelectasis and pooling of secretions in dependent lung segments. Because position influences the distribution of blood flow to the lungs, changing body positions alters ventilation/perfusion ($\dot{V}/\dot{Q}$) relationships within the lungs. When a patient is positioned with the compromised lung segment in a dependent position, that lung receives increased blood flow, resulting in increased $\dot{V}/\dot{Q}$ mismatch and impaired gas exchange.[4] Therefore, if pulmonary contusions or pneumonia are present, positioning the patient with the good lung down improves oxygenation by limiting $\dot{V}/\dot{Q}$ mismatch and improving gas exchange. Improved oxygenation and a reduction in the number of patients with postoperative fever have been documented in humans when side-to-side turning is used.[5]

Frequent position changes in conjunction with comfortable bedding also help reduce the risk of pressure sores, edematous limbs, and muscle and joint stiffness. Repositioning is a simple physical rehabilitation technique that should be employed in all immobile patients.

Postural Drainage

Postural drainage is the use of changes in body position to allow gravity to aid in the removal of tracheobronchial secretions from different lung segments. This method of thoracic physical rehabilitation prevents pooling of respiratory secretions in the lungs, enhances drainage of the periphery of the lung, accelerates clearance of mucus, and increases the functional residual capacity of the lungs.[6] The patient must be positioned so that segmental bronchi are vertical to the affected lung to allow movement of secretions into the larger airways. After secretions reach the mainstem bronchi and trachea, a cough will aid in their removal. Postural drainage is most effective when used in conjunction with percussion and vibration to loosen thick airway secretions.

In human patients, 11 postural drainage positions are used to drain 14 lung segments.[7] Figure 23-1 illustrates seven postural drainage positions that can be used to drain specific areas in the lungs of the canine patient.[8] The duration of postural drainage therapy depends on the number of lung segments requiring drainage, the amount of secretions produced, and the patient's tolerance for the procedure. In general, 5 to 10 minutes per position is necessary for this therapy to be effective. Because

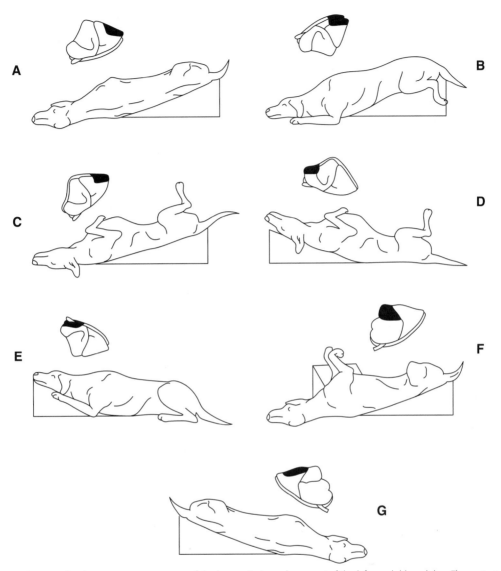

Figure 23-1   Positions for draining various portions of the lungs. **A,** Lateral segment of the left caudal lung lobe. The patient is in left lateral recumbency with the hind end elevated 40 degrees. **B,** Left and right caudal dorsal lung fields. The patient is in sternal recumbency with hind end elevated 40 degrees. **C,** Left and right caudal ventral lung fields. The patient is a dorsal recumbency with the hind end elevated 40 degrees. **D,** Left and right cranial ventral lung fields. The patient is in dorsal recumbency with the front end elevated 40 degrees. **E,** Left and right cranial dorsal lung fields. The patient is in sternal recumbency with the front end elevated 40 degrees. **F,** Right middle lung lobe. The patient is in dorsal recumbency. A pillow has been placed under the left side of the thorax so that the right side is higher than the left side. The hind end is elevated 40 degrees, and the front end is rotated one-quarter turn to the right. **G,** Lateral segment of the right caudal lung lobe. The patient is in left lateral recumbency with the hind end elevated 40 degrees. (From Manning A, Ellis D, Rush J: Physical therapy for critically ill veterinary patients. I. Chest physical therapy, *Compend Contin Educ Pract Vet* 19:680, 1997.)

exercise is superior to postural drainage for mobilization of respiratory secretions, ambulatory patients should be encouraged to walk for 5 to 10 minutes, three to four times a day.[6] Postural drainage is indicated in injured patients with pulmonary contusions, atelectasis, or altered consciousness, and those patients that are immobile secondary to injuries.

Percussion

Chest percussion (coupage) is performed by rhythmically striking the patient's chest wall with cupped hands over the affected lung segments (Figure 23-2). With this technique, a mechanical shock wave is applied to the chest wall and transmitted to the lungs to dislodge

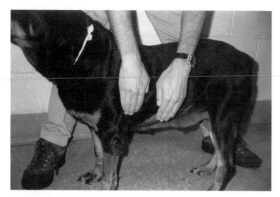

Figure 23-2   Chest percussion is performed by striking the chest wall with cupped hands over the affected lung segments. The goal is to help break up secretions to larger airways so that they may be expelled by coughing or other means.

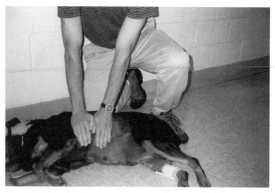

Figure 23-3   After percussion, vibration (shaking of the chest wall) is performed to move the dislodged secretions toward larger airways. Vibration is performed only during exhalation. Both hands are placed on the same side of the chest over the affected lung segment. With arms straight and locked, the therapist vigorously shakes the chest wall. Vibration is performed on four to six consecutive breaths following each episode of percussion.

secretions from bronchial walls. The goal of percussion, in combination with vibration, is to move secretions from small to larger airways where they can be cleared by a cough or postural drainage techniques. Percussion is performed throughout both inspiration and expiration. The amount of force used is determined by patient tolerance to the procedure and the patient's medical problem. Correct hand form and positioning over the affected lung segment are more important than the amount of force used. Only affected lung segments should be percussed because normal lung does not benefit from percussion. The rate of percussion should be steady and the therapist should proceed in a circular motion over the affected area.[9] Erratic percussion, that is, frequent stops and starts, should be avoided. Generally, percussion should be sustained for 3 to 4 minutes followed by vibration. Three to four periods of percussion are generally adequate for each postural drainage position. Percussion is not recommended for those patients that produce little or no sputum with a cough.[10]

Vibration

After each period of percussion, vibration (shaking of the chest wall) is performed to move the dislodged secretions toward larger airways (Figure 23-3). Unlike percussion, which is performed during both inspiration and exhalation, vibration is performed only during exhalation. The technique is performed with both hands placed on the same side of the chest over the affected lung segment. With arms straight and locked, the therapist simultaneously contracts all of his or her

muscles from the hands to the shoulder and vigorously shakes the chest wall. A mechanical vibrator may also be used. Vibration is performed on four to six consecutive breaths following each episode of percussion. Any indication for postural drainage is an indication for percussion and vibration.

Contraindications for Postural Drainage, Percussion, and Vibration

Although most patients tolerate chest physical rehabilitation, critically injured patients may be at risk for complications. In human patients, postural drainage has been associated with transient decreases in oxygen saturation of arterial blood (SaO_2), and percussion can potentiate cardiac arrhythmias.[10,11] Animals with pulmonary contusions often have some degree of hypoxia and should be supplemented with oxygen before and during these techniques. If oxygen desaturation occurs, SaO_2 values generally return to pretreatment values within minutes of position changes and the conclusion of percussion. Animals with chest trauma are at risk for cardiac arrhythmias secondary to traumatic myocarditis. Chest percussion in these animals may precipitate an arrhythmia or cause an existing arrhythmia to worsen. Continuous electrocardiographic monitoring is recommended before and during chest physical rehabilitation. Other injuries in which chest physical rehabilitation is contraindicated are listed in Box 23-1.

> ■ ■ ■ **BOX 23-1** Contraindications for Chest Physical Rehabilitation in Critically Injured Patients
>
> ■ Flail chest or rib fractures
> ■ Pneumothorax
> ■ Platelet count <30,000 platelets/μl
> ■ Areas with open wounds
> ■ Subcutaneous emphysema of the neck or thorax
> ■ Pain
> ■ Unstable cardiovascular condition

Exercise

Exercise is superior to chest physical rehabilitation in reducing atelectasis, mobilizing secretions from the lung periphery, and preventing pooling of secretions in the lungs. Exercise enables deep breathing, which improves ventilation and expiratory flow. Exercise has also been shown to improve sympathetic activity, which increases ciliary beat frequency and decreases mucus viscosity.[12,13] In addition to the respiratory benefits, early mobilization reduces many of the musculoskeletal complications associated with prolonged immobility.

Ambulatory patients should be encouraged to stand and walk for short periods of time (5 to 10 minutes) every 4 to 6 hours. Weak but ambulatory animals can be supported with slings or harnesses. Nonambulatory patients should be assisted to stand for a few minutes every 4 to 6 hours in conjunction with changes in body position.

Clinical Applications of Physical Rehabilitation for the Critically Injured Patient

Soft Tissue Trauma and Orthopedic Injuries

Trauma to soft tissue structures such as skin and muscle may be confined to a limited area or may be extensive. Extensive bruising, swelling, and pain may result from injury. Initial treatment should consist of immobilization, cryotherapy for 10 to 20 minutes every 4 hours, and comfortable bedding. If open wounds are evident, protective bandaging should be applied. Animals should be repositioned at least every 4 to 6 hours to prevent dependent edema from forming in the limbs and to prevent lung atelectasis. If the extremities are injured, the involved limbs should be elevated above the level of the heart to promote drainage and reduce edema. Bandaging the limb can prevent or reduce edema by compressing lymphatics and blood vessels to limit fluid accumulation in the interstitium. Bandages of cast padding and reusable elastic bandage should be applied beginning with the distalmost aspect of the extremity.[8] Bandages may need to be changed several times daily to allow inspection of the area and for physical rehabilitation.

After acute inflammation has resolved, warm compresses or warm water baths may be used. If the animal is capable, restricted exercise is encouraged beginning 48 hours after the initial insult. If spinal cord or orthopedic injuries prevent the patient from ambulation, but permit movement of the limb, gentle passive ROM exercises should be initiated. The limb and all joints should be cycled through their full ROM 10 times, four to six times daily. ROM exercises may be performed in conjunction with massage therapy. If fractures are present, ROM exercises should be withheld until appropriate fixation of the fracture. After surgical stabilization of fractures, cryotherapy should be applied to reduce inflammation, pain, and muscle spasms. Following resolution of the acute inflammatory period, application of warm compresses may be beneficial to help relieve pain and muscle spasms. Passive ROM of the joints above and below the fracture site and massage therapy of the soft tissues are usually initiated 1 to 4 days after surgery if the patient permits.[14] Physical rehabilitation techniques to prevent contracture formation include encouraging ambulation, active and passive ROM exercises, and stretching affected joints and muscles. Massage may be used to break down adhesions, reduce muscle spasm, and limit edema. If severe contractures have already formed, ROM exercises can be combined with serial casting or splinting. The use of casts or splints allows joints and muscles to be stretched for prolonged periods of time. Moderate contractures may be treated by splinting the area for 20 to 30 minutes, four times daily, in conjunction with ROM exercises and massage. Severe contractures may require placement of a cast or splint for 2 to 3 days. At the end of this period, the area is reexamined, and another cast or splint is placed as necessary.

Head Trauma

Patients that have sustained head trauma may have impaired consciousness and usually benefit from both chest and musculoskeletal physical rehabilitation. Depressed consciousness may cause abnormal breathing patterns such as hyperventilation, hypoventilation, irregular respiration, or a Cheyne-Stokes breathing pattern (apnea alternating with hyperpnea). Abnormal breathing patterns may lead to reduced tidal volume, functional residual capacity, and lung compliance, allowing respiratory secretions to accumulate. Comatose or stuporous animals are unable to mobilize secretions because of depressed cough and uncoordinated swallowing mechanisms. Atelectasis due to immobility contributes to respiratory complications. Respiratory physical rehabilitation should be initiated in these patients as soon as they are stable. The therapist should assist the patient to cough and use postural drainage, percussion and vibration techniques within 48 hours of presentation or as the animal's condition permits. Care should be taken when placing these patients in a head-down postural drainage position. If increased intracranial pressure or ongoing hemorrhage are suspected, head-down positions should be avoided.

Comatose or stuporous patients often exhibit abnormal trunk and limb posture. The limbs may be held in rigid extension or flexion or may be limp. As soon as the patient's condition allows, musculoskeletal physical rehabilitation should be initiated to prevent muscle and joint contracture. A combination of frequent position changes, massage, and passive ROM exercises should be employed.

Pulmonary Contusions

Chest physical rehabilitation is frequently used in human patients with pulmonary contusions. In patients with traumatic chest injuries, chest physical rehabilitation is believed to exert its greatest effect on the smaller airways rather than the larger airways.[15,16] Before initiating chest physical rehabilitation, chest radiographs should be taken and evaluated for the presence of pneumothorax, flail chest, or rib fractures that would preclude percussion and vibration. Chest ra-

diographs should also be used to identify contused lung segments so that the therapist may choose the proper postural drainage positions and apply percussion and vibration over the appropriate area.

REFERENCES

1. Halar EM, Bell KR: Contractures and other deleterious effects of immobility. In Delisa JA, Gans BM, Bockenek WL, editors: *Rehabilitation medicine: principles and practice*, Philadelphia, 1988, JB Lippincott.
2. Spector SA et al: Architectural alterations of rat hind limb skeletal muscle immobilized at different lengths, *Exp Neurol* 76:94-110, 1982.
3. Smaldone GC, Messina MS: Flow limitation, cough, and patterns of aerosol deposition in humans, *J Appl Physiol* 59:515-520, 1989.
4. Wheeler SL: Care of respiratory patients. In Slatter D, editor: *Textbook of small animal surgery*, ed 2, Philadelphia, 1993, WB Saunders.
5. Gibb KA, Carden DL: Atelectasis, *Emerg Med Clin North Am* 2:371-378, 1983.
6. Ciesla ND: Chest physical therapy for patients in the intensive care unit, *Phys Ther* 76:609-625, 1996.
7. Frownfelter D: Postural drainage. In Frownfelter D, editor: *Chest physical therapy and pulmonary rehabilitation*, St. Louis, 1987, Mosby.
8. Manning AM, Ellis DR, Rush JE: Physical therapy for critically ill veterinary patients. I. Chest physical therapy, *Comp Cont Educ Pract Vet* 19:675-689, 1997.
9. Frownfelter D: Percussion and vibration. In Frownfelter D, editor: *Chest physical therapy and pulmonary rehabilitation*, St. Louis, 1987, Mosby.
10. Connors AF et al: Chest physical therapy: the immediate effect on oxygenation in acutely ill patients, *Chest* 78:559-564, 1980.
11. Hammon WE, Connors AF, McCaffree DR: Cardiac arrhythmias during postural drainage and chest percussion of critically ill patients, *Chest* 102:1836-1841, 1992.
12. Baldwin DR et al: Effect of addition of exercise to chest physiotherapy on sputum expectoration and lung function in adults with cystic fibrosis, *Respir Med* 88:49-53, 1994.
13. Oldenburg FA et al: Effects of postural drainage, exercise, and cough on mucous clearance in chronic bronchitis, *Am Rev Respir Dis* 120:739-745, 1979.
14. Hodges CC, Palmer RH: Postoperative physical therapy. In Harari J, editor: *Surgical complications and wound healing in the small animal patient*, Philadelphia, 1993, WB Saunders.
15. MacKenzie CF et al: Changes in total lung/thorax compliance following chest physical therapy, *Anesth Analg* 59:207-210, 1980.
16. Ciesla ND, Klemic N, Imle PC: Chest physical therapy for the patient with multiple trauma, *Phys Ther* 61:202-205, 1981.

Chapter 24

Physical Rehabilitation for Geriatric and Arthritic Patients

Robert A. Taylor, Darryl L. Millis, David Levine, Caroline P. Adamson, John Bevan, and Denis Marcellin-Little

Providing care for the aging dog has long been a challenge in veterinary medicine. Medical and surgical advances in veterinary medicine are increasing the life span of our canine companions. A variety of changes may occur over time with the aging process and can prove to be a challenge in the diagnosis and management of dogs with multiple medical conditions. Accurate assessment and diagnosis are important when designing a rehabilitation program for the geriatric patient. The patient should also be reassessed on a regular basis to design and deliver the most accurate and beneficial plan of care.

This chapter will discuss the effects of aging, medical considerations, common neurologic and musculoskeletal conditions in the aging dog, quality-of-life issues, management of pain, nutritional considerations, and general management of the arthritic patient.

Aging in Dogs

The term *geriatric* is defined as relating to elderly people. The World Health Organization defines *middle-age* as being 45 to 59 years, *elderly* as being 60 to 74 years, and *aged* as being 75 years and older.[1] No such groupings have been proposed in dogs, although Table 24-1 describes the ages at which dogs are considered to become "geriatric" and are likely to develop diseases associated with aging.[2] Aging itself is not a disease. A variety of factors, including genetics, environment, and nutrition play a role in the aging process. For example, smaller dog breeds live longer than larger breeds, and mixed-breed dogs have a longer life expectancy than purebred dogs. Obese animals have a shorter life span than nonobese animals.[3] Those dogs that are neutered live longer than those that are not neutered. Pets that live inside also live longer than those that are housed outside.[4]

There are multiple changes that occur as a result of the aging process in dogs, as outlined in Box 24-1. Most of these conditions are chronic (endocrinopathies, hepatic disease, renal disease, cardiac insufficiency) and require lifelong treatment and exceptional owner compliance. In addition, it is important for the therapist to understand the effects these diseases have on function and activities of daily living. For example, hypothyroidism may cause lethargy in the dog and could easily be mistaken for arthritis and inactivity. It is important for the owner to make routine appointments with a veterinarian for patient monitoring and modification of the treatment plan, as necessary.[4]

Common to all of these effects of aging is the fact that these changes are progressive and irreversible. These changes may be hastened by stress, environment, genetics, effects of disease, malnutrition, and lack of exercise.

Medical Considerations

The effects of aging have been documented in human beings, and similar processes are thought to occur in dogs. Quite often, owners of geriatric dogs attribute specific changes in behavior and lifestyle, such as a decreased appetite, a change in sleeping patterns, or decreased activity, to their pet becoming arthritic, or merely succumbing to old age. Although a component of these changes could be the aging process, the presence of concurrent neuromuscular or metabolic diseases

■ ■ ■ **Table 24-1** Typical Ages at Which Various-Size Dogs May Be Considered Geriatric

	Weight	Age (mean ± standard deviation)
Small dogs	0-20 lb	11.48 ± 1.86
Medium dogs	21-50 lb	10.19 ± 1.56
Large dogs	51-90 lb	8.85 ± 1.38
Giant dogs	>90 lb	7.46 ± 1.27

■ ■ ■ **BOX 24-1** Effects of Aging in Dogs

Metabolic effects
- Decreased metabolic rate
- Decreased immune competence
- Decreased phagocytosis and chemotaxis (decreased ability to ward off infections)
- Autoantibodies and autoimmune diseases develop

Physical effects
- Percentage of body weight represented by fat increases
- Skin becomes thickened, hyperpigmented, and less elastic
- Footpads hyperkeratinize and claws become brittle
- Muscle, bone, and cartilage mass are lost, with possible development of arthritis
- Lungs lose elasticity, fibrosis occurs, and pulmonary secretions become more viscous
- Vital capacity is diminished
- Cough reflex and expiratory capacity decrease
- Urinary incontinence frequently develops
- Cardiac output may decrease
- Number of cells in the nervous system decreases

should also be considered. In any aged animal, diagnosis and treatment of concurrent systemic diseases are necessary for the success of a rehabilitation program aimed at managing a disorder such as osteoarthritis (OA). The increased likelihood of multiple conditions being present in a geriatric dog warrants a thorough medical evaluation before a rehabilitation program is designed. A complete medical history, including previous medical diagnoses and treatments, may help determine the origin of the patient's primary problem and identify any previous or concurrent diseases that may affect the success of rehabilitation. In conjunction with the history, performing a thorough physical examination and obtaining a diagnostic database may confirm the presence of concurrent diseases.

Multiple disease processes in older animals, such as those listed in Table 24-2, can cause nonspecific signs that mimic or exacerbate those of other conditions, such as OA.

These signs include weakness, lethargy, and exercise intolerance. Treatment of concomitant diseases before the implementation of a rehabilitation program allows the patient to be in the best condition to appropriately respond to rehabilitation and allows the clinician to provide the most accurate prognosis. If the concurrent disease requires long-term treatment, frequent adjustments of the medical therapy and the rehabilitation program may be required to reach the goals of each treatment. For example, some of the most common systemic diseases in older animals are endocrine disorders and neoplasms. Those conditions that have associated neuromusculoskeletal involvement, such as hyperadrenocorticism, hyperparathyroidism, osteosarcoma, insulinoma, and hypothyroidism, can interfere with the implementation of a successful rehabilitation program and accurate assessment of the patient's progression during the program. Thus understanding the pathophysiologic mechanisms is important not only for the successful treatment of the concurrent disease but also for the development of a rehabilitation plan tailored to the needs and weaknesses of the individual patient. Also, constant communication between the veterinarian, therapist, and owner is required to accurately assess whether a poor or unexpected response to the program requires a change in the program itself or modification of the treatment of the concurrent disease processes.

Common Musculoskeletal and Neurologic Considerations

A list of common geriatric diseases is outlined in Box 24-2. However, the most significant systems related to rehabilitation care are the musculoskeletal and nervous systems.

Muscles and bones tend to atrophy with aging, with resultant loss of muscle and bone mass. Muscle function is diminished as a result of increasing fibrosis, muscle fiber atrophy, and reduced oxygen transport to muscles. Decreased intestinal absorption of calcium may result in decreased bone mineral content, and cartilage tends to deteriorate as a result of altered biomechanical integrity and loss of tensile strength. The most common problem of the musculoskeletal system in aged dogs is OA, with obesity compounding the effects of arthritis (Figure 24-1).[4] Osteoporosis, or reduction in the quantity of bone, is rarely clinically significant in aging dogs. The pri-

■ ■ ■ **Table 24-2**   Common Conditions of Various Body Systems in Geriatric Dogs

System	Condition
Cardiovascular disorders	Cardiomyopathy
	Endocardiosis
	Arrhythmias
	Heartworm disease
	Pericardial disease
	Systemic hypertension
	Endocarditis
Upper respiratory tract disorders	Laryngeal paralysis
	Brachycephalic respiratory syndrome
	Laryngeal/pharyngeal neoplasia
	Bronchomalacia
	Collapsing trachea
Lower respiratory tract disorders	Pneumonia
	Neoplasia (primary vs. metastatic)
	Pleural effusion
	Pulmonary edema
	Bronchitis
	Pneumothorax
Gastrointestinal disorders	Malabsorptive disease (inflammatory bowel disease)
	Protein-losing enteropathy
	Neoplasia (adenocarcinoma, lymphoma)
Hepatobiliary disorders	Hepatic parenchymal disease (chronic hepatitis, cirrhosis, neoplasia, toxic hepatitis)
	Biliary tract abnormalities (pancreatitis, bile duct neoplasia, cholelithiasis, cholecystitis)
Endocrine disorders	Hyperparathyroidism
	Thyroid neoplasia
	Insulinoma
	Diabetes mellitus
	Hypothyroidism
	Hyperadrenocorticism
	Hypoadrenocorticism
	Pheochromocytoma
	Thymoma
	Hypoparathyroidism
Urinary tract disorders	Renal failure
Hematologic and immunologic disorders	Anemia (regenerative vs. nonregenerative)
	Neoplasia (lymphoma, hemangiosarcoma, leukemia)
	Hemostatic disorders
	Immune-mediated polyarthritis
	Systemic lupus erythematosus

■ ■ ■ **BOX 24-2**   Common Geriatric Conditions in Dogs

- Diabetes mellitus
- Obesity
- Cardiovascular disease
- Degenerative joint disease
- Cataract(s)
- Cancer
- Dental disease
- Hypothyroidism
- Urolithiasis
- Hyperadrenocorticism
- Anemia
- Urinary incontinence
- Hepatopathies
- Chronic renal disease

mary importance of senile osteoporosis is its influence on fracture healing. Callus formation is slower in older animals, and fractures require additional healing time. This increases the likelihood of delayed or malunions, muscle atrophy, and disuse osteoporosis. Neoplasia involving the musculoskeletal system, though less common in some breeds of dogs, must also be considered. Malignant primary bone tumors are the most common and include osteosarcoma, chondrosarcoma, fibrosarcoma, and hemangiosarcoma (Figure 24-2).[4]

Several conditions affecting the nervous system also affect aging dogs. In addition to disk disease, degenerative conditions such as degenerative myelopathy and neoplasia may occur in older dogs (Figure 24-3). Cognitive dysfunction is a common issue in aged dogs. In addition to loss of house training, these

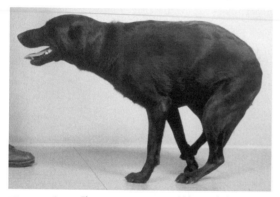

Figure 24-1 The most common problem of the musculoskeletal system in aged dogs is osteoarthritis. Dogs may have difficulty arising, and obesity compounds the effects of arthritis.

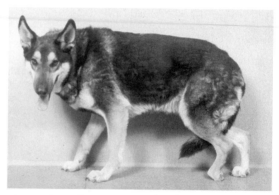

Figure 24-3 Degenerative myelopathy may affect geriatric dogs. The diagnosis is often confounded by the presence of osteoarthritis of multiple joints.

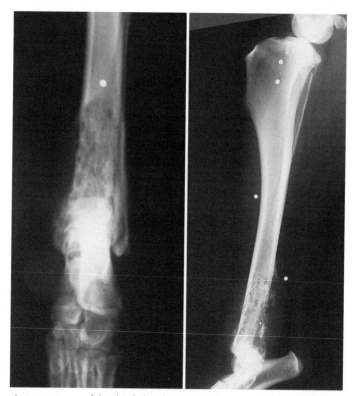

Figure 24-2 Patient with osteosarcoma of the distal tibia that may result in lameness, lethargy, and decreased appetite.

dogs may exhibit signs such as disturbances in sleep and wake cycles, inattention to food or their environment, and inability to recognize familiar people and places. Short-term memory is affected by changes in interneurons that cause a prolonged effect to a stimulus and increased response time to the external environment.[4] This condition may also affect the patient's ability to participate in certain activities of a rehabilitation program.

Maintaining Quality of Life

A geriatric screening program should be implemented as part of a general wellness program for animals 8 years and older. This will allow the veterinarian to target geriatric-related health problems, detect early geriatric disease to implement effective medical care, and offer preventive health-care measures. Client education plays a large role in this process. Owners should be instructed on the normal process of aging, nutrition, appropriate exercise, and bereavement counseling, when indicated. A questionnaire is helpful to provide a baseline for function and may be used to reassess the animal's quality of life over time (Figure 24-4).

The normal process of aging includes changes in muscle tone, hair coat and skin changes, cognitive function changes, and vision and hearing loss. These changes in patients should be assessed, recorded, and addressed as part of the overall treatment program. The initial amount of exercise in the aging dog should be that which is easily tolerated, with increasing amounts added as the rehabilitation program progresses. Low-impact exercise, such as swimming and short, frequent leash walks, should be implemented on a consistent, daily basis. Owners should be aware of changes in water or food consumption, rapid weight loss, abnormal urination or defecation, changes in activity level, and vomiting or diarrhea (Figure 24-5). When appropriate, discussions on support to the owner during the final few weeks of the animal's life and following the death of the animal should be implemented.[1]

Pain Management in the Geriatric Dog

Because aging dogs have a relatively fragile physiologic balance, pain management of geriatric dogs should rely as much as possible on therapeutic options with minimal physiologic impact. For example, geriatric people and dogs are more sensitive to the gastrointestinal side effects of antiinflammatory medications than younger people and dogs. Nonsteroidal antiinflammatory drugs should therefore be used with caution in geriatric dogs. The pain management options with minimal physiologic risks include, but are not limited to, low-impact, low-intensity exercises, massage, heat, and slow-acting disease-modifying osteoarthritic agents. In patients with severe pain, such as may be present with neoplasia, opioid drugs may be prescribed, or transcutaneous fentanyl patches may be applied for sustained delivery of medication. Although these patches may be helpful in the short term, they are rarely used over extended periods of time because of the cost and other factors involved with prolonged treatment.

Nutritional Considerations

The weight management of geriatric patients is particularly important because obesity is one of the most common conditions in geriatric patients. Because of decreased muscle mass and the possible presence of OA in geriatric dogs, excess weight may predispose aging dogs to critical and potentially irreversible ambulatory difficulties. One study has also demonstrated that a 25% restriction in food intake increased median life span and delayed the onset of signs of chronic disease in those dogs.[3] In that study, 48 Labrador retrievers were paired, with one dog in each pair fed 25% less food than its pair-mate from 8 weeks of age until death. Body composition was measured annually until 12 years of age. Compared with control dogs, food-restricted dogs weighed less and had lower body fat content and lower serum triglycerides, triiodothyronine, insulin, and glucose concentrations. Median life span was significantly longer for dogs in which food was restricted. The onset of clinical signs of chronic disease generally was delayed for food-restricted dogs.

In addition to restricting calories, adequate protein, minerals, and vitamins must also be present in the diet of the aging patient. Most high-quality commercial diets have adequate nutritional composition to support most phases of life, but some concentrate specifically on aging dogs, and these should be considered. Adequate protein is necessary to help maintain muscle mass, and it should be of adequate composition and quality to support muscle maintenance. Concurrent medical conditions, such as heart disease, renal disease, and liver disease, should also receive consideration because dietary management of these conditions is vital to successful management.

Management of the Geriatric Patient With Osteoarthritis

Joint disease is a common problem, affecting up to 20% of dogs. OA, often referred to as degenerative joint disease (DJD), is a progressive degenerative condition of joints. Many inflammatory mediators are present in OA, including interleukins, prostaglandins, and metalloproteinases. There is a progressive cascade of mechanical and biochemical events in patients with OA, which ultimately lead to cartilage destruction, subchondral bone

FUNCTIONAL QUESTIONNAIRE

Please complete the questions on this form pertaining to your pet's functional abilities to help us monitor its progress.

1 = not able to perform this activity (needs assistance 100% of the time)
2 = moderate assistance to perform activity (needs assistance >50% of the time)
3 = minimal assistance to perform this activity (needs assistance <50% of the time)
4 = independent with activity (no assistance needed)
5 = N/A

Client:_____Patient:_____Date: _____

Medications:_____

How often is (are) medication(s) given? _____

	1	2	3	4	5
1. Able to position itself to urinate?	1	2	3	4	5
2. Able to position itself to defecate?	1	2	3	4	5
3. Able to transfer from lying to sitting and vice versa?	1	2	3	4	5
4. Able to transfer from sitting to standing and vice versa?	1	2	3	4	5
5. Able to transfer from lying to standing and vice versa?	1	2	3	4	5
6. Able to roll over?	1	2	3	4	5
7. Able to scratch behind its ears?	1	2	3	4	5
8. Able to ascend stairs?	1	2	3	4	5
9. Able to descend stairs?	1	2	3	4	5
10. Able to walk up an incline/hill?	1	2	3	4	5
11. Able to get in and out of your car?	1	2	3	4	5
12. Able to get on/off a couch or bed?	1	2	3	4	5
13. Able to run?	1	2	3	4	5
14. Able to jump?	1	2	3	4	5

Figure 24-4   Functional questionnaire to assess and monitor the progress of a geriatric patient.

15. Experienced an increase or decrease in weight?	Increase	Decrease	Same
16. Experienced an increase or decrease in endurance?	Increase	Decrease	Same
17. Have you noticed a change in your pet's temperament/attitude? Y N Please elaborate:	Increase	Decrease	Same

18. What does your pet like to do for fun?
Is he/she able to do that activity? Please elaborate:
19. Has your pet been able to resume normal activities?   Y   N Please elaborate:
20. Able to go on a walk?   Y   N How long? _____ minutes Could your pet walk longer?   Y   N Does anything prevent him/her from taking longer walks?   Y   N If so, what?
21. Do you notice any problems (limping, stiffness) or are the problems worse after taking a walk?   Y   N If yes, how so?
22. Does your pet tire quickly, have to make rest stops, or lag behind during walks?   Y   N Please elaborate:

Figure 24-4   Cont'd

Continued

23. Does your pet seem to be in pain?   Y   N

What makes you think this?

24. Is there anything your pet CAN do now that it was NOT able to do before?   Y   N
Please explain:

LAMENESS SCALE		
0 = Normal stance	0 = No lameness	0 = No lameness
1 = Slightly abnormal stance (partial weight-bearing)	1 = Lameness barely perceptible	1 = Lameness barely perceptible
2 = Moderately abnormal stance (toe-touch weight-bearing)	2 = Lameness obvious, but not severe	2 = Lameness obvious, but not severe
3 = Severely abnormal stance (holds limb off the floor)	3 = Severe lameness	3 = Severe lameness
4 = Unable to stand	4 = Partial or complete non–weight-bearing lameness	4 = Partial or complete non–weight-bearing lameness

25. Does your dog walk or trot with a limp? (Please select degree of lameness according to the chart below)

Degree of lameness (standing)   Degree of lameness (walk)   Degree of lameness (trot)

Score: _____   _____   _____

26. Are there any other problems that you have noticed that have not been covered in this form?

27. Additional comments:

Figure 24-4   Cont'd

sclerosis, synovial membrane inflammation, and periarticular osteophytes.

Patients with OA have decreased quality of life, limited activity, reduced performance, muscle atrophy, pain and discomfort, and joint stiffness with decreased ROM.[5-7] As OA progresses, a vicious cycle of pain, reduced activity level, joint stiffness, and loss of strength occurs (Figure 24-6).

Veterinarians are approached frequently to treat arthritic patients. Traditional management of dogs with OA has included antiinflammatory and analgesic drugs, changes in lifestyle, and surgical management. More recent advances in the management of OA include weight loss, therapeutic exercise, and physical modalities to reduce the severity of clinical signs and the reliance on medications to control pain and discomfort.[8,9] Management of the arthritic patient involves a number of modalities and must be tailored to each patient and owner. Weight control, physical rehabilitation, and medication are the main components for OA management. Cooperation among the veterinarian, therapist, veterinary technician, and owner is vital to carry out an appropriate management program. Regular monitoring of achievements is essential to help with decision-making for further treatment and maintaining enthusiasm for the program. Some of the benefits of a complete program include increasing muscle strength and endurance, increasing joint ROM, decreasing pain, and improving performance, speed, quality of movement, and function.

Much of the pain associated with OA has been attributed to synovitis. The goal of treatment is to provide adequate analgesia to reduce the severity of clinical signs, which will allow the patient to be active and undergo therapeutic exercise and weight loss. These treatments are important to accomplish an increase in muscle strength and joint function, maintain an acceptable quality of life, control pain and discomfort, slow the progression of disease, and promote repair of damaged tissue when possible.

Surgical treatment focuses on correcting joint disease to prevent further joint degeneration. Early intervention to stabilize a cruciate ligament rupture, remove an osteochondritis dissecans lesion, repair an articular fracture, perform a triple pelvic osteotomy to reduce hip subluxation associated with hip dysplasia, and correct angular limb deformities to avoid abnormal stresses on joints are all surgical procedures that help slow the degenerative process (Figure 24-7). Salvage treatments for end-stage OA include arthrodesis of a joint,

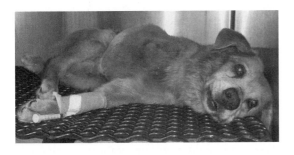

Figure 24-5   Owners should be aware of changes in water or food consumption, rapid weight loss, abnormal urination or defecation, changes in activity level, and vomiting or diarrhea, especially after a major illness or surgery. This dog developed sepsis after an amputation for osteosarcoma.

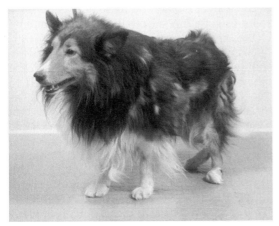

Figure 24-6   As osteoarthritis progresses, a vicious cycle of pain, reduced activity level, joint stiffness, and loss of strength occurs. The resulting weakness and pain may mimic a neurologic condition.

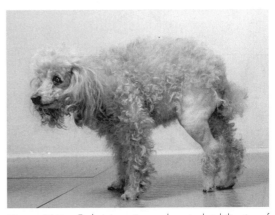

Figure 24-7   Early intervention and surgical stabilization of the stifle joint of dogs with a ruptured cranial cruciate ligament may reduce the progression of osteoarthritis.

especially the carpus and tarsus, and total hip replacement (Figure 24-8).

Medical treatment of OA is multifaceted and includes antiinflammatory medications, weight reduction, controlled exercise, physical modalities, alteration of the environment, and OA disease-modifying agents. Veterinarians must impress on owners that the management of chronic OA is a lifelong commitment and is hard work. It is critical to evaluate patients on a regular basis and provide feedback and encouragement to owners. Management of the arthritic patient should be approached in a logical, stepwise progression.

Antiinflammatory Agents

OA is classified as a noninflammatory joint disease because of the relatively low number of inflammatory cells in the synovial fluid. However, many inflammatory mediators, degradative enzymes released as a result of cell membrane injury (cytokines, leukotrienes, metalloproteinases), and inflammatory cells are intricately involved in a cascade of events leading to the deterioration of articular cartilage. Inflammatory products are produced through enzymatic action (phospholipase A2) on cell membrane phospholipids to produce arachidonic acid. Cyclooxygenase (COX) and lipoxygenase (LOX) act on arachidonic acid to produce prostaglandins, leukotrienes, and related products known as eicosanoids.

Nonsteroidal antiinflammatory drugs (NSAIDs) have been the foundation for medical management of OA, particularly in advanced cases. NSAIDs inhibit the COX enzyme, thereby decreasing inflammatory mediators and reducing pain associated with OA. Two isoforms of the COX enzyme have been identified, COX-1 and COX-2. COX-1 is a constitutive enzyme and is normally produced in physiologic amounts in many tissues. It has protective functions, such as protection of the gastric mucosa, maintaining renal perfusion, and maintaining normal platelet function. The inhibition of the COX-1 enzyme by traditional NSAIDs is believed to be responsible for the adverse side effects of gastric ulceration, prolonged bleeding time, and decreased renal perfusion.

The COX-2 enzyme is inducible, and its production increases in response to inflammation. Traditionally, NSAIDs have inhibited both COX-1 and COX-2 enzymes. The identification of the two COX isoforms has resulted in research to develop products that selectively inhibit the inducible "bad" COX-2 enzyme, while sparing the constitutive COX-1 enzyme. Selective inhibition of COX-2 with preservation of COX-1 should reduce the adverse effects associated with the GI tract and kidneys.

NSAIDs that are frequently used in veterinary medicine include deracoxib, carprofen, etodolac, meloxicam, aspirin, phenylbutazone, piroxicam, and meclofenamic acid. Acetaminophen with or without codeine is occasionally used in dogs, but should never be used in cats. COXIB-class drugs are those that are diarylheterocyclic compounds that preferentially and irreversibly bind the COX-2 enzyme and are relatively COX-1 sparing. Deracoxib is a COXIB-class drug that is approved for use in veterinary medicine. Carprofen, etodolac, and meloxicam also have some preferential selectivity to inhibit mainly COX-2.

Although no NSAID has been conclusively shown to clearly be more efficacious than the others, treatment with deracoxib resulted in the greatest increase in weight-bearing as measured with a forceplate in one study that compared a number of NSAIDs in the same dogs with mild to moderate OA of the stifle joint.[10] Some dogs did not respond to one or more drugs, and not all dogs responded to all drugs equally, but all dogs responded to at least one of the drugs. However, veterinarians are frequently reluctant to perform trial treatments to evaluate the efficacy of various NSAIDs in a particular patient to determine which provides the best clinical improvement.

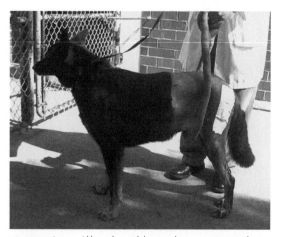

Figure 24-8   Although total hip replacement is a salvage procedure for end-stage osteoarthritis of the hip joint, dogs can have a high quality of life following surgery and rehabilitation.

Two-week trials of various NSAIDs with adequate patient evaluation should be performed to determine which medication provides the best response. A washout period between drugs is recommended if the patient will not be in excessive pain during the washout period. It is important to have the owners also evaluate the response to treatment because they may evaluate the patient in the home environment where the patient must negotiate various obstacles and situations that are not present in a veterinary clinic.

Caution must be used when using any NSAID because of the potential for side effects. Before prescribing any medication, the patient's physiologic state, especially liver and kidney function, should be assessed. It is important to educate the owners regarding potential side effects.

Certain forms of polyunsaturated fatty acids (PUFA), especially omega-3 fatty acids, may reduce the production of certain eicosanoids, especially the more potent inflammatory 5-series leukotrienes, and help reduce inflammation. Some humans with rheumatoid arthritis respond to treatment with PUFAs. Further controlled clinical trials are needed to document the role these products have in the treatment of OA. Tepoxalin is a new medication that is a lipoxygenase inhibitor, but it is also a COX-1 inhibitor.

Oral or injectable corticosteroids are frequently prescribed for patients with OA. Steroids are excellent antiinflammatory drugs and result in clinical improvement in patients. However, their use as a quick fix in lieu of other modalities should be avoided because of the possible long-term adverse effects on cartilage and other body systems. For example, glycosaminoglycan (GAG) synthesis of cartilage is reduced 30% in patients receiving prednisone. Although veterinarians may feel pressured to provide quick results, client education is critical to emphasize that management of OA is a lifetime endeavor.

Slow-Acting Disease-Modifying Osteoarthritic Agents

Agents thought to alter the course of OA are termed slow-acting disease-modifying osteoarthritic agents because it is thought that they improve the health of the articular cartilage or synovial fluid. These agents may be more beneficial in early OA than in end-stage OA. Nutraceuticals are nutritional supplements

believed to have a positive influence on cartilage health by providing precursors necessary for repair and maintenance, and they may also alter the pathophysiology of OA and its progression.

Glucosamine and chondroitin sulfate (CS) are routinely combined as disease-modifying agents. Glucosamine is a precursor to the disaccharide units of GAGs, which comprise part of the proteoglycan (PG) articular cartilage matrix. Studies have shown that glucosamine helps to improve cartilage metabolism and upregulates PG synthesis. CS is the predominant GAG found in articular cartilage. Extracellular and intracellular mechanisms are stimulated by CS to produce GAG and PG. CS also competitively inhibits degradative enzymes found in cartilage and synovium.

Polysulfated glycosaminoglycans (PSGAGs) are available and administered as an intramuscular injection. Studies have indicated that PSGAGs reduce the production of metalloproteinases and increase production of hyaluronic acid and GAGs. In addition, they improve stifle ROM, clinical use of the limb, and the health of the synovium in dogs recovering from experimental cranial cruciate ligament transection and stifle stabilization surgery.[11]

Hyaluronic acid (HA) is a nonsulfated GAG and a major component of synovial fluid and cartilage. HA is available as an intraarticular injection and helps increase synovial fluid viscosity, reduce inflammation and prostaglandin production, and scavenge free radicals. Some patients may benefit from periodic administration of HA.

Obesity

Obesity is strongly associated with the development of OA in people and likely contributes to the progression of OA in dogs.[12] For example, heavy people are 3.5 times more likely to develop OA than light people, and loss of 5 kg decreases the odds of developing OA by over 50%.[13] Additionally, weight loss results in less joint pain and a decreased need for medication to treat OA.[14] Weight reduction of 11% to 18% of the initial body weight of obese dogs resulted in significant improvement of hindlimb lameness associated with hip OA in one study.[15] Another study of obese dogs with hip dysplasia indicated that there is a significant increase in weight-bearing as measured with a force plate following weight loss. In addition, the owners felt that weight loss resulted in significant improvement in a number of areas in the home environment.[16]

In addition to restricting intake of the normal diet and eliminating treats, prescription diets are available that can help achieve and maintain ideal body weight. In general, a goal is to reduce fat composition to 20% to 25% of an animal's total body weight. Clinically, the ribs should be easily palpable, and there should be a "waist" when the animal is viewed from above and the side.

Physical Rehabilitation Modalities

It is generally believed that mild to moderate exercise and training in normal humans and dogs do not cause OA by themselves, but articular cartilage may undergo biochemical, histologic, and biomechanical changes.[17-20] Most studies of moderate running have indicated that there is no injury to articular cartilage with this form of activity, assuming that there are no abnormal biomechanical stresses acting on the joints. Heavy training programs, however, result in changes that may predispose to the development of OA.[21-23]

Controlled therapeutic exercise is a valuable, but underused, form of treatment for patients with OA. Arthritic humans participating in controlled, low-impact exercises have improved function and reduced pain and need for medication.[24,25] The goals of therapeutic exercise should be to reduce body weight, increase joint mobility, and reduce joint pain through the use of low-impact exercises designed to strengthen supporting muscles. Muscle disuse results in atrophy and weakness. Because muscles act as shock absorbers for joints, strengthening periarticular muscles may help protect joints. Mild weight-bearing exercise also helps stimulate cartilage metabolism and increases nutrient diffusion. Exercise may also increase endogenous opiate production and relieve OA pain.

An exercise program must be tailored for the condition of each patient and to each owner (Figure 24-9). An improper program could hasten the progression of OA. Overloading joints should be minimized by performing activities such as walking and swimming until weight loss occurs. Unrealistic demands placed on the owner will likely

---

Guidelines for an Osteoarthritis Home Care Program

Osteoarthritis tends to follow a course of exacerbation and remission. During a period of aggravation, do not force exercise. Low-impact exercises, such as leash walking and swimming are ideal.

One sign of osteoarthritis is stiffness, especially in the morning. Begin the day by taking time to warm up the joints. This can be done using warm water bottles, hot packs, heating wet towels in the microwave (comfortable enough for you to tolerate onyour own skin), or using a bathtub/whirlpool (~85 degrees) for 15 to 20 minutes.

Following warm-up, apply passive range of motion to the affected joints. Slowly flex and extend the joints—DO NOT force beyond a comfortable range. Fifteen to twenty SLOW repetitions are sufficient. This allows for decreased stiffness and increased motion in the joints.

Continue throughout the day taking the dog on several short walks (at least three) with long rest periods in between. Let the patient set the time and distance. Begin walking 10 to 15 minutes at a time, gradually increasing the time and length. Multiple short walks are more beneficial than 1 or 2 long walks. Note any discomfort, increased fatigue or stiffness, or refusal to go any further. Should this occur, cut the previous level of activity in half and continue from there.

Differentiate between muscle soreness and joint pain:
• Muscle soreness—painful upon palpation of muscle groups
• Joint pain—painful when flexing or extending a joint

As tolerance and endurance improve, activities to further improve mobility, reduce pain, and increase muscle strength may be added. Some ideas may be to incorporate ramps, inclines, or stairs into the walking program in incremental amounts. Once again, let the patient set the boundaries.

Following exercise, a period of cool-down is necessary. Massage and use a bag of frozen vegetables or an ice pack on the joints for 15 to 20 minutes to minimize any postexercise swelling that may occur.

No antiinflammatory medications should be given for the first day when beginning a rehabilitation program. The antiinflammatory effect may mask painful joints associated with exercise progression. After a day, if no joint pain is noticed, medications may be given 1 hour before exercise. Withhold medication again as exercise is increased to be certain that the medication is not masking excessive pain.

Osteoarthritis treatment is a lifelong commitment. If rehabilitation is discontinued, any benefits gained will likely be lost.

Figure 24-9 Sample home exercise for an arthritic patient.

decrease compliance, and the physical condition of the owner must be considered. Joint instability should be corrected before initiating an exercise program. Exercise programs must be tailored to account for the typical course of exacerbations and remissions of OA. The animal should not be forced to exercise during times of exacerbation of the arthritic condition because inflammation may increase. In preparation for exercising, warming and stretching affected muscle groups and joints during a warm-up period is recommended.[26,27] Tissue warming promotes blood flow to the area, promotes tissue and collagen extensibility, and decreases pain, muscle spasms, and joint stiffness. Heat is contraindicated if swelling or edema are present in the limb or joint. Heating agents such as moist or dry hot packs, circulating warm water blankets, and warm baths typically heat the skin and subcutaneous tissues to a depth of 1 to 2 cm. Another physical agent used for heating is therapeutic ultrasound (US). Ultrasound frequencies of 1 and 3 MHz in continuous mode produce thermal and nonthermal effects. The effects are related to the treatment time, intensity, frequency, and area being treated. Tissue heating may penetrate to 5 cm, much deeper than with superficial heating modalities. Nonthermal effects include increased cell membrane permeability, calcium transport across the cell membrane, removal of proteins and blood cells from the interstitial spaces, and nutrient exchange. Any stretching should be done during the latter part of warming or immediately after. Massage also has been used to increase blood flow to muscles to warm up the area before activity, and to decrease stiffness after activity.

Electrical stimulation of muscle also appears to be of benefit when treating dogs with OA. Transcutaneous neuromuscular stimulation (TENS) was applied to the stifle joint of dogs with experimentally induced OA. Peak vertical force was significantly increased after TENS application in these dogs.[28]

Controlled leash walking, walking on a treadmill, jogging, swimming, and going up and down stairs or ramp inclines are excellent low-impact exercises (Figure 24-10). The length of the exercise should be titrated so there is no increased pain after activity. Also, it is better in the early phases of training to provide three 20-minute sessions than one 60-minute session. Walks should be brisk and purposeful, minimizing stopping. Avoiding sudden bursts of activity will help avoid acute

inflammation of arthritic joints. Swimming and walking in water are some of the best activities for dogs. The buoyancy of water is significant and limits the impact on the joint while promoting muscle strength and tone and joint motion. Training in an underwater treadmill may increase peak weight-bearing forces by 5% to 15% after therapy, which is comparable to achievements obtained using medication in many patients (Figure 24-11).

Controlled exercise must be titrated so that there is no increase in pain after the activity. If joint pain is perceived to be greater after exercising, the length of the activity should be decreased by half. When stepping up the amount of activity, the increase should be approximately 20% and should not be stepped more than once each week. Ideally, antiinflammatory drugs should not be administered immediately before stepping up activity because it is important to determine if the level of exercise is too great and causes pain. The exercise periods should be evenly spaced throughout each day and over the entire week. Training helps maintain an ideal body weight, improves ROM, and increases muscle strength and tone, which helps to stabilize joints.

Following exercise, a 10-minute cool-down period is recommended. A slower paced walk may be initiated for 5 minutes, followed by ROM and stretching exercises. A cool-down massage may help decrease pain, swelling, and muscle spasms. Finally, cryotherapy (cold packs or ice wrapped in a towel) may be applied to painful areas for 15 to 20 minutes to control postexercise inflammation. Application of cold decreases blood flow, inflammation, hemorrhage, and metabolic rate.

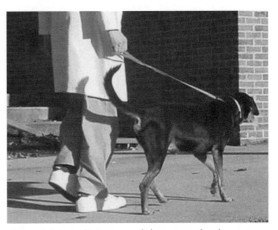

Figure 24-10 Going up and down an inclined ramp is an excellent low-impact exercise. A handicap access ramp also makes it easier to get into buildings.

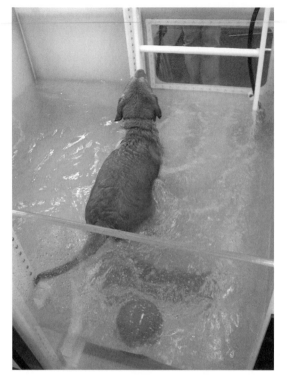

Figure 24-11   Training in an underwater treadmill may significantly increase weight-bearing comparable to achievements obtained using medication in many patients.

Environmental Modifications

Altering the environment may be helpful for dogs with moderate to severe arthritis. The principles for dogs are similar to those for arthritic humans. Whenever possible, animals should be moved from a cold, damp outdoor environment to a warm, dry inside environment. A soft, well-padded bed or waterbed should be provided. A circulating warm-water blanket under the blankets provides heat that may reduce morning stiffness. Provide good footing to avoid slipping and falling. Minimize stair climbing through the use of handicapped ramps and keeping pets on ground floors. Steps are negotiated more easily if they are wider, have a gradual rise, and are spaced farther apart. Portable ramps are available to assist patients getting in and out of vehicles. Avoid overdoing activities on the weekends, and prevent excessive play with other pets because arthritic animals may attempt to keep up, and in the process, become more lame and painful. In some instances, however, play with other animals stimulates activity and provides a welcome break in the exercise routine.

Rehabilitation for the Patient With Neoplasia

Geriatric patients with neoplasia may benefit from specific rehabilitation programs. For example, fibrosis of the skin and subcutaneous tissue may result from radiation therapy. When such fibrosis involves limb tissues, the ROM of a joint may be limited and ambulation may be more difficult. A gentle massage of the affected region and ROM exercises may help limit the impact of that fibrosis. It is particularly critical to develop a comprehensive pain management program in cancer patients because the chronic pain associated with some neoplasms negatively affects the quality of life of patients and may lead to anorexia or decreased ambulation. In addition to all the conventional strategies used for pain management, fentanyl patches may be used to provide pain relief in the short term. Palliative radiation therapy may also be used to provide pain relief in a limb with osteosarcoma. Although the majority of patients respond positively to three or four sessions of palliative radiation therapy generally spaced a week apart, the likelihood of fracture of the affected bone increases after the therapy. The rehabilitation programs of geriatric cancer patients are designed to be gentle, low-intensity exercises and manipulation to minimize the stress to the patient.

Summary

The optimal rehabilitation of geriatric patients involves a thorough initial patient assessment, focusing on the identification of underlying musculoskeletal and metabolic disorders, weight management, OA management (if necessary), environmental modifications that promote low-stress activities, and patient assessment by the veterinarian at regular time intervals to monitor patient progress.

REFERENCES

1. Hoskins JD: Geriatrics, *Vet Clin North Am Small Anim Pract* 27:1273-1614, 1997.
2. Goldston RT: Geriatrics and gerontology, *Vet Clin North Am Small Anim Pract* 19:1-202, 1989.
3. Kealy RD et al: Effects of diet restriction on life span and age-related changes in dogs, *J Am Vet Med Assoc* 220:1315-1320, 2002.
4. Goldston RT, Hoskins JD: *Geriatrics and gerontology of the dog and cat*, Philadelphia, 1995, WB Saunders.
5. Bromiley MW, Ulbrich M: *Physiotherapy in veterinary medicine*, ed 1, Oxford, 1995, Blackwell Scientific.

6. Downer AH, Spear VL: Physical therapy in the management of long bone fractures in small animals, *Vet Clin North Am* 5:157-164, 1975.

7. Millis DL, Levine D: The role of exercise and physical modalities in the treatment of osteoarthritis, *Vet Clin North Am Small Anim Pract* 27:913-930, 1997.

8. Minor MA, Gewett JE, Webel RR: Exercise and disease related measures in patients with rheumatoid arthritis and osteoarthritis. *Arthritis Rheum* 32:1396, 1988.

9. Nicholas JJ: Physical modalities in rheumatological rehabilitation, *Arch Phys Med Rehabil* 75:994, 1994.

10. Millis DL, Loonam JE, Evans M: Comparison of carprofen and etodolac for the management of stifle osteoarthritis: a pilot study, *Proc Vet Orthoped Soc Annu Mtg,* Steamboat Springs, Colo, 2003.

11. Millis DL et al: Effect of polysulfated glycosaminoglycan on articular cartilage in a Pond-Nuki model of osteoarthritis, *Vet Surg* 27:293, 1998.

12. Felson DT, Zhang Y, Anthony JM: Weight loss reduces the risk for symptomatic knee osteoarthritis in women, *Ann Intern Med* 116:535, 1992.

13. Schrager M: Slimming down reduces arthritis risk. *Physician Sportsmed* 23:22, 1995.

14. McGoey BV, Deitel M, Saplys RJ: Effect of weight loss on musculoskeletal pain in the morbidly obese, *J Bone Joint Surg* 72B:323, 1990.

15. Impellizeri JA, Tetrick MA, Muir P: Effect of weight reduction on clinical signs of lameness in dogs with hip osteoarthritis, *J Am Vet Med Assoc* 216:1089-1091, 2000.

16. Burkholder W, Hulse DA: *Signs of osteoarthritis can be improved with weight loss and exerciser,* St. Louis, 2002, Nestle Purina Pet Care.

17. Felson DT: The epidemiology of knee osteoarthritis: results from the Framingham osteoarthritis study, *Semin Arthritis Rheum* 20:42, 1990.

18. Jurvelin J et al: Effect of physical exercise on indentation stiffness of articular cartilage in the canine knee, *Int J Sports Med* 7:106-110, 1986.

19. Kiviranta I et al: Moderate running exercise augments glycosaminoglycans and thickness of articular cartilage in the knee joint of young beagle dogs, *J Orthop Res* 6:188-195, 1998.

20. Newton PM et al: The effect of lifelong exercise on canine articular cartilage, *Am J Sports Med* 25:282-287, 1997.

21. Arokoski J et al: Softening of the lateral condyle articular cartilage in the canine knee joint after long distance (up to 40 km/day) running training lasting one year, *Int J Sports Med* 15:254-260, 1994.

22. Hallett MB, Andrish JT: Effects of exercise on articular cartilage, *Sports Med Arthrosc Rev* 2:29-37, 1994.

23. McKeag DB: The relationship of osteoarthritis and exercise, *Clin Sports Med* 11:471, 1992.

24. Kovar PA, Allegrante JP, Mackenzie CR: Supervised fitness walking in patients with osteoarthritis of the knee: a randomized, controlled trial, *Ann Intern Med* 116:529, 1992.

25. Lewis C: Arthritis and exercise. In Biegel L, editor: *Physical fitness and the older person: a guide to exercise for health care professionals,* ed 1, Rockville, Md, 1984, Aspen Systems.

26. Halbertsma JP, van-Bolhuis AI, Goeken LN: Sport stretching: effect on passive muscle stiffness of short hamstrings, *Arch Phys Med Rehabil* 77:688-692, 1996.

27. Magnusson SP: Passive properties of human skeletal muscle during stretch maneuvers: a review, *Scand J Med Sci Sports* 8:65-77, 1998.

28. Johnston KD et al: The effect of TENS on osteoarthritic pain in the stifle of dogs, *Proc 2nd Int Symp Phys Therapy Rehabil Vet Med,* Knoxville, Tenn, August 2002.

■ C h a p t e r   2 5

■ Putting It All Together: Principles of Protocol Development

■ Caroline P. Adamson, David Levine, Darryl L. Millis, and Robert A. Taylor

A protocol is simply a treatment plan developed to reflect the rehabilitation needs of the patient. Although many patients receive similar injuries and surgical repairs, slightly different needs require changes in the protocol.

There are several reasons to consider developing basic protocols for common conditions and implementing them. Using an established protocol helps to standardize of treatment, allows for several people to provide the therapy, and helps to avoid omissions from a standard treatment plan. The following factors influence protocol development and are important to consider:
1. Nature of the injury
2. Type of surgical repair
3. Anticipated result and prognosis
4. Wound healing and tissue repair
5. Patient/owner compliance

Nature of the Injury

Acute injuries have different needs in a protocol because there is more inflammation and tissue damage than occur in a chronic condition. Some exercises or treatments, such as heat application, may actually increase inflammation. Conversely, heat application may be indicated in chronic conditions in which joint motion is restricted.

Tissue healing progresses through various phases, and attention must be paid to the timing of rehabilitation activities in relation to tissue healing. There are three stages of tissue healing:
1. *Inflammatory (acute) phase:* Signs include swelling, redness, pain, heat upon palpation, and loss of function. Range of motion (ROM) may result in guarding as a result of

pain. This pain arises from increased tissue swelling and tension from effusion and the presence of inflammatory mediators (histamine, prostaglandins, and bradykinins) in the tissues that irritate nerve endings. This stage begins within seconds of the initial insult and has a typical duration of 5 days.
2. *Fibroblastic (subacute) phase:* Progressively decreasing signs of inflammation occur, and pain is usually felt near end ranges of motion and when tissues are stressed beyond normal levels of tolerance. In this stage, new collagen and granulation tissue are formed and capillaries begin to grow into the injured area. Caution should be used when applying rehabilitation techniques during this stage because tissues are easily reinjured. This phase may last up to 6 weeks in tissues with low blood perfusion (e.g., tendons), but typically lasts 2 to 3 weeks.
3. *Remodeling/maturation (chronic) phase:* Inflammation has fully resolved and connective tissues begin to mature in this phase. Scar tissue remodels and is easily aligned according to lines of stress early in this stage. However, if scar maturation occurs before proper remodeling, there may be limitations in function as a result of decreased tissue mobility and extensibility. Average duration for this stage of tissue healing may be 6 months to 1 year, depending on the type of tissues involved, the age of the animal, and the severity of tissue damage.

Type of Surgical Repair

There are many options available for the surgical and nonsurgical management of most

426

orthopedic and neurologic injuries or conditions. For example, a middle-age Labrador retriever with a ruptured cranial cruciate ligament may have the stifle stabilized with one of several different techniques. These may include extracapsular stabilization with large sutures, intracapsular repair using an autograft, fibular head transposition, tibial plateau leveling osteotomy (TPLO), or, in some cases, no surgical repair. Each of the procedures progress through wound healing differently, influencing the stability of the knee and the ability to tolerate certain rehabilitation procedures. With an extracapsular repair, after the inflammation produced by the surgical procedure is resolved, the knee is stable and can undergo early rehabilitation. Intracapsular techniques using autogenous graft tissue require protection of the graft during incorporation because these tissues weaken for a period of time after surgery, and then regain some strength over a period of time.

The rehabilitation plan or protocol will differ based on the actual procedure used and the condition of the tissues and patient. For example, there may be separate protocols for TPLO recovery and extracapsular stabilization, but both plans may share many components. The actual protocol and progression of the patient may be heavily influenced by factors such as the body and cardiovascular condition of the patient, other concurrent conditions (especially the presence of cruciate ligament disease in the contralateral stifle), and the degree of osteoarthritis in the stifle. Other aspects may differ based on the actual procedure performed.

Anticipated Results and Prognosis

A particular protocol or treatment plan might be more appropriate for a field trial competitor as compared to a house pet because one patient is a competitive athlete, and the other is a more sedentary individual. The results and prognosis depend, in part, on the intended use of the patient. The prognosis for a particular injury and its surgical repair is also based on the surgeon's skill, the severity of injury, the presence and severity of any preexisting conditions, and the ability of the tissues to heal. For example, a midshaft closed tibia fracture treated with external fixation likely has a better prognosis for full recovery than a complete tear of the medial collateral ligament of the stifle.

Ideally, a complete functional return to preinjury activity is desired. A proposed grading system to measure outcome assessment is as follows:

Grade A: Return to full preinjury activity; no physical limitations; achieves owner's (realistic) expectations; no postactivity disability

Grade B: Returns to near full preinjury activity, for example, a Class A race athlete returns to Class B or C racing; some minor postactivity disability

Grade C: Occasionally able to achieve preinjury activity after significant periods of rest; some remaining disability

Grade D: Some permanent disability; activity limited to occasional recreational exercise

Grade E: Permanent disability, but is able to perform activities of daily living

Grade F: Unable to perform activities of daily living without assistance

In its most basic form, functional outcomes may also be assessed on the basis of an animal's ability to perform at a particular level or complete a daily task. The strategy of performing a task or the time taken to complete a task may also be analyzed. The relationship between impairments to functional capacity and disability must also be addressed in a patient's rehabilitation. Impairments may be easy to measure but may have little effect on an animal's ability to perform a specific function. For example, an animal may have restricted stifle flexion that does not impair its ability to trot. This restriction may, however, have a profound effect on a dog's ability to race. Subjective questionnaires given to the owner may be used to document function in the home environment. Examples of functional mobility include the ability to hold the head up, walking velocity or distance walked in a certain time, ability to groom and scratch, ascending and descending stairs, posturing for elimination, and climbing into a car or onto the couch.

Wound Healing and Tissue Repair

It is vital that wound healing be optimal and that the protocol development team understand the phases of wound healing and the tissue responses to wound healing, especially as they relate to biomechanical properties. Of equal importance is the ability to integrate the temporal aspects of tissue repair into the treatment protocol. For example, in patients with a rupture of the common calcaneal (Achilles) tendon, the limb is usually immobilized for 3 to 4 weeks before stress is applied to the repair. At that point, there is some strength to the healing structure, and gentle, controlled stress in the form of limited protected weight-bearing is allowed. Following TPLO surgery, the tibial osteotomy should undergo significant healing and the tibial tuberosity must undergo sufficient remodeling before moderate to heavy muscle strengthening can be undertaken.

Patient and Owner Compliance

It can be challenging or impossible to rehabilitate an aggressive dog or please an owner with unrealistic expectations or demands. In some situations, economic, time, or physical restrictions of the owner preclude embarking on the optimal rehabilitation protocol for a patient. For example, ROM exercises may be recommended six times daily, but a single owner working 8 hours per day cannot realistically administer these treatments. Conversely, very dedicated owners may overexercise their pets, which may increase lameness or inflammation. In most cases a rehabilitation plan can be designed for even the most challenging patient and owner, but a thorough evaluation of the patient's behavior and the owner's home situation must be performed and the limitations incorporated into an effective rehabilitation program.

The Five Stages of Protocol Development

Using a consistent method, the veterinarian and therapist should develop general rehabilitation protocols for patients with a particular medical condition and evaluate the unique features of the practice, as well as the resources available for rehabilitation, including the training of the personnel available to help with patient care (Figure 25-1).

Stage 1: Develop a Sense of the Patient Care Team's Current Statistics

It is important to determine the types of cases that are treated in the practice, the signalment of typical patients, the treatments administered, and the outcome of the patients. For example, if 10 dogs with cranial cruciate deficient stifles are presented for treatment, what is the outcome? A practice that is treating cra-

nial cruciate ligament rupture with extracapsular fabella-tibial suture stabilization, with a patient population of 20 patients treated in the past year and consisting of 80% medium to large breeds and 20% small breeds, may have different results than a practice using the same surgical procedure to treat 100 patients in the past year with a patient population consisting of 40% large breeds and 60% small breeds. How well are the patients doing at 1 week, 6 weeks, 12 weeks, and 1 year after surgery and rehabilitation? What prognosis is typically given to the owner? In stage 1 of protocol development, it is important to objectively evaluate the various types of cases that are treated and the typical outcome. For example, some specialty practices may handle more complicated cases that have somewhat less complete recovery than would be expected with routine cases. Although recovery statistics published by others can be useful, it is important to objectively examine your own results. This will help identify areas for improvement and help define the treatment plan for a patient.

Stage 2: Establish Outcome Goals

Based on the injury, form of treatment, and follow-up, establish outcome goals for the procedures performed in your hospital. For example, one goal would be for a patient that has had tibial plateau leveling osteotomy surgery for cranial cruciate ligament rupture to be rehabilitated and ready for competition 12 weeks after surgery. More specifically, goals throughout the rehabilitation program might take into account milestones throughout the program, such as toe touching with ambulation at the time of suture removal, grade 2 weight-bearing lameness 1 month after surgery, full use of the limb with only a grade 1 lameness when rising in the morning 3 months after surgery, and full use of the limb at 6 months.

Another example of an outcome goal would be to have a patient with an intervertebral disk rupture and no motor function, but good deep pain perception, be able to stand, ambulate with assistance, and urinate on its own within 4 weeks after surgery.

Stage 3: Examination of Capabilities and Resources

In this stage, the available resources and the rehabilitation team are evaluated and developed. Adequate funding and other resources, such as space and equipment, that can be com-

Stage 1. Analysis of the patient care team's current statistics of recovery.

Procedure:_____

Patient population:_____

Number of cases and years treatment performed:_____

Percentage of patients with:

Excellent_____ Good_____ Fair_____ Unacceptable_____
outcomes.

Stage 2. Establish outcome goals.

Goal 1:_____

Goal 2:_____

Goal 3:_____

Stage 3. Examination of capabilities and resources.

Space considerations:_____

Personnel available for rehabilitation:_____

Present equipment:_____

Future equipment purchases:_____

Stage 4. Individual patient assessment.

Medical disease requiring rehabilitation and its medical/surgical treeatment:_____

_____

Physical examination:_____

Rehabilitation evaluation:_____

Documentation:_____

Stage 5. Development of a specific patient protocol.

Patient and procedure:_____

Rehabilitation outcome goal(s)/owner's goal(s):_____

Rehabilitation capabilities and resources:_____

Patient current assessment:_____

Patient protocol:_____

Figure 25-1   Five stages of protocol development.

mitted to the effort must be identified. Basic supplies, such as hot packs and cold packs and a space to perform therapeutic exercises, are essential. A neuromuscular electrical stimulation unit and therapeutic ultrasound unit are also valuable pieces of equipment. A ground treadmill and therapy pool allow a great deal of rehabilitation possibilities. The most valuable resource may be the person performing the therapy.

The person(s) who will provide the therapy (physical therapist, physical therapist assistant, veterinarian, or veterinarian technician) must be identified. Personnel must have appropriate training and the desire to provide animal rehabilitation. There should be adequate time provided for rehabilitation services, and the therapist should not become burdened with other duties that interfere with rehabilitation. Having a dedicated person(s), adequate space, and equipment will ensure that a credible and regular program will be developed and implemented. For example, using a veterinary technician when he/she is not busy in surgery to provide physical rehabilitation usually does not work well. One can begin the most basic aspects of physical rehabilitation with a full-time or part-time dedicated person in the practice (PT, PTA, DVM, Veterinary Technician) and add personnel, equipment, and modalities as the effort grows.

Stage 4: Patient Assessment

This is an extremely important stage and reflects the uniqueness of each patient afflicted with the same condition as another patient. The American Physical Therapy Association's Guide to Practice (2001) describes the integration of five major elements of patient management. These elements include examination, evaluation, diagnosis, prognosis, and intervention. Keeping these elements in mind, the ultimate goal of these guidelines is to provide the best quality of care for each patient. Appropriate patient assessment allows the treatment team to choose the most appropriate plan of care and to maximize the patient's outcome.

Examination refers to the thorough screening of a patient and includes the history, appropriate tests, and review of body systems. Evaluation is the clinical judgment made by the physical therapist based on the history and examination. A physical therapy diagnosis is directed more at neuromusculoskeletal deficiencies than at a specific medical condition or disorder. For example, a veterinarian's medical diagnosis may be a ruptured cranial cruciate ligament, while the therapist may make a physical therapy diagnosis of muscle atrophy, movement dysfunction, and pain and inflammation. A prognosis is a prediction of the level of expected improvement and how long it will take to reach those levels. Goals are established as part of the plan of care along with expected outcomes, level of predicted improvement, and interventions to be used, including duration and frequency. The interventions are the actual treatment techniques and procedures used to improve a patient's condition, based on the diagnosis. It is especially important to consider whether the condition is an acute presurgical condition or a chronic injury in which various tissues have already undergone deleterious changes. The steps in patient assessment are listed:

1. *The nature of the condition and surgical repair, if applicable:* There are different rehabilitation demands for extracapsular stabilization procedures for cranial cruciate ligament rupture as compared to the tibial plateau leveling osteotomy procedure. For example, the person(s) providing the rehabilitation must be aware of the date of surgical repair, the severity of the condition, and the method of repair for each patient.

2. *Physical examination:* It is important to evaluate each patient's general health status. A 24-lb inactive obese diabetic patient may have a greater incidence of postoperative problems and delayed wound healing, for example.

3. *Rehabilitation evaluation:* It is important to perform a thorough, objective assessment to allow the therapist to develop an appropriate rehabilitation protocol and to chart patient progress. Goniometry, limb circumference, wound healing, ROM, gait analysis, and other parameters are used to assess the patient. This level of assessment is necessary to properly identify rehabilitation problems and help to eliminate treatment failure. Reevaluation at regular intervals, coupled with a knowledge of the expected and appropriate response to treatment, helps to set a reasonable timeline for return to function. For example, if a patient is slow to recover from a condition, one should be suspicious of an inappropriate treatment protocol for that particular procedure or, perhaps more important, the development of a new condition or complication or a missed diagnosis. As with all evidence-based practice, it is our responsibility to perform a thorough evaluation and to provide appropriate, effective, and comprehensive quality of care to our animal patients, as well as a reasonable prognosis for the owner.

4. *Documentation:* Each portion of the patient assessment and protocol implementation should be documented. This provides a legal record of patient evaluation and treatments performed, is useful to track the progress of the patient or lack thereof, and allows for more than one person to provide

the rehabilitation without question of what treatments have been performed to date. By measuring, assessing and reevaluating, the therapist is able to determine how the animal is progressing or regressing and change the treatment plan as appropriate. Is the chosen intervention nearing the outcome goals? Are changes in the plan of care necessary? This information is vital when improving or changing protocols, while providing evidence of the benefits to the patient and justifying the continued need for treatment to the owner. Documentation chronicles objective data for teaching and research, charts patient progress or lack thereof, provides continuity of care, addresses medical-legal issues, and displays proof of success.

Stage 5: Specific Patient Protocol

Using the information previously developed, a customized protocol can be designed and implemented for each patient. Because of differences in underlying medical conditions and patient characteristics, it is inappropriate to have a strict chronologically based protocol to increase activities and exercises. Rather, it is best to have increases in activity based on the achievement of certain milestones, such as touching the limb to the ground.

In addition, minimal and maximum tolerances to milestone-based progression of the patient must be estimated, based on the stage of tissue healing and the typical responses of average patients. For example, even if a dog is trotting with minimal lameness 8 days after extracapsular stabilization of a cranial cruciate ligament rupture, step 5 activities are not initiated because the stage of tissue healing is not advanced enough to withstand the additional stresses of these activities. Conversely, some patients require some encouragement and prodding to advance to higher levels of performance. Progress that is too slow may result in excessive fibrosis of periarticular structures, joint stiffness, and muscle atrophy. If there is no pain, pathologic reason, or complications to result in delayed progression, some increase in the level of activity may be in order.

Sample Protocol

1: Patient and Procedure

The patient is a 7-year-old hunting/athletic female Labrador retriever with rupture of the cranial cruciate ligament.

A tibial plateau leveling osteotomy was performed. The anticipated surgical results are a healed osteotomy in 7 to 9 weeks.

2: Outcome Goal

This dog is a candidate for Master Hunter with an anticipated return to competition in 12 weeks.

3: Rehabilitation Capabilities and Resources

Currently the practice has a veterinary technician dedicated to rehabilitation and a physical therapist available for consultation. In addition, the practice has heat and cold modality capabilities, an exercise area, and neuromuscular electrical stimulation.

4: Patient Assessment

The dog is a middle-aged healthy female Labrador retriever.

Initial limb assessment indicated a 6-cm difference in limb circumference between the affected and unaffected sides, a painful scar, and mild joint effusion. There was subjective muscle atrophy of the semimembranosus, semitendinosis, and quadriceps muscle groups.

5: Patient Protocol

First week: Emphasis on antiinflammatory control
- Passive range of motion (PROM) and ice packs to the region of the incision tid
- Gentle massage of the limb sid
- Short leash walks at a very slow gait on a flat surface three times daily

Second week: Emphasis on early limb use
- ± Ice packs and PROM, scar massage
- Neuromuscular electrical stimulation of the hamstring and quadriceps muscle groups
- Leash walks for 10 minutes twice or three times daily
- Begin sit-to-stand exercises

Third week: Emphasis on improved limb use
- Patient is reassessed
- Sit-to-stand exercises continue
- Leash walks 20 to 40 minutes ± use of leg weights
- Decline walking (walking down a gentle slope) if possible

Fourth and fifth weeks: Emphasis on muscle strengthening

- Continued muscle strengthening and development with sit-to-stand exercises and short episodes of trotting
- Leash walks for 20 to 40 minutes twice daily with proprioception redevelopment (unbalance while walking)

Sixth week: Emphasis on muscle-specific therapeutic exercises

- Reassessment of stability and limb
- Muscle-specific therapeutic exercise, such as incline walking, stairs, swimming, figure-eight walking and jogging, dancing

Tenth to twelfth weeks

- Reassessment and release from rehabilitation program

Development of a Canine Rehabilitation Facility

Paul Shealy

Although there are many factors that have contributed to the recent interest and popularity of veterinary rehabilitation, awareness of the merits of physical rehabilitation by the pet-owning public and their demand for more of these services has largely driven the emergence of this endeavor. The evolution of the status of pets in the household and the growing demand by pet owners for advanced care have promoted the expansion of veterinary services. The educated public knows the value of optimal medical services for human beings and expects similar if not better care for their pets. Small animal physical rehabilitation is an exciting, developing field of veterinary medicine. Interestingly enough, humans have served as models for animal rehabilitation, and the value and efficacy of physical therapy is well documented in the medical literature for humans. Recent and ongoing veterinary scientific research documents the benefits of small animal physical rehabilitation. It is now clear to those engaged in providing veterinary rehabilitation that historical postoperative and conservative management protocols are suboptimal. The advent of incorporating physical rehabilitation into veterinary practice is the result of the pursuit of optimal animal care. The differences in clinical outcomes are exhibited by the patient, are perceived by the owner, and are progressively being recognized by the veterinary profession.

Considerations

The decision to engage in providing new services in practice follows a feasibility study. To determine if establishing rehabilitation services is feasible, a number of important factors

should be considered. The feasibility study should include at least the following factors:

■ *Patient survey:* It is important to establish a need for this service. The practice should determine the projected numbers of cases of musculoskeletal trauma, neurosurgical cases, and other conditions for which rehabilitation should be indicated. One should establish a minimum number of patients per day in order to justify a full-time effort.

■ *Cost assessment:* The costs of the new facility or equipment, including purchase, setup, marketing, and advertising costs, should be included.

The mission and size of a practice may be a consideration. Progressive practices already offering advanced medicine and surgery to which their clientele have become accustomed may find layering on additional compatible services consistent with continued growth. Although preexisting services may aid in providing additional services, professional and technical staff must be willing to embrace new concepts. The profile of the practice must also be able to provide the cases amenable to physical rehabilitation. General practices with a reputation for orthopedic and neurologic services, and referral centers composed of board-certified surgical and neurological specialists, would be expected to generate an appropriate caseload for physical rehabilitation.

The profile of the owner is as important as the practice profile. Owner compliance includes the owner's commitment to either inpatient or outpatient rehabilitation of the pet as well as the additional costs for these services. In our experience, owner compliance has not been an issue even after the costs of diagnostic and surgical procedures. Owners inherently value the concept of physical

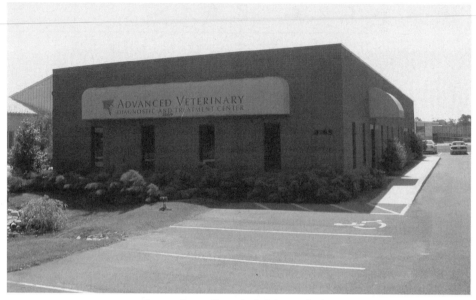

Figure 26-1   Physical rehabilitation facility.

rehabilitation, client compliance depends on proper communication of therapeutic protocols by the attending veterinarian. Overall, owners' perception of value is high for physical rehabilitation when they are informed of the availability of these services and properly educated.

The expected support of the veterinary community through direct referrals to a physical rehabilitation center is an important consideration for the professional and financial support of a facility. Gaining the confidence and support of other practices requires professional due diligence, the acceptance of a new and developing field by colleagues, and trust that patients will return to their practice at the termination of their rehabilitation care.

A crucial consideration is cost. The costs include time, education, design and preparation of existing facilities, physical plant expansion or construction, equipment purchase, staffing, marketing, and other factors. The capital outlay for this venture is in direct proportion to the size and scope of services that the center wishes to provide. As with all services provided in practice, a return on investment should be recognized if physical rehabilitation is not to be considered an added-value service or loss leader. The notoriety of establishing physical rehabilitation services should not prevail over standard proforma financial assumptions or expectations.

In order for veterinary rehabilitation to survive as a stand-alone entity, it must produce a positive cash flow and should be more than a loss leader or a revenue-neutral venture. There should be at least an 18% profitability ratio to justify the effort.

Competency in the science and application of physical rehabilitation is a prerequisite to providing legitimate rehabilitation services. The time involved in developing legitimate competency may be a barrier to establishing a facility. Recruitment of personnel trained in human physical therapy is ideal and provides the necessary staffing as well as a means of cross-training existing personnel as support staff.

Space is almost always a limiting factor in veterinary facilities. Extra, nonproductive space is often not present in existing veterinary facilities. Whether existing space is available or additional space is generated through renovation or separate facility construction, the same professional appearance and appeal required of progressive, traditional veterinary facilities should be considered. Additionally, function should follow appearance. To provide adequate rehabilitation services, a reception and waiting area, patient assessment area, treatment area including room for aquatic equipment, patient housing (particularly for in-house cases), an outdoor exercise area for office space, storage, and owner parking must be considered (Figures 26-1 to 26-7).

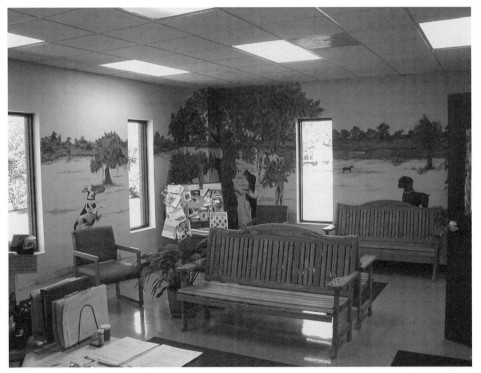

Figure 26-2   Combined reception and waiting area.

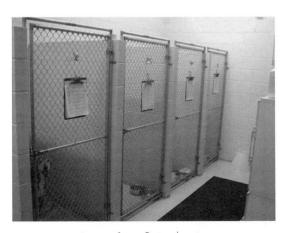

Figure 26-3   Patient housing.

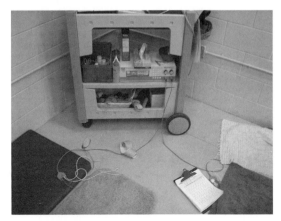

Figure 26-4   Patient assessment area.

Rehabilitation Staff

Physical therapy programs for humans generally provide little or no instruction in nonhuman anatomy or treatment, and the curricula of veterinary schools do not typically include instruction in physical rehabilitation practices. Therefore it is essential that these two fields communicate and collaborate to provide appropriate veterinary care. Both the American Veterinary Medical Association (AVMA) and the American Physical Therapy Association

(APTA) officially address the practice of veterinary physical rehabilitation. In a position statement the AVMA states, "Veterinary physical therapy performed by a non-veterinarian should be performed under the supervision of, or referral by, a licensed veterinarian who is providing concurrent care." The APTA states that the association "endorses the position that physical therapists may establish collaborative, collegial relationships with veterinarians for the purpose of providing physical therapy services or consultation. Physical therapists are the provider of choice for the provision of physical therapy services regardless of the client."

Each state has its own veterinary and physical therapy practice acts that must be adhered to. Obtaining a written practice act for each field is essential to ensure that the rehabilitation staff in the state where the clinic is located meets all legal guidelines. Some physical therapy practice acts use the word "humans" to describe the clients a physical therapist may treat. In these states, the physical therapist should contact the state board to obtain further information and advice regarding veterinary physical rehabilitation.

To establish a rehabilitation staff, a veterinarian and physical therapist are necessary. The veterinarian must provide a diagnosis for the patient and refer potential patients to a physical therapist. Physical therapists are trained in physical evaluation and treatment of human beings. Additional knowledge of variations in animal anatomy should be obtained through self-study or continuing education programs. Evaluations of new patients and establishing a treatment plan should be performed by the veterinarian and physical therapist. Hiring a full-time physical therapist or having one available on a consultation basis is essential. After a physical therapist establishes a treatment plan, the therapist or a physical therapist assistant, who is generally qualified to perform most treatments, ensures the proper delivery of modalities such as ultrasound, electrical stimulation, heat, and cryotherapy. It would be appropriate for the consulting physical therapist to reevaluate the patient every week, or if the patient does not follow the typical course of rehabilitation, to determine if a change in treatment should be made.

Alternatively, veterinarians may obtain a physical therapy degree to provide necessary services. A certified veterinary technician may be beneficial in providing rehabilitation by adding his or her knowledge of animal anatomy, medications, and disease processes. The technician could be an excellent reference for the physical therapist for day-to-day issues with patients.

For patients that stay at the facility (inpatients) during their rehabilitation treatment, ancillary staff will be needed to care for basic needs such as walking, feeding, and the delivery of medications. Veterinary technicians, assistants, or kennel personnel skilled in the handling of postsurgical and painful animals are best suited for this care.

When scheduling, answering phones, and daily paperwork become excessive for the current staff, an additional receptionist should be considered. Using existing office staff for this purpose may be cost effective.

Equipment

The most important tools for a therapist are the hands they use to evaluate and treat patients. Especially in the treatment of animals, therapists must be gentle and yet exploratory in their palpation of the patient. They also must be reassuring and safe when handling these patients.

An initial challenge for most rehabilitation efforts is equipment selection and purchase. It is advisable to purchase core equipment, then add new devices as the practice grows.

Basic Equipment

- Goniometry/tape measure
- Cold/heat packs
- Ultrasound/electrical stimulation devices
- Therapeutic exercise equipment
- Treadmill
- Aquatic device
- Stairs

Rehabilitation efforts can begin with very little equipment. Passive range of motion (PROM), massaging, icing, heating, many other therapeutic activities, and gait training may all be accomplished without much expense. Ice packs, frozen packaged peas, or water frozen in a Styrofoam cup, hot packs or a wet towel warmed in a microwave, and a therapeutic mat are basic equipment to get started. To document a thorough evaluation, a tape measure and goniometer are useful. Some patients may be aggressive with treatment, and therefore a muzzle should be

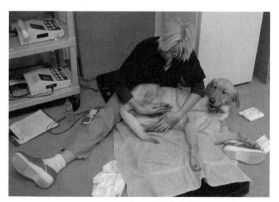

Figure 26-5   Physical rehabilitation.

employed when trying new modalities or activities on patients, especially on patients known to be aggressive.

To be able to work with animals that are unable to create a muscle contraction or require strengthening of a particular muscle group, a neuromuscular electrical stimulation device is an important purchase. To elicit a muscle contraction, a small neuromuscular electrical stimulator (NMES) may be used. If the goal is to provide pain relief, a transcutaneous electrical nerve stimulator (TENS) may be effective. Some companies make electrical stimulation machines that have the ability to deliver multiple waveforms from one piece of equipment. These machines are ideal and can be purchased with more than one channel to allow multiple areas to be stimulated. Along with the machines, electrode pads and ultrasound gel will be needed to deliver the modality to the patient.

An ultrasound machine is useful to accelerate healing in newly injured or postoperative patients. It may also be used to provide deep heating to muscles or joint capsules, and also for more effective stretching of tissues. Ultrasound may also be effective in the treatment of tendinitis and bursitis.

When a patient is treated soon after surgery or injury, weight-bearing activities may be limited so that the healing of tissues is not compromised. To continue strengthening, a pool or other body of water used for aquatic activities is recommended. The buoyancy provided by the water also makes exercise easier for animals that have pain with weight-bearing. The patient can move its legs through a greater range of motion than is tolerable with land activities. Ideally, the water temperature should be maintained between 85° and 90° F. Some patients may have difficulty swimming and may require assistance or a flotation vest for support.

An underwater treadmill is another aquatic modality for rehabilitation of patients. The underwater treadmill allows the animal to work on ambulatory skills with the benefit of reduced weight-bearing. The animal ambulates against the resistance of water, which can increase muscle strength, while moving the legs through a normal gait sequence that carries over to walking abilities.

Another valuable piece of aquatic equipment is a heated whirlpool. Placing the patient in heated water allows for the heating of a large number of sites simultaneously. This provides sensory analgesia and increased tissue elasticity. If larger dogs are treated, a hoist with sling is useful to lift the patient into the whirlpool and support it at the appropriate level in the water.

A land treadmill is useful in providing a stable walking surface for ambulatory patients. Inclines may be adjusted to increase the difficulty, target certain muscle groups, and increase the load on the hindlimbs.

Less costly equipment that is useful in rehabilitation includes walking slings, cuff weights to add resistance, thermal wraps, inflatable cuffs (water wings), theraband for strength training, a backpack to add weight for limb placement and strengthening, physioballs and physiorolls for therapeutic activities, cavaletti rails for limb placement, balance board for therapeutic activities, and a pull cart with harness for resistance with ambulation.

If the patients are boarding at the facility, including outpatients, kennels or cages will be required. An appropriate waiting area for owners requires space and furnishings.

Documentation should be kept up to date and forms will be necessary for evaluations, daily treatments, home care instructions for owners, and notes to doctors informing them of procedures performed and results attained.

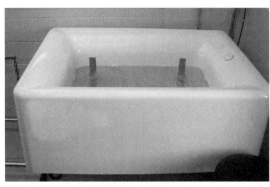

Figure 26-6 Whirlpool.

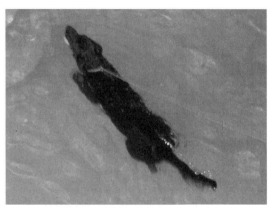

Figure 26-7 Aquatic therapy.

Costs

As with any new service or business, there are startup, fixed, and variable costs. These include facility, equipment and furnishings, staff, administrative, utilities, supplies, and marketing costs.

Modifying or using existing square footage, construction of additional square footage, or designing and constructing a free-standing building may provide the facility to house physical rehabilitation. The scope of rehabilitation services will determine the required space. The cost of construction varies geographically and cannot be accurately estimated in this chapter. Obviously, costs are greatest for designing and building a free-standing facility. For our facility, a recently constructed building was leased, and the interior finishing was performed by subcontract labor at our expense and under our supervision.

Payroll costs vary based on the type and number of employees. Small animal physical rehabilitation is more labor-intensive than human physical therapy, and this must be considered. Professionals trained in human physical therapy may be willing to accept lower remuneration consistent with the economic realities of the veterinary profession. However, consulting physical therapists charge by the hour and may be $30.00 per hour or higher. Daily rates may be negotiated if a contracted number of days can be established that would equate with budgeted labor costs. Compensation for a full-time physical therapist may range from $35,000 to $50,000 plus benefits (12% to 27% of salary). Compensation for a full-time physical therapist assistant may range from $25,000 to $27,000 plus benefits. A compensation package for a full-time veterinarian trained in physical rehabilitation would be expected to be $30,000 to $50,000 plus benefits. Certified veterinary technicians may be trained to provide some therapy, but assisting the therapist or therapist assistant with care with a growing or large caseload would best maximize the use of these staff members. Also, separate or shared assistants, kennel help, and a receptionist may be beneficial to operate the facility. The compensation for these staff members varies regionally.

Administrative costs will be commensurate with the size and intensity of the rehabilitation facility. The founder or owner of the facility may choose to perform these duties, or the use of existing staff already engaged in these duties may prove satisfactory and cost effective. The therapist may provide some or all of these duties, and compensation could be based on profit sharing as an incentive to key staff. Associated costs include computer hardware and software.

In an existing or expanded facility, the utility costs can be allocated to physical rehabilitation by estimation or calculated based on the increase in actual costs. In a separate or free-standing facility these costs would be actual costs. Depending on the services provided, water for hydrotherapy and electricity for heating water will substantially alter the utility costs. Telephones are essential, and Internet services are also highly desirable.

Supplies required are similar to other businesses and include office supplies and supplies unique to providing veterinary physical rehabilitation services, including but not limited to ultrasound gel, electrical stimulation pads, documentation forms, textbooks and other educational items, uniforms, pool chemicals, paper and janitorial products, and disinfectants. Miscellaneous but related costs include a working relationship or service contract with pool professionals for care of aquatic equipment.

Marketing is an important foundation to introduce new services. The development of a logo to project an image is the basis for producing business cards and stationary with letterhead. These can be developed and produced inexpensively with specific computer software. Professionally designed and produced materials may cost several thousand dollars. Brochures highlighting the facility and the merits and application of physical rehabilitation can also be produced inexpensively with specific computer software. Professionally designed and produced brochures may be more costly, but image is very important and the additional costs may be justified. Using the local media to produce press releases can be beneficial to educate the public and promote the merits of physical rehabilitation for small animals. Open-house events are a creative mechanism to showcase the facility and educate veterinary colleagues and the pet-owning public. Continuing education lectures by veterinary and physical therapy staff should be developed and given to veterinarians, as well as to dog clubs, enthusiasts, and associations. Production of videos for owners and veterinarians is an excellent marketing and educational strategy. In our facility, certificates for completing physical rehabilitation, including digital images of the patient engaged in therapy, are provided to owners. Other promotional ideas have included bandanas and leashes displaying the facility logo. Together these items foster owner satisfaction and thus promotion through their interaction with other pet owners.

Projections

As with any business venture, a business, plan, including projections of income and expenses, is an intelligent, sound practice. The development of fees for services not traditionally provided by the profession must be done without historically proven accessions. Regional differences in the costs and expectations of veterinary care will directly influence fee schedules. Income sources are derived from patient evaluation and protocol development by the physical therapist, charges for therapeutic modalities, medical boarding of patients, and ancillary charges such as disposables, drug administration, and additional care that is required. Treatment protocols can be charged on an itemized basis, or therapy packages can be developed to include both surgery and rehabilitation over a specific time.

Expenses include direct, general, and administrative expenses, as well as interest expense and depreciation/amortization. Direct expenses are composed of therapist, therapist assistant, and technician salaries and supplies. General and administrative expenses include payroll taxes, rent, utilities, and miscellaneous expenses.

Standard accounting principles are used to determine profit/loss statements and subsequent cash flow statements. These may be simple P/L statements or produced in a more complex form to provide a better understanding of operations.

Outcome Assessment

Measurements taken at intervals during treatment are the best source of outcome assessment. The information obtained during an initial evaluation will help determine the best course of action for the rehabilitation program of each patient, and reassessment on a timely basis will help guide treatment and create outcome data.

Some objective measurements that can be made include limb girth to measure either swelling or overt muscle mass, goniometric measurements of joint motion, circumference and depth of wounds, and weight-bearing by using scales, a force plate, observation, or pressure on soft surfaces.

Various scales have been created to help evaluate patients, including a neurologic patient grading scale, orthopedic lameness scales, and pain assessment scales. The numeric scores of these scales are used to assess and reassess patients and can be used to monitor progress. Subjectively assessing the patient's overall attitude throughout treatment can also indicate improvement.

Creating an evaluation form that addresses assessment criteria and other pertinent patient information will ensure that the desired criteria are adequately monitored and appropriate data are collected during the rehabilitation process. These measurements also create data for possible clinical studies and research projects, and they provide information regarding the efficacy of animal rehabilitation. In our facility, we provide each owner with a form to evaluate the facility, staff, services, and the owner's perceived benefit of physical rehabilitation to the pet.

Reflections on Small Animal Rehabilitation

The field of veterinary rehabilitation is dynamic, but the future is uncertain. A number of compelling issues need resolution. These include the following:

■ Developing a working relationship between the AVMA and APTA
■ Developing guidelines regarding who performs and provides rehabilitation
■ Encouraging veterinarians and veterinary surgeons to use rehabilitation in their practices
■ Allowing rehabilitation to develop as a "stand-alone" profit center in veterinary medicine

Owner compliance for physical rehabilitation remains very high. In fact postoperative physical rehabilitation for orthopedic and neurologic patients is the standard of care at our facility. Owners inherently value physical rehabilitation and understand the need for these services in the care and rehabilitation of their pets. Complementary to compliance, owner satisfaction is extremely high, based on direct interaction with owners and the results of the owner evaluation forms. Patient care and recovery have reached higher levels of achievement with greater staff involvement. Additionally, the associated professional staff promote the expansion of staff knowledge regarding physical rehabilitation.

Milestones in the continued development of small animal physical rehabilitation include a more global acceptance by the veterinary profession, scientific publications establishing credibility of rehabilitation in animals, and promoting the use of physical rehabilitation for conditioning and weight loss presurgically and postsurgically and for nonsurgical orthopedic and neurologic cases.

The future and continued development of veterinary physical rehabilitation is very exciting. As the benefits of physical rehabilitation steadily accumulate and are acknowledged, those patients entrusted to the care of the veterinary profession will benefit. Establishing a veterinary physical rehabilitation facility is not for everyone, but it is the responsibility of the profession to accept scientifically based and documented treatments that improve the quality of life of animals.

Joint Motions and Ranges

Joints	Joint motions	Normal range of motion for dogs (degrees)
Forelimb Joints		
Shoulder (including scapular motion)	Flexion	30-60
	Extension	160-170
	Abduction	40-50
	Adduction	40-50
	Internal rotation	40-50
	External rotation	40-50
Elbow	Flexion	20-40
	Extension	160-170
	Hyperextension or overextension	
Radioulnar	Pronation	40-50
	Supination	80-90
Carpus (Wrist)	Flexion	20-35
	Hyperextension	190-200
	Radial or medial deviation	5-15
	Ulnar or lateral deviation	10-20
Hip	Flexion	55
	Extension	160-165
	Abduction with a flexed hip	120 (Stifle at 90)
	Adduction with a flexed hip	65 (Stifle at 90)
	Abduction with an extended hip	85
	Adduction with an extended hip	63
	Internal rotation	55
	External rotation	50
Stifle (knee)	Flexion	45
	Extension	160-170
Talocrural, tarsocrural, ankle	Flexion	40
	Extension	170

NOTE: Presently, the tendency is to call the straight joint position 180° rather than 0° being established. Range of motion is expressed in degrees unless noted otherwise.

Goniometry of the Forelimb and Hind Limb

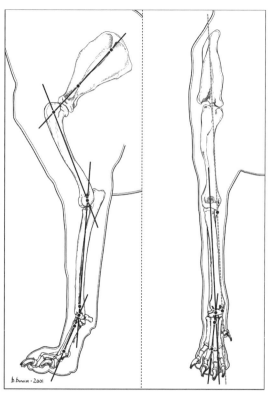

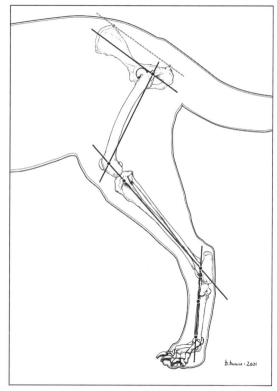

Figure 1   Goniometry of the forelimb. Carpal flexion and extension are measured as the angles formed by the long axis of metacarpal bones III and IV and the line joining the cranial to caudal midpoint of the antebrachium at the level of the ulnar styloid process and the lateral humeral epicondyle. Elbow flexion and extension are measured as the angles formed by the line joining the cranial to caudal midpoint of the antebrachium at the level of the ulnar styloid process and the lateral humeral epicondyle and a line joining the lateral epicondyle to the point of insertion of the infraspinatus muscle on the greater tubercle of the humerus. Shoulder flexion and extension are measured as the angles formed by the line joining the lateral humeral epicondyle and the point of insertion of infraspinatus muscle and the spine of the scapula. Carpal varus and valgus are measured as the angles formed by the long axis of metacarpals III and IV and the long axis of the medial border of the radius.

Figure 2   Goniometry of the hind limb. Tarsal flexion and extension are measured as the angles formed by the long axis of metatarsal bones III and IV and the long axis of the tibial shaft. Flexion and extension of the stifle joint are measured as the angles formed by the long axis of the tibial shaft and the line joining the lateral femoral epicondyle and greater trochanter. Hip joint flexion and extension are measured as the angles formed by the line joining the lateral femoral epicondyle of the femur and greater trochanter and a line joining the tuber sacrale and Ischiadicum

The figures and Table 1 used by permission from Jaegger G, Marcellin-Little DJ, Levine D: Reliability of goniometry in Laborador retrievers, *Am J Vet Res* 63: 979-986, 2002

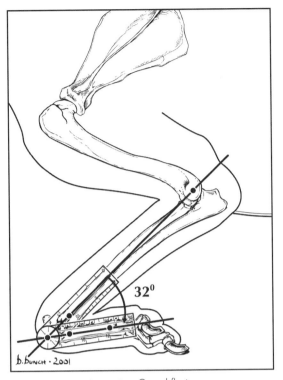

Figure 3   Carpal flexion.

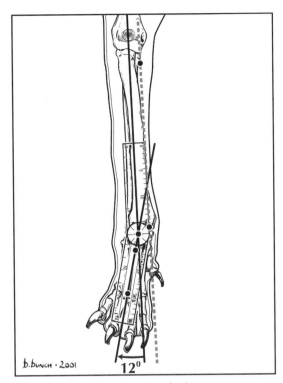

Figure 5   Carpal valgus.

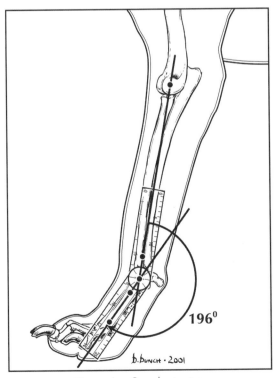

Figure 4   Carpal extension.

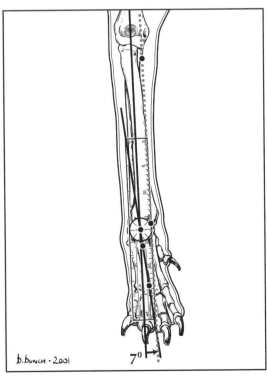

Figure 6   Carpal varus.

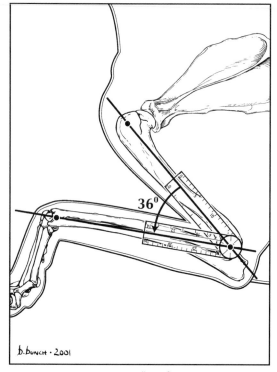

Figure 7 Elbow flexion.

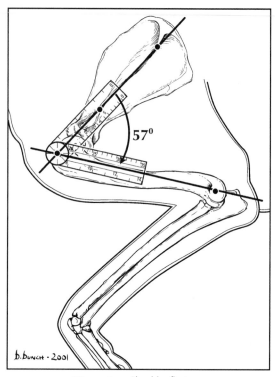

Figure 9 Shoulder flexion.

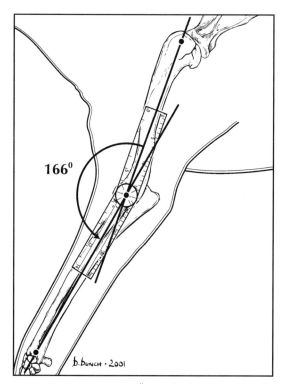

Figure 8 Elbow extension.

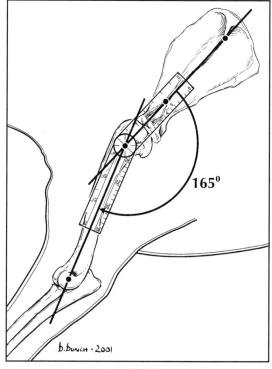

Figure 10 Shoulder extension.

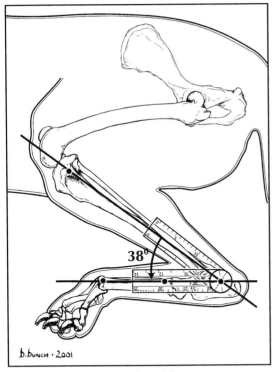

Figure 11   Tarsal flexion.

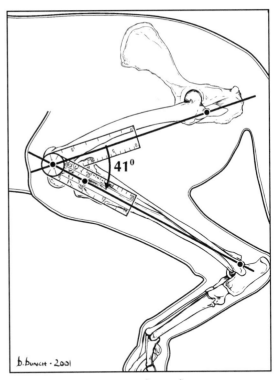

Figure 13   Stifle joint flexion.

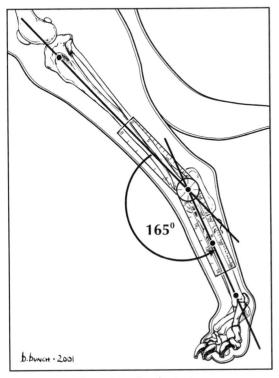

Figure 12   Tarsal extension.

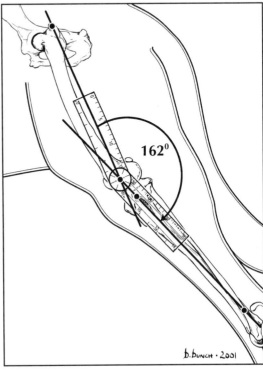

Figure 14   Stifle joint extension.

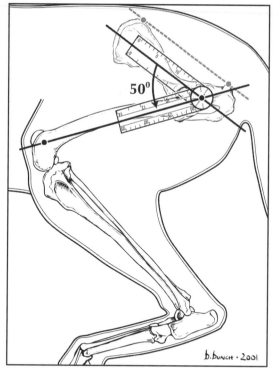

Figure 15   Hip joint flexion.

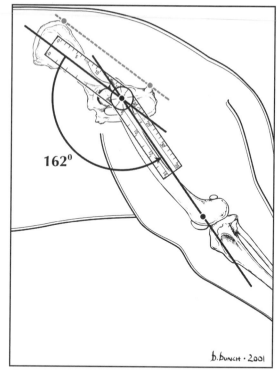

Figure 16   Hip joint extension.

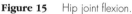

■ ■ ■ **Table 1**   Range of motion (degrees) of various appendicular joints measured by goniometry in 16 healthy Labrador Retrievers

Joint	Position	Mean	SD	95% CI of the mean	Median
Carpus	Flexion	32	2	31-34	32
Extension	196	2	194-197	196	
Valgus	12	2	11-13	12	
Varus	7	1	6-8	7	
Elbow	Flexion	36	2	34-38	36
Extension	165	2	164-167	166	
Shoulder	Flexion	57	2	54-59	57
Extension	165	2	164-167	165	
Tarsus	Flexion	39	2	37-40	38
Extension	164	2	162-165	165	
Stifle	Flexion	42	2	40-43	41
Extension	162	3	160-164	162	
Hip	Flexion	50	2	48-52	50
Extension	162	3	160-164	162	

CI = Confidence interval.

Appendix 2

Comparative Myology of the Dog*

Muscle	Correlated human muscle	Joint action in the forelimb	Main cranial, dorsal, or proximal attachment	Main caudal, ventral, or distal attachment	Fiber direction from proximal to distal attachment (listed in order of importance)	Innervation
Forelimb						
Trunk to Forelimb						
Cutaneous trunci	No correlate; however, like the platysma in the neck	None: Twitch the skin over the scapular and shoulder area	In the superficial fascia of the dorsal, lateral, and ventral walls of thorax and abdomen	Medial side of the forelimb		Lateral thoracic nerve
Trapezius						
Cervical	Upper trapezius	Elevate the scapula cranially and dorsally; abduct the forelimb	Median or mid-dorsal raphe of the neck and supraspinous ligament	Dorsal aspect of the spine of the scapula	Caudoventral	Accessory nerve Cranial XI
Thoracic	Lower trapezius	Depress the scapula; abduct the forelimb	Supraspinous ligament and dorsal spinous processes of T3-T8 or T9	Middle part of the spine of the scapula	Cranioventral	Accessory nerve Cranial XI
The fibrous band in between the cervical and thoracic parts is in the position of the middle trapezius.						
Rhomboideus		Elevate the scapula and forelimb; pull the scapula to the trunk				Ventral rami of cervical spinal nerves
Rhomboideus capitis: two parts		Elevate the scapula and forelimb; pull the scapula to the trunk	Nuchal crest of the occipital bone	Cranial dorsal border of the scapula	Craniodorsal	
Rhomboideus cervicis	Rhomboid minor	Elevate the scapula and forelimb; pull the scapula to the trunk	Median fibrous raphe of neck, spinous processes of T1-T3	Caudal (base) of the scapula, medially and laterally	Craniodorsal	
Rhomboideus thoracis	Rhomboid major	Joint action in the forelimb	Spinous process of T4-T7	Caudal (base of scapula, medially and laterally)	Craniodorsal	
Serratus ventralis	Serratus anterior	Carry the trunk and shoulder forward and back, support the trunk, depress the scapula	Transverse processes of C3-C7 and ventral ribs 1-7 or 8	Medial scapula, dorsal one third	Craniodorsal and cranioventral	Ventral rami of cervical spinal nerves and long thoracic nerve

Muscle		Action	Origin	Insertion	Direction	Nerve
Brachiocephalicus: two parts	Two parts are divided by a fibrous cla-vicular intersection					Accessory nerve Ventral rami of cervical spinal nerves
Cleidobrachialis	Anterior deltoid	Extend the shoulder; advance the forelimb	Ventral aspect of the clavicle	Cranial surface, distal third of the humerus, between the biceps brachii medially and the brachialis laterally	Distomedial	
Cleidocephalicus—neck muscle		Draw the head to the side; extend the neck	Dorsal aspect of the clavicle	Cranial half mid-dorsal fibrous raphe and nuchal crest of occipital bone	Dorsocranial	
Superficial pectoral: two parts—						
Descending pectoral portion	Part of pectoralis major	Adduct the shoulder, prevent abduction in weight-bearing; extend the shoulder; draw trunk sideward	Ventral sternum, most cranial aspect (ventral to the transverse pectoral muscle)	All but most distal part of crest of greater tubercle of humerus	Distolateral	Cranial pectoral nerves
Transverse pectoral portion	Part of pectoralis major	As above, plus flex or extend shoulder, depending on position	Ventral sternum, cranial half dorsal to the descending pectoral muscle	All but most distal part of crest of greater tubercle of humerus	Distolateral	Cranial pectoral nerves
Deep pectoral	Part of pectoralis major	Flex the shoulder; move the trunk cranially during weight-bearing; support the trunk with the serratus ventralis	Ventral aspect of the sternum, dorsal to the superficial pectoral muscle cranially	Major portion—lesser tubercle of humerus, aponeurosis to the greater tubercle and crest of humerus Caudal portion—medial brachial fascia	Craniodisto-lateral	Caudal pectoral nerves
Latissimus dorsi	Latissimus dorsi	Flex the shoulder; draw the trunk cranially in weight-bearing; adduct the	Thoracolumbar fascia from spinous processes of most caudal seven or	Teres major tuberosity on the humerus and teres major tendon; joins tip of the	Craniolatero-distal	Thoracodorsal nerve

Continued

Muscle	Correlated human muscle	Joint action in the forelimb	Main cranial, dorsal, or proximal attachment	Main caudal, ventral, or distal attachment	Fiber direction from proximal to distal attachment (listed in order of importance)	Innervation
Forelimb—Cont'd						
		shoulder; support the trunk	eight thoracic and lumbar vertebrae; most caudal two or three ribs	muscle cutaneous trunci laterally		
Shoulder: Within Forelimb						
Deltoideus: two parts	Deltoid			The two parts of the deltoid blend near the shoulder joint and attach to the deltoid tuberosity		
Spinous head	Posterior deltoid	Shoulder flexion	Scapular spine, blending with the infraspinatus		Distolateral	Axillary nerve
Acromial head	Middle deltoid	Shoulder abduction	Acromion		Laterodistal	Axillary nerve
Infraspinatus	Infraspinatus	Shoulder flexion or extension depending on position; shoulder abduction and lateral rotation; stabilize lateral shoulder	Infraspinous fossa	Lateral side of the greater tubercle of the humerus	Laterodistal	Suprascapular nerve
Teres minor	Teres minor	Shoulder flexion and lateral rotation	Infraglenoid tubercle	Infraglenoid tuberosity of the humerus	Laterodistal	Axillary nerve
Supraspinatus	Supraspinatus	Extend the shoulder; stabilizes and prevents collapse of the shoulder	Supraspinous fossa, wider and larger than the infraspinatus	Greater tubercle of the humerus by a thick tendon	Distally on the cranial aspect of the shoulder, then medially	Suprascapular nerve
Subscapularis	Subscapularis	Adduct, extends and stabilizes the shoulder medially	Subscapular fossa	Lesser tubercle of the humerus	Craniodistal	Subscapular nerve
Teres major	Teres major	Shoulder flexion and medial rotation	Caudal angle and border of the scapula and caudal subscapularis	Teres major tuberosity of the humerus	Cranial and then distal	Axillary nerve

Coracobrachialis	Shoulder adduction and extension	Coracoid process of the scapula	Crest of the lesser tubercle of humerus, proximal to teres major tuberosity	Distolateral	Musculocutaneous nerve
Biceps brachii— one head	Shoulder extension and elbow flexion; some passive stability in weight-bearing, preventing shoulder flexion	Supraglenoid tubercle of the humerus	Ulnar tuberosity on proximal cranial ulnar; Radial tuberosity on proximal cranial radius (weaker part)	Distomedial	Musculocutaneous nerve
Brachialis	Elbow flexion	Proximal third of the lateral humerus (brachialis groove)	Ulnar tuberosity on proximal cranial ulnar	Distolateral	Musculocutaneous nerve
Triceps brachii— three heads	Elbow extension; helps tense the antebrachial fascia				Radial nerve
Long head	Elbow extension, shoulder flexion	Caudal border of the scapula	Olecranon tuber or tuberosity	Caudodistal	
Lateral head	Elbow extension	Tricipital line of the humerus—covers the accessory head	Olecranon tuber, lateral to long head	Caudodistal	
None	Elbow extension	Neck of the humerus	Olecranon tuber, between lateral and medial heads	Caudodistal	
Medial head	Elbow extension	Crest of lesser tubercle near teres major tuberosity	Olecranon	Caudodistal	
Anconeus	Elbow extension; helps tense the antebrachial fascia	Lateral supracondylar crest; lateral and part of medial epicondyles of the humerus	Lateral surface, proximal end of ulna	Caudal	Radial nerve
None	Elbow extension; chief tensor of the antebrachial fascia	Fascia covering the latissimus dorsi; very thin	Olecranon and the medial fascia of the forearm	Distolateral	Radial nerve
Cranial and Lateral Forearm or Antebrachium					
Brachioradialis	Supination; rotation of the radius dorsolaterally	Lateral supracondylar crest of the humerus; thin and inconstant muscle	Distal fourth of the radius	Medial then distal	Radial nerve

Continued

Muscle	Correlated human muscle	Joint action in the hindlimb	Main cranial, dorsal or proximal attachment	Main caudal, ventral, or distal attachment	Fiber direction	Innervation
Cranial and Lateral Forearm or Antebrachium—Cont'd						
Extensor carpi radialis	Extensor carpi radialis longus and brevis	Carpal extension; elbow flexion	Lateral supracondylar crest	Small tuberosities on dorsal bases of MCs II and III		Radial nerve
Common digital extensor	Extensor digitorum communis	Extension of digits II-V; carpal extension	Lateral epicondyle of the humerus	Extensor processes of the distal phalanges of digits II-V	Distomedial	Radial nerve
Lateral digital extensor	None	Extension of digits III-V; carpal extension	Lateral epicondyle of the humerus	Proximal ends, all phalanges III-V; extensor processes of distal phalanges of III-V	Distomedial	Radial nerve
Ulnaris lateralis	Extensor carpi ulnaris	Carpal ulnar deviation or abduction; weak carpal flexion	Lateral epicondyle of the humerus	Lateral aspect, MC V; accessory carpal bone	Distolateral	Radial nerve
Supinator	Supinator	Supination; elbow flexion	Lateral epicondyle of the humerus	Cranial surface, proximal fourth of the radius	Distomedial	Radial nerve
Caudal and Medial Forearm or Antebrachium						
Pronator teres	Pronator teres	Pronation, elbow flexion	Medial epicondyle of the humerus	Medial border of the radius between middle and proximal thirds	Distolateral	Median nerve
Flexor carpi ulnaris: two parts	Flexor carpi ulnaris	Carpal flexion, carpal abduction	Proximally the ulnar head is more cranial and distally the humeral head is more cranial			Ulnar nerve
Ulnar head			Caudal border and medial surface of the olecranon	Accessory carpal bone		
Humeral head			Medial epicondyle of the humerus	Accessory carpal bone		
Flexor carpi radialis	Flexor carpi radialis	Carpal flexion	Medial epicondyle of the humerus	Palmar aspect of proximal metacarpals I and II		Median nerve

Muscle	Action	Origin	Insertion		Nerve
Superficial digital flexor	Flexion of PIP and MCP of II-V; carpal flexion	Medial epicondyle of the humerus and medial border of radius	Palmar surface, base of middle phalanges of II-V		Median nerve
Deep digital flexor: three parts Humeral head	Flexion of digits; carpal flexion	Medial epicondyle of the humerus—radial, deep, and medial bellies	For all three heads: palmar surface of the base (proximal end) of the distal phalanx of digits II-V and a weak tendon to digit I		Median nerve to radial head, deep and medial parts of humeral head
Ulnar head	None	Proximal three-fourths of caudal border of the ulna			Ulnar nerve to ulnar head and lateral part of humeral head
Radial head	None	Middle third, medial border of the radius			
Pronator quadratus	Pronation	Medial surface of the ulna, caudal to the interosseous membrane	Caudal surface of the radius except proximal and distal ends	Distomedial	Median nerve
Hindlimb *Caudal Thigh Muscles* Biceps femoris: two or three heads—longest and widest thigh muscle in the hindlimb	Cranial—hip and stifle extension Caudal—stifle flexion, tarsocrural extension, hip (hindlimb) abduction	Sacrotuberous ligament and ischiatic tuberosity	Patella; patellar ligament and cranial border of tibia via fascia lata and crural fascia; tibial body via crural fascia; calcaneal fascia; calcaneal tuberosity	Distocranio-lateral	Sciatic nerve
Caudal crural abductor muscle	Stifle flexion and hip (hindlimb) abduction with caudal biceps femoris muscle	Sacrotuberous ligament near ischiatic tuberosity	Via crural fascia to the digital extensor	Distocranio-lateral	Sciatic nerve

Continued

Muscle	Correlated human muscle	Joint action in the hindlimb	Main cranial, dorsal or proximal attachment	Main caudal, ventral, or distal attachment	Fiber direction	Innervation
Hindlimb—Cont'd						
Semitendinosus	Semitendinosus	Hip and tarsocrural extension; stifle flexion	Ischiatic tuberosity	Medial tibial body and calcaneal tuberosity via crural fascia	Distocranio-medial	Sciatic nerve
Semimembranosus: two bellies	Semimembranosus	Hip extension Femoral belly—stifle extension Tibial belly—stifle flexion or extension, depending on stifle position	Ischiatic tuberosity	Medial lip, distal shaft, caudal rough surface of the femur—distal to pectineus muscle; medial aspect, proximal part, medial tibial condyle	Distocranio-medial	Sciatic nerve
Medial Thigh Muscles						
Sartorius	Sartorius					
Cranial part		Hip flexion, stifle extension	Iliac crest, thoraco-lumbar fascia	Patella, with rectus femoris	Distocaudal	Femoral nerve
Caudal part		Hip flexion, stifle flexion	Cranial VIS, adjacent ventral ilium	Cranial border, medial tibia, with gracilis		
Pectineus	Pectineus	Hip or hindlimb adduction	Body of pubis, iliopubic eminence to pubic tubercle	Medial lip, distal shaft, caudal rough surface of the femur, proximal to semimembranosus	Distocaudal	Obturator nerve
Adductor: two parts, which may or may not be distinguishable	Adductors magnus, brevis, and longus	Hip or hindlimb adduction, hip extension	Entire symphysis pelvis via symphysial tendon, adjacent ischiatic arch, ventral pubis and ischium	Entire lateral lip of the caudal rough surface of the femur	Distocranio-lateral	Obturator nerve
Lateral Thigh Muscles						
Tensor fasciae latae	Tensor fascia lata / tensor fasciae latae	Tense the fascia lata, hip flexion, stifle extension	Cranial VIS and adjacent ilium (=tuber coxae), aponeurosis of	Via fascia lata, connects to biceps femoris and quadriceps femoris	Distocaudal	Cranial gluteal nerve

			middle gluteal muscle	muscle to patella	
Superficial gluteal	Gluteus maximus	Hip extension, hip or hindlimb abduction	Lateral border of sacrum, caudal 1 or 1st vertebra of the tail, sacrotuberous ligament, cranial DIS via deep gluteal fascia	Third trochanter, fusing with aponeurosis of tensor fasciae latae—synovial bursa deep to attachment in one third of dogs	Caudolatero-distal	Caudal gluteal nerve
Middle gluteal	Gluteus medius	Hip extension, abduction, internal rotation	Crest and gluteal or lateral surface of the ilium	Greater or major trochanter	Caudolatero-distal	Cranial gluteal nerve
Piriformis—may actually be part of the middle gluteal or deep gluteal muscle	Piriformis	Hip extension	Lateral surface of S3 and C1	Greater trochanter with middle gluteal muscle	Caudolatero-distal	Caudal gluteal nerve
Deep gluteal	Gluteus minimus	Hip extension, abduction, internal rotation	Body of ilium, ischiatic spine	Greater trochanter, cranial aspect	Caudodistal	Cranial gluteal nerve
Cranial Thigh Muscles						
Iliopsoas	Iliopsoas	Hip flexion				Ventral rami of lumbar and femoral nerves
Psoas major	Psoas major	Hip flexion, vertebral column flexion, lumbar spine extension with ventral tilting of the pelvis	Transverse processes and bodies of the lumbar vertebrae	Lesser trochanter with the iliacus	Caudoventro-lateral	
Iliacus	Iliacus	Hip flexion	Smooth ventral surface of the ilium	Lesser trochanter with the psoas major	Caudoventro-lateral	
Quadriceps femoris	Quadriceps femoris	See actions below				
Rectus femoris	Rectus femoris	Stifle extension, hip flexion	Lateral ilium, cranial to the acetabulum—bursa occasionally deep to this attachment	Tibial tuberosity	Distocranio-lateral	Femoral nerve

Continued

Muscle	Correlated human muscle	Joint action in the hindlimb	Main cranial, dorsal or proximal attachment	Main caudal, ventral, or distal attachment	Fiber direction	Innervation
Cranial Thigh Muscles—Cont'd						
Vastus lateralis	Vastus lateralis	Stifle extension	Proximal part of the lateral lip of the caudal rough surface of the femur	Tibial tuberosity—bursa usually deep to tendon attachment	Distocranio-medial	Femoral nerve
Vastus intermedius	Vastus intermedius	Stifle extension	Lateral side of the proximal femur, with the vastus lateralis	Tibial tuberosity	Distocranio-medial	Femoral nerve
Cranial Thigh Muscles						
Vastus medialis	Vastus medialis	Stifle extension	Medial side, proximal end of the cranial femur; proximal end, medial lip, caudal rough surface of the femur	Tibial tuberosity—bursa usually deep to tendon attachment	Distocranio-lateral	Femoral nerve
Articularis genu	Articularis genu	Stifle extension; tenses the proximal pouch of the stifle joint capsule	Cranial surface of femur, proximal to the trochlea	Tibial tuberosity		Femoral nerve
Craniolateral Muscles of the Leg or Crus						
Cranial tibial	Anterior tibialis/tibialis anterior	Talocrural flexion; rotates the hindpaw so the plantar surface of the paw faces medially	Extensor groove and adjacent articular margin of tibia, lateral edge of the cranial border of the tibia	Plantar surface of base of MT I and II after coursing deep to the crural extensor retinaculum	Distomedial	Deep peroneal nerve
Long digital extensor	Extensor digitorum longus	DIP and PIP extension II–V, talocrural flexion	Extensor fossa on the femur lateral to the trochlea	Extensor processes on the dorsum, distal phalanges of digits II–V coursing deep to the crural and tarsal extensor retinacula	Distomedial	Peroneal nerve

Muscle	Homolog	Action	Origin	Course	Insertion	Nerve
Extensor digiti I longus	Extensor hallucis longus and part of the extensor digitorum longus	Digit II extension, digit I extension	Cranial border of the fibula between proximal and middle third of the interosseous membrane cranial to the peroneus brevis	Distomedial	Fascia and tendon of the lateral digital extensor of MTP joint II; aponeurosis of the metatarsus, rudiment of digit I or hallux	Deep peroneal nerve
Lateral digital extensor	Peroneus tertius	Digit V extension and abduction	Proximal third of the fibula		Extensor process on the dorsum of digits V coursing deep to the crural and tarsal extensor retinacula	Superficial peroneal nerve
Peroneus longus	Peroneus longus	Talocrural flexion, rotates the hindpaw so the plantar surface of the paw faces laterally	Lateral tibial condyle, proximal fibula, lateral collateral ligament of the stifle, which then attaches to the lateral femoral epicondyle	Distal on the leg then medial on the plantar hindpaw	Fourth tarsal bone/quartal bone, plantar aspect of the base of the MTs after coursing deep to the abductor digiti V muscle	Common peroneal nerve, deep peroneal nerve
Peroneus brevis	Peroneus brevis	Talocrural flexion	Lateral surface of the distal two thirds of the fibula and tibia	Distal and slightly medial	Proximal end of MT V in a common sheath with the extensor digitorum lateralis after coursing deep to the lateral collateral ligament of the ankle	Superficial peroneal nerve
Caudal Muscles of the Leg						
Popliteus	Popliteus	Stifle internal rotation/leg internal rotation	Lateral condyle of the femur	Distomedial	Proximal third caudal surface of tibia, with a sesamoid at the muscle–tendon junction	Tibial nerve

Continued

Caudal Muscles of the Leg—Cont'd

Muscle	Correlated human muscle	Joint action in the hindlimb	Main cranial, dorsal or proximal attachment	Main caudal, ventral, or distal attachment	Fiber direction	Innervation
Gastrocnemius: two heads	Gastrocnemius—two heads	Talocrural extension; stifle flexion	Medial and lateral supracondylar tuberosities of the femur; each tendon has a sesamoid bone or fabella that articulates with a femoral condyle	Dorsal surface of the calcaneal tuberosity by the common calcaneal tendon to provide the largest portion of the tendon		Tibial nerve
Superficial digital flexor	Flexor digitorum brevis	MTP and PIP joints of II-V; stifle flexion, talocrural extension	Lateral supracondylar tuberosity of the femur	Calcaneal tuberosity and bases of middle phalanges digits II-V		Tibial nerve
Deep digital flexor	Flexor digitorum longus	Digit flexion; talocrural extension by both parts	See each part separately below	Two heads join at the distal tarsals and then attach to the plantar surface of the base of distal phalanges I-V	Distomedial	Tibial nerve
Lateral digital flexor (flexor hallucis longus)	Flexor hallucis longus		Caudolateral border of the proximal two thirds of tibia, proximal half of fibula, and adjacent interosseous membrane	Before joining the medial digital flexor muscle, the tendon is bound in a groove at the sustentaculum tali		
Medial digital flexor (flexor digitorum longus)	Flexor digitorum longus		Caudomedial border of the tibia, popliteal line head of the fibula	Tendon lies on the caudomedial side of the tibia before joining the lateral digital flexor muscle		
Caudal tibial	Posterior tibialis/tibialis posterior	Rotation of the hindpaw so the plantar paw faces medially; talocrural extension	Medial proximal fibula	Medial ligamentous masses of the tarsus after coursing as a very thin tendon, lying cranial to	Distomedial	Tibial nerve

Muscle	Action	Origin	Insertion		Innervation
			medial digital flexor at the talocrural joint		
Deep Dorsal Muscles of the Neck					
Splenius	Extension, ipsilateral side bend, and ipsilateral rotation of the neck, raising the head and neck, stabilization of T1	Spinous processes of T1-T2, ligamentum nuchae cranial to T1, median dorsal raphe of cervical spine, by aponeurosis of cranial part of thoracolumbar fascia, extending to T5-T6	Mastoid part the temporal bone with the longissimus capitis, dorsal nuchal line of occiput, at times to the wing of the atlas	Cranioventral	Dorsal rami of cervical nerves
Deep Ventral Muscles of the Neck					
Scalenus: two parts	Ipsilateral side bend of the neck, pulls the neck down, inspiration				Ventral rami of cervical and thoracic spinal nerves
Supracostal scalenus—superficial part (two or three parts)		Lateral surfaces of ribs 1-9	Transverse processes of C4 and C5 and sometimes C3	Craniomedio-dorsal	
Primae costae scalenus—deep part (three parts)		As three portions from the cranial border of rib 1	Superficial part to transverse process of C3 through C5; two deep parts to transverse processes of C6 and C7	Craniomedio-dorsal	
Longus capitis	AO flexion, pulls the neck down	Caudal surfaces of the transverse processes of cervical vertebrae	Ventral surface of the basioccipital bone of the skull	Cranial	Ventral rami of cervical spinal nerves
Longus colli	Neck flexion, pulls the neck down	Ventral convex surfaces of T1-T6 vertebrae	Ventral border of the wing of C6 and the transverse process of C7	Cranial Craniomedial	Ventral rami of cervical spinal nerves
		Ventral borders of transverse processes of C6-C3	Ventral aspect of the next cranial vertebra	Craniomedial	

Continued

Muscle	Correlated human muscle	Joint action in the hindlimb	Main cranial, dorsal or proximal attachment	Main caudal, ventral, or distal attachment	Fiber direction	Innervation
Deep Ventral Muscles of the Neck—Cont'd						
			Ventral surface of the angle of cranial ribs	Ventral aspect of the atlas		
Lateral and Ventral Thoracic Wall Muscles						
External intercostals	External intercostals	Draw ribs together, breathing	Caudal border of a rib	Cranial border of the next caudal rib	Caudoventral	Intercostal nerves
Internal intercostals	Internal intercostals	Draw ribs together, breathing	Extending from the vertebral column to the distal ends of the rib—cranial border of a rib	Caudal border of the next cranial rib	Cranioventral	Intercostal nerves
Muscles of the Abdominal Wall and Diaphragm						
Rectus abdominis	Rectus abdominis	Flexion of the spine, bring pelvis forward (i.e., posterior pelvic tilt); abdominal press functions—expiration, urination, defecation, parturition; support of abdominal viscera	Sternum, rib 1, and 1st costal cartilage, and a fleshy attachment on the sternal portion of the 9th costal cartilage	Pecten ossis pubis, between the two iliopectineal eminences	Caudal	Intercostal, costoabdominal, ilioinguinal nerves, medial branches
External abdominal oblique: abdominis two parts	External oblique abdominis	Flexion of the spine, ipsilateral side bend, functions of abdominal press, contralateral rotation of the spine, support of abdominal viscera	Last ribs, thorocolumbar fascia	Linea alba, cranial pubic ligament	Caudoventral	Intercostal nerves 3 or 4-12, costoabdominal, iliohypogastric and ilioinguinal nerves, lateral branches
Internal abdominal oblique: abdominis three parts	Internal oblique abdominis	Flexion of the spine, ipsilateral side bend, functions of abdominal press, support of abdominal viscera	Thoracolumbar fascia caudal to rib 12 with the pars lumbalis	Rectus abdominis and linea alba	Cranioventral	Caudal intercostal nerve and medial branches of the costoabdominal, iliohypogastric, and ilioinguinal nerves

Muscle	Action	Origin	Insertion	Direction	Nerve
Transversus abdominis	Abdominal press, support of abdominal viscera	Costal cartilage of rib 8, transverse process of L7, and tuber coxae	Linea alba	Ventral	Caudal intercostal nerve and medial branches of the costoabdominal nerve
Diaphragm	Inspiration, support of abdominal viscera	Ventral surfaces of lumbar vertebrae, ribs, and sternum	Central tendon	Craniomedial	Phrenic nerve, ventral rami of C5-C7
Deep Dorsal Muscles of the Neck and Trunk					
Iliocostalis system: two parts	Ipsilateral side bend; stabilizes the spine, expiration by pulling the ribs caudally				Dorsal rami of thoracic and lumbar nerves
Iliocostalis thoracis		Cranial borders of vertebral ends of ribs 2-12	Costal angles of the ribs, transverse process of C7	Cranial	
Iliocostalis lumborum		Pelvic surface of the wing of the ilium, the iliac crest, and the intermuscular septum between the iliocostalis and longissimus muscles	Lumbar vertebrae and last 5 ribs	Cranioventral	
Longissimus System: three parts—extent is from the iliac crest to C7					
Longissimus thoracis et lumborum: two parts—strongest muscle of the trunk in the thoracic and lumbar region	Extension of the spine, raising the cranial portion of the body from the pelvis; stabilizes the spine, raises the caudal body with the hindlimbs			Craniolateral	Dorsal rami of thoracic and lumbar nerves
Longissimus thoracis		Spinous processes and supraspinous ligament of thoracic vertebrae	Medial tendons to the accessory processes of T6-T13 and caudal ends of transverse processes of T1-T5		

Continued

Longissimus System: three parts—extent is from the iliac crest to C7—Cont'd

Muscle	Correlated human muscle	Joint action in the hindlimb	Main cranial, dorsal or proximal attachment	Main caudal, ventral, or distal attachment	Fiber direction	Innervation
				Lateral tendons to the groove adjacent to the costal tubercle of ribs 6-13 Cranially, both attach to the costal tubercles of ribs 1-5		
Longissimus lumborum	Longissimus lumborum		Iliac crest and ventral surface of the ilium, supraspinous ligament of lumbar vertebrae	Dorsal aspects and cranial articular processes of lumbar vertebrae, disk of lumbosacral joint		
Longissimus cervicis	Longissimus cervicis	Extension of the neck, ipsilateral side bend and rotation	Spinous processes and supraspinous ligament of cranial thoracic and caudal cervical vertebrae	Transverse processes of cranial cervical vertebrae		Dorsal rami of cervical and thoracic nerves
Longissimus capitis	Longissimus capitis	AO extension, ipsilateral side bend and rotation	Transverse processes of T1-T3, caudal articular processes of C3-C7	Mastoid process of the temporal bone, united with splenius at the level of the atlas		Dorsal rami of cervical nerves

Transversospinalis System—joins one or more vertebrae
Transversus spinalis

Muscle	Correlated human muscle	Joint action in the hindlimb	Main cranial, dorsal or proximal attachment	Main caudal, ventral, or distal attachment	Fiber direction	Innervation
Spinalis et semispinalis thoracis et cervicis: two parts	Spinalis and semispinalis thoracis	Neck extension, raises the neck, stabilizes the spine	Dorsal aspect of the longissimus thoracis muscle, spinous processes and accessory processes of cranial lumbar vertebrae and C7-T6 and mammillary processes of T13-L2, iliac crest,	Thoracis portion—spinous processes of thoracic vertebrae Cervicis portion—spinous processes of C2-C5 vertebrae	Craniomedial	**Dorsal rami** Dorsal rami of thoracic nerves Dorsal rami of cervical nerves

Muscle	Comparable muscle	Action	Origin	Insertion	Direction	Innervation
Spinalis et semispinalis thoracis—lateral			spinous processes of T13-S2			Dorsal rami of cervical nerves
Spinalis cervicis—medial	Spinalis cervicis					
Semispinalis capitis: two parts	Semispinalis capitis	Neck extension, ipsilateral side bend, stabilize the neck				Dorsal rami of cervical, thoracic, and lumbar nerves
Multifidus: three parts	Multifidus	Stabilize the vertebral column			Craniomedial	
Multifidus lumborum	Multifidus lumborum		Dorsal sacrum, mammillary processes of L7-T12	Spinous processes of T9-L6		Dorsal rami of lumbar and thoracic nerves
Multifidus thoracis	Multifidus thoracis		Mammillary and transverse processes of T3-T11	Spinous processes of T7-T8		Dorsal rami of thoracic nerves
Multifidus cervicis	Multifidus cervicis		Articular process of T2	Spinous process of axis		Dorsal rami of cervical nerves
Muscles of the Tail						
Sacrocaudalis dorsalis lateralis	None	Tail extension or lifting, ipsilateral side bend	Aponeurosis of the longissimus, mammillary processes L1-L6 and Cd1-Cd8 articular processes of the sacrum	Mammillary processes of Cd vertebrae Continuation of the longissimus muscle	Caudomedial	Dorsal rami of caudal nerves
Sacrocaudalis dorsalis medialis	None	Tail extension or lifting, ipsilateral side bend	Spines and dorsolateral aspects of cranial vertebrae	Dorsolateral aspects of caudal vertebrae	Caudolateral	Dorsal rami of caudal nerves

Continued

Muscles of the Tail—Cont'd

Muscle	Correlated human muscle	Joint action in the hindlimb	Main cranial, dorsal or proximal attachment	Main caudal, ventral, or distal attachment	Fiber direction	Innervation
Sacrocaudalis ventralis lateralis	None	Tail flexion, ipsilateral side bend	Ventral surface of L7 and the sacrum, ventral surfaces of transverse processes of Cd vertebrae	Ventrolateral tubercle of more caudal vertebrae	Caudomedial	Ventral rami of caudal nerves
Sacrocaudalis ventralis medialis	None	Tail flexion, ipsilateral side bend	Ventral surface of S3 and Cd vertebrae	Hemal process of the next caudal vertebrae	Caudomedial	Ventral rami of caudal nerves

AA, Atlantoaxial; *AO*, atlantoocipital; *caudal DIS*, caudal dorsal iliac spine; *C*, cervical spinal nerve; *Cd*, caudal; *CN*, cranial nerve; *caudal VIS*, caudal ventral iliac spine; *cranial DIS*, cranial dorsal iliac spine; *cranial VIS*, cranial ventral iliac spine; *Cx*, coccygeal; *L*, lumbar spinal nerve; *MC*, metacarpal bone; *MCP*, metacarpophalangeal joint; *MT*, metatarsal bone; *MTP*, metatarsophalangeal joint; *PIP/DIP*, proximal/distal interphalangeal joint; *S*, sacral spinal joint.

Main Ligament Attachments and Function

Name of Ligament	Correlate human ligament	Proximal Attachment	Distal Attachment	Fiber direction	Motion restricted by ligament/function
Forelimb Shoulder Joint					
Transverse humeral retinaculum	Transverse humeral	Medial side of greater tubercle	Lateral side of lesser tubercle	Transverse/horizontal	Stabilizes the biceps brachii, proximal tendon
Medial glenohumeral	Glenohumeral	Medial lip of glenoid fossa	Greater tubercle	Distal	Stabilizes humeral head, preventing medial dislocation
Lateral glenohumeral	Glenohumeral glenoid fossa	Lateral lip of glenoid fossa	Lesser tubercle	Distolateral	Stabilizes humeral head, preventing lateral dislocation
Elbow Joint					
Medial collateral	Lateral or radial collateral	Humeral medial epicondyle	Radial tuberosity and radius and ulna in the interosseous space by crura	Distal	Limits elbow valgus
Lateral collateral	Medial or ulnar collateral	Humeral lateral epicondyle	Ulna with the annular ligament and area distal to the radial neck	Distal	Limits elbow varus
Radioulnar Joints					
Annular	Annular	Lateral extremity of the radial notch of the ulna	Medial extremity of the radial notch of the ulna	Circular	Stabilizes radial head position
Interosseous	Interosseous	Radius	Ulna	Between ulna and radius	Stabilizes radius and ulna in radioulnar pronation
Radioulnar	Distal radioulnar	Distal, lateral radius	Distal, medial ulna	Transverse	Stabilize the distal radioulnar joint
Carpal Joints					
Flexor retinaculum/ transverse palmar carpal	Transverse carpal	Accessory carpal and styloid process of radius	Palmar projections of radius and proximal carpals	Transverse	Two layers stabilize tendons of the superficial and deep digital flexors
Short radial collateral	Radial collateral of the wrist				
Straight part		Tubercle proximal to radial styloid process	Medial radial carpal	Distal	Valgus deviation
Oblique part		Radial styloid process	Palmomedial surface of radial carpal	Distal	Valgus deviation

Ligament	Attachment	Attachment	Direction	Function
Short ulnar collateral	Ulnar styloid process	Ulnar carpal	Distal	Varus deviation
Dorsal radiocarpal	Dorsolateral radius	Dorsoproximal ulnar carpal	Distolateral	Carpal flexion
Palmar carpal	Palmar aspect of radius, ulna, and carpals	Distally on the carpals and metacarpals	Distal, distolateral, distomedial	Carpal extension
Digital Joints				
Collaterals of the MCP joints	Distal ends of metacarpals	Proximal ends of proximal phalanges	Vertical in weight-bearing	Medial and lateral MCP joint motion
Collaterals of the PIP joints	Distal ends of proximal phalanges	Collateral tubercles on the proximal ends of the middle phalanges and distal phalanges in digit I	Vertical in weight-bearing	Medial and lateral PIP motion
Collaterals of the DIP joints	Distal ends of middle phalanges	Sides of the ungual crests of the distal phalanx	Caudodistal	Medial and lateral PIP motion
Hindlimb Hip Joint				
Transverse acetabular	One side of acetabular notch	Other side of acetabular notch	Caudal	Completes the acetabular lip to secure femoral head in the acetabulum
Ligament of the femoral head	Fovea in the femoral head	Acetabular fossa	Mediocaudal	Maintains hip reduction
Ligamentum teres or ligamentum capitis femoris				
Stifle Joint				
Cranial	Intercondylar fossa, caudomedial part of the femoral lateral condyle	Cranial intercondylar area of the tibia	Craniodistal	Stifle cranial glide during extension, also internal rotation
Anterior cruciate				
Caudal	Intercondylar fossa, femoral medial condyle	Medial edge, popliteal notch of tibia, caudal to the caudal attachment of the medial meniscus	Caudodistal	Stifle caudal glide during flexion
Posterior cruciate				
Medial collateral	Medial femoral epicondyle	Medial tibial border, distal to the condyle Attaches to the medial meniscus	Distocranial	Stifle valgus and extension
Medial or tibial collateral				
Lateral collateral	Lateral femoral epicondyle	Fibular head and adjacent tibial condyle	Distal (vertical instance)	Stifle varus and extension
Lateral or fibular collateral				

Continued

Name of Ligament	Correlate human ligament	Proximal Attachment	Distal Attachment	Fiber direction	Motion restricted by ligament/function
Stifle Joint—Cont'd					
Patellar ligament	Patellar ligament (patellar tendon)	Quadriceps tendon and patella	Tibial tuberosity	Distal	Transfer force of quadriceps muscle to the tibia
Talocrural Joint					
Medial collateral	Medial or tibial collateral				Stabilization of lateral motion of the tarsus
Long part		Medial aspect of the medial malleolus	Firmly to tarsal I and the central tarsal and loosely to MTs I-II and the talus	Distocranial	
Short part: two parts		Medial aspect of the medial malleolus	1. Tarsal I and MTs, sustentaculum tali (deep to long part) 2. Talus	Distocranial / Caudal	
Lateral collateral	Lateral or fibular collateral				Stabilization of internal motion of the tarsus
Long part		Lateral malleolus	Calcaneus, tarsal IV, and base of MT V	Distocranial	
Short part: two parts		Lateral malleolus	1. Tuber calcanei 2. Talus	Distocaudal Caudodistal	
Tarsus					
Distal extensor retinaculum—distal transverse ligament of tarsus	None	Calcaneus	Surrounds the long digital extensor to attach to the calcaneus	Circular	Secure the long digital extensor muscle
Dorsal ligaments—many, named by connecting bones	Many dorsal ligaments	From one tarsal bone	Another tarsal bone or MT bone	Different for each ligament	Stabilize the dorsal tarsus Limit tarsal extension
Talocalcaneal	Subtalar interosseous	Talus—distal surface	Calcaneus—proximal surface	Near vertical	Stabilize the talocalcaneal articulation
Plantar ligaments—thicker and stronger than dorsal talocrural ligaments	Long and short plantar ligaments				Support the joints of the plantar hindpaw Increase stability Limit dorsiflexion
Medial plantar		Sustentaculum tali; plantar surface	Central tarsal and tarsometatarsal joint capsule	Distolateral	

Ligament		Attachment	Attachment	Direction	Function
Middle plantar—most commonly injured plantar ligament		Body of the calcaneus, plantar aspect	Tarsal bone IV and bases of MTs IV and V	Distal	
Lateral plantar		Caudolateral calcaneus	Long part of lateral collateral ligament of the talocrural joint and base of MT V	Distal	
Digital Joints					
Collaterals of the MTP joints		Distal ends of MTs	Proximal ends of proximal phalanges	Vertical in weight-bearing	Abduction and adduction MTP motion
Collaterals of the PIP joints		Distal ends of proximal phalanges	Collateral tubercles on the proximal ends of the middle phalanges and distal phalanx in digit I	Vertical in weight-bearing	Abduction and adduction PIP motion
Collaterals of the DIP joints		Distal ends of middle phalanges	Sides of the ungual crests of the distal phalanx	Caudodistal	Abduction and adduction PIP motion
Proximal and distal digital annular		One side of phalanx	Other side of phalanx crossing the plantar surface	Mediolateral	Secure the flexor tendons close to the phalanges
Spine					
AO Joint					
Dorsal AO ligament or membrane	Posterior AO	Dorsal edge of foramen magnum	Cranial border of the arch of the atlas	Craniocaudal	AO flexion Punctures are made through this membrane to drain cerebrospinal fluid
Ventral AO ligament or membrane	Anterior AO	Ventral edge of foramen magnum	Body of the atlas	Craniocaudal	AO extension
Lateral AO ligament	Lateral AO	Lateral part of the dorsal arch of the atlas	Jugular process of the occipital bone	Cranioventro-lateral	AO contralateral side bend
AA Joint					
Dorsal AA membrane	Posterior AA	Caudal margins of the sides and body of the atlas	Cranial margin of the same areas of the axis	Craniocaudal	AA contralateral side bend

Continued

Name of Ligament	Correlate human ligament	Proximal Attachment	Distal Attachment	Fiber direction	Motion restricted by ligament/function
AA Joint—Cont'd					
Apical ligament of the dens	Apical	Dens of the axis	Foramen magnum, occipital bone medial to the caudal parts of the occipital condyles	Cranial and craniolateral	Stabilizes the dens
Transverse ligament of the atlas	Transverse portion of the cruciform ligament	Internal surface of the ventral arch of the atlas	Internal surface of the other side of the arch of the atlas	Mediolateral	Stabilizes the dens
Intervertebral Joints					
Ligamentum nuchae/nuchal ligament	Ligamentum nuchae	Caudal part of the spinous process of C2	Tip of spinous process of T1	Craniocaudal	Stabilizes the cervical spine
Supraspinous	Supraspinous	Spinous process, T1 being the most cranial	Each sequential spinous process to Cd3	Craniocaudal	Limits separation of the spinous processes during spine flexion motion
Ventral longitudinal	Anterior longitudinal	Ventral surfaces of bodies of vertebrae, C2 being the most cranial Best developed caudal to the middle thorax	Ventral surfaces of bodies of vertebrae, the sacrum being the most caudal	Craniocaudal	Limits spine extension
Dorsal longitudinal	Posterior longitudinal	Dorsal surfaces of bodies of vertebrae, C2 being the most cranial Heavier than the ventral longitudinal ligament	Dorsal surfaces of bodies of vertebrae, the end of the vertebral canal in the Cd region being the most caudal	Craniocaudal	Limits spine flexion
Interspinous	Interspinous	Cranial border of a spinous process	Caudal border of a spinous process	Craniocaudal	Limits spine flexion
Intertransverse	Intertransverse	Transverse process of a caudal vertebra	Transverse process of an adjacent cranial vertebra	Craniolateral	Limits side bend
Yellow/interarcuate/ligamentum flavum	Ligamentum flavum	Loose thin elastic ligament attached to the arch of a vertebra	Arch of an adjacent vertebra	Craniocaudal	Limits spine flexion
Ligaments of the Ribs					
Ligament of the head		Head of the rib	Lateral part of the intervertebral disk and body adjacent to the disk	Mediolateral	Stabilizes the rib

Ligament				Function
Ligament of the tubercle/dorsal costotransverse ligament	Distal to the articular capsule of the tubercle Strongest	Transverse process of the vertebra corresponding to the rib	Mediolateral	Stabilizes the rib
Ligament of the neck	Neck of the rib	Ventral surface of transverse process and adjacent lateral surface of the body of the vertebra	Medioventral	Stabilizes the rib
Sacroiliac Joint				
Ventral sacroiliac	Sacrum, ventral surface	Ilium, ventral surface	From the sacrum, dorsolateral and medial	Stabilizes the sacroiliac joint, prevents ventral displacement of the sacrum
Dorsal sacroiliac	Caudal dorsal iliac spine	Caudal two thirds of the lateral border of the sacrum or even Cd1	Caudomedial portion and dorsocaudal portion	Stabilizes the sacroiliac joint
Sacrotuberous	Caudolateral apex of the sacrum and Cd1	Lateral angle of the ischiatic tuberosity	Caudolatero-ventral	Stabilizes the sacrum and pelvis Muscle attachment site

AA, Atlantoaxial; *AO,* atlantooccipital; *Cd,* caudal; *DIP,* distal interphalangeal; *L,* lumbar; *MCP,* metacarpophalangeal; *MTP,* metatarsophalangeal; *PIP,* proximal interphalangeal; *S,* sacral.

■ A p p e n d i x 4

Sample Protocols

Darryl L. Millis, David Levine, Robert A. Taylor, and Caroline P. Adamson

The sample protocols in this appendix are designed to address common conditions in patients not experiencing complications. Individual patient characteristics must be considered when designing an individual patient protocol. Furthermore, diagnosis and treatment should be provided by trained personnel.

A: Sample Postoperative Extracapsular Cranial Cruciate Ligament Rupture Repair Rehabilitation Protocol

A sample postoperative rehabilitation protocol is presented that is designed specifically for dogs that have undergone an extracapsular procedure, such as a fabellar-tibial suture technique, for cranial cruciate ligament rupture. This is a working protocol that should be modified according to clinical necessity, efficacy, and each patient's progress within the rehabilitation program. This protocol is not to be rigidly adhered to, but serves as a guide to allow an effective rehabilitation plan of care.

Preoperative Therapy

Whenever possible, it may be beneficial to provide chondroprotective (polysulfated gly-cosaminoglycan by IM injection, but discontinue for at least 24 hours before surgery, and oral glucosamine and chondroitin sulfate) and antiinflammatory therapy (e.g., deracoxib or carprofen) to minimize postoperative inflammation while awaiting surgery. It is also an opportune time to begin training the dog for postoperative exercises. Particularly, acquainting the dog with aquatic therapy is desirable. If a therapeutic pool or whirlpool is to be used,

it is beneficial to acclimate the dog to the pool to determine whether it will be a candidate for aquatic therapy. Some dogs become frantic around water, and it is better to determine if these dogs will not be candidates for aquatic therapy before surgery so that they do not injure themselves postoperatively. It also may be beneficial to acquaint the dog with the ground treadmill, and, if available, an underwater treadmill. The benefits of muscle strengthening and reestablishing knee range of motion (ROM) after an acute tear of the anterior cruciate ligament are well known in humans. The same benefits may also be true in dogs. However, cruciate ligament disease differs in dogs, with most ruptures of the ligament occurring gradually, with the initiation of osteoarthritis already under way by the time of diagnosis. Also, it is well known that encouraging weight-bearing exercise on an unstable stifle will accelerate the progression of osteoarthritis. Therefore strength training in dogs should probably be restricted to non–weight-bearing activities before stifle stabilization. Neuromuscular electrical stimulation and aquatic therapy are two methods of accomplishing some strength training prior to surgery with minimal or no weight-bearing on the unstable stifle.

The patient should also be evaluated before surgery to establish baseline data and to determine a suitable rehabilitation plan for an individual patient. Limb circumference should be determined as an indicator of muscle mass on both the affected and unaffected limbs. ROM (goniometry) should be determined on the affected and unaffected limbs, and gait analysis should be performed to evaluate weight-bearing and the degree of lameness of the affected limb.

Immediate Postoperative Therapy

Immediately after surgery, cryotherapy should be administered while the patient is recovering from anesthesia. Ice packs or other commercial cryotherapy devices may be used around the stifle joint for 15 to 30 minutes. During this time, it may also be beneficial to perform slow, continuous passive ROM to the stifle. It is important that a layer of towel be placed between the skin and the cold pack because the dog will not be awake enough to indicate if the limb is too cold. Following removal of the cold pack, a mild pressure wrap, such as a modified Robert Jones bandage, should be placed to limit swelling and edema. The wrap should keep the stifle and hock in a functional walking position. The bandage may be removed the next morning in preparation for the rehabilitation session. Appropriate analgesic medication should be administered so that the patient is comfortable.

Step 1: Day 1 Postoperative Until Toe-touching

GOALS

The main goals for the first days after surgery include the following:
- Swelling and edema control
- Improving stifle ROM
- Limiting muscle atrophy
- Pain control

Nonsteroidal antiinflammatory medication (e.g., deracoxib, etodolac, or carprofen) should be administered 30 to 60 minutes before the first session of the day. Remove the bandage if one is present. Begin the session with gentle massage of the area, concentrating on edema resolution, muscle relaxation, mobilization of soft tissues near the incision, and gentle mobilization of the patella in all planes. Passive ROM and stretching exercises should follow massage, slowly performing 10 to 20 repetitions. Slow leash walks should be attempted to determine the patient's willingness to touch the toes of the affected limb to the ground. If the patient is willing to toe-touch, the dog is walked very slowly for 5 minutes the first day. Neuromuscular electrical stimulation (NMES) may be applied for 15 minutes, concentrating on the biceps and quadriceps muscle groups. This may be performed as co-contraction if no net joint movement is desired, or with contraction of one muscle group followed by the other. This will help limit muscle atrophy and may provide some analgesia. Follow with cryotherapy for 15 to 20 minutes. If swelling and edema are present, a pressure bandage may be applied. These activities may be performed a total of 2 to 3 times per day, with the exception of the NMES, which should only be administered once daily. Transcutaneous electrical nerve stimulation (TENS), a form of NMES for analgesia, may be applied several times daily, but NMES for muscle strengthening and the attenuation of muscle atrophy should only be administered once daily to prevent muscle soreness.

Most dogs have a comfortable ROM of 60 to 80 degrees of flexion and 120 to 135 degrees of extension during the first few days after surgery. Patients in this category should have ROM performed 2 or 3 times daily, followed by cryotherapy and bandage application if swelling is present. If the patient does not have this ROM, it may be necessary to perform ROM exercises 3 to 5 times daily. If the patient is in considerable pain, the clinician should be contacted to determine if there is a postoperative complication. Dogs in this category may require opioid analgesia.

Heat should not be applied for the first 72 hours because this may increase inflammation, swelling, and edema. Moist heat or therapeutic ultrasound may typically begin on day 4 or 5 after surgery before ROM exercises to warm up tissues, increase tissue elasticity, provide comfort to the patient and for general relaxation of muscles and tissues. Therapeutic ultrasound may also be applied for tissue heating, as long as the patient remains comfortable.

In general, dogs will hold the affected limb in a non–weight-bearing flexed position for 1 to 4 days after surgery. Continue step 1 procedures during this initial period of pain. It is extremely important during this early recovery phase that the dog not be overworked and become more painful following therapy sessions.

The patient should be leash-walked very slowly to encourage weight-bearing. When the dog begins to carry the limb in a more extended position, with the toes held only 1 to 3 inches from the ground, this is an indication that the dog is about to begin toe-touching. Step 2 activities may begin at this point.

Step 2: Early Weight-Bearing

GOALS

The main goals during early weight-bearing are as follows:

- Continue pain control
- Reduce swelling
- Work to return ROM to a more normal state
- Increase toe-touching weight-bearing

Antiinflammatory therapy may continue as long as there are no contraindications, such as diarrhea or vomiting, particularly if there is blood present. The first session may begin with therapeutic ultrasound or hot packs to warm up the tissues. ROM and stretching exercises may continue if full flexion (40 degrees) and full extension (160-165 degrees) have not been achieved.

Toe-touching should be encouraged by gently shifting the dog off balance so that the affected leg begins to touch the ground for balance. This may be performed while standing still or while slowly walking. Dogs should be leash walked very slowly for 5 to 10 minutes to allow an opportunity for weight-bearing. To encourage weight-bearing, it may be beneficial in some dogs to gently push the dog off balance toward the affected limb as the unaffected limb begins the swing phase of gait to encourage toe-touching and greater weight-bearing.

Dogs may also begin work on a ground treadmill. Depending on the prior condition and fitness of the dog, the first rehabilitation session should last 1.5 to 2.5 minutes, at 0.5 mph, on a level surface or with a maximum 1.5-degree grade. Most dogs will begin to toe-touch within the first few seconds, but others may need support and encouragement. Occasionally a dog will resist toe-touching; weight-bearing may be encouraged by lifting the affected foot and advancing it and placing it on the ground during a normal gait cycle on the treadmill. Most dogs will quickly begin to use the limb. As the dog continues to increase weight-bearing activity on the limb, treadmill time may be increased 15 to 30 seconds per day, and the grade increased by 0.5 to 1.0 degree every other day. Treadmill activity may be performed 1 or 2 times per day.

Leash walks may be increased in length and speed as weight-bearing improves. In addition, walking up inclines or hills is beneficial to allow driving from the rear limbs, which improves muscle strength of the rear limbs. A reasonable goal is 10 to 15 minutes of leash walking, with 5 to 10 repetitions up a gently inclined surface. In any case, it is extremely important that the patient not experience increased pain or lameness following the rehabilitation session. Although it is inevitable that this may occur in the occasional patient, it is important that the program not be overly aggressive and that the amount of activity be reduced until the dog is ready to increase the level of activity again without being painful. Cryotherapy may be administered following a session.

Ankle weights placed on the normal unaffected limb may feel strange to the dog and take its mind off of the surgical limb, resulting in use of the affected limb. Another trick is to place a syringe cap on the bottom of the unaffected limb while leash or treadmill walking.

The afternoon session may be preceded by massage, ROM and stretching, or other warm-up activities. To help prevent muscle atrophy, NMES may be performed during the afternoon session every other day. Following this, the dog should be leash walked very slowly for 5 to 10 minutes to encourage weight-bearing. Cryotherapy may follow the session. A third leash-walking session may be added if time permits and the dog tolerates the activity without becoming more lame or sore.

Aquatic therapy may be substituted for NMES following suture removal (day 8-14 after surgery). Caution should be exercised to be certain that the incision is sealed, with no drainage or discharge from the incision, or gaping of the wound edges with gentle pressure applied to the healing incision. In general, swimming is usually too strenuous this early after surgery in many patients. Walking in a pool, tub, or underwater treadmill has the benefits of encouraging use of the limb while walking in a buoyant environment. Water temperature should be approximately 85° F. Dogs may be lifted into the body of water using a sling and lift system, or the dog may be walked into the underwater treadmill or the shallow end of a body of water. Sessions should initially last 2 to 3 minutes, with the dog supported if needed. Dogs should be slowly walked (0.5-1.0 mph) with water at the midthigh to midchest level. The time may be increased 0.5 to 3 minutes each session as the dog improves, but caution is exercised to carefully evaluate soreness and lameness to be certain that activity is not stepped up too rapidly.

By the end of step 2, the dog should be consistently using the limb during every stride at a walk, although lameness will still be apparent. The dog may be intermittently or consistently toe-touching at a trot. Step 3 procedures should now begin.

Step 3: Consistent Weight-Bearing

GOALS

The goals during the consistent weight-bearing phase are as follows:

- Achieve maximum joint ROM
- Improve weight-bearing at a walk and trot

A weight-loss program (Step 5+ activities) may be begun during this phase if necessary. It is generally best to wait for 2 weeks after surgery before initiating a weight-loss program to avoid unintended loss of lean tissue mass.

If normal ROM has not yet been achieved, continue passive ROM and stretching exercises. It may be most beneficial to perform therapeutic ultrasound while simultaneously stretching if tissues seem to be tight or have lost extensibility. In addition, it may be more effective to maintain the stretch while the tissues are cooling. Also perform ROM and stretching if the dog does not have normal stifle extension during walking and trotting.

Following a warm-up activity of leash walking at a moderate pace for 5 minutes, the dog should be walked up inclines or hills for 5 to 10 minutes. When the dog is comfortable going up an inclined surface, the dog may be walked up a flight of steps. Care should be taken to go slowly and encourage full weight-bearing and pushing off with the affected limb. Stair climbing may be alternated with sit-to-stand exercises. The goal of this exercise is to encourage the dog to sit squarely, and then arise from the sitting position by using the affected limb to push off. Initially, 5 to 10 repetitions should be performed, and the amount increased to up to 20 repetitions. It may be helpful to offer a small, low-calorie treat to encourage and train the dog to perform these exercises. Stairs or sit-to-stand activities should be performed two times daily; it may be beneficial to alternate the activities to avoid boredom and to exercise different muscle groups.

During one session per day, the dog may jog slowly for 2 to 5 minutes. If available, underwater treadmill exercise should be continued, with a goal of brisk walking for 15 to 30 minutes twice daily in lieu of stairs or sit-to-stand exercises. Appropriate substitutions of activities should be instituted with the overall goal to increase limb use and prevent lameness or pain as a result of the therapeutic exercises. Swimming for 2 to 5 minutes daily or every other day may also be very beneficial at this stage. Swimming may occur in a large tub, swimming pool, lake, or pond. It is important that the dog be slowly lowered or walked into the body or water, with no explosive leaps into the water to avoid injury to the surgical site. When the dog is bearing significant weight on the affected limb at a trot, step 4 activities may begin.

Step 4: Consistent Weight-Bearing at a Trot

GOALS

The goals while achieving consistent weight-bearing at a trot are as follows:

- Improve ability to use the limb with some speed
- Improve muscle mass and strength
- Improve stamina and endurance

At this point, the dog should be using the limb consistently at a trot. Some mild lameness may be apparent, and prolonged activity may result in worsening of lameness. If lameness worsens following activity, antiinflammatory medication should be administered and the dog should be rested for 1 or 2 days, followed by a return to a reduced level of activity (activity should be 50% to 75% of what it was just before the lameness and then gradually increased over a slower period of time). Trotting activities should initially be encouraged for 5- to 10-minute sessions, twice daily. The speed, length, and frequency of jogging should be increased to 15 to 25 minutes three times daily, as long as pain and lameness do not worsen. At least part of this time should be spent jogging up an inclined surface, such as a hill. Stair climbing and sit-to-stand exercises should continue. If possible, swimming should be offered several times per week, for 10-20 minutes depending on the fitness of the dog. Controlled playing with a ball at a fast trot or slow lope may be substituted for jogging several times per week for 5 to 10 minutes. Caution should be used to avoid sharp turns and jumping up. An occasional day of reduced activity may be beneficial. Step 4 should be continued until the dog willingly trots quickly and with minimal or no lameness.

Step 5: Trotting at Speed With Minimal to No Lameness

GOALS

The goals of step 5 are as follows:

- Continue improving speed at a lope and slow gallop
- Continue improving muscle mass and strength

- Continue improving stamina and endurance
- Return to as normal activity as possible

This step is designed to have dogs return to as normal function as possible. In some situations, other factors, such as advanced osteoarthritis of the affected stifle, cranial cruciate ligament disease in the contralateral limb, or musculoskeletal conditions of other limbs, may preclude the patient from returning to very good or excellent function. Dogs may run up and down hills, inclines, and trot up steps. Swimming may continue for 15 to 20 minutes several times per week if possible. Ball playing may be encouraged with the dog running at a gallop for 3 to 5 minutes initially, working up to 15 to 20 minutes daily. Dogs may jog for prolonged distances. It is important that the level of activity be relatively consistent from day to day, rather than allow vigorous activity for 1 or 2 days per week with little activity for the remainder of the week. Depending on the initial condition of the dog's stifle (degree of osteoarthritis, meniscal injury, cartilage erosions), intermittent antiinflammatory therapy may be necessary.

Step 5+: Weight Loss

GOALS

The goals of this step, which may begin anytime after 2 weeks postoperatively, are as follows:
- Reduce weight to allow a more complete recovery in the affected limb
- Allow greater general stamina and endurance
- Reduce the chance for progressive arthritis in the stifle
- Possibly reduce the chances for rupture of the other cranial cruciate ligament

Beginning with step 3 (early in the postoperative recovery stage), a reducing diet may be instituted using dry food only, or a combination of dry and canned reducing diet. Commercially available weight loss diets are effective aids to weight loss. Weight should be monitored and charted once weekly to document changes and provide incentive to the owner. Treats may consist of ice cubes or raw vegetables. Absolutely no table scraps are allowed. In the home environment, the dog should not be in the room during family meals. The diet should only be offered for short periods of time, 2 or 3 times daily. It is important to feed animals separately if there are several pets in the household, and the patient should not have access to the other pets' food.

Important Considerations

During all of the five steps, particular attention should be paid to any deterioration in the dog's progress. Specifically, attention should be focused on lameness or stiffness following activity. If the patient appears to have stiffness or increased pain or lameness at any time after a therapy session, the level of activity should be decreased and a slower rate of progression should be instituted. It is very important that dogs be as comfortable and pain-free as possible during the rehabilitation period.

It is important to realize that the dog may not be totally normal even with intensive physical rehabilitation. Depending on the condition of the dog's stifle before surgery, there may be permanent arthritic changes which would preclude return to normal function. However, rehabilitation is key in obtaining and maintaining as much function as possible. If the dog does not appear to be making progress, has any complications, or if there are any questions, the patient should be discussed with the clinician to determine an appropriate course of action.

B: Sample Postoperative Rehabilitation Protocol for Tibial Plateau Leveling Osteotomy

A sample postoperative rehabilitation protocol is presented which is designed specifically for dogs that have undergone a tibial plateau–leveling osteotomy (TPLO) procedure for cranial cruciate ligament rupture. This is a working protocol that should be modified according to clinical necessity, efficacy, and each patient's progress within the rehabilitation program. This protocol is not intended to be rigidly adhered to, but serves as a guide to allow an effective rehabilitation plan of care. More attention must be paid to restricted activity because the biomechanics of the stifle are altered, placing additional stress on the patellar ligament and its insertion on the tibial tuberosity. Therefore overuse of the limb before appropriate tissue remodeling often results in patellar ligament desmitis or avulsion of a portion of the tibial tuberosity. Particular attention should be paid to these areas throughout the rehabilitation program to help prevent these problems.

Preoperative Therapy

Whenever possible, it may be beneficial to provide chondroprotective (polysulfated glycosaminoglycan by IM injection, but discontinue for at least 24 hours before surgery, and oral glucosamine and chondroitin sulfate) and antiinflammatory therapy (e.g., deracoxib or carprofen) to minimize postoperative inflammation while awaiting surgery. It is also an opportune time to begin training the dog for postoperative exercises. Particularly, acquainting the dog with aquatic therapy is desirable. If a therapeutic pool or whirlpool is to be used, it is beneficial to acclimate the dog to the pool to determine whether it will be a candidate for aquatic therapy. Some dogs become frantic around water and it is better to determine if these dogs will not be candidates for aquatic therapy before surgery so that they do not injure themselves postoperatively. It also may be beneficial to acquaint the dog with the ground treadmill, and if available, an underwater treadmill. The benefits of muscle strengthening and reestablishing knee range of motion (ROM) following an acute tear of the anterior cruciate ligament are well known in humans. The same benefits may also be true

in dogs. However, cruciate ligament disease differs in dogs, with most ruptures of the ligament occurring gradually, with the initiation of osteoarthritis already under way by the time of diagnosis. Also, it is well known that encouraging weight-bearing exercise on an unstable stifle will accelerate the progression of osteoarthritis. Therefore strength training in dogs should probably be restricted to non–weight-bearing activities before stifle stabilization. Neuromuscular electrical stimulation and aquatic therapy are two methods of accomplishing some strength training prior to surgery with minimal or no weight-bearing on the unstable stifle.

The patient should also be evaluated prior to surgery to establish baseline data and to determine a suitable rehabilitation plan for an individual patient. Limb circumference should be determined as an indicator of muscle mass on both the affected and unaffected limbs. ROM (goniometry) should be determined on the affected and unaffected limbs, and gait analysis should be performed to evaluate weight-bearing and the degree of lameness of the affected limb.

Immediate Postoperative Therapy

Immediately after surgery, cryotherapy should be administered while the patient is recovering from anesthesia. Ice packs or other commercial cryotherapy devices may be used around the stifle joint for 15 to 30 minutes. During this time, it may also be beneficial to perform slow, continuous passive ROM to the stifle. It is important that a layer of towel be placed between the skin and the cold pack because the dog will not be awake enough to indicate if the limb is too cold. Following removal of the cold pack, a mild pressure wrap, such as a modified Robert Jones bandage should be placed to limit swelling and edema. The wrap should keep the stifle and hock in a functional walking position. The bandage may be removed the next morning in preparation for the rehabilitation session. Appropriate analgesic medication should be administered so that the patient is comfortable.

Step 1: Day 1 Postoperative Until Discharge From the Hospital
GOALS

The main goals for the first days after surgery include the following:

- Swelling and edema control
- Improving stifle ROM
- Limiting muscle atrophy
- Pain control

Nonsteroidal antiinflammatory medication (e.g., deracoxib, etodolac, or carprofen) should be administered 30 to 60 minutes before the first session of the day. Remove the bandage if one is present. The limb is palpated to assess sensitivity, skin temperature, muscle atrophy, and edema. Begin the session with gentle massage of the area, including the quadriceps, sartorius, semitendinosus, gracilis, biceps femoris muscles, concentrating on edema resolution, muscle relaxation, mobilization of soft tissues near the incision, and gentle mobilization of the patella in all planes. Passive ROM and stretching exercises to the hip, stifle, and hock (10 repetitions, two to three times per day) should follow massage. Slow leash walks should be attempted to determine the patient's willingness to touch the toes of the affected limb to the ground. Support with a towel or sling should be used to prevent the patient from falling. If the patient is willing to toe-touch, the dog is walked very slowly two to three times per day, for 5 minutes. Follow with cryotherapy for 15 to 20 minutes. If swelling and edema are present, a pressure bandage may be applied. These activities may be performed a total of 2 to 3 times per day.

Most dogs have a comfortable ROM of 60 to 80 degrees of flexion and 120 to 135 degrees of extension during the first few days after surgery. Patients in this category should have ROM performed 2 or 3 times daily, followed by cryotherapy and bandage application if swelling is present. If the patient does not have this ROM, it may be necessary to perform ROM exercises 3 to 5 times daily. If the patient is exceptionally painful, the clinician should be contacted to determine if there is a postoperative complication. Dogs in this category may require opioid analgesia.

Heat should not be applied for the first 72 hours because this may increase inflammation, swelling, and edema. Moist heat may typically begin on day 4 or 5 after surgery before ROM exercises to warm up tissues, increase tissue elasticity, provide comfort to the patient, and general relaxation of muscles and tissues.

In general, dogs will hold the affected limb in a non–weight-bearing flexed position for 1 to 4 days after surgery. Continue step 1 procedures during this initial period of pain. It is extremely important during this early recovery phase that the dog not be overworked and experience increased pain after therapy sessions.

The patient should be leash-walked very slowly to encourage weight-bearing. When the dog begins to carry the limb in a more extended position, with the toes held only 1 to 3 inches from the ground, this is an indication that the dog is about to begin toe-touching. Patients usually reach this point 1 or 2 days after surgery and may be discharged to the owner's care. The owner should be instructed to provide support to the dog with a towel or sling when walking to prevent slipping and injury. If a bandage has been applied to provide support or help alleviate swelling and edema, the owner should be instructed on proper bandage care (check toes twice daily for swelling, keep clean and dry, place a plastic bag over the bandage when walking outside and remove the bag when the dog is indoors).

Step 2: Discharge From the Hospital to 3 Weeks After Surgery

GOALS

The main goals during the early postoperative period are as follows:
- Continue pain control
- Reduce swelling
- Work to return ROM to a more normal state
- Increase weight-bearing at a walk

The dog may return to the clinic for outpatient therapy or the owner may provide initial care in the home environment. Appropriate analgesic medication, ROM and stretching exercises, and cryotherapy are continued as appropriate. Moist heat (in the form of moistened towels) may typically begin on day 4 or 5 after surgery before ROM exercises to warm up tissues, increase tissue elasticity, provide comfort to the patient, and general relaxation of muscles and tissues. Slow leash walks are continued (with support if needed) for short distances with the dog on a short leash. The dog should be monitored for any pain or stiffness, and if present, the leash walks should be shortened.

For the first week after surgery, massage of the area may be performed before passive ROM and after leash walks. Passive ROM, 10 to 15 repetitions, should be performed slowly before leash walks. Short walks should be performed for 5 to 10 minutes on a short leash, three times per day. Ice should be applied for 15 minutes after passive ROM and walks.

For weeks 2 and 3 after surgery, therapeutic activities should progress as the patient's condition allows. At this point, it is likely that passive ROM and massage may be discontinued. However, if stifle extension or flexion is not normal or near normal, these activities should continue. The length of the leash walks is increased to 10 to 20 minutes, three times per day. The distance of the walks should also be accordingly increased. The amount of activity is limited by the dog's response and tolerance to treatment. If there is increased fatigue, soreness or discomfort with the increase in time and distance walked, revert to the previous level of activity until those signs resolve, and begin increasing again from that point at a slower rate. Reevaluation of the patient should be performed at week 3, including assessing thigh circumference, ROM, gait, palpation of the stifle, and pain.

Client education should also include the time frame for tissue and bone healing. Owners should also receive proper instructions regarding how to walk their pet, perform passive ROM and stretching activities, and how to apply cryotherapy and heat therapy. Explosive activities, such as running, jumping, or playing must be avoided.

Owners should also be instructed regarding signs of potential complications or problems, such as persistent edema, acute pain, change in use of the affected limb, licking the incision site, or drainage, excessive swelling or pain at the incision. An appointment should be made for suture removal 10 to 14 days after surgery. A follow-up appointment should be scheduled 3 weeks after surgery.

Step 3: Weeks 3 to 5 After Surgery

GOALS

The goals during the intermediate postoperative phase are as follows:
- Achieve maximum joint ROM
- Increase endurance and strength
- Improve weight-bearing and proprioception

A weight-loss program (step 5+ activities) may be begin during this phase if necessary. It is generally best to wait for 2 to 3 weeks after surgery before initiating a weight-loss program to avoid unintended loss of lean tissue mass.

If normal ROM has not yet been achieved, continue passive ROM and stretching exer-

cises. It may be most beneficial to perform therapeutic ultrasound while simultaneously stretching if tissues seem to be tight or have lost extensibility. In addition, it may be more effective to maintain the stretch while the tissues are cooling. Also perform ROM and stretching if the dog does not have normal stifle extension while walking.

Slow leash walk therapeutic exercise should progress to 20 to 30 minutes three times daily or as the patient will tolerate. Functional strengthening may begin with sit-to-stand activities, 10 repetitions, three times daily. The exercises are more easily performed by backing the dog into a corner with the operated leg against the wall. It may be helpful to offer a small, low-calorie treat to encourage and train the dog to perform these exercises. The goal of this exercise is to encourage the dog to sit squarely, and then arise from the sitting position by using the affected limb to push off.

Neuromuscular reeducation may also be instituted by placing the rear limbs on a balance board or walking on a trampoline, couch cushion, or inflatable mattress. In addition, walking in a figure 8 pattern or walking circles to the left and right help encourage use of the limb and improve proprioception.

Step 4: Weeks 6 to 8 After Surgery

GOALS

The goals at this stage are as follows:
- Improve ability to use the limb while trotting
- Continue improving muscle mass and strength
- Continue improving stamina and endurance

Radiographs should be made to confirm bone healing of the osteotomy site and to reassess the patient. If the osteotomy is not yet fully healed, return to step 3 activities. If healing is progressing as expected, the intensity and duration of therapeutic activities may be increased. Leash walks may be performed on a longer leash for 30 to 40 minutes, three times per day or as tolerated by the patient. The patient may weave through cones at a walk. Trotting may be performed on a longer lead in a straight line with no sharp turns or cuts. In addition, dogs may be trotted in a figure 8 pattern, with no sharp turns.

To strengthen rear limb muscles, patients may walk up and down an inclined surface or ramp and slowly ascend and descend stairs, 5 to 10 stairs, two to three times per day. Tug-of-war may be carefully instituted, although caution should be used to not perform this activity too frequently, and it should be avoided in dogs with aggressive tendencies. Dancing on the rear limbs may also be used to help strengthen rear limb muscles. Neuromuscular reeducation and balance activities should be continued. Swimming may be instituted, but caution should be used so that there is not an explosive or sudden entry into water. Swimming should be offered several times per week, for 5 to 20 minutes, depending on the fitness of the dog.

At this point, the dog should be using the limb consistently at a trot. Some mild lameness may be apparent, and prolonged activity may result in worsening of lameness. If lameness worsens following activity, antiinflammatory medication should be administered and the dog should be rested for 1 to 2 days, followed by a return to a reduced level of activity (activity should be 50% to 75% of what it was just prior to lameness, and then gradually increased over time). An occasional day of reduced activity may be beneficial.

Step 5: Weeks 9 to 12 After Surgery
GOALS

The goals of step 5 are as follows:
- Continue improving speed at a more rapid gaits
- Continue improving muscle mass and strength
- Continue improving stamina and endurance
- Return to the prior level of activity at the end of 12 weeks

This step is designed to have dogs return to as normal function as possible. Final radiographs are made between 9 and 12 weeks to be certain that healing of the osteotomy is complete. Reassessments are made at this time to determine the patient's progress, and to alter the rehabilitation plan to optimize the recovery. In some situations, other factors, such as advanced osteoarthritis of the affected stifle, cranial cruciate ligament disease in the contralateral limb, or musculoskeletal conditions of other limbs, may preclude the patient from returning to very good or excellent function.

Therapeutic exercises continue as before. In addition, other activities may be added, such as trotting in a zigzag pattern and running in a straight line. Strap-on leg weights may be added to the affected limb (0.5-1 lb to begin with). Swimming may continue for 15 to 20 minutes several times per week if possible. It

is important that the level of activity be relatively consistent from day to day, rather than allow vigorous activity for 1 or 2 days per week with little activity for the remainder of the week. Depending on the initial condition of the dog's stifle (degree of osteoarthritis, meniscal injury, cartilage erosions), intermittent antiinflammatory therapy may be necessary.

Step 5+: Weight Loss
GOALS

The goals of this step, which may begin anytime after 3 weeks postoperatively, are as follows:
- Reduce weight to allow a more complete recovery in the affected limb
- Allow greater general stamina and endurance
- Reduce the chance for progressive arthritis in the stifle
- Possibly reduce the chances for rupture of the other cranial cruciate ligament

Beginning with step 3, a reducing diet may be instituted using dry food only, or a combination of dry and canned reducing diet. Commercially available weight loss diets are effective aids to weight loss. Weight should be monitored and charted once weekly to document changes and provide incentive to the owner. Treats may consist of ice cubes or raw vegetables. Absolutely no table scraps are allowed. In the home environment, the dog should not be in the room during family meals. The diet should only be offered for short periods of time, 2 or 3 times daily. It is important to feed animals separately if there are several pets in the household, and the patient should not have access to the other pets' food.

Important Considerations

During all of the five steps, particular attention should be paid to any deterioration in the dog's progress. Specifically, attention should be focused on lameness or stiffness following activity. If the patient appears to have stiffness or increased pain or lameness at any time after a therapy session, the level of activity should be decreased and a slower rate of progression should be instituted. It is very important that dogs be as comfortable and pain-free as possible during the rehabilitation period.

It is important to realize that the dog may not be totally normal even with intensive physical rehabilitation. Depending on the condition of the dog's stifle before surgery, there may be permanent arthritic changes which would preclude return to normal function. However, rehabilitation is key in obtaining and maintaining as much function as possible. If the dog does not appear to be making progress, has any complications, or if there are any questions, the patient should be discussed with the clinician to determine an appropriate course of action.

Expected outcomes at the end of rehabilitation include the following:

1. A stifle that is free of inflammation
2. Full ROM of the stifle
3. Equal muscle development between the affected and unaffected limbs
4. Complete healing of the osteotomy
5. Slowed progression of osteoarthritis
6. Function of limb better than before surgery

C: Sample Postoperative Femoral Head and Neck Ostectomy Rehabilitation Protocol

The keys to a successful outcome following femoral head and neck ostectomy (FHO) are adequate analgesia in the perioperative and postoperative period and active motion of the pseudoarthrosis. In addition to a properly performed FHO to remove the entire femoral neck and any sharp bone spurs, initiation of immediate postoperative rehabilitation is important. Placing an ice pack over the area during recovery helps to control swelling and also provides some analgesia. Slowly flexing and extending the pseudoarthrosis while the patient is recovering from anesthesia, similar to a passive ROM machine, appears to help encourage early active use of the limb in the postoperative period. Passive ROM continues during the recovery from anesthesia until the patient indicates discomfort by turning the head toward the limb, tensing the muscles of the limb, or vocalizing.

The reason for performing the FHO must be considered in assessing the progression of the patient and designing the rehabilitation program. For example, if the FHO has been performed because of a fracture of the acetabulum in a previously healthy joint, the recovery may be prolonged, sometimes requiring several weeks to have reasonable weight-bearing on the limb. However, if the FHO has been performed because of moderate to severe osteoarthritis of the coxofemoral joint secondary to hip dysplasia, much soft tissue remodeling has already occurred, such as thickening of the joint capsule and periarticular fibrosis, and formation of the pseudoarthrosis has already begun. Animals may place substantial weight on the limb during the first week, particularly if the patient was very painful before surgery.

Step 1: Day 1 Postoperative Until Toe-touching

One of the most critical factors in the early rehabilitation of the FHO patient is to provide adequate analgesia. A multimodal approach to pain control is used, especially during the first several days. Combinations of injectable opioid medications or prolonged release forms of fentanyl, in additional to nonsteroidal antiinflammatory drugs are beneficial.

The rehabilitation session may begin with gentle massage of the region, followed by very gentle passive ROM and stretching exercises, especially hip extension. Opportunities for weight-bearing with off-balance exercises and slow leash walks are encouraged. The session ends with cryotherapy. These activities should be repeated 3 to 4 times per day.

Step 2: Early Weight-Bearing

Analgesics, nonsteroidal antiinflammatory drugs, massage, passive ROM and stretching are continued. For patients in which acute inflammation has subsided and that have restricted ROM, application of hot packs or therapeutic ultrasound may be beneficial.

Slow leash walks up inclined surfaces are encouraged to build gluteal muscle mass and to encourage active extension of the hip joint. For patients that have delayed weight-bearing, placing a syringe cap under the contralateral foot often encourages active use of the affected limb. Ground treadmill walking is also a useful activity to initiate weight-bearing because the belt helps to move the limb caudally and create active-assisted extension of the hip. Underwater treadmill activity has similar benefits to ground treadmill walking, with the added benefit of unloading the limb as a result of the buoyancy effect of water. Cryotherapy is administered at the end of the rehabilitation session to help reduce inflammation.

Step 3: Consistent Weight-Bearing

Analgesics, nonsteroidal antiinflammatory drugs, and massage are continued if needed. Passive ROM, stretching, hot packs, and therapeutic ultrasound may be continued.

Dogs are walked at a medium fast speed up an inclined surface. Sit-to-stand exercises are initiated to develop gluteal muscles, while minimizing full extension of the hip joint if the animal is still painful. Walking up a flight of stairs may be added to help develop power in the rear limbs and actively extend the hips to a greater degree. Dancing exercise is a more advanced exercise that may be added to encourage muscle strengthening with the hip fully extended.

Light jogging may be initiated at this stage for 3 to 5 minutes per day. Swimming is added to the exercise routine 3 to 5 times per week if possible. Active use of the rear limbs is encouraged during swimming by tossing a toy some distance from the dog and having the dog swim to the toy and retrieve it. Although swimming helps to develop rear limb muscle strength, full hip extension is generally not achieved with swimming.

Step 4: Consistent Weight-Bearing at a Trot

ROM and stretching are continued if needed. Fast walks and jogging up inclined surfaces or hills are initiated to continue with gluteal muscle development. Climbing several flights of stairs may be alternated with sit-to-stand exercises. Aquatic therapy, dancing, and playing ball under controlled conditions with increasingly longer distances and times are continued. Pulling weights is a method of strength training to increase power to the rear limbs. It is important to keep the dog's head in a raised position to encourage driving off the rear limbs.

Step 5: Trotting at Speed With Minimal to No Lameness

By this time in the rehabilitation program, ROM and stretching will probably not be needed. Fast walks up inclined surfaces, stairs, and sit-to-stand exercises are continued. Dogs may run up hills, trot up stairs, continue swimming, and have prolonged jogging as long as lameness is not exacerbated with the increased level of activities. Vigorous ball playing may be introduced to increase speed and power.

D: Sample Postoperative Rehabilitation Protocol for Distal Femoral Physeal Fractures

Before initiating any rehabilitation protocol, it is essential that the surgeon is certain of the stability of the repair. Appropriate analgesia and anti-inflammatory medications are instituted in the perioperative period. Cryotherapy is applied for 20 minutes to the affected area immediately after surgery while recovering. After cryotherapy has been applied, the limb is placed in a 90-degree stifle flexion sling for 2 to 4 days to prevent hyperextension of the stifle in the immediate postoperative period.

After the sling has been removed, gentle ROM and stretching exercises are performed, especially stifle flexion. If the animal still has a tendency toward hyperextension of the stifle, a dynamic non–weight-bearing sling (e.g., a Robinson sling) is applied using elastic material. This sling may be removed twice daily for rehabilitation sessions.

It is critical that these patients have early, active use of the limb with flexion and extension of the stifle. Although passive ROM exercises are beneficial, active flexion and extension are necessary to prevent fracture disease and quadriceps contracture. Encourage opportunities for weight-bearing with off-balance exercises and slow leash walks. If the patient is not actively bearing weight by the fifth day after surgery and there is no obvious reason why, a syringe cap may be placed on the bottom of the contralateral foot to act as an irritant; this usually results in weight-bearing on the affected limb. Another option, if the patient is leash trained, is to have the dog walk on a ground treadmill. Extreme caution should be exercised, however, because young dogs and puppies may be frightened and if sudden movements or falls occur, the repair may be damaged. Sessions may be repeated 2 to 3 times daily, followed by cryotherapy.

If the ROM is not near normal by 10 days, heat or therapeutic ultrasound may be applied prior to ROM exercises. ROM and stretching should be continued for a full 3 to 4 weeks because fibrous tissue continues to mature and undergo contracture during this time frame and may result in decreased ROM if exercises are not continued.

As the patient is able, slow walks up inclined surfaces will encourage active use of the quadriceps and gluteal muscles. Some puppies may not be leash trained, but will usually follow the owner or therapist up the incline, particularly if a treat or favorite toy is offered. Ground treadmill activity may be continued if the patient is amenable. Swimming may be initiated in a pool, whirlpool, or bathtub. This is excellent as a form of non–weight-bearing active exercise that encourages active flexion and extension of the stifle.

As the patient continues to progress and bear weight on the limb, climbing stairs, performing sit-to-stand exercises, dancing, and light jogging may be introduced. Before initiating these higher level exercises, it is important to radiograph the healing fracture to be certain that adequate healing is occurring and that the implants are stable. Generally, these activities may be introduced between 2 and 3 weeks after repair. Cryotherapy is performed after sessions to help reduce inflammation.

In general, the patient is walking on the limb very well by 2 weeks. Joint ROM should be near normal with minimal joint effusion present. Failure to initiate adequate rehabilitation very early in the postoperative period may result in permanent loss of motion or a stiff stifle. Active use of the limb is extremely important to prevent these complications.

E: Sample Thoracolumbar Intervertebral Disk Rupture Rehabilitation Protocol

The expected time course for recovery following surgery for intervertebral disk rupture depends a great deal on the animal's condition before surgery. Perhaps the most important prognostic indicator is the presence or absence of deep pain sensation to the rear limbs. If deep pain is present, and the patient has some motor function, the chances for recovery to a functional house pet are very good to excellent. Conversely, if deep pain sensation has been absent for more than 48 hours, the chances for functional recovery are relatively poor. Although some cases may eventually regain some function, the tissue changes that occur as a result of disuse are serious, and may be irreversible.

Step 1: Immediately Postoperatively to Supporting Weight

The surgical approach to the spinal cord is quite extensive, and multiple muscles are elevated from the articular facets of the vertebrae. Cryotherapy of the incision site and underlying tissues may be beneficial to reduce inflammation and swelling in this area. Depending on the surgeon and the severity of injury to the spinal cord and the surgeon, corticosteroids may be administered to help reduce the effects of swelling and inflammation on the spinal cord. Because the patient may not be ambulatory for a period of time, ROM exercises should be performed to all of the joints of the rear limbs. Massage of the rear limb muscles may help to relax the muscles in cases with upper motor neuron lesions, while tapotment of the muscles may be beneficial to help maintain muscle tone in cases with lower motor neuron lesions.

Neuromuscular electrical stimulation to the rear limb muscles is helpful to attenuate muscle atrophy if lower motor neuron signs are present. Standing exercises are instituted the day after surgery to encourage neuromuscular re-education of the muscles responsible for maintaining normal standing posture and to strengthen these muscles to allow weight-bearing, and ultimately, ambulation.

It is also extremely important to provide excellent nursing care to dogs that are recumbent and unable to shift body positions without assistance. Care of the recumbent dog includes being certain that the patient is on a soft bed, is turned every 4 hours to help prevent decubital ulcers, is kept clean to avoid urine scalds, can easily reach food and water (offering these every few hours is important), and providing bladder care to be certain that the bladder does not become overdistended, especially if an upper motor neuron lesion is present. Because patients will knuckle over on the dorsum of the feet, these areas must be evaluated on a daily basis to be certain that there are no excoriations or abrasions. Protective boots may be placed on the feet, which helps to protect them from injury and helps to position the foot in a more correct standing position.

Step 2: Supporting Weight to Initial Motor Function

Passive ROM exercises are continued, as are standing exercises. The patient should be placed in a standing position with all four limbs placed squarely under the dog to provide stability. The therapist then helps to balance the patient to prevent it from falling to the side. If the patient begins to weaken and collapse, the therapist pulls the dog into a standing position again. This will help to strengthen the back and limb muscles in preparation for ambulation. Standing in water is very beneficial because the buoyancy of the water helps the patient to maintain a standing position, even if weakness is present. The buoyancy of the water also gives the animal more time to maintain a standing position if the patient loses its balance, allowing a split second of time to readjust the limbs before falling. Standing in water is especially useful if the patient is a large or giant breed of dog. When a dog is able to stand without assistance, even for a few seconds, gentle force may be applied to the wings of the iliums to increase muscle strengthening and to provide neuromuscular reeducation.

Swimming is excellent to encourage early motor function. Many patients will make minimal attempts to move their limbs when on dry ground, even if supported by an attendant. Many of these patients will make some crude motor movements while floating in the water, even if those motions are weak and uncoordinated. This form of initial motor activity is important for neuromuscular reeducation and to help maintain muscle mass.

Walking while supported in a sling is the next step to encourage gait patterning and strengthening. The back is a critical component to help the dog support its weight, and to initially help the patient to shift a large amount of the body weight to the forelimbs while the rear limbs are recovering coordination and strength. Because a hemilaminectomy is the typical surgical procedure to remove herniated disk material, and the muscles on one side undergo extensive dissection, neuromuscular electrical stimulation to the weak side of the back may be beneficial.

Step 3: Initial Motor Function to Good Motor Function With Proprioceptive Deficits

Swimming is continued to help with muscle strengthening and gait retraining. In addition, walking on a ground treadmill with the therapist positioned to assist gait and correct placement of the foot when it is advanced helps with gait training and is a vital functional activity.

Balancing activities, to help enhance proprioceptive training may be instituted when motor function is recovered to the point that some gait patterning has returned. Proprioceptive exercises are those that facilitate rapid muscle contractions, focusing on closed kinetic chain exercises and improving dynamic stability. Such exercises include use of a balance board, weight shifts, standing on a therapy roll while it is rocked back and forth, varying the speed of ambulation, incorporation of zig-zags when walking or trotting, figure 8s patterns, circles to the right and left, and walking on trampolines or other unstable surfaces.

Step 4: Good Motor Function with Proprioceptive Deficits to Near Normal Gait

Swimming and treadmill walking are continued to enhance gait training and muscle strengthening. Increasing the speed and length of treadmill walking will help challenge patients to achieve a higher level of functioning. Stair climbing may be added as another functional activity that should be mastered. In addition, negotiating stairs helps with proprioceptive training, as well as strength training of the rear limb muscles.

Balancing activities are continued as in step 3. To further help with proprioceptive training, patients may be walked over rails placed on the ground, or raised Cavaletti rails. Rear limb muscle strengthening may be further enhanced with sit-to-stand exercises. Jogging may be added as the patient regains proprioceptive functioning to allow work at higher speeds.

Step 5: Near Normal Gait to Normal Gait

The other activities in previous steps may be continued. The length of time spent swimming is increased to improve endurance and muscle strengthening. In addition, jogging on the treadmill and jogging up and down small stairs may be added to encourage proprioceptive challenges at higher speeds. Walking over raised Cavaletti rails is continued, and if the patient is able, they may negotiate the rails while jogging. Playing ball is added as an activity as the patient nears return to a normal gait.

A Glossary of Terms in Physical Rehabilitation

Accessory joint motions See arthrokinematic joint motions.

Active assisted range of motion Occurs when some degree of muscle activity assists joint range of motion activities.

Active range of motion The motion of a joint that may be achieved by active muscle contraction.

Activities of daily living Activities involved in self-care, communication, and mobility. Examples are dressing, shaving, and other skills necessary for independent living.

Aerobic activity/conditioning The performance of exercise to increase endurance.

Aerobic capacity A measure of the ability to perform work or participate in activity over time using a body's oxygen uptake, delivery, and energy release mechanisms.

Affective Relating to the expression of emotion; for example, affective disorder.

Afferent Proceeding from the peripheral to the central nervous system.

Airway clearance techniques A broad group of activities used to manage or prevent consequences of acute and chronic lung diseases and impairments, including those associated with surgery.

Algometer (pressure) An instrument for measuring the degree of sensitivity to a painful stimulus.

Ambulation Walking, with or without the use of assistive devices.

Amplitude The maximum difference between an alternating current's peak and average values.

Anaerobic threshold The point during exercise at which a person cannot supply enough oxygen to meet the demands of the body.

Anterior: In front; ventral

Approximation Bringing together two joint surfaces.

Arrhythmia An irregular or abnormal heart rhythm.

Arthrokinematic joint motion Describing the motion of a joint without regard to the forces producing that motion or resulting from it; describing the structure and shape of joint surfaces. Examples of these motions are glide (slide), roll, spin, distraction or traction, and compression or approximation.

ASIF Association for the Study of Internal Fixation.

Assistive, adaptive, supportive, and protective devices A variety of implements or equipment used to aid individuals in performing tasks or movements.

Atelectasis Airlessness of the lungs due to failure of expansion or resorption of air from the alveoli.

Athermal Not using heat, describing, for example, a modality such as pulsed ultrasound.

Atlantoaxial luxation Occurs when instability of the joint allows the axis to luxate dorsally, relative to the atlas, and compress the spinal cord. Congenital in some toy breeds of dogs.

Autogenic drainage Airway clearance through the patient's own efforts (such as coughing).

Balance The ability of an individual to maintain the body in equilibrium with gravity both statically (e.g., while stationary) and dynamically (e.g., while walking).

Ballistic stretching A form of stretching in which a series of quick movements are used to stretch the muscles and connective tissues.

Beam nonuniformity ratio (BNR) Regarding therapeutic ultrasound, compares the maximal intensity from the transducer to the average intensity. This ratio should be low (between 2 and 6) to indicate that the energy distribution is relatively uniform.

Biofeedback A training technique that enables an individual to gain some element of voluntary control over muscular or autonomic nervous system functions using a device that produces auditory or visual stimuli.

Biomechanical Describing the action of forces on the body, especially as they affect the musculoskeletal system.

Body mechanics The interrelationships of the muscles and joints as they maintain or adjust posture in response to environmental forces.

Carpal hyperextension A problem of the carpal joints in which the palmar carpal ligaments and palmar carpal fibrocartilage are damaged and the dog develops a palmigrade stance.

Case management The coordination of patient care or client activities.

Cauda equina syndrome A progressive neurologic syndrome characterized by lumbar pain, fecal and urinary incontinence, and possible progressive neurologic deficits caused by soft and hard tissue proliferation associated with lumbosacral intervertebral disk disease.

Caudal In animals, a directional term meaning toward the tail.

Caudal cervical stenotic myelopathy See cervical spondylomyelopathy.

Cervical spondylomyelopathy A disorder caused by abnormal development of the cervical vertebrae resulting in compression of the spinal cord. Relatively common in Great Danes and Doberman pinschers. Sometimes also called caudal cervical stenotic myelopathy or wobbler syndrome.

Chondroprotectant Various compounds that are proposed to have a positive effect on the health and metabolism of chondrocytes and synoviocytes.

Cicatrix Scar; the fibrous tissue replacing the normal tissues destroyed by injury or disease.

Circulation The passage of blood through the heart, blood vessels, organs, and tissues; it also describes the oxygen delivery system.

Client An individual, business, agency, or other organizational entity receiving consultative services.

Clinical indications The patient factors (symptoms, impairments, deficits, and so forth) that suggest that a particular kind of care (examination, intervention) would be appropriate.

Closed kinetic chain exercise Exercise with foot fixed against a resistance.

Coaptation device A bandage, splint, or cast which is used to immobilize joints and tissues.

Compression therapy Treatment using devices or techniques that decrease the density of a part of the body through the application of pressure.

Compressive joint motion Compressive or approximation accessory movements of joint surfaces.

Conduction Transmission of electrical energy.

Conduction velocity The speed at which electrical energy is transmitted.

Consultation The provision by a physical therapist or veterinarian of a professional, expert opinion or of advice.

Continuous passive motion (CPM) The use of a device that allows a joint (such as the knee) to be exercised without the involvement of the patient, often in the early postoperative period.

Contracture, joint Inability to move a joint through its full range of motion.

Contrast bath Alternately immersing the patient or body part in cold and hot water, most appropriate during the early subacute phase of tissue healing.

Cosmesis A concern in therapeutics, especially in surgical operations, for the appearance of the patient.

Cranial In relation to animals, a directional term indicating toward the head.

Cranial cruciate ligament (CCL) Analogous to the anterior cruciate ligament in humans.

Cranial nerve One of the 12 paired nerves (such as olfactory and optic) that emerge from or enter the brain.

Critical inquiry The process of applying the principles of scientific methods to read and interpret professional literature, participate in research activities, and analyze patient care outcomes, new concepts, and findings.

Cryokinetics The combination of cryotherapy with motion (passive, active-assisted, active) to facilitate normal, pain-free movement and to promote reduction of edema.

Cryotherapy Therapeutic application of cold (such as ice).

Cyanosis A bluish or purplish discoloration of the skin or mucous membranes due to a severe oxygen deficiency.

Cyclooxygenase (COX)   An enzyme that is necessary for the production of prostaglandins from arachidonic acid. Two forms of the enzyme are recognized, COX-1 and COX-2. COX-2 is produced in response to inflammation.

Debridement   Excision of contused and necrotic tissue from the surface of a wound. *Autolytic:* Self-debridement, that is, removal of contused or necrotic tissue through the action of enzymes in the tissue. *Sharp:* Debridement using a sharp instrument.

Deficit   A shortfall in amount or quality. *Developmental:* Difference between expected and actual (lower) performance in an aspect of development (e.g., motor). *Receptive:* A shortfall in the skills involving reception (e.g., in vision, in hearing).

Degenerative lumbosacral stenosis   A condition in which soft tissue and bony changes, possibly in conjunction with abnormal motion of the lumbosacral joint, impinge on the nerve roots of the cauda equina.

Degenerative myelopathy   A poorly understood neurologic condition associated with progressive motor weakness caused by progressive spinal cord degeneration.

Developmental delay   The failure to reach expected age-specific performance in one or more areas of development (such as motor or sensory-perceptual).

Diagnosis   A label encompassing a cluster of signs and symptoms, syndromes, or categories. It is also the decision reached as a result of the diagnostic process, which is the evaluation of information obtained from the patient examination organized into clusters, syndromes, or categories.

Discospondylitis   An infection of the intervertebral disk and adjacent vertebral bodies, resulting in an inflammatory response surrounding the associated spinal cord or nerve roots.

Dislocation   A disturbance or disarrangement of the usual relationship of bones as they enter into the formation of a joint.

Distraction joint motion   Distraction or traction motions are tensile (pulling apart) movements between bones.

Dolorimeter   A device to measure pain.

Dorsal   In animals, a directional term meaning toward the spine.

Dressing   A material (such as a topical agent or gauze) applied to a lesion.

Duty cycle   Refers to the percentage of time that ultrasound is emitted during one pulse period. Duty cycle = pulse duration (time on)/the pulse period (time on + time off).

Dynamometry   Measuring the degree of muscular power.

Dyspnea   Shortness of breath; subjective difficulty or distress in breathing frequently manifested by rapid, shallow breaths; usually associated with serious disease of the heart or lungs.

Edema   An accumulation of fluid, often occurring as part of the inflammatory process after trauma.

Efferent   Sending information away from the central nervous system.

Effusion   The escape of fluid into a body part or tissue.

Electrical device   An instrument or modality that applies electrical current to biologic tissue for pain control, tissue healing, or muscle dysfunction; an instrument that records electrical activity from excitable tissues of the body for purposes of neuromuscular diagnosis, education, or relaxation.

Electrical stimulation   Treatment through the application of electricity. *Functional:* The application of electrical stimulation to particular peripheral nerves to allow paretic and paralyzed muscles to make functional and purposeful movements.

Electrogoniometry   The measurement of the movement of a joint using an electrical potentiometer.

Electromyography (EMG)   The recording of the electrical activity of a muscle.

Electrophysiologic   Concerned with the electrical activity of various body tissues or systems.

Electrophysiologic testing   The process of examining the relationships of body functions to electrical phenomena, such as the effects of electrical stimulation on the tissues, the production of electrical currents by organs and tissues, and the therapeutic use of electrical current.

Electrotherapeutic modalities   A broad group of therapeutic physical agents (e.g., neuromuscular electrical stimulation, iontophoresis).

Endurance   The ability to perform work over time.

Environmental, home, and work barriers   The physical impediments that keep individuals from functioning optimally in their surroundings, including safety hazards (such as throw rugs or slippery surfaces), access problems (such as narrow doors or high steps), and home design (such as a multiple-story environment).

Evaluation   A dynamic process in which the physical therapist makes clinical judgments based on data gathered during the examination.

Evoked potentials   The electrical signals recorded from a sensory receptor, nerve, muscle, and so forth, of the central nervous system that has been stimulated, most often by electricity (e.g., auditory evoked potentials).

Examination   The process of obtaining a patient history, performing relevant systems reviews, and selecting and administering specific tests and measures.

Excursion   Movement within the body, with return to the original state implied (e.g., excursion of the diaphragm).

Extracapsular suture stabilization   A procedure used to stabilize cranial cruciate deficient stifles using sutures of various materials to span from the caudal aspect of the stifle to the tibial crest.

Exudation   The process of expressing material through a wound, usually characterized as oozing.

Fibrocartilaginous embolic myelopathy (FCE)   A poorly understood phenomenon in which fragments of intervertebral disk material embolize and create regional vascular compromise to the spinal cord.

Fibrotic myopathy   Fibrosis and contracture of skeletal muscle secondary to trauma.

Field trails   A sporting event where dogs compete in hunting, retrieving, or pointing competition.

Fluidotherapy   "Dry whirlpool"; the application of dry heat through a fluidotherapy machine.

Force plate   A plate embedded in the floor used to measure the force that an individual exerts when walking.

Fragmented medial coronoid process (FCP)   A condition in which the medial coronoid process of the proximal ulna becomes fragmented, possibly due to elbow incongruency or osteochondrosis.

Frequency   The number of cycles per second, expressed as hertz (Hz). Ultrasound and neuromuscular electrical stimulation units generally have various frequency settings.

Function   The special, normal, or proper action of any part or organ; the action specifically for which an individual or thing is fitted or employed; an act, process, or series of processes that serve a purpose; to perform an activity or to work properly or normally.

Functional limitation   A restriction of the ability to perform a physical action, activity, or task in a typically expected, efficient, or competent manner.

Gait   The manner in which a person walks, characterized by rhythm, cadence, step, stride, and speed.

Glide joint motion   Shear or sliding motions of opposing articular surfaces.

Goal   The long-term statement(s) that define the patient's expected level of performance at the end of the rehabilitation process: the functional outcomes of therapy, indicating the amount of independence, supervision, or assistance required and the equipment or environmental adaptation necessary to ensure adequate performance. Desired outcomes may be stated as long-term or short-term as determined by the needs of the patient and the setting.

Goniometry   *Manual:* The measurement of the movement of a joint by manual methods. *Electrical:* See electrogoniometry.

Graded forces   A term used in manual therapy to denote the application by the physical therapist of varying amounts of pressure on the patient's body.

Hansen's type I disk   An acute explosive intervertebral disk herniation.

Hansen's type II disk   A chronic progressive intervertebral disk herniation.

Herniated disk   The protrusion of one of the spinal disks into an opening in the spinal cord, thereby compressing the nerve root.

Hertz (Hz)   Cycles per second.

History   An account of past and present health status that includes the identification of complaints and provides the initial source of information about the patient. The history also suggests the patient's ability to benefit from physical therapy services.

Home, environmental, or architectural barriers   The physical impediments (such as stairs or slippery surfaces) that restrain or obstruct an individual's ability to function in the usual environment.

Hubbard tank   A shallow tank made of stainless steel, Plexiglas, or tile, for administering hydrotherapy.

Hydrodynamic   Concerned with the flow of liquids.

Hydrotherapy   Treatment with external water.

Hygroma   Seroma, hematoma associated with the olecranon.

Hypertrophic osteodystrophy A developmental disease of rapidly growing large- and giant-breed dogs characterized by metaphyseal new bone formation.

Hypomobility/hypermobility Abnormally low or high movement or ability to move (as of a joint).

Impairment A loss or abnormality of physiologic, psychological, or anatomical structure or function.

Infrared heat A therapy using thermal radiation with a wavelength greater than that of the red end of the visible spectrum.

Infraspinatus contracture Fibrotic contracture of the infraspinatus muscle causing a gait abnormality. Contracture of the infraspinatus muscle limits full extension of the shoulder and causes the affected forelimb to be abducted.

Innervation The supply of nerve fibers to a part of the body, such as an organ.

Integrity The characteristic of being whole or fully functional.

Intensity Refers to the rate of energy delivery per unit area.

Intervention The purposeful and skilled interaction of the physical therapist with the patient, using various methods and techniques to produce changes in the patient's condition.

Intervertebral disk disease A common condition, especially in chondrodystrophic breeds of dogs, in which protrusion or extrusion of an intervertebral disk causes pain, weakness, and varying degrees of neurologic dysfunction.

Iontophoresis Use of continuous direct electrical current to enhance the transdermal administration of medication.

Ischemia Local anemia due to mechanical obstruction (mainly arterial narrowing) of the blood supply.

Jack Local irritation, seroma, or chronic periostitis associated with mechanical interference between the forelimbs and hindlimbs.

Joint integrity The conformance of the joints to expected anatomic, biomechanic, and kinematic norms.

Joint mobility The ability to move a joint; takes into account the structure and shape of the joint surface as well as characteristics of tissue surrounding the joint.

Kinematic Having to do with the possible motions of a part or all of the human body.

Kinesthesia The awareness of the body's or a body part's movement.

Knocked-up toe Abnormal carriage of the toes due to avulsion or rupture of the deep digital flexor tendon.

Lateral splint Splint fashioned from casting material applied to the lateral aspect of the leg.

Laxity Looseness, as in laxity of a joint.

Lipoxygenase (LOX) An enzyme that converts arachidonic acid to leukotrienes.

Loading The force placed on a body part (such as a foot or the feet); used often in describing the employment of an assistive device.

Lure coursing A sporting event where sight hounds chase lures pulled by a rope or cord.

Lymphatic Concerned with the lymph nodes and vessels, which form a system for collecting fluid from the tissues and adding it to the venous blood system.

Maceration Softening by the action of a liquid.

Magnetic fields energy, pulsed A therapy using the intermittent application of energy produced by magnetic fields.

Manipulation A therapeutic movement, usually of small amplitude, accomplished at the end of the available range of motion but with the anatomical range at a speed over which the patient has no control.

Manual therapy A broad group of skilled hand movements used by the physical therapist to mobilize soft tissues and joints for the purpose of modulating pain, increasing range of motion, and so forth.

Mechanical Caused by or derived from machinery; habitual, routine, automatic; related to, controlled, or affected by physical forces (such as a traction device). *Biomechanical:* The physical structure, forces, and movements in the human body.

Medial buttress Periarticular fibrosis and swelling of the medial aspect of the distal femur associated with chronic stifle instability and cranial cruciate deficiency.

Meniscal release Involves cutting the medial meniscus just caudal to the medial collateral ligament. Used in conjunction with the TPLO procedure.

Mentation A mechanism of thought or mental activity.

Metabolic Concerned with metabolism, the sum of all physical and chemical changes that take place within an organism; all energy and material transformations that take place within living cells.

Microvolt One millionth of a volt.

Mobilization A therapeutic movement accomplished within the available range of motion at a speed that the patient cannot control.

Modality(ies) Physical agent(s), including, but not limited to, thermal, acoustic, light, mechanical, or electrical energy, applied to produce therapeutic changes in biologic tissue.

Monkey muscle Long head of the triceps.

Motor function The ability to learn or demonstrate the skillful and efficient assumption, maintenance, modification, and control of voluntary postures and movement patterns. *Fine:* Refers to relatively delicate movements. *Gross:* Refers to larger-scale movements.

Multisegment motion Simultaneous movement of several parts of the body.

Muscle length The length of the muscle during various stages of tension (from resting at full extension through the contractile range); in conjunction with joint integrity and connective tissue extensibility, muscle length determines flexibility.

Muscle performance The capacity of a muscle to do work (force × distance).

Nerve root compression A squeezing of one of two bundles of nerve fiber emerging from the spine; frequently caused by a herniated disk.

Nervous system The brain, spinal cord, nerves, and ganglia. *Central nervous system:* The brain and spinal cord. *Peripheral nervous system:* The system of nerves in the extremities.

Neural Having to do with a nerve or nerves.

Neuromotor development The acquisition and evolution of movement skills throughout the life span.

Nonvolitional Involuntary, not controllable.

Nutraceutical Nondrug substances that are produced in a purified or extracted form and are administered orally to provide compounds required for normal body structure and function with the intent of improving health and well-being.

Objective A measurable behavioral statement of an expected response or outcome; something worked toward or striven for; a statement of direction or desired achievement that guides actions and activities.

Open kinetic chain exercises Exercises with the foot not fixed against a resistance.

Orthosis A device (such as a splint or brace) that supports weak or ineffective joints or muscles.

Osteochondrosis A growth-related disease of the cartilage. The primary problem is failure of endochondral bone formation that allows the articular cartilage to irregularly develop and often tear. A cartilage flap is referred to as osteochondrosis dissecans.

Osteokinematic joint motion Primary motion of a joint and the movement of bones as a whole, such as occurs with stifle flexion and extension.

Osteoporotic Pertaining to or characterized by a porous condition of the bones; refers to a reduction in the quantity of bone or atrophying skeletal tissue.

Oxygen consumption The amount of oxygen inspired minus the amount of oxygen exhaled.

Oxygen saturation The degree to which oxygen is present in a particular substance.

Outcome The result of physical therapy management expressed in five areas: prevention and management of symptom manifestation, consequences of disease (impairment, disability, and/or role limitation), cost-benefit analysis, health-related quality of life, and client satisfaction. A successful outcome includes improved or maintained physical function when possible, slows functional decline where the status quo cannot be maintained, and/or is considered meaningful by the client.

Outcomes analysis A systematic examination of patient outcomes in relation to selected patient variables (e.g., age, sex, diagnosis, interventions performed); outcomes analysis may be used in quality assessment, economic analysis of practice, and so forth.

Pain A disturbed sensation causing suffering or distress.

Palpation Examination using the hands (such as palpation of the spleen).

Panosteitis A growth-related problem of immature rapidly growing dogs. It is characterized by intramedullary deposition of bone and a shifting leg lameness.

Paraffin bath A superficial heat treatment using paraffin wax and mineral oil.

Passive range of motion Motion across a joint with no muscle contraction.

Pathomechanical Describing a disturbance in function not resulting from disease.

Pathophysiologic Describing the functional changes that accompany a particular disease or syndrome.

Pathway A conduction route for nerve impulses. *Sensory pathway:* A conduction route for nerve impulses from the sense organs.

Patient One who is being treated for an illness or injury; an individual receiving health care.

Percussion (mechanical) A diagnostic procedure in which the clinician taps a body part with a finger or rubber-headed hammer to estimate its density.

Performance battery A set of tests designed to measure a patient's ability to function in a particular area(s).

Peripheral circulation The movement of blood through the extremities.

Peripheral vascular Concerned with the blood vessels of the extremities.

Phonophoresis The use of ultrasound to enhance the delivery of topically applied medications through the skin.

Photosensitivity Sensitivity of the skin to light, usually due to the action of certain drugs (or plants, or other substances).

Phototherapy Treatment using the application of light. *Ultraviolet:* Light therapy using rays with wavelengths beyond the violet end of the visible spectrum.

Physical agent A form of mechanical, radiant, thermal, acoustic, or electrical energy that is applied to biologic tissues in a systematic manner to achieve a therapeutic effect; a therapeutic modality used to treat physical problems.

Physical function The measurement of physiologic, biomechanical, social, and psychological performance in practical or goal-oriented terms.

Physical therapist A licensed health professional who offers services designed to preserve, develop, and restore maximum physical function.

Physical therapist assistant An educated health care provider who performs physical therapy procedures and related tasks that have been selected and delegated by the supervising physical therapist.

Physical therapy aide A nonlicensed worker, trained under the direction of a physical therapist, who performs designated routine physical therapy tasks.

Physiologic joint motion See Osteokinematic motion.

Planes (midline and segmental) Imaginary flat surfaces drawn through the body; the midline plane bisects the body vertically, while segmental planes are drawn at various angles.

Posterior Relating to the back or dorsal side.

Postural drainage Placing the body in a position that causes fluid to drain from the lungs.

Postural reactions The adjustments of the body to gravity required for normal performance; the ability to alter the position of the head, trunk, and extremities to balance one's body with gravity.

Posture The alignment and positioning of the body in relation to gravity, center of mass, and basis of support.

Posturography Procedures to test standing posture, balance, and equilibrium sense.

Power Work produced per unit of time.

Presenting problem The specific dysfunction that causes a client to seek attention or intervention (that is, the chief complaint).

Proactive Seizing the initiative; responding actively rather than passively; performing an action with the idea of influencing events.

Prognosis The determination of the level of maximal improvement that might be attained by the patient and the amount of time needed to reach that level.

Proprioception The reception of stimuli from within the body (such as from muscles or tendons); includes position sense (the awareness of the joints at rest) and kinesthesia (the awareness of movement).

Prosthesis An artificial device, often mechanical or electrical, used to replace a missing part of the body.

Pulses The dilations of arteries (occasionally veins or vascular organs) that correspond to the beating of the heart.

Quadriceps tiedown A disability characterized by an inability to fully flex or extend the stifle following a fracture of the femur.

Range of motion Describes the space, distance, or angle through which a patient can move a joint or series of joints.

Recurvatum An angular limb deformity where the affected joint is excessively hyperextended. The most common form is genu recurvatum, in which the stifle joint is abnormally hyperextended.

Reepithelialization Skin growth to replace skin loss due to a wound or other injury.

Referral A recommendation that a patient seek service from another health care provider or resource.

Reflex A stereotyped reaction to a variety of sensory stimuli.

Reflex inhibition A situation in which sensory stimuli decrease reflex activity or the voluntary activation of muscle.

Rehabilitative   Concerned with restoration of a patient to full or at least improved function.

Remediation   The act or process of providing some degree of relief for a patient's clinical problems.

Respiration   A term that refers primarily to the exchange of oxygen and carbon dioxide across a membrane into and out of both the lungs and cells.

Respiratory quotient   The ratio of the carbon dioxide that the body tissues give off to the amount of oxygen that they absorb.

Righting   Adjusting or restoring the body to a desired position.

Robert Jones bandage   A soft, padded bandage to limit tissue swelling and joint motion.

Robinson sling   A bandage used to allow only toe touching of the rear leg. Sometimes called a Humane Society bandage.

Roll joint motion   Involves one bone rolling on another, such as the femoral condyles rolling on the tibial plateau.

Schroeder-Thomas splint   A splint consisting of a metal hoop and stirrups used to immobilize fractures.

Screening   Determining the need for further examination or consultation by a physical therapist or for referral to another health professional.

Sensory   Having to do with sensations or the senses; includes peripheral sensory processing (such as sensitivity to touch) and cortical sensory processing (such as two-point and sharp/dull discrimination).

Sensory integration   The ability to integrate information from the environment in order to produce normal movement outputs.

Sequential casting   A process in which the patient is casted several times, with each cast less restrictive than the previous one.

Sequelae   Aftereffects of a disease or injury.

Serosanguineous   Containing both serum and blood.

Serous   Like serum, watery.

Somatosensory   Having to do with the sensations received in the skin and deep tissues.

Somatosensory deficit   A shortfall in the reception of sensations in the skin and deep tissues.

Spatial average intensity   In reference to therapeutic ultrasound, the total output (in watts) of the transducer divided by the transducer surface area (in cm²).

Spatial peak intensity   The greatest intensity anywhere within the therapeutic ultrasound beam.

Spin joint motion   Joint surface motions that result in continual contact of a single area of articular cartilage on adjacent articular cartilage within a joint.

Spinal curve   An abnormal curvature of the spinal column (e.g., S curve, kyphosis).

Splinting, dynamic   Functional splinting that aids in the movements initiated by the patient and/or controls the plane and range of motion.

Spoon splint   A plastic or metal splint shaped like a spoon used to immobilize or support the limb.

Sprain   A joint injury without dislocation or fracture involving possible ligament or tendon rupture.

Stopper bone   Accessory carpal bone.

Strain   Injury from overuse or improper use.

Strengthening, active assistive   A form of strength-building exercise in which the physical therapist applies resistance through the range of motion of the patient's active movement.

Strengthening, resistive   Any form of active exercise in which a dynamic or static muscular contraction is resisted by an outside force. The external force may be applied manually or mechanically.

Sympathetic disturbance   A malfunction in the sympathetic part of the autonomic nervous system, which governs smooth muscle and the contraction of blood vessels.

Symptom magnification scale   An examination tool used to elicit descriptions of levels of pain.

Syndrome   The aggregate of signs and symptoms associated with any morbid process that together constitute the picture of a known disease.

Synergy   The capability of properly grouping movements in order to perform acts that require special adjustments.

Systems review   A brief or limited examination that provides additional information about the patient's general health to help the physical therapist formulate a diagnosis and select an intervention program.

Telemetry   The science of measuring a quantity, transmitting the results to a distant station, and then interpreting, indicating, and recording the results.

TENS (transcutaneous electrical nerve stimulation)   The use of electrical current to stimulate cutaneous and peripheral nerves via electrodes on the skin's surface.

Tests and measures General methods and techniques used to conduct an examination.

Therapeutic exercise A wide range of activities designed to increase strength, improve cardiovascular fitness, increase flexibility, enlarge range of motion, or otherwise increase the body's functional capacity.

Thermal Using heat, as in a thermal agent, for its therapeutic effects.

Thermistor A device for determining temperature; may be extremely small and may also be used to establish and maintain temperature.

Thermography A process of measuring temperature by means of a registering thermometer, one form of which records every temperature variation and registers its rise and fall on a circular temperature chart turned by clockwork.

Thermotherapy The therapeutic application of heat.

Tibial plateau leveling osteotomy (TPLO) A corrective osteotomy technique used in the treatment of cranial cruciate ligament disease.

Tilt table/standing table Two kinds of tables used to bring patients from a supine to a vertical position in a deliberate manner.

Tissue Collection of similar cells and the intercellular substances that surrounding them.

Topical agent An ointment, medication, or similar material applied to the skin for its therapeutic effect.

Torque A force that produces rotation or twisting of a part on its axis.

Traction The therapeutic use of tension created by a pulling force. *Mechanical:* The use of tractive forces to produce a combination of distraction and gliding to relieve discomfort and increase tissue flexibility; also called passive mobilization.

Treatment One or more interventions used to cure or ameliorate a disease or pathologic condition or otherwise produce changes in the patient's health status; the sum of the therapies offered to a patient during a complete episode of care.

Triage An initial review of a patient or prospective patient to determine the need for further treatment.

Triple pelvic osteotomy (TPO) A surgical procedure involving osteotomies of the ilium, ischium, and pubis and rotation of the acetabulum to increase dorsal coverage of the head of the femur for the treatment of hip dysplasia.

Turgor Fullness, swelling.

Ulcer A break in the skin surface or in a mucous membrane with loss of tissue, usually accompanied by inflammation. *Decubitus ulcer:* Bedsore. *Vascular insufficiency ulcers:* Lesions caused by occlusion of a blood vessel or other vascular disorder.

Ultrasound A diagnostic or therapeutic technique using high-frequency sound waves. Used therapeutically, ultrasound produces heat. *Pulsed ultrasound:* The application of therapeutic ultrasound at frequent predetermined levels.

Vasopneumatic compression device A device intended to decrease swelling by "milking" fluid away from an area, such as an inflatable sleeve strapped around a patient's swollen extremity.

Velpeau sling A bandage used to secure the forelimb to the thorax, used for immobilization of the shoulder.

Ventilation The movement of a volume of gas into and out of the lungs.

Ventral In animals, a directional term meaning toward the belly.

Vestibular Describing the sense of balance located in the inner ear.

Vital signs Heart rate, blood pressure, temperature, and respiration rate.

Volitional Intentional, as in controlled movement.

Volumetric displacement The amount of a fluid that leaves a container (of any size) following the introduction of a part or all of the body.

Wellness A concept that embraces a proactive, positive approach to good health. Wellness advocates seek to increase a person's level of health as a preventative measure to guard against future disease.

Wobbler syndrome See cervical spondylomyelopathy.

Work conditioning An intensive, goal-oriented treatment program designed specifically to restore an individual's systemic neuromusculoskeletal functions (strength, endurance, movement, flexibility, and motor control) and cardiopulmonary functions.

Zoonosis The transmission of a disease from an animal or nonhuman species to humans.

Index

A

A delta fibers
  autonomic nervous system theory of acupuncture and, 341
  gate theory of acupuncture and, 339
Abdominal wall muscles, attachments, actions, and innervations for, 460
Abducent nerve, 199, 199t
Abduction, 54
Absorption, therapeutic ultrasound and, 324
Accessory joint motion, 50, 215, 216
Acetabular fracture secondary to automobile trauma, 370-371
Acetabular ligament anatomy, 75
Acetaminophen for osteoarthritis in geriatric dogs, 420
Acetylcholine receptors, effects of immobilization on, 127-128
Achilles tendon injury, 385, 385f
ACL. *See* Anterior cruciate ligament.
Actin in muscle contraction, 160-161, 161f
Actinomyces species, 401
Active assisted range of motion, 229
  clinical application of, 235
Active assisted standing exercise, 246-247
  with carts and slings, 247, 247f
  using exercise rolls, 247-248, 248f
Active range of motion, 230
  for cervical intervertebral disk disease, 389
  clinical application of, 235-241
  for musculoskeletal injuries, 405t
Activities of daily living in outcomes assessment, 221
Acupressure, 343
Acupuncture, 337-354
  clinical application of, 345
  conditions treated with, 342
  literature review regarding
    in dogs, 341-342
    in humans, 338-341, 340f
  location and individual action of points in, 348t, 348-349, 349f, 350t-353t
  for neurologic and vertebral disease, 347
  for peripheral neuropathy, 348
  technique, equipment, and instrumentation for, 343f, 343-345, 344f
  terminology specific to, 337-338, 339f

The letter t denotes table, f denotes figure, b denotes box.

Acupuncture points, 337-338
  location and individual actions of, 348t, 348-349, 349f, 350t-353t
  selection of, 345-346, 346f
Adduction, 54
  assessment of before massage therapy, 315, 315f
Adenosine diphosphate in muscle contraction, 160-161, 161f
Adenosine monophosphate in muscle energy systems, 162
Adenosine triphosphate
  in muscle contraction, 160-161, 161f
  in muscle energy systems, 162, 163
Adequan for osteoarthritis, 174-175
Adhesion
  massage therapy and, 307
  stretching techniques and, 236
Administrative costs, development of rehabilitation facility and, 438
ADP. *See* Adenosine diphosphate.
Adrenocorticotropic hormone, decreased output of due to massage therapy, 305
Age factors, in immobilization and remobilization, 118
  of bone, 118, 150
Aged, defined, 411
Aggrecan, effects of immobilization on, 116
Aggression by dog, 33-34, 34f, 35f
Aging, 411, 412b, 412t. *See Also* Geriatric patient.
  maintaining quality of life during, 414-415, 416f-418f, 419f
  medical considerations in, 411-412, 413t
  muscular contraction and, 125
  musculoskeletal and neurologic systems and, 411-412, 413t
Air mattress, standing or walking on, 253-254, 254f
Alternative and complementary veterinary medicine. *See Also* specific types.
  guidelines for adopted by American Veterinary Medical Association, 2
  regulatory and practice issues for, 6
    collaborative relationships with veterinarians in, 10-11
    referral guidelines in, 7-8
    reimbursement and remuneration for services in, 12
    risk management in, 11-12
    state practice acts in, 8-10
    veterinarian-client-patient relationship in, 6-7

Methylprednisolone
  effects of on immobilized ligaments and tendons, 144
  for spinal cord injury treatment, 400
Methylsulfonylmethane for osteoarthritis, 174
Microcurrent therapy, 345
Middle-age, defined, 411
Mineralization of supraspinatus tendon, 356
MMP2. *See* Gelatinase.
Mobility, massage therapy and, 307
Mobility cart
  for active assisted standing exercise, 247, 247f
  for dynamic ambulation activities, 252f, 252-253
Model Practice Act of American Veterinary Medical
    Association, 5-6
Monocyte, 108
Mononuclear cells, arthritis-related changes in, 193t
Monosynaptic stretch response, 237
Motion
  cryotherapy combined with, 277
  of joint, 38-39, 49-56, 53b, 54b, 441
    aquatic therapy and, 274, 274t
    evaluation of in outcomes assessment, 215f, 215-216
    in gait evaluation, 182
    in limbs and spine, 41f, 42f, 51-55
    maintained joint postures *versus,* 56
    normal and ranges of, 56, 441
    pelvic, 55-56
    shape of articular surfaces in, 49-51
    during trot, 208, 209f
  planes of, 38, 39f
Motion analysis of gait, 208-210, 209f, 210f
  in outcomes assessment, 213-214
Motor neuron lesion, neurologic assessment of, 199-200,
    200f
Motor unit, muscular, 161
  point location in
    for acupuncture, 337
    for electrical stimulation, 300
Mouth in assessment of body language, 32
Movement, voluntary, assessment of in neurologic
    examination, 193
Moxibustion, acupuncture and, 343
MRI. *See* Magnetic resonance imaging.
MRS. *See* Magnetic resonance spectroscopy.
MSM. *See* Methylsulfonylmethane.
Mugwort plant, acupuncture and, 343
Muscle
  adaptation of to increased mechanical stress,
    133-135
  aging of, 412
  anatomy and physiology of, 58-68, 105, 106f
    of forelimb, 59, 60f, 61f, 62f, 63f, 64f, 65f, 66f
    of hindlimb, 59-64, 67f, 68f, 69f, 70f, 71f, 72f, 73f, 74f,
      75f
    of trunk and neck, 64-68, 76f, 77f, 78f, 79f, 80f, 81f
  atrophic
    due to disuse and immobilization, 125-128, 126f, 165
    neurogenic, 129f, 129-130
    palpation for in orthopedic and neurologic
      examination, 183f, 183-184
    related to fracture, 132
  attachments, actions, and innervations for, 447-464
  biopsy of, 124
  effects of arthritis on, 133
  effects of cranial cruciate ligament injury on, 130-132,
    131f, 132f
  effects of fracture on, 132
  effects of hip conditions on, 130-133, 131f, 132f
  effects of massage on, 306f, 306-307

Muscle (*Continued*)
  effects of neuromuscular electrical stimulation on
    enzymes of, 294-295
  effects of remobilization on, 133
  energy systems of, 162f, 162-163
  evaluation of in outcomes assessment, 217f, 217-223,
    218f, 219f, 220f
  exercise physiology and, 160-161, 161f
  factors effecting contraction of, 124-125
  functional excursion of, 228
  healing of, 105-107, 106f
  injury to, evaluation of in outcomes assessment,
    222-223
  neurogenic atrophy of, 129f, 129-130
  neuromuscular electrical stimulation-related fatigue of,
    296
  palpation of
    in forelimb, 89-90
    in hindlimb, 92-95
    in trunk, 98
  pennate *versus* fusiform, 161
  range of motion of, 228. *See Also* Range-of-motion
    exercise.
  response of to disuse and immobilization, 125-128, 126f
    medications effect on, 135-137
  spastic due to spinal cord injury, 404-405
  specific gravity of, 264
  stretching techniques on, 236
  tissue healing rates for, 102t
Muscle fibers
  anatomy of, 105, 106f
  effects of aging on, 125
  effects of disuse and immobilization on, 125-127
  effects of neuromuscular electrical stimulation on, 295
  effects of training on
    endurance, 134
    strength, 134
  recruitment of in electrical stimulation, 293-294
  response of to musculoskeletal conditioning, 163
  types of, 123-124
Muscle mass
  arthritis and, 133
  loss of
    due to bedrest or spaceflight, 128
    following cranial cruciate ligament resection, 130-131
  measurement of in outcomes assessment, 217f, 217-
    221, 218f, 219f, 220f
Muscle soreness, massage therapy for, 309, 309b
Muscle spasm
  cryotherapy for, 281
  massage therapy for, 306, 320-321, 321f
  therapeutic ultrasound for, 333
Muscle strain, 105
Muscle strength
  cryotherapy's effect on, 281
  effects of disuse and immobilization on, 126
  measurement of in outcomes assessment, 221-222
  muscle anatomy and, 59
Musculoskeletal system
  bone of. *See* Bone.
  cartilage of. *See* Cartilage.
  critical injury to, 404-405, 405t
  effects of aging on, 412-414, 413b, 414f
  exercise physiology and, 160-167
  joints of. *See* Joint.
  ligaments of. *See* Ligaments.
  muscles of. *See* Muscle.
  tendons of. *See* Tendons.
Musculotendinous junction, 161